MW00685386

Diagnostic Imaging in Clinical Cardiology

Diagnostic Imaging in Clinical Cardiology

Edited by

João A C Lima MD FACC
Associate Professor of Medicine
Johns Hopkins School of Medicine, and
Director of Transesophageal and Stress Echocardiography
The Johns Hopkins Hospital
Baltimore
Maryland
USA

MARTIN DUNITZ

First published in the United Kingdom in 1998 by
Martin Dunitz Ltd
The Livery House
7–9 Pratt Street
London NW1 0AE

A CIP catalogue record for this book is available from the British Library

ISBN 1-85317-309-6

Composition by Scribe Design, Gillingham, Kent, UK
Printed and bound in Spain by Grafos, S.A. Arte sobre papel

Dedication

This book is dedicated to Sandy, Michael and Jonathan, for unconditional love and support of a very intense academic life

Contents

List of contributors

Marvin L Appel MD PhD
Department of Anesthesiology and Critical Care Medicine, The Johns Hopkins Hospital, 600 N Wolfe Street, Baltimore, MD 21287, USA.

James Ayd RDCS
Department of Anesthesiology and Critical Care Medicine, The Johns Hopkins Hospital, 600 N Wolfe Street, Baltimore, MD 21287, USA.

Albert Andrew Burton MD
Division of Cardiology, The Johns Hopkins Hospital, 600 N Wolfe Street, Baltimore, MD 21287, USA.

Edmundo J Nassri Câmara MD
Associate Professor, Universidade Federal da Bahia, Brazil

John B Chambers MA MD FRCP
Senior Lecturer in Cardiology and Head of Echocardiography, Department of Cardiology, Hunt House, Guy's Hospital, Thomas Street, London SE1 9RT, UK.

Henry H Chong MD
Fellow in Cardiology, Division of Cardiology, University of Maryland School of Medicine, University Center, 22 South Green Street, Baltimore, MD 21201–1595, USA.

Mary C Corretti MD
Assisstant Professor of Medicine, Gudelsky Tower 3K17, University of Maryland, Division of Cardiology, 22 South Green Street, Baltimore, MD 21201–1595, USA.

Zahi A Fayad PhD
Assistant Professor of Medicine and Radiology, The Cardiovascular Institute and Department of Radiology, Mount Sinai School of Medicine, New York, NY, USA.

Victor A Ferrari MD
Associate Director, Cardiac Noninvasive Laboratory and Assistant Professor of Medicine and Radiology, Cardiovascular Division, Department of Medicine, University of Pennsylvania Medical Center, 3400 Spruce Street, Philadelphia, PA 19104–4283, USA.

Nicholas J Fortuin MD
Professor of Medicine, The Johns Hopkins University School of Medicine, 10755 Falls Road, Lutherville, MD 21093, USA.

Norbert Goebel MD
Chief of Comuted Tomography, Institute of Diagnostic Radiology, City Hospital Triemli, Zurich, Switzerland.

Markus Hauser MD
Attending Physician, Division of Diagnostic Radiology, Department of Medical Radiology, University Hospital, Zurich, Switzerland.

Eugenie S Heitmiller MD
Department of Anesthesiology and Critical Care Medicine, The Johns Hopkins Hospital, 600 N Wolfe Street, Baltimore, MD 21287, USA.

Rolf Jenni MD
Professor and Chief of Echocardiography, Division of Cardiology, Department of Internal Medicine, University Hospital, Zurich, Switzerland.

Edward K Kasper MD
Division of Cardiology, The Johns Hopkins Hospital, 600 N Wolfe Street, Baltimore, MD 21287, USA.

Mark D Kelemen
Division of Cardiology, The Johns Hopkins Hospital, 600 N Wolfe Street, Baltimore, MD 21287, USA.

Philip Kilner
Magnetic Resonance Unit, Royal Brompton Hospital, Sydney Street, London SW3 6NP, UK.

Elizabeth Klodas MD
Division of Cardiology, The Johns Hopkins Hospital, 600 N Wolfe Street, Baltimore, MD 21287, USA.

Christopher M Kramer MD
Division of Cardiology, Allegheny General Hospital, 320 East North Avenue, Pittsburgh, PA 15212, USA.

João A C Lima MD FACC
Associate Professor of Medicine, Johns Hopkins School of Medicine, and Director of Transesophageal and Stress Echocardiography, The Johns Hopkins Hospital, 600 N Wolfe Street, Baltimore, MD 21287, USA.

Harold I Palevsky
Associate Professor of Medicine and Director, Pulmonary Vascular Diseases Program, Pulmonary and Critical Care Division, Department of Medicine, University of Pennsylvania Medical Center, 3400 Spruce Street, Philadelphia, PA 19104–4283, USA.

Ted Plappert CVT
Cardiovascular Division, University of Pennsylvania, Gates Building, 3400 Spruce Street, PA 19104–4283, USA.

Gary D Plotnick MD
Professor of Medicine and Director of Echocardiography, Division of Cardiology, University of Maryland School of Medicine and Associate Professor of Medicine, Johns Hopkins School of Medicine, Baltimore, MD 21224, USA.

Wendy S Post MD MS
Division of Cardiology, The Johns Hopkins Bayview Medical Center, 4940 Eastern Avenue, Baltimore, MD 21224, USA.

Simon Ray MD MRCP
Consultant Cardiologist, Department of Cardiology, Wythenshawe Hospital, Southmoor Road, Manchester M23 9LT, UK.

Jon Resar
Division of Cardiology, The Johns Hopkins Hospital, 600 N Wolfe Street, Baltimore, MD 21287, USA.

James W Roberts MD
Division of Cardiology, The Johns Hopkins Hospital, 600 N Wolfe Street, Baltimore, MD 21287, USA.

Edward P Shapiro MD FACC
Associate Professor of Medicine, Division of Cardiology, The Johns Hopkins Bayview Medical Center, 4940 Eastern Avenue, Baltimore, MD 21224, USA.

Martin St John Sutton FRCP
Cardiovascular Division, University of Pennsylvania, Gates Building, 3400 Spruce Street, PA 19104–4283, USA.

Scott Takeda MB BS
Research Fellow, Department of Cardiology, Hunt House, Guy's Hospital, Thomas Street, London SE1 9RT, UK.

Jennifer W Tanio MD
Division of Cardiology, The Johns Hopkins Hospital, 600 N Wolfe Street, Baltimore, MD 21287, USA.

Gustav K von Schulthess MD PhD
Professor and Director, Division of Nuclear Medicine, Department of Medical Radiology, University Hospital, Zurich, Switzerland.

Chris Ward MD FRCP
Consultant Cardiologist, Department of Cardiology, Wythenshawe Hospital, Southmoor Road, Manchester M23 9LT, UK.

James L Weiss MD
Division of Cardiology, The Johns Hopkins Hospital, 600 N Wolfe Street, Baltimore, MD 21287, USA.

Susan E Wiegers MD
Cardiovascular Division, University of Pennsylvania, Gates Building, 3400 Spruce Street, PA 19104–4283, USA.

Preface

The main objective of this text is to provide the clinical cardiologist or internist with the necessary knowledge of the appropriate utilization of cardiac imaging for the solution of clinical problems. Commonly, imaging texts are written along the lines of different modalities and emphasize the value of specific imaging technologies for the clinical problem at hand. This book was conceived from a different angle. We asked clinical cardiologists with extensive background in cardiac imaging to describe the tests they use, and what types of information they seek when facing patients with specific cardiac conditions. Therefore, the two requirements I used to select contributors to this text were hands on involvement in clinical cardiology, and extensive knowledge of cardiac imaging and its utilization in medicine. The text is faithful to its original intent.

The topics covered by the text were also chosen with the clinical cardiologist and internist in mind. The vast majority of cardiac imaging studies in clinical practice are performed to assess the consequences of known or suspected heart disease to left ventricular structure and function. In this regard, the two initial chapters, dedicated to left ventricular function and hypertrophy respectively, are designed to address these most common clinical questions. Coronary artery disease and its effects on the heart, which represent the second most common reason for cardiac imaging studies in industrialized countries, are approached in the second part of the text. Cardiac imaging is crucial to the adequate management of ischemic heart syndromes. However, this text emphasizes noninvasive cardiac imaging and therefore does not cover coronary angiography in depth. On the other hand, the recent development of intravascular ultrasound has brought the noninvasive cardiologist to the catheterization laboratory working side by side with interventionists in cases of unstable coronary syndromes. Chapter 3 was conceived to address this need for joint effort on the approach to diverse ischemic syndromes requiring intravascular imaging for better diagnosis and treatment.

The impact of ischemia on left ventricular function is discussed both in the acute and chronic settings. Patients with documented or suspected acute myocardial infarction or ischemia have benefited enormously from echocardiography which can be performed serially and at the bedside if necessary. More recently, the advent of magnetic resonance imaging and the possibility of placing noninvasive myocardial markers by this technique (tissue tagging), has generated important knowledge on the architectural changes undergone by the left ventricle after acute and chronic infarction. Finally, the text does not cover the large body of existing knowledge relative to the utilization of nuclear techniques in ischemic heart disease. While the authors were free to choose their preferred modality of approach to the different clinical conditions, the paucity of data on nuclear imaging in this text merely reflects individual preferences of the authors, and the fact that such techniques can be presently substituted by exercise or pharmacologically induced stress echocardiography.

Cardiac imaging techniques represent the cornerstone of diagnostic modalities in patients with known or suspected valvular heart disease. The advent of doppler echocardiography has placed cardiac ultrasound as the modality of choice in patients with valvular heart disease and is used routinely to quantify the degree of aortic stenosis, the effect of mitral valvuloplasty on mitral valve area, and to detect and estimate the magnitude of mitral regurgitation. The third section, Chapters 6 through 9, is dedicated to valvular heart disease and its effects on the heart. The fourth section discusses the utilization of cardiac imaging to address the most common problems involving primary myocardial and pericardial diseases. These two types of cardiac disease processes were grouped in the fourth section because they often generate similar diagnostic dilemmas. Cardiac imaging plays a crucial role in differentiating the diverse types of primary myocardial problems from acute and chronic pericardial disease.

An equally important group of cardiac imaging applications is discussed in the last section of our text. As treatment for congenital heart disease improves, more and more patients with congenital heart problems survive into adulthood, requiring sophisticated cardiac care. Most of these patients are followed by echocardiography traditionally, and more recently by MRI. Similarly, in patients with stroke, the possibility of cardioembolism has been recognized with increasing frequency. This results largely from the advent of transesophageal echocardiography, which has enabled cardiologists and internists to identify cardiac sources of emboli and gain important insight into the etiology of this frequently devastating disease. In addition, cardiac imaging applications to the detection of cardiac tumors and aortic dissection are well established in medical practice, as is the utilization of echocardiography during cardiac surgical procedures and in patients with chronic pulmonary disease. They comprise the topics addressed in the last section of this text, and represent an important part of the everyday activity of cardiologists primarily dedicated to imaging.

The book would not have been completed without the significant administrative support of offices on both sides of the Atlantic. Kathleen Lensch and Joseph Wassil were crucial in the organization of text and selection of echocardiographic images for diverse chapters respectively. In England, the administrative efforts of Jenny Cranwell were crucial to the completion of this project, as was the fastidiousness of Tanya Wheatley, my project editor, in the overall management of the project. Finally my appreciation to Alan Burgess from Martin Dunitz Ltd for helping me realize the vision of a novel approach to the transmission of knowledge on cardiac imaging to clinical cardiologists.

João A. C. Lima, MD FACC
Assistant Professor of Medicine and Radiology,
Johns Hopkins School of Medicine, and
Director of Transesophageal and Stress
Echocardiography, The Johns Hopkins Hospital.

1

Noninvasive approaches to the evaluation of left ventricular function

Elizabeth Klodas and James L Weiss

Introduction

The bedside clinical assessment of left ventricular function is notoriously poor.[1,2] However, accurate evaluation of both systolic and diastolic properties of the left ventricle is of paramount importance in guiding patient therapy, determining prognosis, and following the course of cardiac disease.[3–5] Although left ventriculography via cardiac catheterization has traditionally been considered the gold standard for quantification of function,[6] this technique is limited by the fact that the three-dimensional ventricle is viewed in two dimensions, significantly hampering accuracy, and that repeat measurements, often required for patient management, are impractical.

Several noninvasive techniques have been developed for quantification of left ventricular function, and these have in many respects surpassed angiography in terms of accuracy and ease of applicability. The present chapter outlines the current noninvasive modalities employed to assess left ventricular function, concentrating on echocardiography, nuclear imaging, electron beam computed tomography, and magnetic resonance imaging. The evaluation of both systole and diastole is reviewed, and the relative merits and shortfalls of each technique are discussed.

General considerations

During contractions, the left ventricle undergoes complex changes in shape and size.[7–14] Not only is there thickening of the ventricular walls, resulting in diminution of cavity size, but also significant longitudinal shortening (from base to apex), rotation about the long axis, tilting perpendicular to the long axis, translation from side to side, as well as rotation of the apex with respect to the base. Furthermore regional variability of these motions has been documented not only in diseased but also in normal hearts, adding to the difficulties encountered in accurately tracking cardiac motion. From a practical standpoint, this means that imaging modalities are subject to spatial limitations in following myocardial segments during the cardiac cycle. Inaccurate tracking may result in incorrect volume determinations, leading to false conclusions regarding global function as well as misjudgments regarding segmental motion.

Furthermore, no measure of left ventricular systolic function can be viewed in isolation. Aside from pathologic states such as ischemia and ventricular hypertrophy, preload, afterload, contractile state, and heart rate all influence ventricular function, and contribute to the variability of quantitative assessments.[15–18] Any change in measured values must therefore be interpreted not only with the test's variability in mind, but also with the clinical state of the patient factored in. Another confounder not to be overlooked is the presence of ventricular interdependence, with right ventricular events influencing the function of the left ventricle.[19–21]

The quantitative parameters of diastolic function are influenced by hemodynamic status, heart rate, rhythm, systolic ventricular performance, and age of the patient.[22] This again underscores the need to interpret all quantitative data in the context of patient status, and to recognize that changes in those data do not necessarily represent irreversible alterations in ventricular function but potentially reversible changes in clinical state.

Electrocardiography

Often overlooked for this purpose, standard 12-lead electrocardiography may be extremely helpful in the evaluation of systolic ventricular performance. Although other ECG findings are nonspecific, the presence of an *entirely normal 12-lead electrocardiogram* virtually ensures the presence of normal systolic function (95% likelihood).[23] This point should be kept in mind before going on to further testing, especially if the purpose of the evaluation is determination of ejection fraction.

Electrocardiographic findings are insensitive and nonspecific for the evaluation of diastolic function, and although false positive rates are low, electrocardiographic criteria for the diagnosis of left ventricular hypertrophy display relatively poor sensitivity (< 60%).[24]

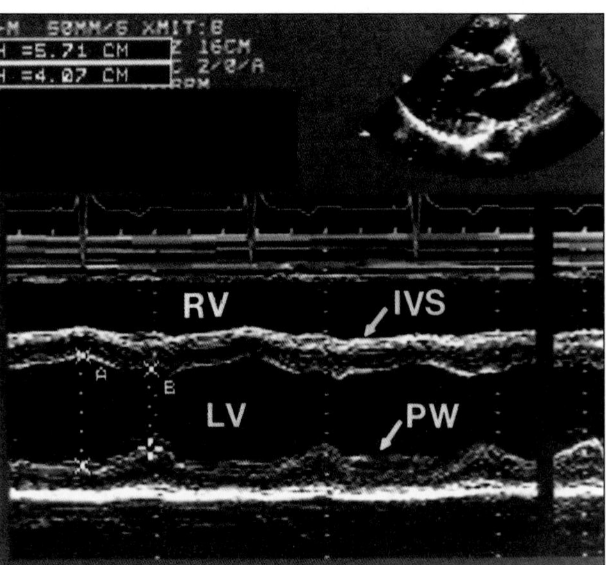

Figure 1.1
M-mode echocardiogram of left ventricular (LV) illustrating measurement of end-diastolic and end-systolic dimensions. The M-mode tracing is obtained using two-dimensional guidance, in either the parasternal long-axis (shown) or short-axis (not shown) view. The end-diastolic measurement (A) is made at the Q wave of the simultaneous electrocardiogram, and the end-systolic measurement (B) is made at the point of greatest posterior wall excursion. All measurements are made from leading edge to leading edge. IVS, interventricular septum; PW, posterior wall; RV, right ventricular cavity.

Echocardiography

Echocardiography is the most widely used noninvasive imaging modality employed to assess cardiac function and anatomy. The equipment is portable, no exposure to ionizing radiation is required, noninvasive assessment of cardiac hemodynamics is easily accomplished, and, with the advent of the transesophageal approach, virtually any patient regardless of body habitus or clinical state can be imaged successfully. Echocardiography, however, is highly operator dependent, and obtaining accurate information by this technique requires not only skilled technicians, but also knowledgeable interpreters. From a practical standpoint, this probably constitutes echocardiography's greatest limitation as an imaging modality.

Global systolic function

Assessment of systolic function depends primarily upon determination of end-diastolic volumes (EDV) and end-systolic volumes (ESV) and obtaining an ejection fraction (EF) by the formula:

$$EF = \frac{EDV - ESV}{EDV} \qquad (a)$$

Various methods for the derivation of these volumes exist, and all rely upon assumptions regarding ventricular geometry.

One of the simplest methods employs M-mode derived ventricular diameters (*D*) in the minor axis.[25] EDV is obtained by cubing the end-diastolic diameter (EDD) and ESV is obtained by cubing the end-systolic diameter (ESD) from a single cardiac cycle (Fig. 1.1). The ejection fraction is then derived as:

$$EF = \frac{EDD^3 - ESD^3}{EDD^3} \qquad (b)$$

Several assumptions are inherent in the cubed method, including that the minor axes of the left ventricular are of identical length, that the long axis of the left ventricle is twice the length of the measured minor axis, and, most significantly, that the single tomographic view examined is representative of all myocardial segments. The cubed method, therefore, is limited by overestimation of volumes when the heart assumes a more spherical shape (dilated cardiomyopathy, valvular regurgitation), and by significant inaccuracies (under- or overestimation of ejection fraction) in the presence of asymmetric wall motion. Although correlation with angiographic volumes is only modest ($r = 0.64–0.89$),[25–28] in view of ease of utility, the cubed method remains a widely applied method to quantitate left ventricular function. However, in the presence of regional wall motion abnormalities or septal asynergy, this method is highly inaccurate and should not be employed.[29]

The Teicholz method[27] also employs minor axis diameters, but attempts to correct for left ventricular shape by employing the following formula for volume (V) determinations:

$$V = [7.0/(2.4 + D)] \times D^3 \qquad \text{(c)}$$

Volumes derived by this method have been found to correlate well with angiographic estimates of LV geometry,[27,30] and although the formula is cumbersome, most commercially available ultrasound systems are equipped with an analysis package capable of automatically computing EF using the Teicholz method. The presence of regional asynergy again results in inaccurate EF determinations using this approach.

As an attempt to better represent multiple levels of the left ventricle, Quinones et al developed a method wherein the diameters employed represented an average of several diameters as viewed during two-dimensional imaging: two from the parasternal long-axis view, three from the 4-chamber, and three from the 2-chamber view, both at end-systole and end-diastole.[31] The fractional shortening of the long axis was also incorporated, and could be calculated based upon change in long-axis length during systole (L), or estimated based upon apical function.

$$\text{EF} = [(\text{mean EDD}^2 - \text{mean ESD}^2)/\text{mean EDD}^2] \qquad \text{(d)}$$
$$+ [1 - ([\text{mean EDD}^2 - \text{mean ESD}^2]/\text{mean EDD}^2)] \times (L)$$

or

$$\text{EF} = [(\text{mean EDD}^2 - \text{mean ESD}^2)/\text{mean EDD}^2]$$

+ 0.15 if the apex contracts normally
+ 0.05 if the apex is hypokinetic
+ 0.00 if the apex is akinetic
− 0.05 if the apex is dyskinetic

Because multiple separate measurements must be made and averaged, this method is cumbersome, and despite its ability to partially account for regional dysfunction, is not widely employed. It should be noted that this method is not based on determination of volumes and should not be employed for this purpose.

The single plane area/length method (Fig. 1.2) developed for angiography can be applied to echocardiography during apical two-dimensional imaging as follows:

$$V = 0.85(A)^2/L \qquad \text{(e)}$$

In general, this method should be employed when only one apical view is obtainable since it is less accurate than the biplane method of disks (see below).[29]

The volumetric method which best incorporates regional function is the method of disks, sometimes referred to as the modified Simpson's method. This consists of defining the left ventricular cavity as the sum of a series of stacked disk volumes (Fig. 1.3). The cavity is traced from the mitral annulus back to the mitral annulus along the endocardial border, excluding the papillary muscles both in end-systole and end-diastole, and computer software automatically divides the traced cavity into a finite number of disks and sums their calculated volumes. Ejection fraction is then calculated according to formula (a). Although this method may be performed in 'single plane' (whereby the left ventricular cavity is traced only in the 4-chamber apical view), the 'biplane' (left ventricular cavity traced in the orthogonal 4-chamber and 2-chamber apical views, measurements averaged) is superior, especially if regional wall motion abnormalities are evident.[29]

The number of disks employed is not standardized, although in normal ventricles the lower limit for the number of disks under which significant volumetric errors occur has been established at four.[32] Currently, most automated systems divide the ventricle into 20 equal sections. The method of disks requires good endocardial border definition, thus limiting its applicability in some patients. However, many of the geometric assumptions that hamper the other abovementioned methods are avoided and excellent correlation with true volumetric data is possible ($r = 0.97$),[33] thus making the biplane method of disks the method of choice from a practical standpoint whenever highly accurate quantitation of ventricular volumes and ejection fraction are required.

Integrated backscatter analysis (automated border detection (ABD) or acoustic quantitation (AQ)) automatically differentiates tissue from blood on the basis of differences in the amplitude of reflected ultrasound (Fig. 1.4). This can be employed to instantaneously define left ventricular volumes according to various computerized algorithms, allowing for automated determination of not only cardiac volumes and ejection fractions, but also filling and ejection rates, as well as time to peak filling.[34–37] Relatively operator-independent instantaneous quantitation of volumes and function is therefore possible, irrespective of cavity shape and regional function, making this method very attractive and user friendly. However, excellent endocardial definition must be present on the baseline image, gain settings must be optimized for tracking the endocardium, and care must be taken to avoid foreshortened views. Automatic quantitation is available only on the most recent echocardiographic equipment, and has not yet to date replaced the quantitative methods outlined above.

Three-dimensional echocardiography, a recent development in the field of cardiac ultrasound, can also be employed to evaluate left ventricular function. Several methods for three-dimensional reconstruction of two-dimensional images exist, and image acquisition must be gated to the electrocardiogram as well as to respiratory phase. Volumes determined by three-dimensional echocardiography have been

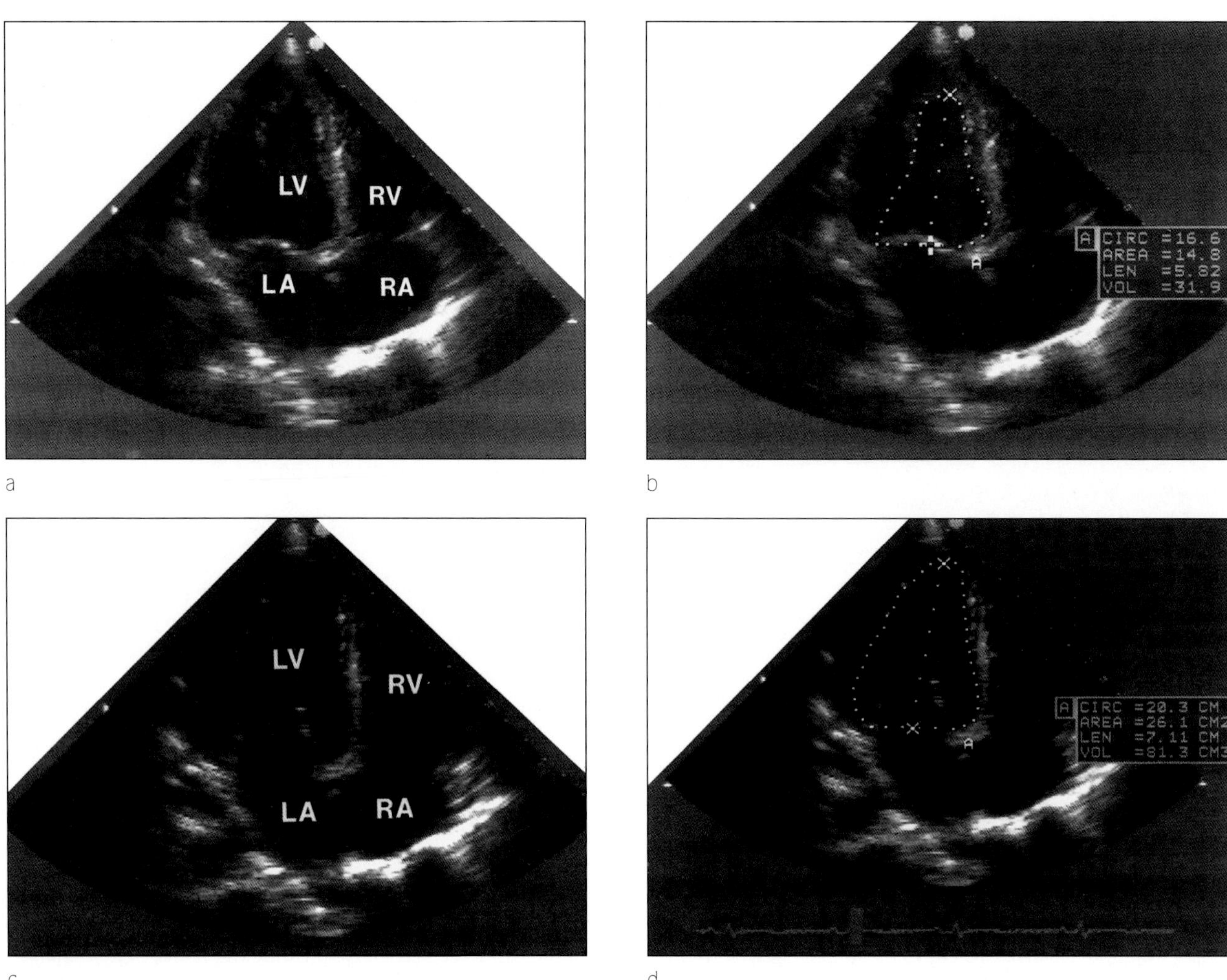

Figure 1.2
Single-plane area/length method of calculating left ventricular (LV) volume in systole (a and b) and diastole (c and d). The ventricular cavity is traced along the endocardial surface from mitral annulus back to the mitral annulus, excluding the papillary muscles. Cavity length is measured from the apical endocardium to the midpoint of the mitral valve plane. Computer software available on most echocardiographic equipment then automatically calculates the ventricular volumes and resultant ejection fraction. RV, right ventricle; LA, left atrium; RA, right atrium.

found to correlate well with actual measured volumes in vitro (r = 0.97–0.98),[38,39] and since no geometric assumptions are required to determine volumes or ejection fractions, this method may become the echocardiographic gold standard for quantification of left ventricular function. Presently, however, three-dimensional echocardiography is principally employed in the research setting, and current approaches are laborious.

Another method to determine ejection fraction is visual estimation. During review of the entire echocardiographic study, the interpreter estimates a numerical value for the ejection fraction, based upon integration of all views provided. When performed by experienced readers, these estimates correlate well with radionuclide ejection fractions (r = 0.82–0.96),[40,41] and are usually adequate for clinical purposes. Although intraobserver variability in interpretation appears to be acceptable, interobserver variability may be substantial, thus limiting the suitability of this technique for following left ventricular function in instances where small changes in EF might be considered clinically significant.

Irrespective of which method of quantitation is chosen, it is important that the same method be used in the same patient over time for comparison purposes. Because each

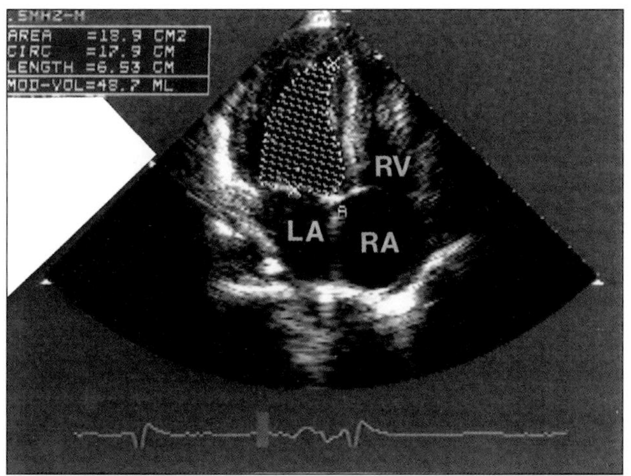

a

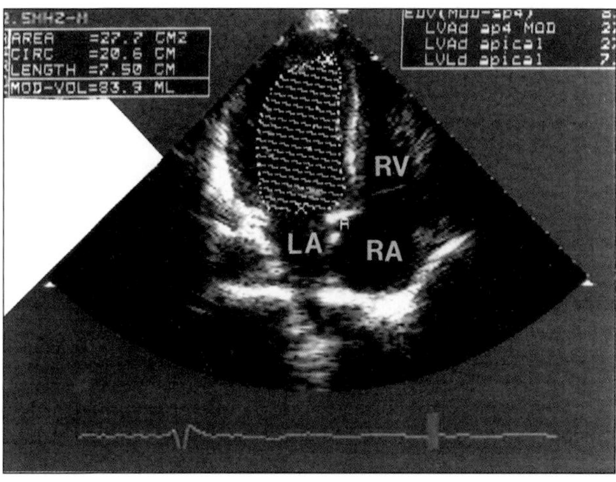

b

Figure 1.3
Biplane method of disks as used to determine left ventricular volumes and ejection fraction. (a) A tracing in systole; (b) tracing in diastole. For the area/length method, the ventricular cavity is traced along the endocardial surface from mitral annulus back to the mitral annulus, excluding the papillary muscles. The volumes and ejection fraction are automatically calculated on-line by the equipment's computer. RV, right ventricle; RA, right atrium; LA, left atrium.

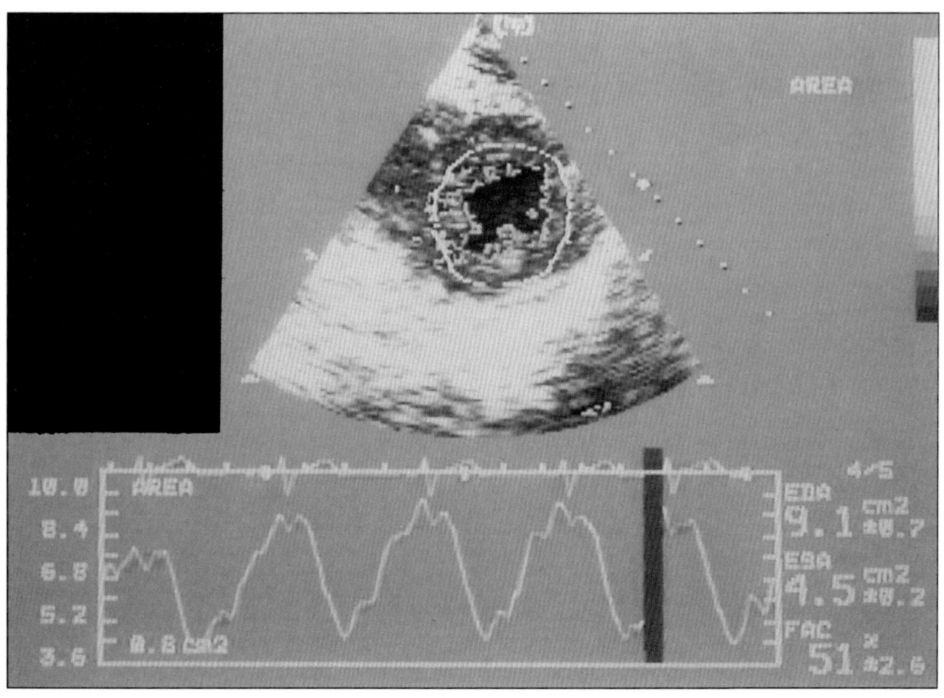

Figure 1.4
Automated endocardial border detection within selected region of interest in short-axis view of left ventricle. Tracking of area change with time lends itself to analysis of both systolic and diastolic parameters of ventricular function.

approach makes different assumptions regarding ventricular geometry, the various methods will not yield identical volumes or ejection fractions.[42] Ideally, when a value is reported, the method used to obtain the measurement should also be specified.

Myocardial mass

Myocardial mass may be estimated from M-mode measurements, with the same inherent geometric assumptions as for volume determinations (Fig. 1.5). Therefore,

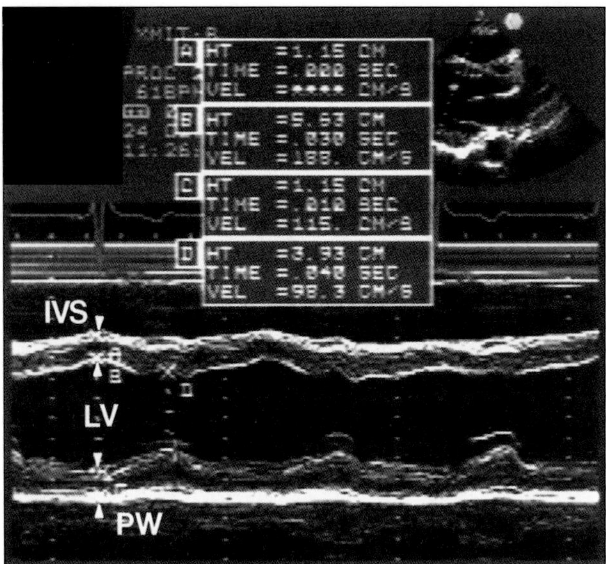

Figure 1.5
M-mode measurements used to calculate myocardial mass. All diastolic measurements are obtained at the onset of the Q wave of the simultaneous electrocardiogram. Distances are measured from leading edge to leading edge. Although the systolic ventricular cavity diameter has been measured in this illustration (dimension D), this value is not required for the determination of myocardial mass using the Penn convention. IVS, interventricular septum; LV, left ventricle; PW, posterior wall.

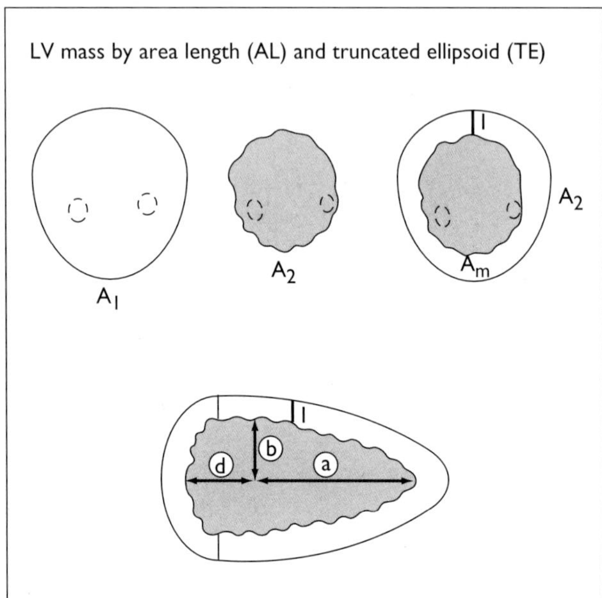

Figure 1.6
Two-dimensional method of calculating myocardial mass by the area/length (AL) technique. Reprinted with permission from Schiller et al.[29]

mass estimates using the M-mode technique will be most accurate in symmetric ventricles of normal shape.[27] According to the Penn convention, mass is estimated at end-diastole, using the measurements of septal thickness (ST), posterior wall thickness (PWT), and left ventricular internal diameter (LVID) as follows:

$$\text{LV mass} = 0.8\,\{1.04[(\text{ST} + \text{PWT} + \text{LVID})]^3 - \text{LVID}^3\} + 0.6\text{ g} \qquad \text{(f)}$$

where 1.04 is the specific gravity of myocardium and 0.8 is a correction factor added since anatomic weight would otherwise be overestimated by approximately 20%.[43]

The area/length two-dimensional method (Fig. 1.6) has been found to be reliable in human studies,[44] and is preferred to the M-mode method according to the American Society of Echocardiography Committee on Standards.[29] For a more detailed discussion regarding left ventricular mass determinations by echocardiography, see Chapter 2.

Regional systolic function

Although assessment of global ventricular function is important from a prognostic and management perspective, delineation of regional function may be of critical importance in patients with ischemic heart disease. For example, in patients with chest pain but nondiagnostic electrocardiograms, the presence or absence of regional wall motion abnormalities by echocardiography may be used to affect acute management decisions. Furthermore, the exploding field of stress echocardiography depends upon assessment of regional function before and during stress in order to accurately define the anatomic location and extent of reversible ischemia.

Regional function evaluation is standardized according to the American Society of Echocardiography.[29] The left ventricle is divided into 16 segments (Fig. 1.7): 6 at the base, 6 at midventricular level, and 4 at the apex. Each segment is then judged visually according to the degree of systolic myocardial thickening (*not* motion) as normal or hypercontractile (score = 1), hypokinetic (score = 2), akinetic (score = 3), dyskinetic (score = 4), or aneurysmal (score = 5). Adding the scores for all the segments and dividing by 16 yields a 'wall motion score index', which has been shown to be associated with prognosis.[45] Wall thickening rather than endocardial motion is preferentially assessed since it is less likely to be affected by rotation or translation, and it is more sensitive and specific for the presence of ischemia or infarction.[46] Furthermore, it is less likely to be abnormal in other settings of abnormal wall motion (conduction abnormalities, following

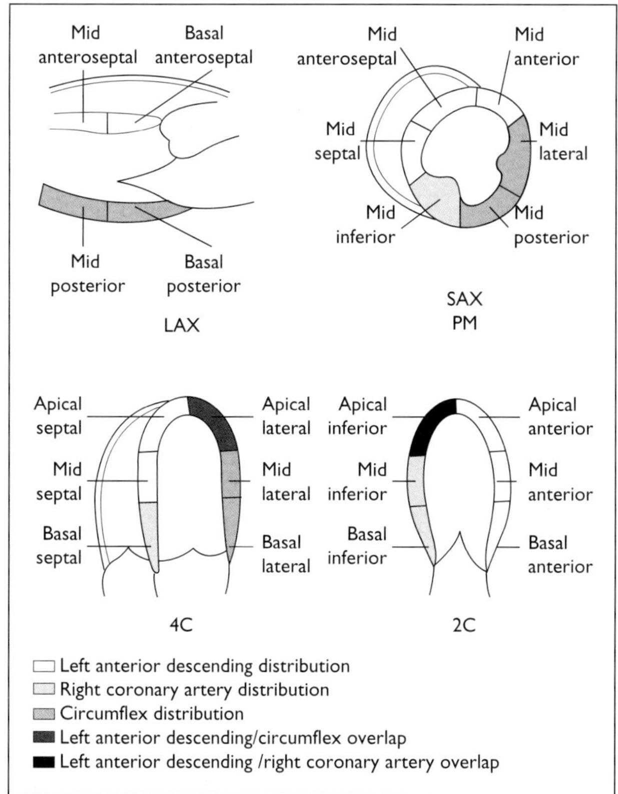

Figure 1.7
Sixteen-segment regional wall motion model of the left ventricle with the corresponding coronary artery distributions. Reprinted with permission from Segar et al.

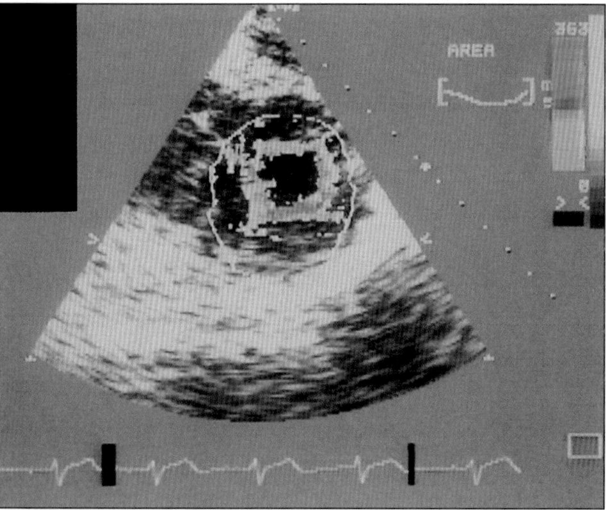

Figure 1.8
Computer-aided quantification of systolic wall motion and thickening. Systolic circumferential motion is represented by a color map which depicts timing of contraction (yellow, early; blue, late) and degree of contraction (color map thickness at any radius point).

pericardiotomy, in patients with right ventricular overload).[47,48] Clearly, assessment of regional wall motion is subjective and qualitative, relying upon visual determination of per cent thickening, and as such requires not only adequate visualization of segments by the sonographer, but also substantial experience on the part of the interpreter. Computer-aided quantification of wall motion and thickening (Fig. 1.8) is now possible with newer echocardiographic equipment, and appears promising from the standpoint of reducing subjectivity.

Doppler evaluation of systolic function

Doppler echocardiography can be used to determine stroke volume (SV) and cardiac output (CO) noninvasively. The flow rate through a circular orifice with a cross-sectional area *A*, is obtained by multiplying that area by the time-integrated velocity of flow through the orifice:

$$\text{flow} = A\ (\text{cm}^2) \times \text{velocity (cm/s)} \times \text{time (s)} = \text{cm}^3 \qquad (g)$$

where *A* may be calculated as

$$(\text{orifice diameter})^2 \times \pi/4 \qquad (h)$$

In echocardiography, the orifice most frequently utilized is the left ventricular outflow tract (LVOT), the diameter of which is measured directly from two-dimensional images, and velocity of blood flow during systole is time-integrated using pulse wave Doppler technology (Fig. 1.9). The calculated flow through the LVOT is stroke volume, and cardiac output is calculated by multiplying SV by the heart rate. Attention must be paid to careful measurement of the LVOT diameter since any errors will be squared, significantly affecting the accuracy of the measurement, and Doppler beam orientation must be nearly parallel to flow to avoid underestimating time-integrated velocity. Performed properly, however, Doppler assessment of cardiac output is reproducible, and correlates well with invasive data.[49–51]

Doppler interrogation of the mitral regurgitation (MR) signal can also be used to determine dP/dT, thus providing noninvasive assessment of myocardial contractility (Fig. 1.10).[52] This is particularly useful in patients with severe MR, wherein systolic function may appear normal despite the presence of irreversible myocardial damage. In the context of severe MR, a normal dP/dT is reassuring that following corrective surgery systolic function will be preserved.[53]

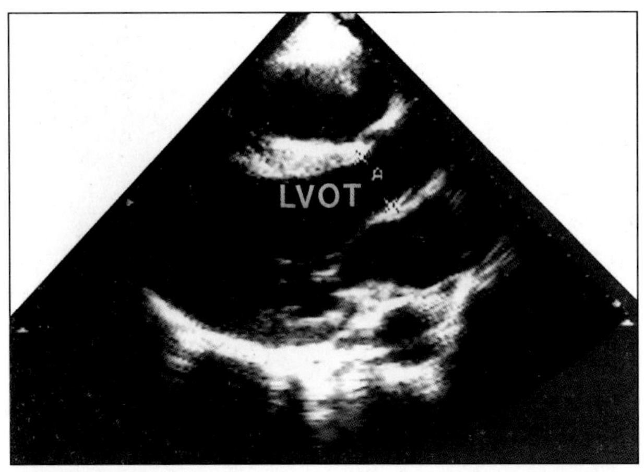

a

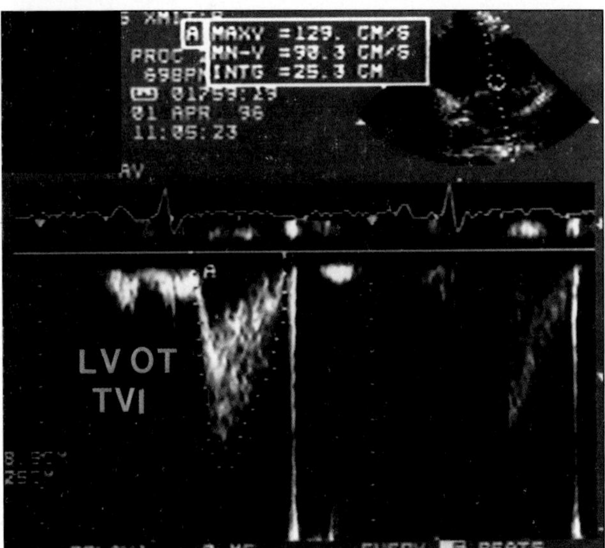

b

Figure 1.9
Determination of cardiac output using Doppler echocardiography. Measurements required for calculation include left ventricular outflow tract (LVOT) diameter as assessed from the parasternal long-axis view (A), and the LVOT time velocity integral (TVI) obtained by pulse wave Doppler from the apical 5-chamber view.

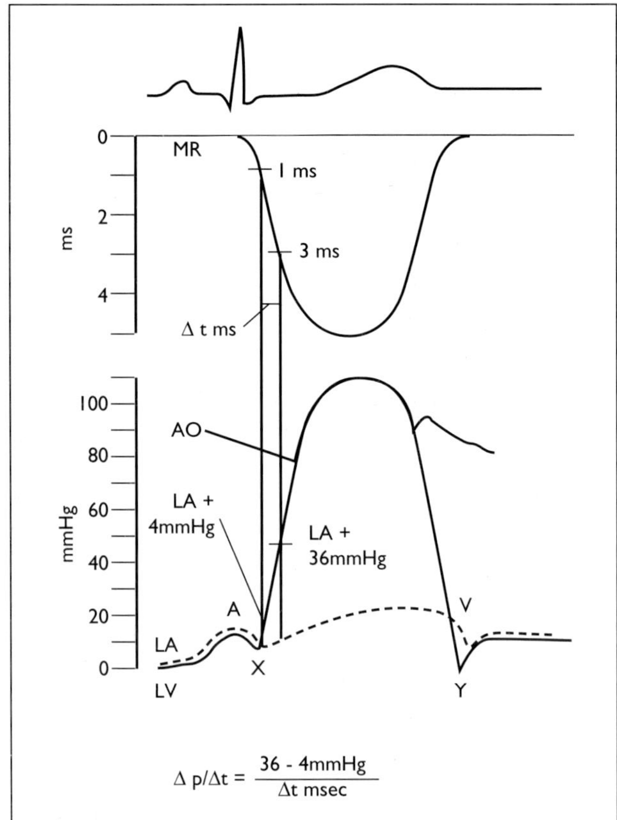

Figure 1.10
Method of calculating left ventricular d*P*/d*t* by Doppler echocardiography. T, time taken for the mitral regurgitant velocity to rise from 1 to 3 m/s; P, magnitude of rise in left ventricular pressure when mitral regurgitant velocity rises from 1 to 3 m/s, about 32 mmHg because left atrial pressure does not significantly rise during this period. LV d*P*/d*t* = 32/*t* in ms × 100 mmHg/s. MR, mitral regurgitation; AO, aortic; LA, left atrial; LV, left ventricular. Reprinted with permission from Pai et al.[53]

Diastolic function

Diastolic dysfunction is an early manifestation of cardiac disease, and an important contributor to cardiac morbidity. In some instances, diastolic dysfunction may be the only underlying pathophysiologic process, yet may result in significant signs and symptoms. Indeed, a significant proportion of patients with congestive heart failure have symptoms on the basis of diastolic dysfunction alone.[54]

Doppler echocardiography has emerged as the preferred method to noninvasively assess diastole, and comprehensive evaluation involves pulsed wave Doppler sampling of mitral and pulmonic vein inflow signals. Mitral inflow interrogation allows for characterization of left ventricular isovolumic relaxation time (IVRT), early diastolic filling (E wave), rapidity of pressure equalization between left ventricle and left atrium during early filling (deceleration time), and evaluation of atrial contribution to filling (A wave) (Fig. 1.11). Pulmonic inflow signals, on the other hand, are evaluated from the standpoint of relative forward flow during ventricular systole (S) and early diastole (D), and velocity and duration of reversed flow during atrial contraction (AR) (Fig. 1.12).

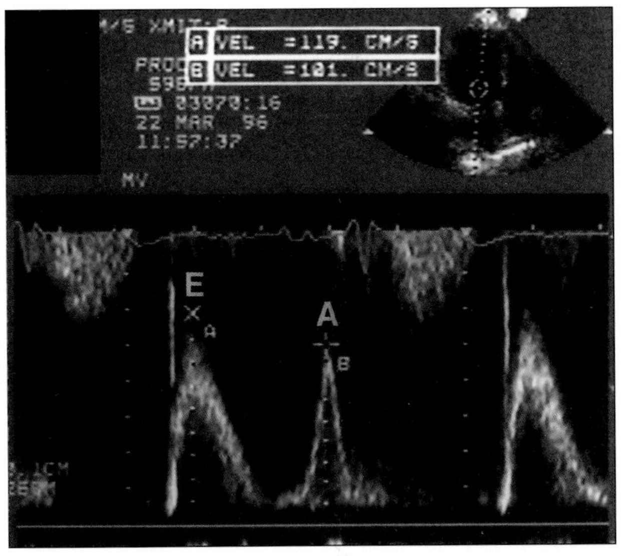

a

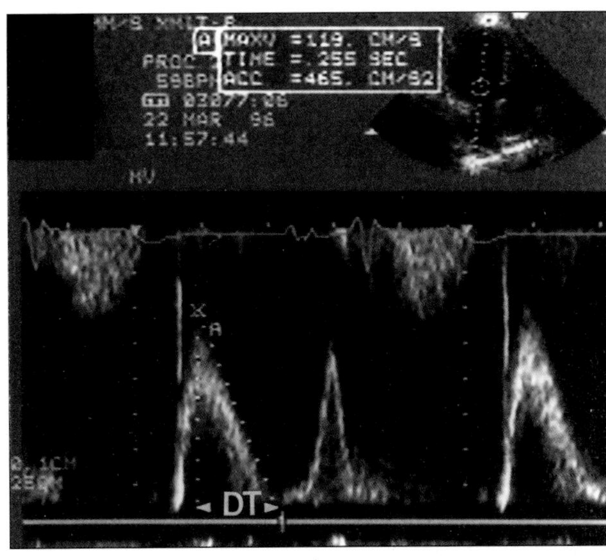

b

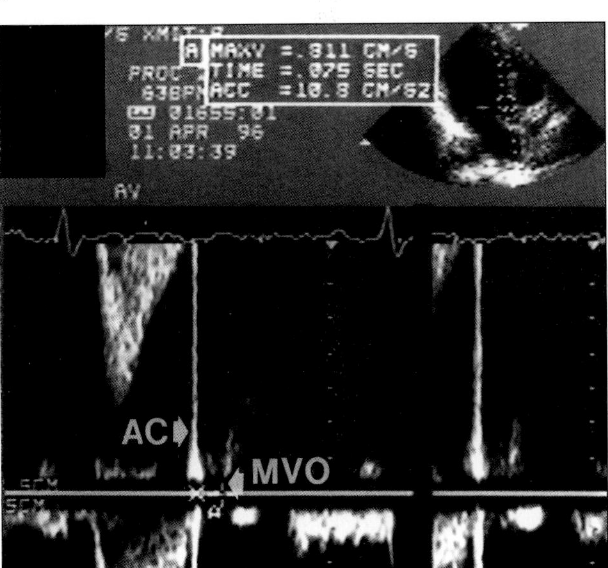

c

Figure 1.11
Components of mitral inflow pulsed wave Doppler signal utilized to assess left ventricular diastolic function. The E wave represents early diastolic filling, while the A wave represents left ventricular filling resulting from atrial contraction. The deceleration time (DT) measures the time interval from peak early filling to equalization of pressure between left atrium and left ventricle. The isovolumic relaxation time may be measured noninvasively by determining the time interval aortic valve closure (AC) and mitral valve opening (MVO).

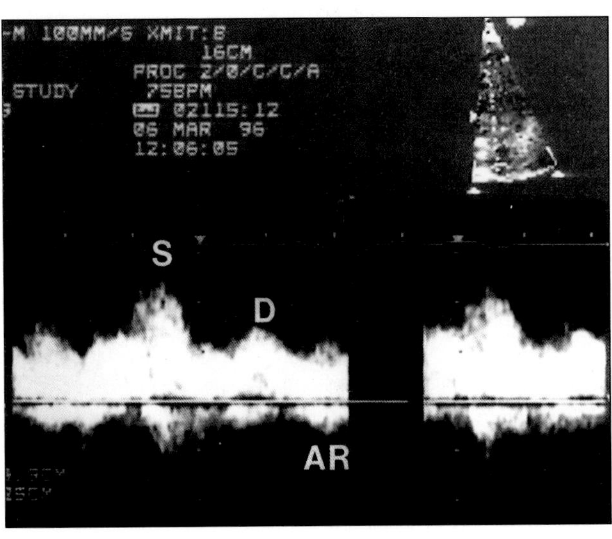

Figure 1.12
Components of pulmonic vein pulsed wave Dopper signal used to help assess diastolic function. S, forward flow from pulmonary vein into the left atrium during ventricular *systole* (atrial diastole); D, forward flow from pulmonary vein into the left atrium during ventricular *diastole* (mitral valve open); AR, reverse flow from left atrium back into the pulmonary vein during atrial contraction (*atrial reversal*).

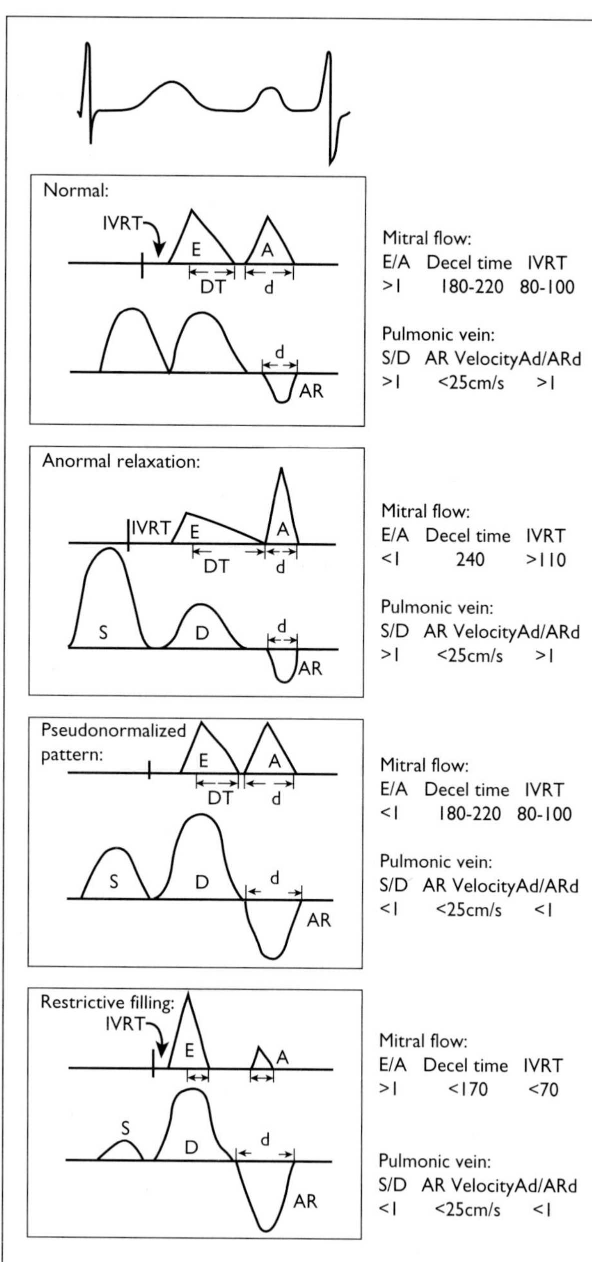

Figure 1.13
Summary of flow patterns across the mitral inflow and pulmonic veins as seen under normal conditions, and in the settings of abnormal relaxation, pseudonormalization, and restrictive filling. Ad, duration of mitral A wave; ARd, duration of pulmonic atrial reversal signal. (See text for explanation.)

It has become apparent that several remarkably distinct patterns of flow across these orifices are possible, and they have been conventionally labeled as 'normal', 'relaxation abnormality', 'pseudonormalization', and 'restrictive filling' (Fig. 1.13). These patterns represent a continuum of diastolic abnormalities, with 'relaxation abnormality' being the first, most common, and mildest perturbation seen.[55,56] It should be emphasized that diastolic flows through the mitral valve and pulmonic veins are influenced by ventricular preload, afterload, heart rate, electrocardiographic PR interval, as well as intrinsic myocardial relaxation and compliance parameters.[55] Therefore, although the labels may imply a myocardial process, various extrinsic factors may be responsible for the diastolic flow abnormality, and the abnormality may therefore be dynamic and potentially reversible.

Compared to the 'normal pattern', 'relaxation abnormality', is characterized by a low-amplitude E wave and a prominent A wave, while 'restrictive filling' is defined by the presence of a very large E wave, and a diminutive A wave. While left ventricular end-diastolic pressures (LVEDP) are characteristically normal when 'relaxation abnormality' is present, they are usually elevated when the 'restrictive filling' pattern is seen.

The existence of the 'pseudonormal pattern' (a pattern which results from the combined existence of impaired ventricular relaxation with moderate elevations in end-diastolic pressures) underscores the necessity of sampling inflow not only across the mitral valve, but also within the pulmonary vein, as pulmonary vein flow abnormalities may be the only clue to elevated LVEDPs. The normal pattern of pulmonary venous flow is that of larger systolic than diastolic antegrade signals, associated with normal wedge pressures. When systolic forward flow is normal, but the diastolic flow is absent or nearly absent, abnormally low wedge pressure is suggested (<8 mmHg), indicating reduction in preload.[57] In the absence of MR, the presence of a systolic forward flow velocity that is lower than diastolic forward flow velocity indicates elevated wedge pressure (generally >20–25 mmHg) (Fig. 1.14). Another recently described method to determine if LVEDP is elevated involves measuring the durations of mitral inflow A wave and pulmonic vein atrial reversal signals (Fig. 1.15).[58] If the A wave duration is shorter than the atrial reversal duration, an elevated LVEDP may be assumed.

Several pitfalls are possible during Doppler investigation of left ventricular diastolic function.[56] Proper placement of the pulsed wave Doppler sample volume at the mitral leaflet tips and 1–2 cm into the pulmonic vein is critical to obtaining accurate flow information. Significant changes in flow parameters occur when the sample volume is placed closer to the mitral annulus or at the orifice of the pulmonary vein, and inaccurate technique may result in inaccurate conclusions regarding the status of diastolic function. With normal aging, and in the presence of most cardiac disease states, mitral inflow patterns may become consistent with relaxation abnormality. Therefore, in patients over 65 years of age, or in any patient suspected of having myocardial disease, if a normal mitral inflow pattern is observed, pseudonormalization must be ruled out. Significant aortic regurgitation will shorten deceleration

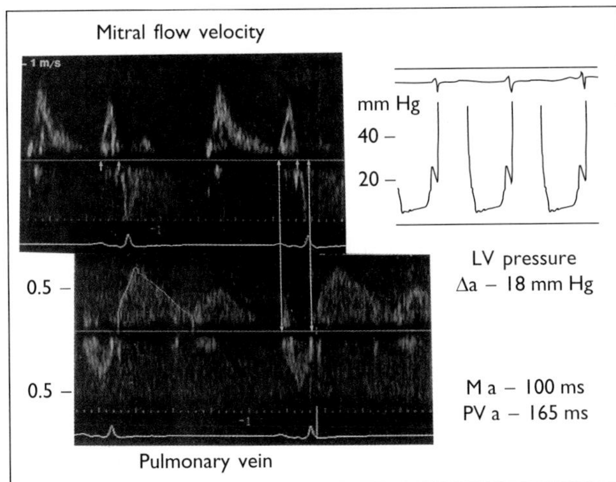

Figure 1.14
Illustration of markedly decreased systolic pulmonic venous forward flow in a patient with markedly elevated left ventricular end-diastolic pressure. Reprinted with permission from Rossvoll and Hatle.[58]

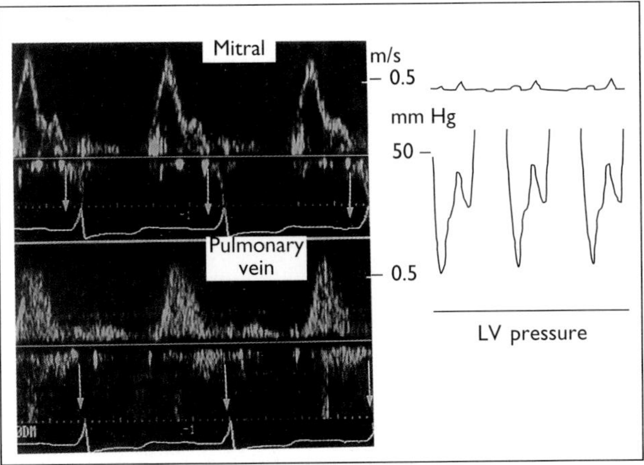

Figure 1.15
Elevated left ventricular end-diastolic pressure as suggested by disproportionately increased pulmonic vein atrial reversal flow duration (as compared to mitral A wave flow duration). Reprinted with permission from Rossvoll and Hatle.[58]

times and may result in mitral inflow patterns which appear restrictive. In this setting, it should be recognized that this diastolic abnormality may be due to the valve lesion alone, and does not necessarily imply intrinsic myocardial diastolic dysfunction. Atrial fibrillation results in loss of the A wave, and the E wave velocity and pulmonic vein inflows become variable and therefore difficult to interpret. The presence of a rapid heart rate or first degree atrioventricular block may result in overlap of the E and A waves complicating interpretation of their relative magnitudes. Finally, more than trivial mitral stenosis will produce significant alterations in values for all parameters used for the assessment of left ventricular diastolic function. In the presence of significant mitral valve disease, therefore, Doppler assessment of left ventricular diastolic events is inaccurate, and should not be pursued.

Radionuclide assessment of ventricular function

Gated radionuclide angiography

Despite recent advances in other noninvasive methods, radionuclide angiography (RNA) remains the gold standard for quantitative assessment of global ventricular function. This technique may be applied to almost all patients, irrespective of body habitus or underlying illness, and provides reproducible, accurate, and relatively operator-independent measurements.[59–62] Although patients are exposed to ionizing radiation, the total body dose is minimal and does not preclude repeated or frequent testing.[63]

Gated blood pool scanning requires labeling of the blood pool with technetium and computer acquisition of a series of gamma camera images gated to the R wave of the patient's electrocardiogram (Fig. 1.16). Determination of function relies upon the quantitation of count rate changes, which are proportional to volume changes, within the ventricular cavity over time. Because count data are employed, all quantitative measurements are independent of ventricular geometry, and do not rely upon any mathematical assumptions as to ventricular shape.[64,65] Although segmental function may be assessed by gated RNA, not all myocardial segments are well seen owing to significant structural overlap, and the major strength of this technique lies in its accurate quantitation of global function.

Assessment of ventricular function is performed both qualitatively and quantitatively. Inspection of all views allows for limited assessment of regional wall motion (Fig. 1.17).[63] It should be noted that RNA allows an exceptionally good view of the lateral wall and exercise RNA has been shown to be superior to exercise perfusion imaging in assessment of circumflex coronary artery disease.[66] During assessment of regional wall motion, overall global function should be estimated to verify the accuracy of the computer-generated results.

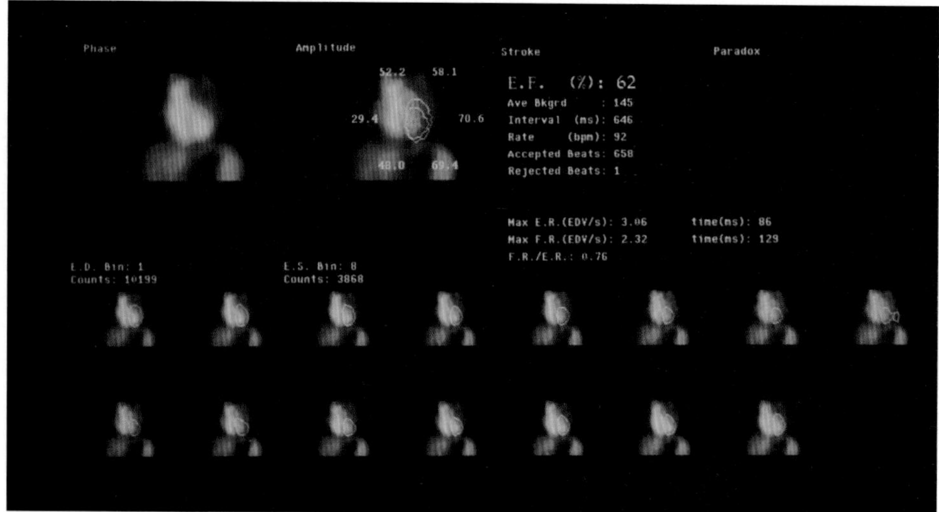

a

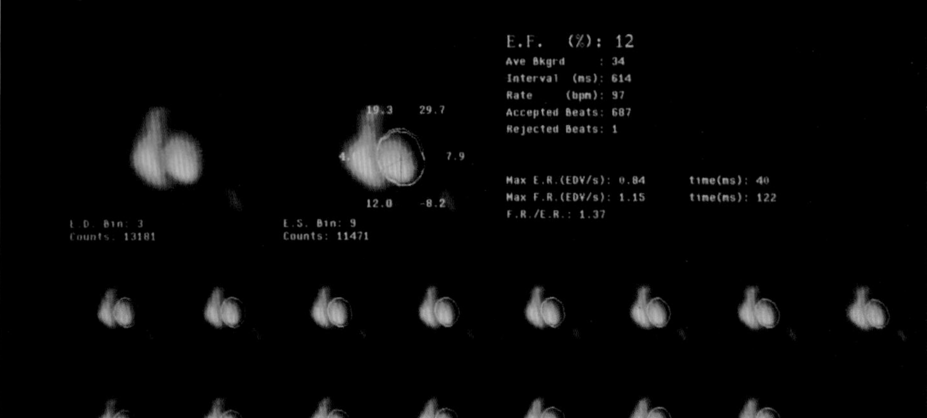

b

Figure 1.16
Assessment of left ventricular function by gated radionuclide angiography in a patient with normal (a) and severely abnormal (b) function. Although quantitation of regional ejection fractions is possible, gated radionuclide angiography is best employed to assess global function.

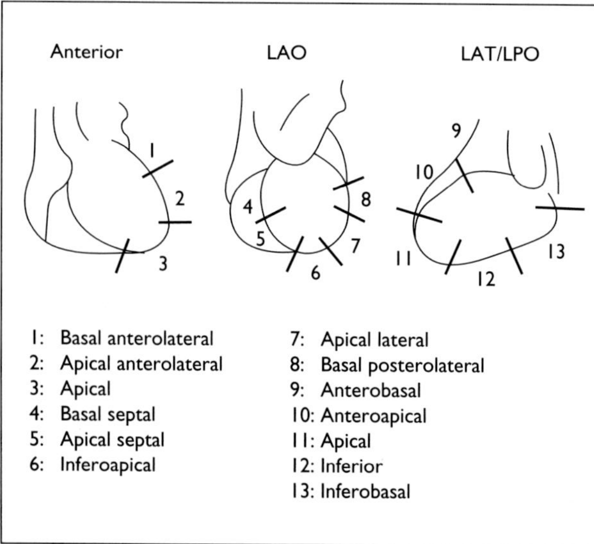

Figure 1.17
Wall motion segments as seen via three commonly obtained views during radionuclide angiography. Note that the true inferior wall is only seen in the lateral projection. Reprinted with permission from Johnson.[63]

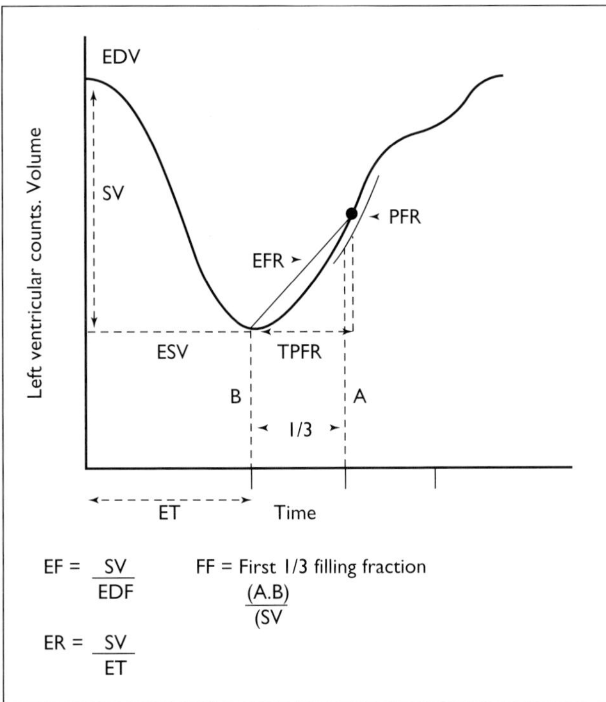

Figure 1.18
Left ventricular time activity curve showing phases of the cardiac cycle and how peak filling rate (PFR) and time to peak filling (TPFR) are calculated. EDV, end-diastolic volume; ESV, end-systolic volume; SV, stroke volume; ET, ejection time; ER, ejection rate; EFR, early filling rate. Reprinted with permission from Johnson.[63]

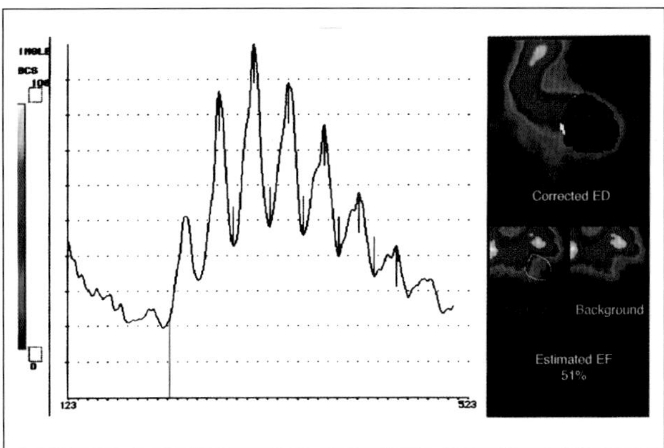

Figure 1.19
First pass time activity curve used to determine left ventricular ejection fraction. Each sawtooth oscillation represents an individual cardiac cycle, and the ejection fraction is calculated from the sum of selected end-diastolic counts (peaks) and systolic counts (troughs), corrected for background activity. Reprinted with permission from Johnson.[63]

Radionuclide imaging is not as widely utilized as echocardiography for the assessment of diastole. The time activity curve generated over the course of the cardiac cycle can demonstrate the phases of diastole at relatively slow heart rates (Fig. 1.18). However, as the R–R interval shortens, these phases become less distinct and accurate assessment of diastole becomes difficult. Two diastolic indices that have been widely studied are peak filling rate (akin to mitral E wave by echocardiography), and time to peak filling.[67] At heart rates < 100 beats/min the normal value for peak filling rate is greater than 2.5 EDV and time to peak filling is less than 180 ms.

First pass studies

With different instrumentation (a multicrystal camera) and different tracer handling (bolus injection), 'first pass' radionuclide angiograms are also possible. This methodology relies upon the tracking of the tracer bolus as it passes through the ventricular cavities immediately following injection to rapidly determine end-diastolic and end-systolic counts. Although temporal resolution with this technique is excellent, only a few beats are investigated, spatial resolution is poor, and only one view is acquired, precluding detailed regional wall motion assessment. However, acquisition time is rapid, often less than 30 s.

Determination of the left ventricular EF depends upon temporal separation of the tracer bolus between the two ventricles. Therefore, interference with the integrity of the bolus will affect the accuracy of systolic function assessment.[63] Poor injection technique, arrhythmias, pulmonary hypertension, atrial septal defect, and significant tricuspid or mitral regurgitation will all result in inaccurate left ventricular EF estimates, and under these circumstances gated radionuclide imaging should be employed.

As the bolus passes through the left ventricule, a sawtooth appearing time activity curve is generated (Fig. 1.19), with peaks representing end-diastole and troughs representing end-systole.[68] Counts from the peaks and troughs are summed, and the EF is obtained as for gated radionuclide studies. Assessment of left ventricular systolic function by first pass techniques has been validated against angiography and proven to be accurate and reproducible.[69,70] When the tracer employed is technetium 99m sestamibi, the first pass technique allows for assessment of both function and perfusion with the same bolus injection, providing complementary prognostic information in patients with heart disease at little additional cost.[71]

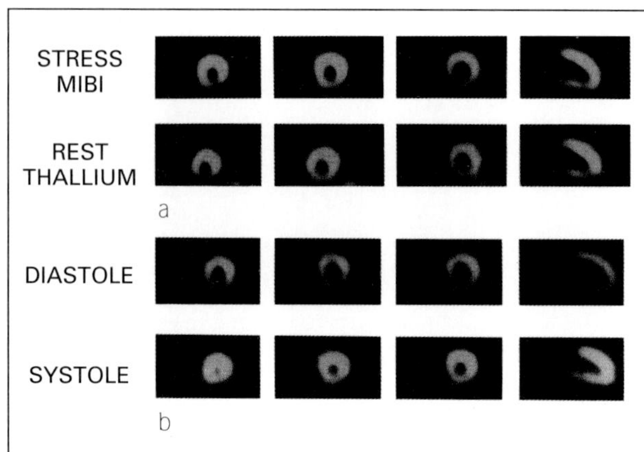

Figure 1.20
Nuclear perfusion study using a stress sestamibi-rest thallium-201 protocol. This patient displays a mild, nonreversible defect in the inferior wall, suggesting diaphragmatic attenuation or inferior infarction. Gated SPECT study showing corresponding systolic and diastolic images from the same patient. Note that wall motion is preserved in the inferior wall, which suggests that attenuation is responsible for the nonreversible perfusion defect. Reprinted with permission from Chua et al.[73]

Gated perfusion imaging

During acquisition of technetium 99m sestamibi perfusion images, data collection can be gated to the patient's ECG such that 8 frames per cardiac cycle are obtained. At the tradeoff of increasing imaging time, gating allows for qualitative cine loop review of left ventricular systolic function and wall thickening (best detected as brightening of the wall during systole).[72–74] Programs have also been developed for quantitation of both global and regional EFs using this technique.[72,75] Because a separate multicrystal camera is not required, this method of assessing LV systolic function is becoming widely utilized, especially in combination with perfusion imaging. Furthermore, computer reconstruction of the images permits quantitative and qualitative assessment of left ventricular systolic and diastolic performance in three dimensions. Accurate estimation of systolic ventricular function using gated perfusion imaging is hampered when severe perfusion defects are present (e.g. following transmural myocardial infarction), as tracer is not taken up by these segments, and they are therefore difficult to visualize. A major application of gating lies in its ability to aid in the discrimination between true mild perfusion defects and imaging artifact (breast or diaphragmatic attenuation) (Fig. 1.20).

Other applications

Reduced left ventricular cavity thallium activity in association with a perfusion defect on ungated tomographic perfusion

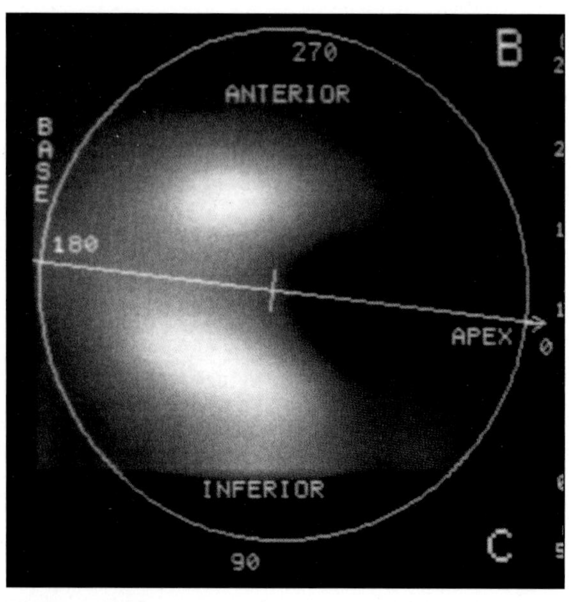

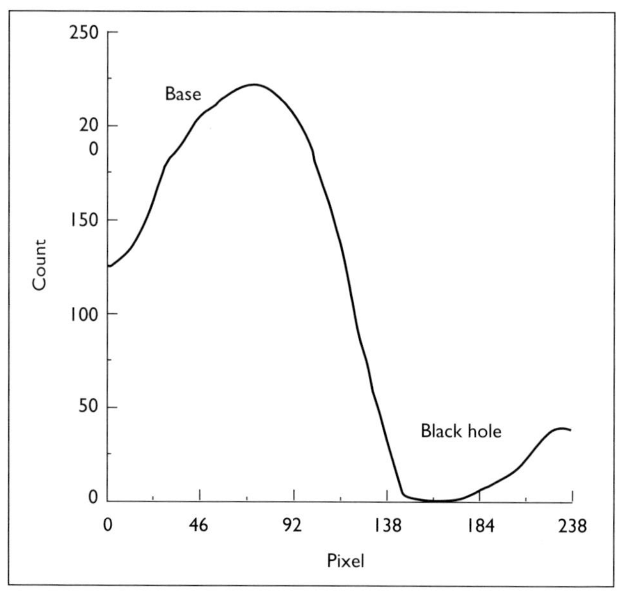

Figure 1.21
(a) Mid long-axis single photon emission computed tomographic slice from a patient with a left ventricular aneurysm illustrating the 'black hole sign'. (b) Linear count profile through the left ventricular cavity from base toward the apex. The highest activity corresponds to the basilar intracavitary activity. The lowest activity represents the black hole region. ANT, anterior; INF, inferior. Reprinted with permission from Civelek et al.[76]

images (the 'black hole' sign) (Fig. 1.21), has been found to be correlated with the presence of a left ventricular aneurysm,[76] and the relative degree of cavity opacification in general may be directly related to global left ventricular function. Reconstruction of tomographic radionuclide angiograms[77] and ambulatory monitoring of systolic function with miniature gamma cameras[78,79] have been pursued largely in the research setting. Bedside nuclear imaging is also possible with portable cameras, and allows for assessment of ventricular function or perfusion in patients who are too ill to be transported to an imaging laboratory and/or in whom other portable imaging modalities have failed. From a practical clinical standpoint, however, beside nuclear imaging is rarely required in a setting where transthoracic and transesophageal echocardiography is available. Radionuclide imaging is poorly suited to measurement of left ventricular mass.

Electron beam computed tomography

Traditional, and even spiral, computed tomography systems have been inadequate for cardiac imaging because the time required for the camera to rotate about the patient has been too prolonged to allow temporal resolution of phases of the cardiac cycle. The advent of electron beam computed tomography (EBCT, ultrafast CT, cine CT), has overcome this limitation, by apparatus design whereby an electron beam, rather than the camera unit, rotates around the patient, allowing for images to be acquired within 50 msec, with an interscan interval of 8 msec[80].

During scanning, the imaging table is positioned such that transverse short axis views and long axis views (comparable to those obtained by echocardiography) are acquired. Eight to 10 simultaneous parallel cross-sectional gated slices of the LV can be obtained, and to encompass the entire heart, with a slice thickness of 8 mm, it normally requires two complete short axis acquisitions. The long axis study typically requires only eight levels (one acquisition). Nonionic contrast is injected, typically 60–90 ml per imaging sequence, not to exceed 3 ml/kg patient weight[81,82].

Volumetric analysis of any cardiac chamber is easily performed by tracing end diastolic and end systolic endocardial borders at each level. Scanner software then calculates chamber volumes and stroke volumes for each level, with global chamber volumes being determined via level summation[83]. This allows for volume assessment which is geometry independent. Excellent correlation has been documented between volumes obtained by EBCT and those from biplane cineangiography and with ventricular cast volumes[84–86]. Ejection fraction is then determined in the standard fashion using the formula:

$$EF = \frac{EDV - ESV}{EDV}$$

One drawback of this method is that planimetry of each level is time consuming, requiring approximately 30 min to complete all levels. However, the resultant measurements are highly accurate and reproducible, and correlate well with radionuclide angiography ($r = 0.94$).[87] Three-dimensional reconstruction of the images is possible, and provides yet another venue by which left ventricular function may be evaluated. Geometry-independent, tomographic, volumetric analysis possible with both EBCT and magnetic resonance imaging (see below) represents the great advantage of these techniques, which probably outperform two-dimensional echocardiography and angiography in terms of accuracy and reproducibility.

Cross-sectional imaging as provided by EBCT, allows for qualitative assessment of regional wall motion.[88] Furthermore, owing to excellent spatial resolution and with appropriate computer software, EBCT easily lends itself to quantitative assessment of regional function capable of providing numerical and graphical displays of regional contractility.[89]

Cardiac output measurements may be obtained by multiplying (EDV–ESV) by heart rate (as in echocardiography or nuclear imaging), or may be determined by time density analysis of a contrast bolus, akin to the indicator dilution techniques employed in angiography. Excellent correlation has been noted between EBCT-determined time density cardiac output measurements and thermodilution measurements over a wide range of values ($r = 0.92$).[90]

Assessment of diastole may be accomplished by changing the scanning parameters to increase the number of images obtained during early diastole. The optimal sequencing is affected by heart rate and needs to be individualized. As heart rates increase, the reliability of the measurements is affected by the temporal resolution limits of the scanner (maximum frame rate of 17 images per second).[91] The diastolic filling curve is generated by planimetry of the chamber cavity at each time sequence, allowing assessment of time to peak filling, filling fraction, and time to peak filling rate[88] (Fig. 1.23), and these measurements have been found to agree with radionuclide angiography values.[91]

Measurement of myocardial mass is easily accomplished by tracing of the endocardial and epicardial borders,

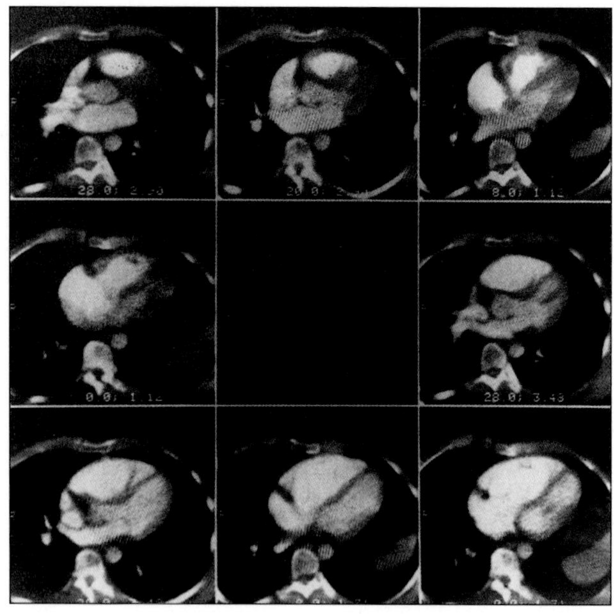

a

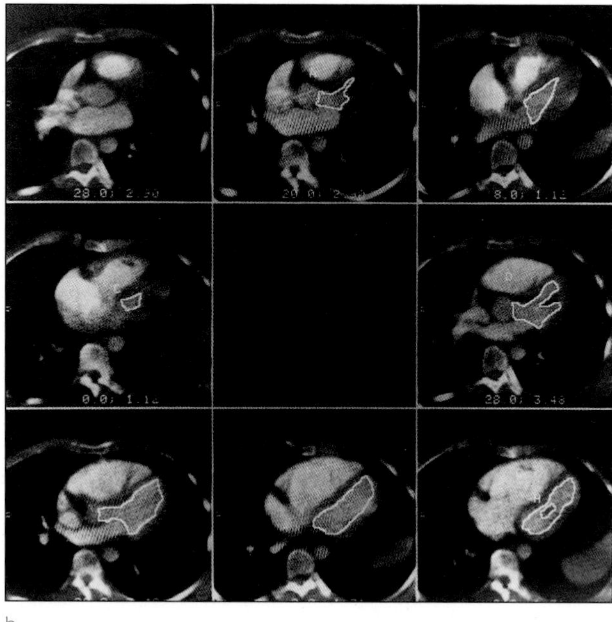

b

Figure 1.22
Four level EBCT scan in the long axis (a). The left ventricular end-systolic images for each contiguous slice are displayed left-to-right as the first four images. The corresponding end-diastolic images for contiguous slices are displayed left-to-right in the second four images. The same four level EBCT (b) with closed irregular circles are traced by computerized planimetry, outlining the left ventricular cavity–endocardium interface. Areas calculated for each slice are used to derive the volume of each slice. Reprinted with permission from MacMillan et al.[83]

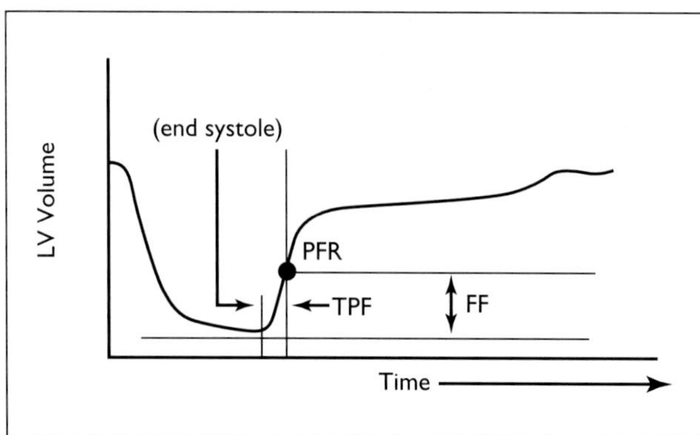

Figure 1.23
Diastolic indices as assessed by EBCT. PFR, peak filling rate (maximal slope of the early filling curve); TPF, time to peak filling; FF, filling fraction (the percentage of the total diastolic filling that has occurred by the time of peak filling). (From: Rumberger JA. Use of ultrafast computed tomography to assess early diastolic filling in man. In: Stanford W, Rumberger JA (eds). *Ultrafast Computed Tomography in Cardiac Imaging*. (Futura: Mount Kisco, 1992) 161–75 with permission.

subtracting the ventricular cavity volume, and multiplying the result by the specific gravity of the myocardium.[88] Mass determinations as obtained by this method display excellent correlation with autopsy data (r = 0.99).[92]

Although EBCT is an excellent imaging modality, in terms of both accuracy and reproducibility, the need for contrast infusion, and lack of availability in many medical centers has limited its applicability. Furthermore, lack of portability of the system is an issue, precluding imaging of patients who are severely ill. From a technical standpoint, functional quantitation cannot be performed unless scanning is properly triggered from the R wave of the ECG tracing. Cardiac arrhythmias, particularly atrial fibrillation, result in improper triggering precluding quantitative analysis.[88] Finally, radiation exposure is required and, for a complete cardiac study, is comparable to that received from a standard abdominal CT.[93]

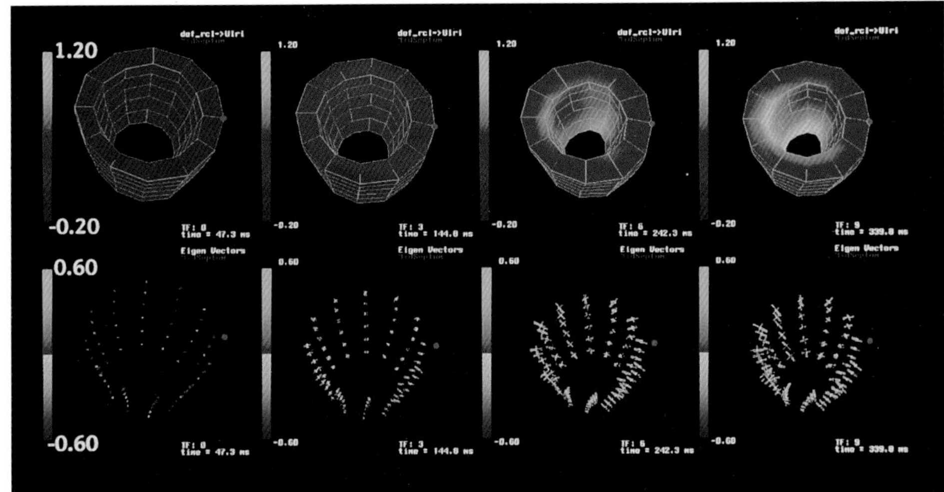

a

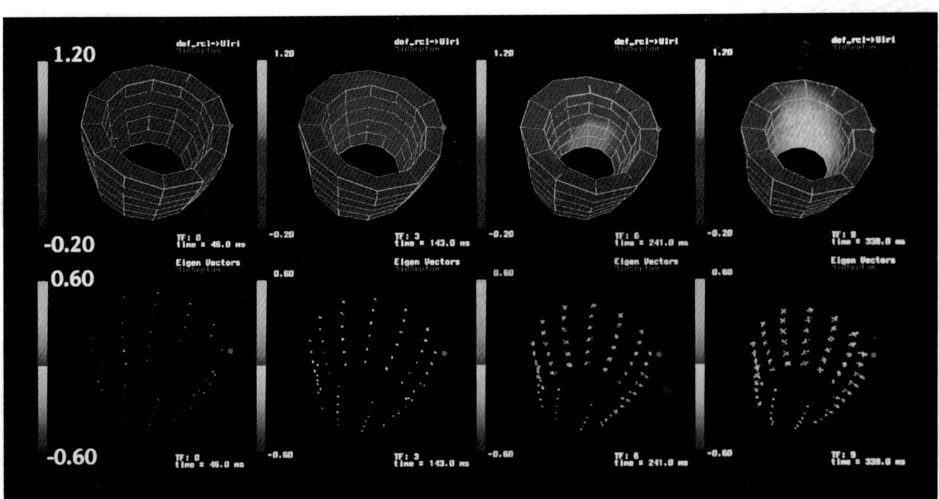

b

Figure 1.24
Three-dimensional reconstructions of normally (a) and abnormally (b) contracting human left ventricles using MRI. Normal contraction velocity is represented in red/orange. In (b), the inferior wall is akinetic.

Magnetic resonance imaging (MRI)

Like computed tomography, magnetic resonance (MR) imaging of the heart relies upon the obtaining of tomographic sections, which may be reconstructed to provide three-dimensional images (Fig. 1.24). Unlike CT, because of high intrinsic contrast between blood and myocardial tissue in the MR image, intravenous dye is not required. Furthermore, due to the inherent three-dimensional nature of MRI, any imaging plane can be obtained, and there is no radiation exposure during scanning.[88] However, scanning times are significantly longer, requiring as many as 64–126 cardiac cycles per tomographic image, resulting in total examination times of 15–20 min.[94] Artifacts due to patient movement, including respiration, are much more apparent than for EBCT, and may significantly reduce image quality and the accuracy of MR measurement of ventricular function. These motion artifacts can be eliminated with breath-hold segmented imaging, as shown in Figure 1.25.

Recently, high-speed modifications have been introduced, the most promising of which appears to be echoplanar imaging (EPI). This is a single-shot imaging method wherein all information regarding a single cardiac image may be obtained in approximately 40 ms.[95] This reduces the time required for a complete functional heart study to less than 10 s, allowing for elimination of respiratory motion via breath holding. Although very attractive, echoplanar imaging has not yet found its way into routine clinical use owing to the substantial technical requirements

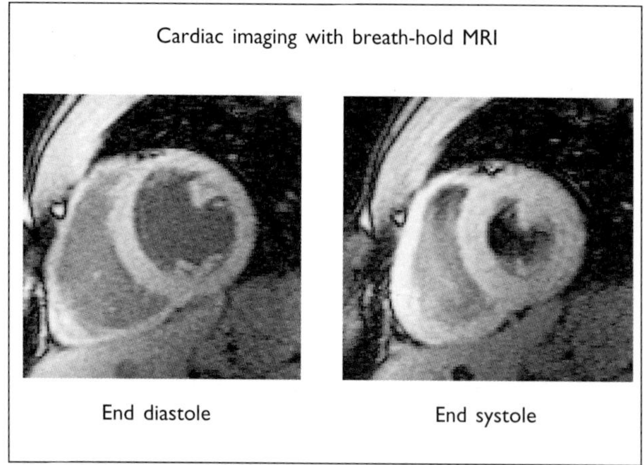

Figure 1.25
Breath-hold segmental MRI imaging of the human left ventricle during diastole (A) and systole (B).

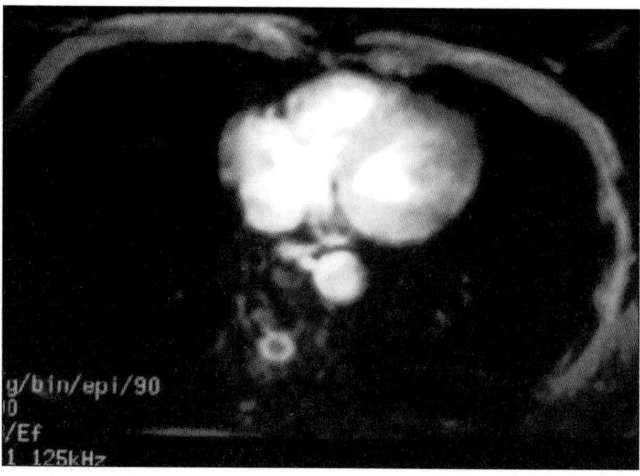

Figure 1.26
Echoplanar imaging via the single shot method. Note the loss of signal in the septal and posterior regions of the ventricle due to magnetic field heterogeneities.

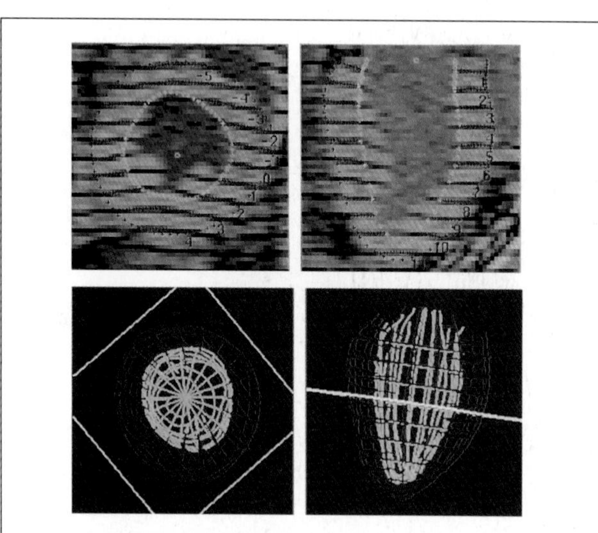

Figure 1.27
Left ventricular volume determination by MRI. Endocardial contours are drawn in contiguous MR sections and the enclosed blood pool areas are added to provide the end-diastolic and end-systolic volumes, allowing calculations of ejection fractions.

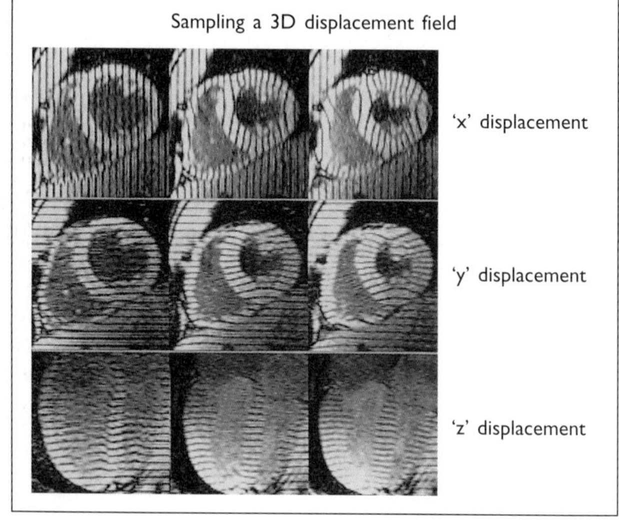

Figure 1.28
Myocardial tagging for the assessment of regional ventricular motion. Thickening, and also rotation and torsion may be tracked because the grid lines may be applied in three dimensions.

for MR hardware and software, and remains available at a limited number of institutions. Also, magnetic field heterogeneities cause loss of signal in some regions of the heart for single-shot EPI. This can be seen in the septal and posterior regions of the left ventricle in Figure 1.26.

As described for EBCT, absolute volumes of the left ventricle can be measured by drawing the endocardial contours in contiguous MR sections and adding the enclosed blood pool areas. Summation of these areas provides the end-diastolic and end-systolic volumes required to calculate EF (Fig. 1.27). Correlation of MR volumes with those obtained during nonsimultaneous contrast ventriculography have been very good with correlation coefficients ranging from 0.84 to 0.98,[96,97] while correlation of ejection fraction with those obtained by ventriculography and radionuclide angiography range from 0.83 to 0.98.[98,99]

In order to shorten examination times, monoplane or biplane long-axis imaging may be employed, and volumes and EF assessed as for echocardiography.[100] Not surprisingly, these methods have been shown to be less accurate and less reproducible than multisection MRI.[94]

Assessment of regional function may be accomplished as with EBCT. However, MRI is also uniquely capable of myocardial tagging through superimposition of a magnetic grid on the MR image (Fig. 1.28). The intersections of the grid lines serve as fixed reference points in the myocardium, such that not only thickening, but also rotation and torsion are tracked.[94] Furthermore, three-dimensional tagging grids may be applied, such that long-axis contraction can also be evaluated.[101,102] The precision of tag detection has been estimated to be 0.1–0.2 mm. Whether the increased accuracy of wall motion characterization by the MR tagging method has clinical implications remains to be proven.[94]

MRI appears to be excellent for determination of myocardial mass, both in normal ventricles and those deformed by acute infarction.[103–105] Correlation with autopsy data even in abnormal hearts has been excellent ($r = 0.94–0.98$), and MR may become the noninvasive standard for quantification of left ventricular mass.[106]

Overall, MRI may prove eventually to be the noninvasive gold standard and procedure of choice for quantitation of left ventricular systolic function, both global and regional, and as the examination length shortens, general availability improves, and patient tolerance issues are overcome, this technique will be likely to become more acceptable and practical outside of the academic setting.

Summary

The choice of imaging modality for the assessment of left ventricular function depends upon availability, practicality, and expertise of each laboratory performing the studies. By and large, echocardiography remains the cornerstone technique. It is widely and readily available, relatively inexpensive, and excellent for qualitative assessment of left ventricular function (global and regional, systolic and diastolic). Echocardiography is also an excellent technique for quantitative information, but only if meticulous attention is paid to the acquisition and interpretation of data.

Radionuclide angiography, although potentially supplanted by EBCT or MRI in the future, continues to be regarded as the gold standard for quantitation of global ventricular function. From a practical standpoint, if patient management requires numeric quantitation of systolic function, radionuclide angiography should be considered the test of choice.

Electron beam computed tomography and magnetic resonance imaging are potentially more accurate and more reproducible than either echocardiography or nuclear imaging. However, owing to availability limitations and intrinsic procedural constraints, these techniques are less likely to be encountered in the routine clinical setting.

References

1 Ghali JK, Kadakia S, Cooper RS et al: Bedside diagnosis of preserved versus impaired left ventricular systolic function in heart failure. *Am J Cardiol* 1991; **67**: 1002–6.

2 Marantz PR, Tobin JN, Wassertheil-Smoller S et al: The relationship between left ventricular systolic function and congestive heart failure diagnosed by clinical criteria. *Circulation* 1988; **77**: 607–18.

3 Mock MB, Ringvist I, Fisher LD et al: Survival of medically treated patients in the coronary artery surgery study (CASS) registry. *Circulation* 1982; **66**: 562–8.

4 Dougherty AH, Naccarelli GV, Gray EL et al: Congestive heart failure with normal systolic function. *Am J Cardiol* 1984; **54**: 778–82.

5 Topol EJ, Traill TA, Fortuin NJ: Hypertensive hypertrophic cardiomyopathy of the elderly. *N Engl J Med* 1985; **312**: 277–83.

6 Sheehan FH: Cardiac angiography. In: Marcus ML, Schelbert HR, Skorton DJ, Wolf GL, eds, *Cardiac Imaging: A Companion to Braunwald's Heart Disease* (WB Saunders: Philadelphia, 1991); 109–48.

7 Feiring AJ, Rumberger JA, Reiter SJ et al: Sectional and segmental variability of left ventricular function: experimental and clinical studies using ultrafast computed tomography. *J Am Coll Cardiol* 1988; **12**: 415–25.

8 Greenbaum RA, Gibson DG: Regional non-uniformity of left ventricular wall movement in man. *Br Heart J* 1981; **45**: 29–34.

9 Ingels NB, Daughters GT, Stinson EB et al: Measurement of midwall myocardial dynamics in intact man by radiography of surgically implanted markers. *Circulation* 1975; **52**: 859–67.

10 McDonald IG: The shape and movement of the human left ventricle during systole. A study by cineangiography and by cineradiography of epicardial markers. *Am J Cardiol* 1970; **26**: 221–30.

11 Pandian NG, Skorton DJ, Collins SM et al: Heterogeneity of left ventricular segmental wall thickening and excursion in 2-dimensional echocardiograms of normal human subjects. *Am J Cardiol* 1983; **51**: 1667–73.

12 Zerhouni EA, Parish DM, Rogers WJ et al: Human heart: tagging with MR imaging–a method for noninvasive assessment of myocardial motion. *Radiology* 1988; **169**: 59–63.

13 Buchalter MB, Weiss JL, Rogers WJ et al: Noninvasive quantification of left ventricular rotational deformation in normal humans using magnetic resonance imaging myocardial tagging. *Circulation* 1990; **81**: 1236–44.

14 Rogers WJ, Shapiro EP, Weiss JL et al: Quantification of and correction for left ventricular systolic long-axis shortening by magnetic resonance tissue tagging and slice isolation. *Circulation* 1991; **84**: 721–31.

15 Ross J Jr, Braunwald E: The study of left ventricular function in man by increasing resistance to ventricular ejection with angiotensin. *Circulation* 1964; **29**: 739–49.

16 Ross J Jr, Covell JW, Sonnenblick EH: The mechanics of left ventricular contraction in acute experimental cardiac failure. *J Clin Invest* 1967; **46**: 299–312.

17 Katz AM: Regulation of myocardial contractility 1958–1983: an odyssey. *J Am Coll Cardiol* 1983; **1**: 42–51.

18 Mitchell JH, Wallace AG, Skinner NS: Intrinsic effects of heart rate on left ventricular performance. *Am J Physiol* 1963; **205**: 41–8.

19 Olsen CO, Tyson GS, Maier GW et al: Dynamic ventricular interactions in the conscious dog. *Circ Res* 1983; **52**: 85–104.

20 Bemis CE, Serur JR, Borkenhagen D et al: Influence of right ventricular filling pressure on left ventricular pressure and dimension. *Circ Res* 1974; **34**: 498–504.

21 Ross J Jr: Acute displacement of the diastolic pressure volume curve of the left ventricle: role of the pericardium and the right ventricle. *Circulation* 1979; **59**: 32–7.

22 Marcus ML, Dellsperger KC: Determinants of systolic and diastolic ventricular function. In: Marcus ML, Schelbert HR, Skorton DJ, Wolf GL, eds, *Cardiac Imaging: A Companion to Braunwald's Heart Disease* (WB Saunders: Philadelphia, 1991); 24–38.

23 O'Keefe JH, Zinsmeister AR, Gibbons RJ: Value of normal electrocardiographic findings in predicting resting left ventricular function in patients with chest pain and suspected coronary artery disease. *Am J Med* 1989; **86**: 658–62.

24 Romhilt DW, Bove KE, Norris RJ et al: A critical appraisal of the electrocardiographic criteria for the diagnosis of left ventricular hypertrophy. *Circulation* 1969; **40**: 185–95.

25 Pombo F, Troy BL, Russell RO Jr: Left ventricular volumes and ejection fraction by echocardiography. *Circulation* 1971; **43**: 480–90.

26 Fortuin NJ, Hood WP, Sherman ME et al: Determination of left ventricular volumes by ultrasound. *Circulation* 1971; **44**: 575–84.

27 Teicholz LE, Kruelen T, Herman MV et al: Problems in echocardiographic volume determinations: echocardiographic–angiographic correlations in the presence or absence of asynergy. *Am J Cardiol* 1976; **37**: 7–11.

28 Feigenbaum H, Popp RL, Wolfe SB et al: Ultrasound measurements of the left ventricle: a correlative study with angiocardiography. *Arch Intern Med* 1972; **129**: 461–7.

29 Schiller NB, Shah PM, Crawford M et al: Recommendations for quantitation of the left ventricle by two-dimensional echocardiography: American Society of Echocardiography Committee on Standards Subcommittee. *J Am Soc Echocardiogr* 1989; **2**: 358–67.

30 Kronik G, Slany J, Mosslacher H: Comparative value of eight M-mode echocardiographic formulas for determining left ventricular stroke volume. *Circulation* 1979; **69**: 1308–16.

31 Quinones MA, Waggoner AD, Reduto LA et al: A new simplified and accurate method for determining ejection fraction with two-dimensional echocardiography. *Circulation* 1981; **64**: 744–53.

32 Weiss JL, Eaton LW, Kallman CH et al: Accuracy of volume determination by two-dimensional echocardiography: defining requirements under controlled conditions in the ejecting canine left ventricle. *Circulation* 1983; **67**: 889–95.

33 Eaton LW, Maughan WL, Shoukas AA et al: Accurate volume determination in the isolated ejecting canine left ventricle by two-dimensional echocardiography. *Circulation* 1979; **60**: 320–6.

34 Vandenberg BF, Rath LS, Stuhlmuller P et al: Estimation of left ventricular cavity area with an on-line, semiautomated echocardiographic edge detection system. *Circulation* 1992; **86**: 159–66.

35 Gorcsan J III, Lazar JM, Schulman DS et al: Comparison of left ventricular function by echocardiographic automated border detection and by radionuclide ejection fraction. *Am J Cardiol* 1993; **72**: 810–15.

36 Perez JE, Waggoner AD, Barzilai B et al: On-line assessment of ventricular function by automatic boundary detection and ultrasonic backscatter imaging. *J Am Coll Cardiol* 1992; **19**: 13–20.

37 Perez JE, Klein SC, Prater DM et al: Automated on-line quantitation of left ventricular dimensions and function by echocardiography with backscatter imaging and lateral gain compensation. *Am J Cardiol* 1992; **70**: 1200–5.

38 Sapin PM, Schroder KM, Gopal AS et al: Comparison of two- and three-dimensional echocardiography with

cineventriculography for measurement of left ventricular volume in patients. *J Am Coll Cardiol* 1994; **24**: 1054–63.

39 Siu SC, Rivera JM, Guerrero JL et al: Three-dimensional echocardiography: in vivo validation for left ventricular volume and function. *Circulation* 1993; **88**: 1715–23.

40 Amico AF, Lichtenberg GS, Reisner SA et al: Superiority of visual versus computerized echocardiographic estimation of radionuclide left ventricular ejection fraction. *Am Heart J* 1989; **118**: 1259–65.

41 Rich S, Sheikh A, Gallastegui J et al: Determination of left ventricular ejection fraction by visual estimation during real-time two-dimensional echocardiography. *Am Heart J* 1982; **104**: 603–6.

42. Wahr DW, Wang YS, Schiller NB: Left ventricular volumes determined by two-dimensional echocardiography in a normal adult population. *J Am Coll Cardiol* 1983, **1**: 863–8.

43 Devereux R, Alonso D, Lutas E et al: Echocardiographic assessment of left ventricular hypertrophy: comparison to necropsy findings. *Am J Cardiol* 1986; **57**: 450–8.

44 Byrd BF III, Wahr D, Wang Y et al: Left ventricular mass and volume/mass ratio determined by two-dimensional echocardiography in normal adults. *J Am Coll Cardiol* 1985; **6**: 1021–5.

45 Nishimura RA, Tajik AJ, Shub C et al: Role of two-dimensional echocardiography in the prediction of in-hospital complications after acute myocardial infarction. *J Am Coll Cardiol* 1984; **4**: 1080–7.

46 Lieberman AN, Weiss JL, Judgutt BI et al: Two-dimensional echocardiography and infarct size: relationship of regional wall motion and thickening to the extent of myocardial infarction in the dog. *Circulation* 1981; **63**: 739–46.

47 Nieminen M, Parisi AF, O'Boyle JE: Serial evaluation of myocardial thickening and thinning in acute experimental infarction: identification and quantification using two-dimensional echocardiography. *Circulation* 1982; **66**: 174–80.

48 Aurigemma GP, Gaasch WH, Villegas BJ et al: Noninvasive assessment of left ventricular mass, chamber volume, and contractile function. *Curr Probl Cardiol* 1995; **20**: 361–440.

49 Christie J, Sheldahl LM, Tristani FE et al: Determination of stroke volume and cardiac output during exercise: comparison of two-dimensional and Doppler echocardiography, Fick oximetry and thermodilution. *Circulation* 1987; **76**: 539–47.

50 Dittman H, Voelker W, Karsch K et al: Influence of sampling site and flow area on cardiac output measurements by Doppler echocardiography. *J Am Coll Cardiol* 1987; **10**: 818–23.

51 Nicolosi GL, Pungercic E, Cervesato E et al: Feasibility and variability of six methods for the echocardiographic and Doppler determination of cardiac output. *Br Heart J* 1988; **59**: 299–303.

52 Chen C, Rodriquez L, Lethor J et al: Continuous wave Doppler echocardiography for noninvasive assessment of left ventricular *dP/dt* and relaxation time constant from mitral regurgitant spectra in patients. *J Am Coll Cardiol* 1944; **23**: 970–6.

53 Pai RG, Bansal RC, Shah PM: Doppler derived rate of left ventricular pressure rise: its correlation with the postoperative left ventricular function in mitral regurgitation. *Circulation* 1990; **82**: 514–20.

54 Grossman W: Diastolic dysfunction in congestive heart failure. *N Engl J Med* 1991; **325**: 1557–64.

55 Thomas JD, Weyman AE: Echocardiographic Doppler evaluation of left ventricular diastolic function: physics and physiology. *Circulation* 1991; **84**: 977–90.

56 Appleton CP, Hatle LK: The natural history of left ventricular filling abnormalities: assessments by two-dimensional and Doppler echocardiography. *Echocardiography* 1992; **9**: 437–57.

57 Pai RG, Shah PM: Echocardigraphic and other noninvasive measurements of cardiac hemodynamics and ventricular function. *Curr Probl Cardiol* 1995; **20**: 681–772.

58 Rossvoll O, Hatle LK: Pulmonary venous flow velocities recorded by transthoracic Doppler ultrasound: relation to left ventricular diastolic pressures. *J Am Coll Cardiol* 1993; **21**: 1687–96.

59 Brown ML, Vaqueiro M, Clements IP et al: Stability of radionuclide left ventricular volume measurements. *Nuc Med Com* 1988; **9**: 117–22.

60 Jensen DG, Genter F, Froelicher VF et al: Individual variability of radionuclide ventriculography in stable coronary artery disease patients over one year. *Cardiology* 1984; **71**: 255–65.

61 Verani MS, Gaeta J, LeBlanc AD et al: Validation of left ventricular volume measurements by radionuclide angiography. *J Nuc Med* 1985; **26**: 1394–401.

62 Links JM, Becker LC, Shindledecker JG et al: Measurement of absolute left ventricular volume from gated blood pool studies. *Circulation* 1982; **65**: 82–91.

63 Johnson LL: Radionuclide assessment of ventricular function. *Curr Probl Cardiol* 1994; **19**: 591–635.

64 Dehmer GJ, Lewis SE, Hills LD et al: Nongeometric determination of left ventricular volumes for equilibrium blood pool scans. *Am J Cardiol* 1980; **45**: 293–300.

65 Clements IP, Brown ML, Smith HC: Radionuclide measurement of left ventricular volume. *Mayo Clin Proc* 1981; **56**: 733–9.

66 Dilsizian V, Perrone-Filardi P, Cannon RO III et al: Comparison of exercise radionuclide angiography with thallium SPECT imaging for detection of significant narrowing of the left circumflex coronary artery. *Am J Cardiol* 1991; **68**: 320–8.

67 Mancini GBJ, Slutsky RA, Norris SL et al: Radionuclide analysis of peak filling rate, filling fraction, and time to peak filling rate. *Am J Cardiol* 1983; **51**: 43–51.

68 Nichols K, Depuey EG, Gooneratne N et al: First-pass ventricular ejection fraction using a single-crystal nuclear camera. *J Nuc Med* 1994; **35**: 1292–302.

69 Marshall RC, Berger HJ, Costin JC et al: Assessment of cardiac performance with quantitative radionuclide angiocardiography: sequential left ventricular ejection fraction normalized left ventricular ejection rate and regional wall motion. *Circulation* 1978; **57**: 320–9.

70 Marshall RC, Berger, HJ, Reduto LA et al: Variability in sequential measures of left ventricular performance assessed with radionuclide angiocardiography. *Am J Cardiol* 1978; **41**: 531–6.

71 Boucher CA, Wackers FJT, Zaret BL et al: Technetium-99m sestamibi myocardial imaging at rest for assessment of myocardial infarction and first-pass ejection fraction. *Am J Cardiol* 1992; **69**: 22–7.

72 Klodas E, Rogers PJ, Sinak LJ et al: Quantitation of regional ejection fractions using gated tomographic imaging with Tc-99m sestamibi. *J Am Coll Cardiol* 1996; **27**: 215A (abstract).

73 Chua T, Kiat H, Germano G et al: Gated technetium-99m sestamibi for simultaneous assessment of stress myocardial perfusion, postexercise regional ventricular function and myocardial viability: correlation with echocardiography and rest thallium-201 scintigraphy. *J Am Coll Cardiol* 1994; **23**: 1107–14.

74 Najm YC, Timmis AD, Maisey MN et al: The evaluation of ventricular function using gated myocardial imaging with Tc-99m MIBI. *Eur Heart J* 1989; **10**: 142–8.

75 Tischler MD, Niggel JB, Beattle RW et al: Validation of global and segmental left ventricular contractile function using gated planar technetium-99m sestamibi myocardial perfusion imaging. *J Am Coll Cardiol* 1994; **23**: 141–5.

76 Civelek AC, Shafique I, Brinker JA et al: Reduced left ventricular cavitary activity ('black hole sign') in thallium-201 SPECT perfusion images of ateroapical transmural myocardial infarction. *Am J Cardiol* 1991; **68**: 1132–7.

77 Corbett JR, Jansen DE, Lewis SE et al: Tomographic gated blood pool radionuclide ventriculography: analysis of wall motion and volumes in patients with coronary artery disease. *J Am Coll Cardiol* 1985; **6**: 349–58.

78 Tamaki N, Gill JB, Moore RH et al: Cardiac response to daily activities and exercise in normal subjects assessed by an ambulatory ventricular function monitor. *Am J Cardiol* 1987; **59**: 1164–9.

79 Breisblatt W, Weiland F, McLain JR et al: Usefulness of ambulatory radionuclide monitoring of left ventricular function early after myocardial infarction for predicting residual myocardial ischemia. *Am J Cardiol* 1988; **62**: 1005–10.

80 Lipton MJ, Higgins CB, Boyd DP: Computed tomography of the heart: evaluation of anatomy and function. *J Am Coll Cardiol* 1985; **5**: 55s–69s.

81 Stanford W, Galvin JR, Weiss RM et al: Ultrafast computed tomography in cardiac imaging: a review. *Semin Ultrasound CT MRI* 1991; **12**: 45–60.

82 Rumberger JA: Ultrafast computed tomography scanning modes, scanning planes and practical aspects of contrast administration. In: Stanford W, Rumberger JA, eds, *Ultrafast Computed Tomography in Cardiac Imaging* (Futura: Mount Kisco, 1992).

83 MacMillan RM, Rees MR, Maranahao V et al: Comparison of left ventricular ejection fraction by cine computed tomography and single plane right anterior oblique ventriculography. *Angiology* 1986; **37(4)**: 299–305.

84 MacMillan RM, Rees MR: Measurement of right and left ventricular volumes in humans by cine computed tomography: comparison to biplane cineangiography. *Am J Cardiol Imag* 1988; **2**: 214–19.

85 Pietras RJ, Wolfkiel CJ, Veselik K et al: Validation of ultrafast computed tomographic left ventricular volume measurement. *Invest Radiol* 1991; **26**: 28–34.

86 Reiter SJ, Rumberger JA, Feiring AJ et al: Precision of measurements of right and left ventricular volume by cine computed tomography. *Circulation* 1986; **74**: 890–900.

87 Rumberger JA, Behrenbeck T, Sheedy PF II et al: Ultrafast computed tomography. In: Giulaiani ER, Fuster V, Gersh BJ et al, eds, *Cardiology Fundamentals and Practice* (Mosby Year Book: St Louis, 1991); 387–98.

88 Thompson BH, Stanford W: Evaluation of cardiac function with ultrafast computed tomography. *Radiol Clin North Am* 1944; **32**: 537–51.

89 Chomka EV, Brundage B: Left ventricular evaluation by exercise ultrafast computed tomography. In: Stanford W, Rumberger JA, eds, *Ultrafast Computed Tomography in Cardiac Imaging* (Futura: Mount Kisco, 1992); 139–60.

90 Garrett JS, Lanzer P, Jaschke W et al: Measurement of cardiac output by cine computed tomography. *Am J Cardiol* 1985; **56**: 657–61.

91 Rumberger JA, Weiss RM, Fiering AJ et al: Patterns of regional diastolic function in the normal human left ventricle: an ultrafast computed tomographic study. *J Am Coll Cardiol* 1989; **14**: 119–26.

92 Feiring AJ, Rumberger JA, Reiter SJ et al: Determination of left ventricular mass in dogs with rapid acquisition cardiac computed tomographic scanning. *Circulation* 1985; **6**: 1355–64.

93 Rumberger JA: Limitations of ultrafast computed tomography. In: Stanford W, Rumberger JA, eds, *Ultrafast Computed Tomography in Cardiac Imaging* (Futura: Mount Kisco, 1992); 337–9.

94 Pattynama PM, De Roos A, Van der Wall EE et al: Evaluation of cardiac function with magnetic resonance imaging. *Am Heart J* 1994; **128**: 595–607.

95 Cohen MS, Weisskoff RM: Ultra-fast imaging. *Mag Res Imag* 1991; **9**: 1–37.

96 Just H, Holubarsch C, Friedburg H: Estimation of left ventricular volume and mass by magnetic resonance imaging: comparison with quantitative biplane angiocardiography. *Cardiovasc Intervent Radiol* 1987; **10**: 1–4.

97 MacMillan RM, Murphy JL, Kresh JY et al: Left ventricular volumes using cine-MRI: validation by catheterization ventriculography. *Am J Card Imag* 1990; **4**: 79–85.

98 Mogelvang J, Thomsen C, Mehlsen J et al: Left ventricular ejection fraction determined by magnetic resonance imaging and gated radionuclide ventriculography. *Am J Noninvasive Cardiol* 1987; **1**: 278–83.

99 Gaudio C, Tanzilli G, Mazzarotto P et al: Comparison of left ventricular ejection fraction by magnetic resonance imaging and radionuclide ventriculography in idiopathic dilated cardiomyopathy. *Am J Cardiol* 1991; **67**: 411–15.

100 Benjelloun, H, Cranney GB, Kirk AA et al: Interstudy reproducibility of biplane cine nuclear magnetic resonance measurements of left ventricular function. *Am J Cardiol* 1991; **67**: 1413–20.

101 Beyar R, Shapiro EP, Graves WL et al: Quantification and validation of left ventricular wall thickening by a three-dimensional volume element magnetic resonance imaging approach. *Circulation* 1990; **81**: 297–307.

102 Lima JAC, Jeremy R, Guier W et al: Accurate systolic wall thickening by nuclear magnetic resonance imaging with tissue tagging: correlation with sonomicrometers in normal and ischemic myocardium. *J Am Coll Cardiol* 1993; **21**: 1741–51.

103 Keller AM, Peshock RM, Malloy CR et al: In vivo measurements of myocardial mass using nuclear magnetic resonance imaging. *J Am Coll Cardiol* 1986; **8**: 113–17.

104 Maddahi J, Crues J, Berman DS et al: Noninvasive quantification of left ventricular myocardial mass by gated proton nuclear magnetic resonance imaging. *J Am Coll Cardiol* 1987; **10**: 682–92.

105 Shapiro EP, Rogers WJ, Beyar R et al: Determination of left ventricular mass by magnetic resonance imaging in hearts deformed by acute infarction. *Circulation* 1989; **79**: 706–11.

106 Weiss JL, Shapiro EP, Buchalter MB et al: Magnetic resonance imaging as a noninvasive standard for the quantitative evaluation of left ventricular mass, ischemia, and infarction. *Ann NY Acad Sci* 1990; **601**: 95–106.

2

Left ventricular hypertrophy: cardiac imaging techniques

Scott Takeda and John B Chambers

Introduction

Left ventricular hypertrophy has come under increasing interest in the past two decades, with evidence supporting its importance as a prognostic indicator for cardiovascular events and outcome. The clinical management of increased left ventricular mass is outside the scope of this chapter. We will discuss the echocardiographic methods currently used in its assessment, as well as the newer imaging modalities of three-dimensional echocardiography, ultrafast computed tomography and magnetic resonance imaging.

Why measure left ventricular mass?

Left ventricular hypertrophy is an independent risk factor for stroke, myocardial infarction, congestive heart failure and sudden death[1] not only in patients with hypertension or aortic stenosis,[2] but also in those with no evidence of pressure overload.[3]

Left ventricular hypertrophy occurs in approximately 25–30% of all hypertensive patients[4] and is associated with myocardial infarction or death at a rate of 4.6 events per 100 patient years. This is three times the risk in hypertensive patients without left ventricular hypertrophy.[5,6] Even in asymptomatic subjects with normal blood pressure, the relative risk of all-cause mortality increases by 1.5 in men and 2.0 in women for every 50 g/m increment in left ventricular mass indexed to height.[3] The relative risk of sudden death is 1.7 per 50 g/m increment.[3]

Multivariate analysis shows that left ventricular hypertrophy is a stronger independent risk factor in patients with and without coronary artery disease than systolic and diastolic blood pressure, smoking and serum cholesterol concentration.[5,6] The risk conferred by increased left ventricular mass is similar to that from multivessel disease. In black subjects, the 5-year mortality is 16.1% with left ventricular hypertrophy and normal coronary anatomy, compared to 17.6% with multivessel disease and normal left ventricular mass.[7]

The presence of left ventricular hypertrophy may therefore have a number of practical implications. In patients with borderline hypertension it can be used as a criterion for beginning therapy. In patients with established hypertension, it is possible that treatment should be changed to a drug known to induce regression of left ventricular hypertrophy. It could be argued that patients with coronary disease and left ventricular hypertrophy should be investigated and treated more aggressively than those with normal left ventricular mass, although this has not yet been proved to be effective at reducing mortality. The measurement of left ventricular mass is also part of the assessment of patients with valve disease before and after surgery and of patients with suspected hypertrophic cardiomyopathy.

Assessment of left ventricular hypertrophy

M-mode echocardiography

Despite its limitations, M-mode echocardiography is still the most widely used method in clinical practice today (Fig. 2.1). The practical aspects of obtaining an adequate study are worth stressing. The presence of regional wall motion

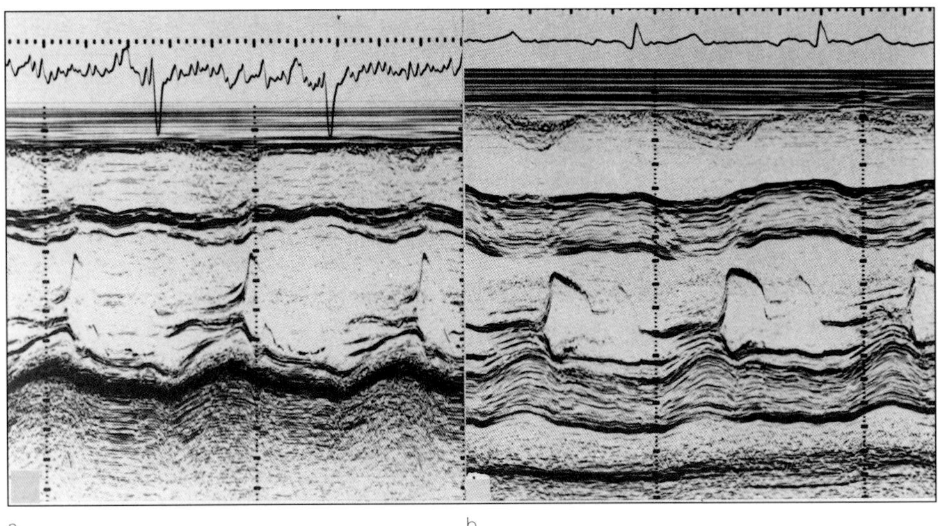

Figure 2.1
M-mode echocardiogram in (a) a normal patient and (b) a patient with chronic renal failure with hypertension inducing marked left ventricular hypertrophy (interventricular septal diameter = 2.2 cm).

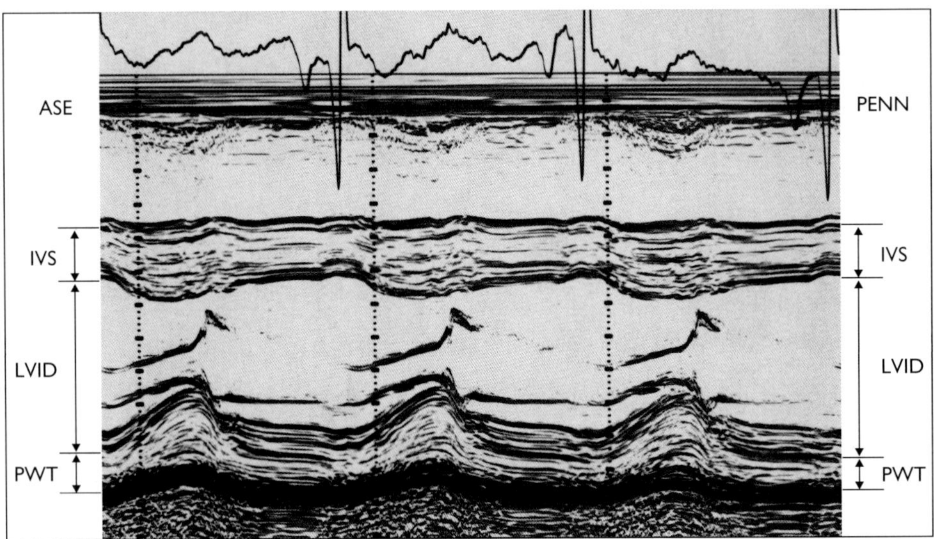

Figure 2.2
M-mode—ASE versus Penn convention. Using the Penn convention (*right*) the thickness of both the septal and free wall endocardial echoes are excluded from the septal (IVS) and posterior wall thickness (PWT) measurements. This contrasts to the 'leading edge to leading edge' convention of the ASE (*left*).

abnormalities must be excluded since M-mode at the base of the heart can only be used to generalize to the whole heart in the presence of symmetrical geometry and motion. Then, the posterior wall and septum must both be aligned perpendicular to the beam. This is not possible in many subjects, especially for the elderly in whom the angle between the septum and aortic root becomes more acute. Much care must be taken to position the patient adequately and control their respiration. The cursor must be positioned just below the tips of the mitral leaflets in either a long-axis or short-axis parasternal view whichever more accurately cuts through the true diameter of the ventricle. Mass may be calculated in diastole or systole although conventionally the diastolic calculation is usually used. For its calculation, septal width (IVS), posterior wall width (PWT) and left ventricular diameter (LVID) must be measured (Table 2.1). The derivation of the widely applied Devereux formula requires the measurements to be made using the Penn convention rather than the more frequently used convention of the American Society of Echocardiography (ASE) (Fig. 2.2). Use of the ASE convention considerably overestimates left ventricular mass.[8] It is important to average a number of

Table 2.1 Normal intracardiac dimensions (cm) in men and women aged 18–72 years, 150–203 cm (59–80 in) in height

	Men		*Women*	
Left atrium	3.0–4.5	$n = 288$	2.7–4.0	$n = 524$
LV diastolic diameter	4.3–5.9	$n = 394$	4.0–5.2	$n = 643$
LV systolic diameter	2.6–4.0	$n = 288$	2.3–3.5	$n = 524$
IV septum (diastole)	0.6–1.3	$n = 106$	0.5–1.2	$n = 109$
Post wall (diastole)	0.6–1.2	$n = 106$	0.5–1.1	$n = 119$

References: Lauer et al;[12] Devereux et al.[11]

consecutive representative cycles usually three to five in view of beat to beat variability. The Devereux formula treats the left ventricle as a cube so that the myocardial volume is the difference between the outer margin defined by the diameter LVID + IVS + PWT and the cavity with diameter LVID. Mass is derived from volume after multiplying by the density of cardiac muscle, 1.04 g/cm^3. By correlating calculated left ventricular mass with angiographic and post-mortem findings, a correction factor 13.6 g was found giving the formula:

$$LV = 1.04 \times [(LVID + PWT + IVS)^3 - (LVID)^3] - 13.6\ g$$

Left ventricular mass must then be indexed to body habitus. This is conventionally performed against body surface area taken from DuBois nomograms although a simplified method may be useful if charts are not available:[9]

$$BSA(m^2) = \frac{\sqrt{Height\ (cm) * Wt(kg)}}{3600}$$

The problem with indexing to body surface area (BSA) is that it may disguise the effect of weight (Wt). Morbid obesity is associated with heart failure and sudden death so apparently normalized indexed left ventricular masses may in fact be pathologic. This is why some authors index to height (Ht) and this method should certainly be adopted in obese subjects.[10]

Left ventricular mass should be considered a continuous variable in terms of its risk of cardiovascular events, but it is still helpful to have a bipartite division into normal and abnormal for clinical characterization. The problem is that mass is dependent not only on body habitus, but a number of other variables such as age, sex, activity, race and Angiotensin Converting Enzyme (ACE) genotype.[11–13] This means that the normal range of each individual may be uncertain. For research studies a carefully matched control population needs to be chosen. In clinical practice, criteria that diagnose hypertrophy in no more than 2.5% of a normal population are reasonable. The gender-specific criteria proposed by Hammond et al are widely used and are >134 g/m^2 for men and 110 g/m^2 for women.[4]

Active athletic individuals may also cause diagnostic confusion. Except in weight lifters, the heart in a trained athlete is slightly dilated and mildly hypertrophied. The septal width is rarely >1.3 cm and probably never >1.6 cm, and the diastolic cavity dimension may be up to 6.2 cm (Table 2.2).[14]

There are a number of problems with left ventricular mass derived from the Devereux formula. The formula was derived in only 34 patients and comparison with mass at post-mortem was by regression equations. However, it is

Table 2.2 Cardiac dimensions (cm) in athletic individuals (95% limits)

	Male (n = *738*)	*Female* (n = *209*)
LA	3.1–4.3	2.8–4.0
LVDD	4.6–6.2	4.1–5.6
IVS	0.8–1.3	0.7–1.0
PW	0.8–1.1	0.6–1.1

Reference: Pelliccia et al.[14] LA, left atrium; LVDD, left ventricular diastolic dimension; IVS, interventricular septum; PW, posterior wall.

well-known that strong correlations are possible even in the absence of adequate agreement.[15] More modern studies now show far better correlations between post-mortem mass and calculated mass using two-dimensional or three-dimensional echocardiography (see below). M-mode dimensions may have limited reproducibility.[16,17] A further problem is that M-mode cannot be applied in subjects with inadequate image quality or those with asymmetric geometry or motion.

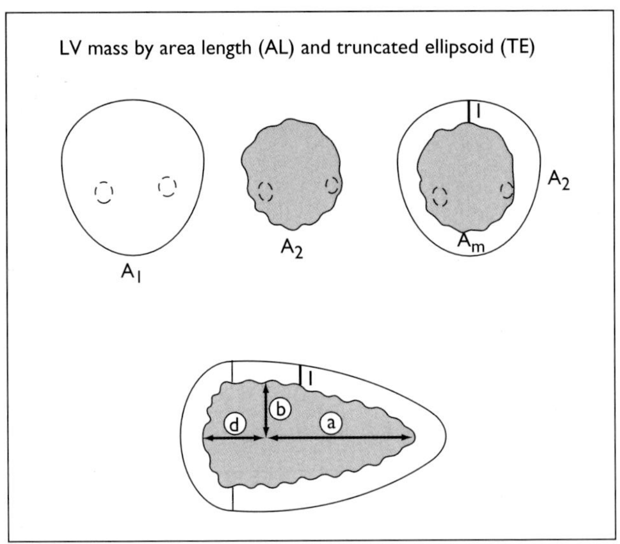

Figure 2.3
Two dimensional left ventricular mass quantification: measurements for the truncated ellipsoid and area length methods.
Upper panel—diagram of the left ventricular short axis at papillary muscle level. A_1, epicardial cross-sectional area; A_2, endocardial cross-sectional area; t, mean wall thickness; *Am*, myocardial cross-sectional area.
Lower panel—diagram of the left ventricle in the apical 4-chamber view showing the major long axis. a, semi-major axis; d, truncated semi-major axis; b, short axis radius. (Adapted from Schiller et al. 1989, ASE recommendations for quantification of the left ventricle by two-dimensional echocardiography.)

2D Echocardiography

Estimation of left ventricular mass by two-dimensional echocardiography has been shown to be more accurate in patients with distorted hearts and grossly abnormal geometry than uni-dimensional M-mode measurements. In a study by Reichek, the correlation between two-dimensional left ventricular mass and anatomical left ventricular mass was higher (R = 0.93, SEE 31 g) than the correlation with M-mode (R = 0.86, SEE 59 g).[18] Collins et al showed that two-dimensional echocardiographic estimates of LV mass were more reproducible than M-mode.[19] This is particularly important as we are now increasingly performing serial studies looking for progression or regression of left ventricular hypertrophy and at changes in left ventricular function following interventions such as valve replacement.

In 1989 to try and foster uniformity and wider use of these techniques, the American Society of Echocardiography (ASE) Committee on Standards published recommendations for quantification of the left ventricle by two-dimensional echocardiography.[20] Despite the logical advantage and recent evidence supporting the use of two-dimensional echocardiography for the estimation of left ventricular mass, it is still surprisingly little used in research or routine clinical practice.

Methods

The ASE defined two anatomically validated methods for quantification of myocardial mass: the area/length and the truncated ellipsoid methods (Fig. 2.3). Both require the determination of the myocardial cross-sectional area at the level of the papillary muscle tips in the short-axis view. This view gives the best definition of the epicardium. The epicardial and endocardial borders are traced to measure cross-sectional areas (A_1 and A_2 respectively). Assuming a circular cross-section, mean wall thickness (t) can be calculated from mean outer (a) and inner (b) radius:

$$t = a - b$$

$$t = \sqrt{\frac{A_1}{\pi}} - \sqrt{\frac{A_2}{\pi}}$$

Both methods then use an apical 4-chamber and 2-chamber view to measure the major long axis (Fig. 2.3).

The area/length method uses the entire major axis whereas the truncated ellipsoid method divides the major axis into two parts at the level of the widest minor axis. These two segments are called the semi-major axis (a) and truncated semi-major axis (d):

Truncated ellipsoid:

$$\text{LVmass} = 1.05\pi\left\{(b+t)^2\left[\frac{2}{3}(a+t) + d - \frac{d^3}{3(a+t)^2}\right] - b^2\left[\frac{2}{3}a + d - \frac{d^3}{3a^2}\right]\right\}$$

Area/length:

$$\text{LVmass} = 1.05\left\{\left[\frac{5}{6}A_1\,(a+d+t)\right] - \left[\frac{5}{6}A_2\,(a+d)\right]\right\}$$

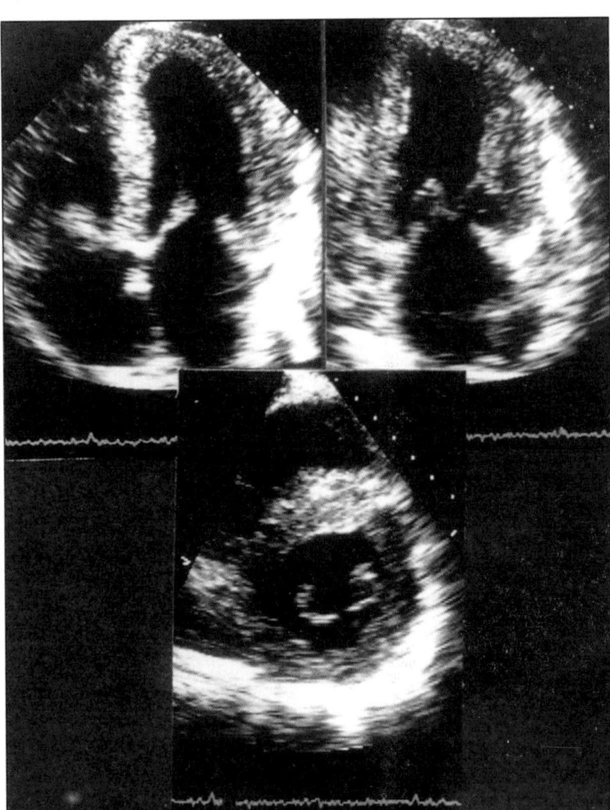

Figure 2.4
Two-dimensional images for calculation of left ventricular mass. The four-chamber and two-chamber apical views (*left and right upper panel*) are used for determination of major long-axis dimensions. Cross-sectional myocardial area is calculated from planimetry of epicardial and endocardial borders in the short axis view at the papillary muscle level (*lower panel*)

The area/length method is therefore a much easier and quicker calculation. If the 4- and 2-chamber views have already been analyzed for left ventricular volume determination, most systems have programs which automatically recall the maximum major axis and use it to calculate LV mass, again facilitating its use in the clinical setting.[21] Both methods show good correlation with anatomic LV mass.[11,22–24]

Although two-dimensional echocardiography is an improvement on M-mode, it still relies on geometric assumptions in calculating left ventricular mass since it generalizes to the whole left ventricle from only two or three sections. This has spawned the search for other newer and more accurate techniques in the assessment of left ventricular mass.

Left ventricular geometry

In looking at the pathophysiology of left ventricular hypertrophy it is important to examine the relationship of left ventricular mass to left ventricular cavity size and to the total hemodynamic load imposed on the left ventricle. Further classification by left ventricular geometry, may refine risk stratification. These geometric patterns are defined by the **relative wall thickness ratio (RWT ratio)**, which is the **thickness of the posterior wall divided by left ventricular radius in diastole**. The patterns develop to normalize wall stress based on the Laplace relationship which states that left ventricular wall stress (*S*) is directly proportional to intracavitary pressure (*P*) and chamber radius (*R*) and is inversely proportional to wall thickness (*Th*):[25]

$$S = P \cdot R / Th$$

The relative wall thickness ratio is remarkably constant in the normal population with a mean value of 0.33 ± 0.06.[26] Reichek and Devereux showed that a relative wall thickness ratio >0.45 at end-diastole is a reliable marker of increased left ventricular pressure (>0.5 is a good indicator of a left ventricular pressure of 180 mmHg or more).[27] Conversely, in left ventricular decompensation or severe left ventricular volume overload without heart failure, this relationship breaks down and there is often a normal relative wall thickness ratio suggesting 'inadequate hypertrophy'. This may play an important role in the progression to LV dysfunction. Studies by Gaasch et al have usefully applied the relative wall thickness ratio to determine left ventricular function and prognosis in aortic regurgitation.[28]

Three main groups of abnormal left ventricular geometry have been described: those with increased left ventricular mass and increased relative wall thickness ratio (>0.45) are considered to have **concentric hypertrophy**, those with increased left ventricular mass and normal relative wall thickness ratio (<0.45) to have **eccentric hypertrophy** and, finally, those with normal left ventricular mass but increased relative wall thickness ratio are said to have '**concentric remodelling**'. Several studies have shown that morbid events are up to four times more likely in subjects with concentric left ventricular hypertrophy.[22] In a recent study by Verdecchia et al even subjects with normal left ventricular mass, but with concentric remodelling, showed an increased incidence of morbid events (2.39 compared to 1.12 per 100 patient years in those with normal geometry).[29] Clinically, it may therefore be important to identify concentric remodelling since early treatment might prevent progression to overt concentric hypertrophy. Those with eccentric hypertrophy also have a significantly increased risk of cardiovascular events, although not as great as those with concentric hypertrophy.

The differences in risk in these geometric patterns of hypertrophy may be explained in part by their differing

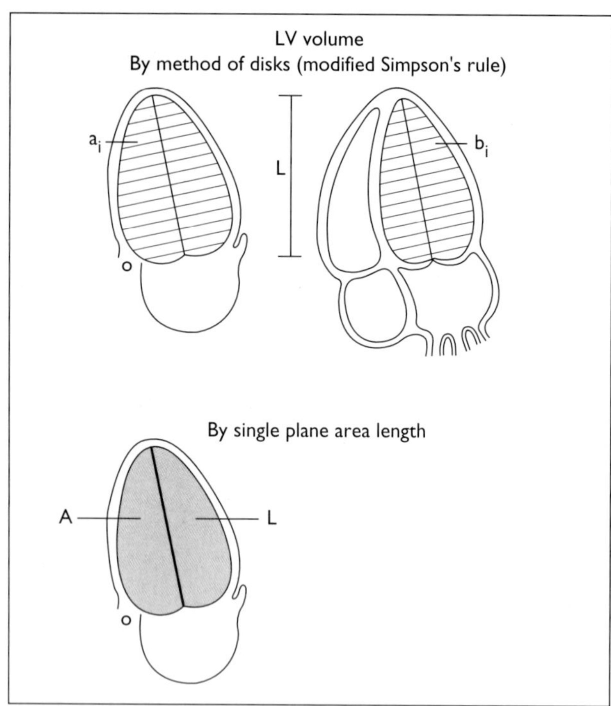

Figure 2.5
Calculation of left ventricular volume.
Top panel—Method of discs. Calculation of volume is from summation of areas from diameters a_i and b_i of discs of equal height; apportioned by dividing left ventricular longest length (L) into equal sections.
Bottom panel—Single plane area length. Useful if only one apical view is obtainable. A, area of left ventricular cavity; L, length of left ventricular cavity.
(Adapted from Schiller et al. 1989, ASE recommendations for quantitation of the left ventricle by two-dimensional echocardiography.)

pathophysiological associations.[23] Concentric hypertrophy is associated with increased peripheral resistance with high systemic arterial pressures, especially during ambulatory monitoring, and also with a reduced plasma volume. In contrast, those with eccentric hypertrophy may be associated with an expanded plasma volume.[30–32]

Relative wall thickness is based on linear dimensions in the face of the left ventricle being a three-dimensional structure. It is however possible to express the volume/mass ratio using two-dimensional echocardiography. Post-mortem studies show a direct relationship between the left ventricular volume/mass ratio and the severity of congestive heart failure before death in patients with hypertrophic hearts.[33,34]

Cavity volume measurements

The guidelines of the ASE suggest two methods for the calculation of left ventricular volumes.[20] The preferred algorithm is the **method of disks or disk summation** (previously known as the modified Simpson's rule) for which linear and area measurements are obtained from paired apical views (both 2- and 4-chamber) that may be considered nearly orthogonal (see Fig. 2.5). It is preferred because it is relatively accurate in geometrically irregular ventricles. When only one apical view is available and the ventricle is not severely deformed, the **single plane area/length** algorithm can be used.

Systolic and diastolic function

Mass represents only the anatomical aspect of the problem of left ventricular hypertrophy, and assessment of systolic and diastolic physiological function is also necessary. In pressure overload, left ventricular hypertrophy is initially beneficial in normalizing systolic wall stress and preserving systolic function. However, it may cause diastolic dysfunction with impaired ventricular relaxation and also reduced coronary vasodilator reserve leading to subendocardial ischemia and systolic ventricular dysfunction.[38] Cuocolo et al studied hypertensive patients with normal systolic function at rest, but who had an abnormal response during exercise.[39] These patients all showed impaired diastolic filling at rest with a blunted augmentation of end-diastolic volume on exercise, suggesting that systolic dysfunction in these patients was secondary to impaired diastolic filling. Potentially abnormal patterns of left ventricular filling may develop early in patients with hypertension even before an increase in left ventricular mass is detected.[38,40] In patients with aortic stenosis, diastolic dysfunction was observed in approximately 50% of patients with normal systolic ejection performance, but was found in 100% of those with depressed systolic function.[41]

Systolic function must be assessed both regionally and globally. Every region corresponding to the arterial supply of the heart is described according to the degree of systolic thickening and the motion of the endocardium:

- normal;
- hypokinetic (the endocardium moves inwards less than 50% of normal);
- akinetic (no motion);
- dyskinetic (motion out of phase with the expected direction).

For research studies, a score can be given to the motion observed in each of 16 segments as defined by the ASE.[24]

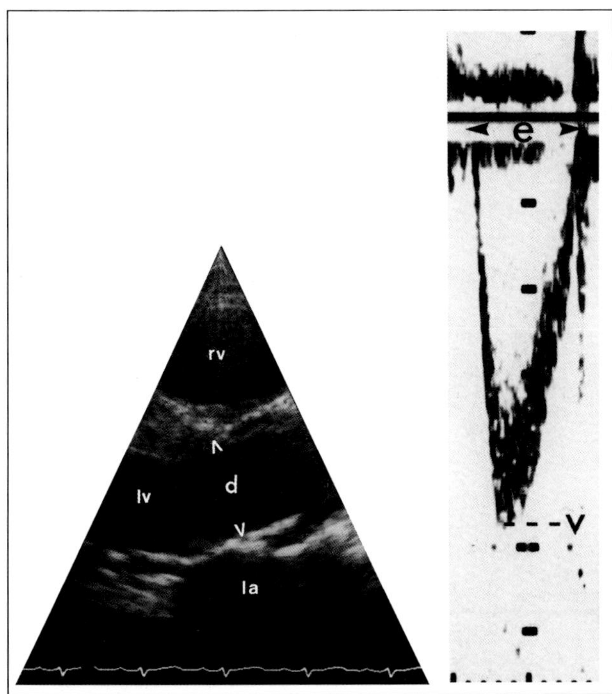

Figure 2.6
Left panel—parasternal long axis view. LA, left atrium; LV, left ventricle; RV, right ventricle; d, left ventricular outflow tract diameter.
Right panel—Pulsed wave Doppler trace from the left ventricular outflow tract. Stroke distance is the planimetered area under the waveform. Stroke volume can be calculated by multiplying stroke distance by the cross-sectional area of the left ventricular outflow tract.

Global measures of function include ejection fraction, stroke volume and end-systolic volume. Ejection fraction is usually estimated by eye, but can also be calculated using on-line computer software from diastolic and systolic volumes as calculated above. End-systolic chamber area or derived-volume alone are relatively more accurate because, for technical reasons, the endocardium is well imaged in systole. The pulsed Doppler sample volume is then turned to record flow through the aortic valve (Fig. 2.6). The waveform is effectively a graph of velocity against time and since distance = speed × time, the area under the waveform represents the distance travelled in one cycle by blood leaving the left ventricle. This is called the systolic velocity integral or 'stroke distance' and when multiplied by the cross-sectional area of the left ventricular outflow tract, it gives the stroke volume. The cardiac output is then the product of stroke volume and heart rate.

Diastolic function is assessed by placing the pulsed Doppler sample in the left ventricular cavity at the level of the tips of the mitral leaflets in their fully-open diastolic position using the 4-chamber view (Fig. 2.7). This gives a record of the phases of diastole: isovolumic relaxation before the mitral valve opens, then early active filling (E); as flow falls after this, the mitral leaflets drift towards the closed position during diastasis (D), and immediately after this the atrium contracts (A). In the normal person, the early velocity (E wave) is higher than the velocity during atrial systole (A wave) and the E descent is 140–220 ms (Table 2.3). There are two main pathological patterns (Fig. 2.8). The first is called the 'slow relaxation pattern' and consists of a low E wave, prolonged E wave deceleration time (and isovolumic relaxation time) with a tall A wave. This pattern is seen in patients with pressure overload or hypertrophied left ventricles. The second pattern is the 'restrictive pattern' which occurs in left ventricular dysfunction from any cause associated with high filling pressures (pulmonary wedge pressure >20 mmHg) or with a fast rate of rise of left ventricular diastolic pressure (as in restrictive myopathy or pericardial constriction). This has a tall E wave, short E deceleration time (and short isovolumic relaxation time) with a small or absent A wave.

These patterns are dependent on loading conditions and drug therapy. It is also important to remember that transmitral velocities do not reflect absolute cavity pressure or even pressure differences. Thus, in the latter stages of early filling, there is a small reversal of pressure difference with the left ventricular cavity pressure higher than left atrial pressure. Blood continues to flow into the ventricle under its own momentum. Similarly the same pattern may be seen with widely different absolute cavity pressures. Thus, if a patient with a slow filling pattern develops a high filling pressure, the transmitral waveform can change to a pattern that is superficially similar to normal. However, this can be differentiated in a number of ways. One method is to time the duration of atrial systole and of pulmonary vein retrograde flow. If the duration of retrograde flow excedes that of atrial systole by more than 30 ms, diastolic dysfunction is likely to be present.[42] Another method is the deceleration time of the A wave.[43] If this is shorter than 70 ms, it is likely that diastolic dysfunction is present; if shorter than 60 ms there is a high chance of abnormality.

The pattern in the elderly may appear abnormal even in the absence of symptoms. Whether these patterns are false positives or whether the left ventricle is strictly abnormal as a result of long-standing mild hypertension or ischemic disease, or is simply behaving pathologically as a result of other age-related changes, is not properly established. The echocardiographer should, however, be aware that the limits of normal do change in the elderly (Table 2.3).

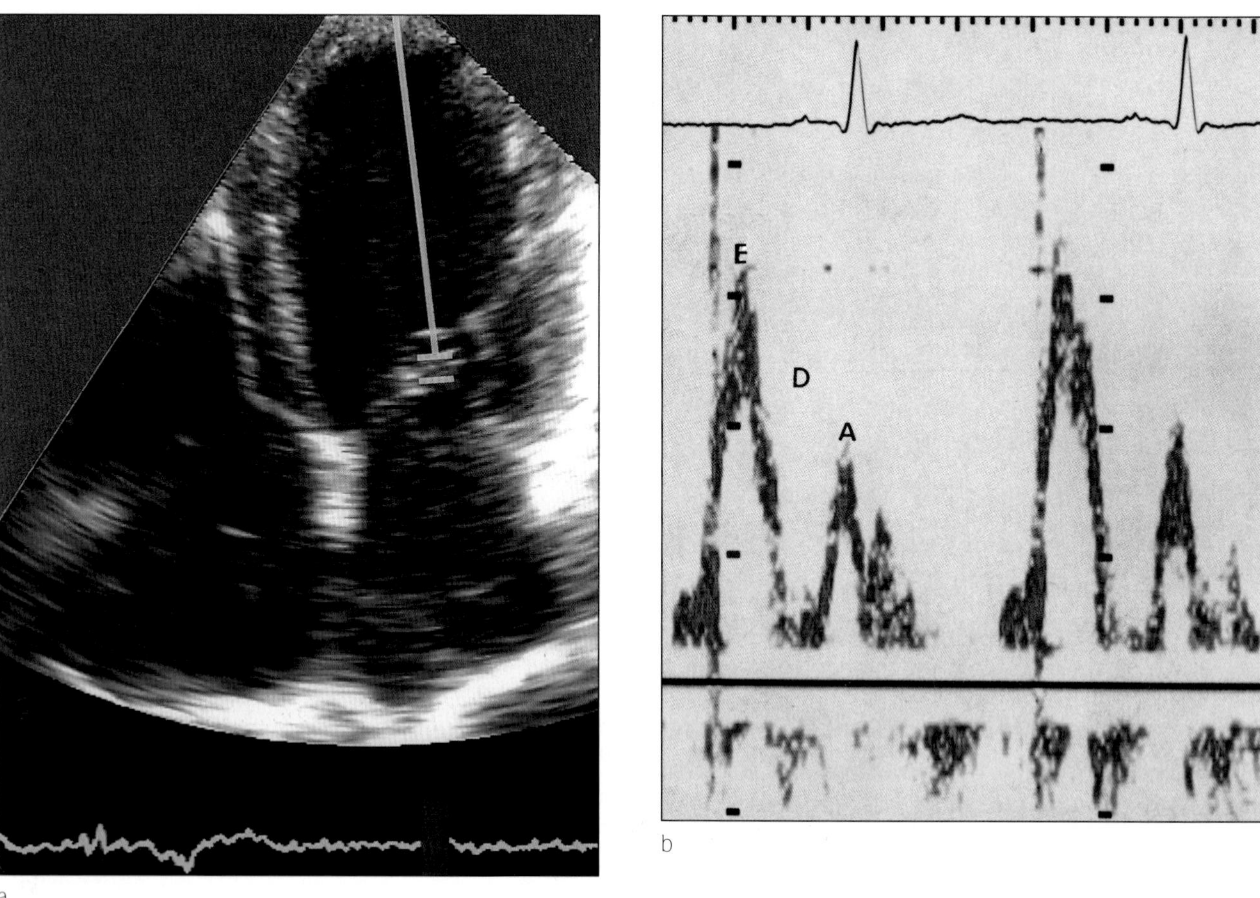

Figure 2.7
(a) Position for sampling the pulsed Doppler mitral valve trace at the level of the leaflet tips in diastole. (b) Pulsed Doppler mitral recording. E, early active filling; D, diastasis; A, atrial contraction.

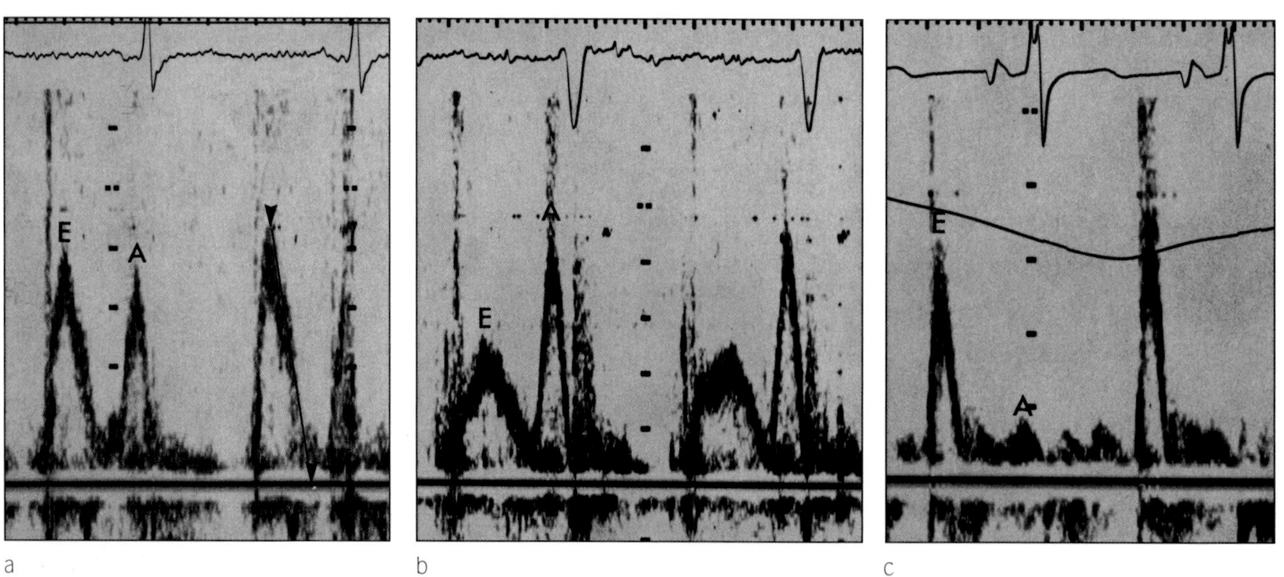

Figure 2.8
Mitral flow patterns. (a) Normal flow pattern. The peak E wave velocity is higher than the peak A wave velocity. The E deceleration time is 140–220 ms. (b) 'Slow relaxation' pattern. The peak E wave velocity is low with reversal of the E/A ratio, and the E wave deceleration time is prolonged. (c) 'Restrictive pattern'. The peak E wave velocity is high, and the deceleration time is short with a small or absent A wave.

Table 2.3 Normal ranges for measures of systolic and diastolic function echocardiography

End-diastolic volume (ml)*	58–166 (male)	49–129 (female)
End-systolic volume (ml)*	3–67 (male)	9–57 (female)
4-chamber area diastole (cm^2)	18.6–48.6	
4-chamber area systole (cm^2)	8.6–30.4	
Doppler		
Mitral valve E (cm/s)	44–100	34–90 (elderly)
Mitral valve A (cm/s)	20–60	31–87 (elderly)
E:A ratio	0.7–3.1	0.5–1.7 (elderly)
Tricuspid valve E (cm/s)	20–50	
Tricuspid valve A (cm/s)	12–36	
E:A ratio	0.8–2.9	
Time intervals		
Mitral E dec time (ms)	139–219	138–282 (elderly)
Mitral A dec time (ms)	>70	
IVRT (ms)	54–98	56–124 (elderly)

References: Pearlman;[61] Kitzman et al;[36] Wahr et al;[37] Van Dam[62]

Other methods of assessing left ventricular mass

3D Echocardiography

Currently used systems reconstruct a three-dimensional image from multiple two-dimensional cross-sectional images taken from long- and short-axis views either randomly or in a predetermined (linear, fan-like or rotational) fashion.[44] However, work is in progress to develop three-dimensional matrix probes.[45] The advantage of random image acquisition is that multiple different non-selected views can be used in a way similar to current two-dimensional techniques and the optimal image used. However, **spatial locating systems** must be used to orientate the random images. The earliest localizing systems used mechanical arms with the transducer held in a mounting system with movable joints. Acoustical or electromechanical locating devices mounted on the ultrasound transducer were later used allowing more freedom of image acquisition.[46–48] Current work using the transesophageal approach has returned to mechanical devices to rotate or occasionally to draw out the probe in carefully controlled increments.

Such scanning techniques using a predetermined acquisition pattern do not require a spatial locating system, and allow the recording of more closely and evenly spaced cardiac cross-sections giving more detailed and precise images. However, movement of transducer and patient can cause significant artifacts and distortions of three-dimensional reconstructions.

Precordial systems have been developed particularly using rotational scanning techniques as only a small window is required and data can be acquired in real time. Roelandt et al developed a rotatable transducer system controlled by software-based steering logic considering both heart cycle variations by ECG-gating and respiratory cycle variation by impedence measurement.[49] Data from the static two-dimensional images is digitally transferred to computer and formatted in correct sequence. Mathematical interpolation is used to create three-dimensional image elements known as 'voxels'. Cardiac structures are then separated from bloodpool and background with computer algorithms to generate the final three-dimensional image (Fig. 2.9). This can be displayed graphically in three ways: as a wire frame, with surface rendering, or with volume rendering. Wire frame display is simple, requires less computer memory and is useful for simple volume calculations. Surface rendering introduces shading to surfaces giving a

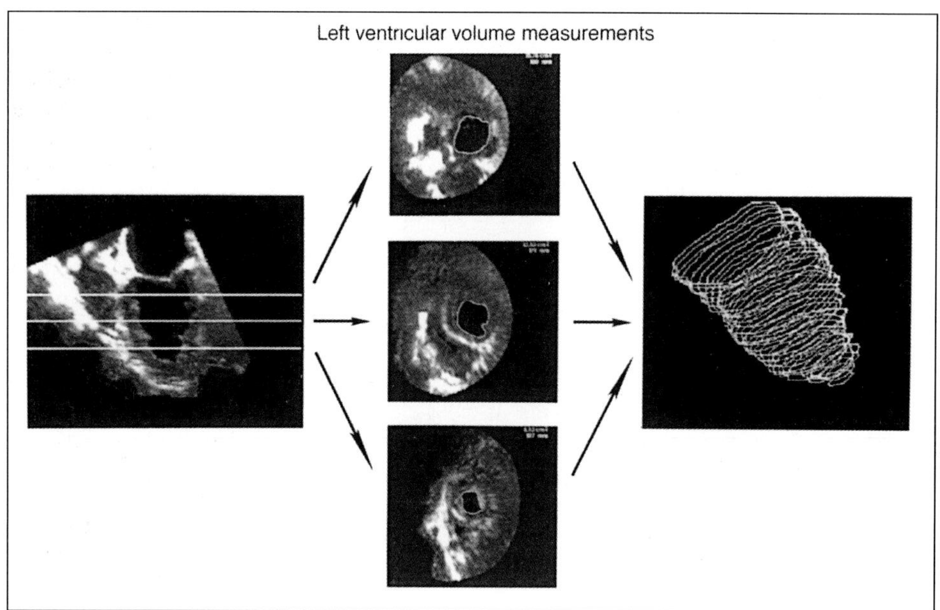

Figure 2.9
Left panel—a long axis cut plane is selected from the three-dimensional dataset. Short axis cut planes (perpendicular to the long axis) at predetermined distance are selected. *Middle panel*—three representative short axis images are shown. For each short axis image the endocardial contour is drawn. *Right panel*—finally all contour lines can be displayed in their spatial orientation and rotated on the screen for better representation. (Reproduced from Roelandt et al. 1995, with permission of the author and the editor of the *British Heart Journal*)

three-dimensional perspective. Volume rendering allows dynamic three-dimensional visualization with maintainance of the gray scale, allowing for example, visualization of valve structure and function.

Current use

Studies have looked at quantification of left ventricular volumes and mass.[50,51] Three-dimensional echocardiographic volume quantification has been shown to be accurate and reproducible, both in symmetric and distorted hearts. Fewer geometric assumptions are made, compared with two-dimensional techniques. Quantification of left ventricular volume and mass is achieved by representing the left ventricle as a composite of geometric figures such as trapezoids or pyramids and using a polyhedral surface algorithm from short-axis cross-sectional views. An advantage is that from the original three-dimensional data set any two-dimensional plane can be selected and reconstructed in cine-loop format thus overcoming the limitations of acoustic access—so called 'anyplane' two-dimensional imaging.

The technique is limited in that left ventricular endocardial borders still need to be traced manually, therefore adding considerably to the time required for image reconstruction. The images themselves are still limited by the resolution of current ultrasound systems.

Ultrafast CT scanning

Ultrafast computed tomographic (CT) scanning provides higher image resolution than echocardiography (Fig. 2.10) and allows a truly tomographic assessment of the left ventricle.[52] It therefore makes fewer geometric assumptions when calculating left ventricular mass. In common with echocardiography, additional information such as stroke volume or cardiac output can be assessed at the same time. It is not limited by poor windows, but morbidly obese subjects may not be able to fit the scanner. The disadvantage is the need for ionizing radiation and intravenous contrast which does not make it as suitable as echocardiography for serial studies.

As a method of assessing left ventricular mass it has been anatomically validated in dogs with good correlation between in vivo, and post-mortem left ventricular mass.[53] It has also been shown to have excellent reproducibility in serial studies and very low inter- and intraobserver error.[54]

Ultrafast CT uses electron beam technology to allow rapid image acquisition which previously limited the use of CT in cardiac imaging. The patient is positioned supine with the scanning table angled 20° to the right in a 15° reverse Trendelenberg position to obtain the optimal short-axis view. Images are obtained at eight levels (8 mm slices) with a minimum of 10 images at each level. The exposure time is only 50 ms per image so gating is not required. Initial

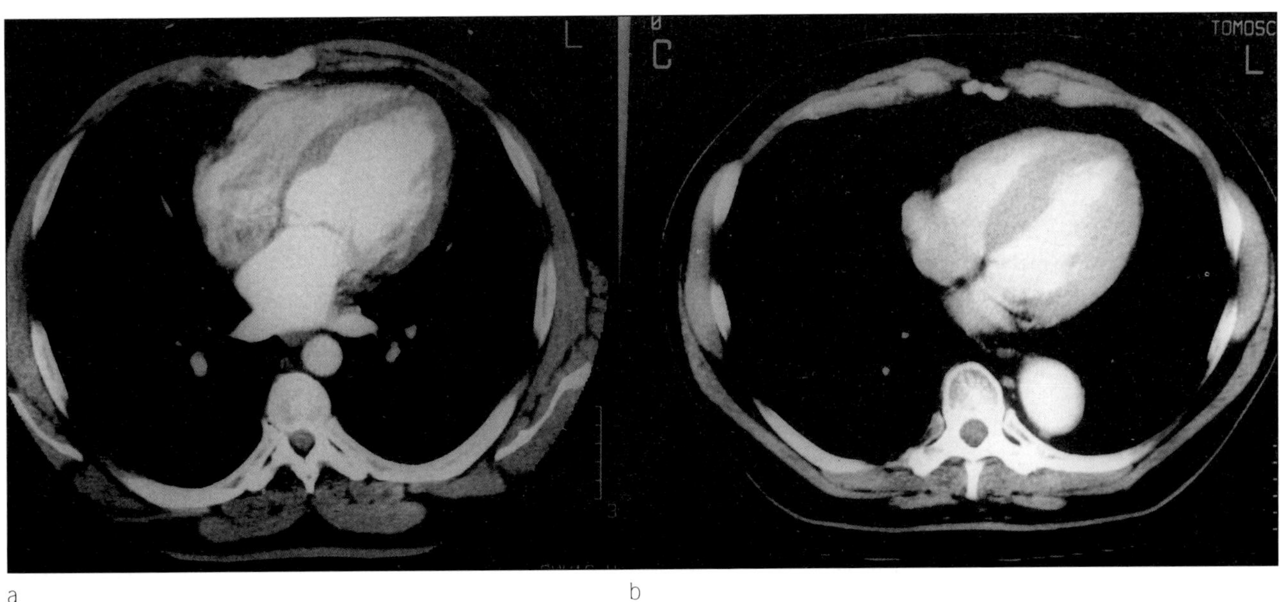

a b

Figure 2.10
Ultrafast CT. Mid-ventricular slices in (a) a subject with normal left ventricular mass and (b) a patient with aortic stenosis and significant left ventricular hypertrophy.
(Figures kindly supplied by Dr S. Rankin, Dept. of Radiology, Guy's Hospital, London, UK.)

localization scans are performed to position the left ventricle and the circulation time calculated to predict peak contrast enhancement of the left ventricle. Current techniques allow scans for left ventricular mass estimation to be done in less than 15 min which is quicker than an echocardiographic study.

Image analysis is performed by tracing the endocardial and epicardial borders to calculate the myocardial area. Slice thickness is fixed and therefore the myocardial volume for each section can be calculated. The apex myocardial volume is calculated by determination of Hounsfield units for myocardium and for adjacent lung and soft tissue. The total left ventricular myocardial volume is calculated by summation of section volumes and multiplied by the density of myocardium (1.04 g/cm^3) to obtain left ventricular mass.[55]

Nuclear magnetic resonance imaging

Magnetic resonance imaging techniques are accurate in estimating left ventricular mass and have been anatomically validated against anatomic mass in cadaver hearts (R = 0.99, SEE = 6.8 g)[55,56] and in vivo in dogs compared to subsequent post-mortem left ventricular mass (R = 0.98, SEE = 6.1 g).[57] Human in vivo studies show good correlation between left ventricular mass determined by magnetic resonance imaging in normal individuals and autopsy-derived normal ranges.[58] It has good reproducibility with extremely low inter- and intraobserver error, allowing accurate serial estimates of left ventricular mass, for example, in assessing response to therapeutic intervention.

Magnetic resonance imaging has several advantages over echocardiography. Image quality is superior and truly tomographic views of the left ventricle can be taken which reduces the reliance on complex geometric assumptions. Magnetic resonance imaging is therefore more accurate in assessing asymmetric hearts, for example in dogs with experimentally induced acute myocardial infarction[59] or in humans with hypertrophic cardiomyopathy.[56] The standard error in all these studies is <10 g for magnetic resonance imaging estimated LV mass compared to echo, which even in ideal conditions has a standard error of >30 g.

Magnetic resonance imaging also has the advantage of not requiring ionizing radiation and is therefore better suited to serial studies than CT scanning. A number of subjects cannot be scanned because of claustrophobia or the presence of implanted metallic devices such as pacemakers or some mechanical heart valves. The cost is higher than for echocardiography. Another drawback is that scan times may sometimes be unacceptably long.

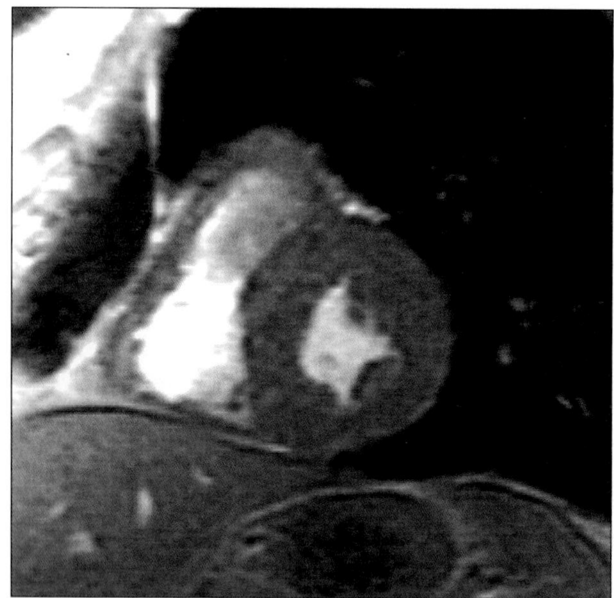

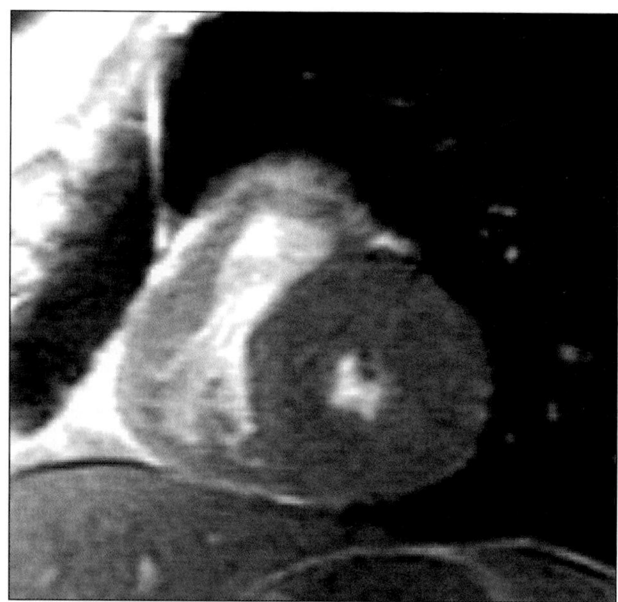

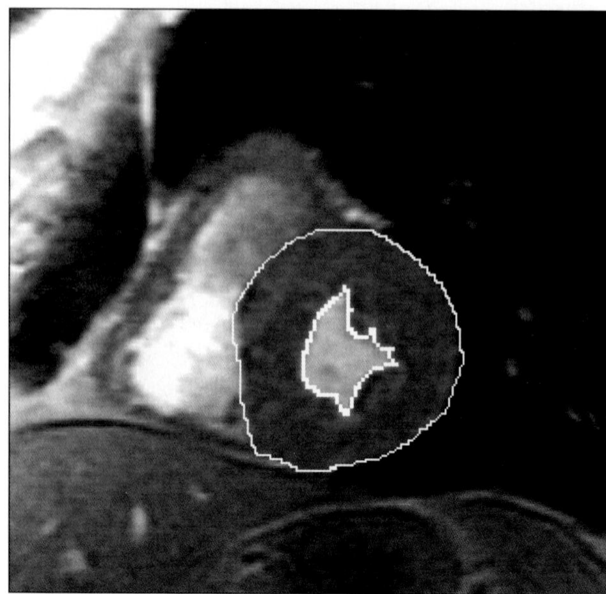

Figure 2.11
Magnetic resonance imaging.
Upper panel—shows a short axis slice in diastole (*left*) and systole (*right*), in a patient with severe left ventricular hypertrophy.
Bottom panel—shows manually traced endocardial and epicardial borders (in diastole) for calculation of slice volume. Left ventricular mass is then calculated by summation of slice volumes using Simpson's rule.
(Figures kind supplied by Dr M. Graves, Addenbrokes Hospital, Cambridge, UK.)

Magnetic resonance imaging scans are ECG gated and use a spin-echo technique with the patient at a 30° tilt in the right anterior oblique position to allow short-axis slices through the left ventricle. Usually 8–10 slices (1 cm thick) are taken with five images at each slice location, incorporating diastolic and systolic images. Image acquisition is normally controlled by R wave triggering so that the first end-diastolic image is taken 4 ms after the R wave. Total scan time is 45–60 min in a patient with a heart rate of 70 beats/min.

End-diastolic images from each slice are divided into a matrix of 256 × 256 pixels or volume elements known as 'voxels'. The voxel volume is determined from phantoms and slice thickness (e.g. 1.6 mm × 1.6 mm × 10 mm). The epicardial and endocardial borders are traced as with other methods (Fig. 2.11). The number of voxels between the two borders is determined to calculate the slice volume. The individual slice volumes are then summed to give total left ventricular volume by Simpson's rule, and then multiplied by the density of myocardium (1.04 g/cm^3) to give left ventricular mass. The calculation can take up to 45 min if done manually.

Recently newer techniques using single-phase cardiac magnetic resonance imaging have reduced the imaging time to under 15 min.[58,60] Here, images at each sequential slice location are obtained at a different phase of the cardiac cycle so that only one or two acquisition sequences (5–10 images) are required instead of a whole acquisition sequence for each slice (50 images). This allows rapid, accurate, reproducible sequential scanning which is ideal for monitoring small changes in left ventricular mass. Magnetic resonance imaging assessment of left ventricular mass is now regarded by many as the 'gold standard' and method of choice in clinical investigations and for serial evaluation of selected patients. Its cost and accessibility, however, still limit its widespread clinical use.

Summary

Assessment of left ventricular hypertrophy is of importance for risk stratification in cardiac disease. For routine clinical work the simple and quick M-mode methods are adequate since the relationship between left ventricular mass and risk is robust. For more detailed routine clinical work, for example to decide whether left ventricular hypertrophy is present in a borderline case or to detect regression of left ventricular hypertrophy, the more accurate two-dimensional methods should be used. For research purposes we believe that magnetic resonance imaging is the 'gold standard'.

Acknowledgements

We thank Dr Sheila Rankin, Head of CT Scanning Guy's and St Thomas' Hospital and Dr Martin Graves, Head of MRI, Addenbrooke's Hospital, Cambridge, UK for their advice, helpful criticism, and for supplying Figures 2.10 and 2.11.

References

1 Kannel WB: Prevalence and natural history of electrocardiographic left ventricular hypertrophy. *Am J Med Supplement* 1983; **3A**: 4–11.

2 Carroll JD, Carroll EP, Feldman T et al: Sex-associated differences in left ventricular function in aortic stenosis of the elderly. *Circulation* 1992; **86**: 1099–107.

3 Levy D, Garrison RJ, Savage DD, Kannel WB, Castelli WP: Prognostic implication of echocardiographically determined left ventricular mass in the Framingham heart study. *N Engl J Med* 1990; **322**: 1561–6.

4 Hammond IW, Devereux RB, Alderman MH et al: The prevalence and correlates of echocardiographic left ventricular hypertrophy among employed patients with uncomplicated hypertension. *J Am Coll Cardiol* 1988; **7**: 639–50.

5 Casale PN, Devereux RB, Milner et al: Value of echocardiographic measurement of left ventricular mass in predicting cardiovascular morbid events in hypertensive men. *Ann Int Med* 1986; **105**: 173–8.

6 Koren MJ, Devereux RB, Casale PN et al: Relation of left ventricular mass and geometry to morbidity and mortality in uncomplicated essential hypertension. *Ann Int Med* 1991; **114**: 345–52.

7 Liao Y, Cooper RS, McGee DL et al: The relative effect of left ventricular hypertrophy, coronary artery disease, and ventricular dysfunction on survival among black adults. *JAMA* 1995; **273**: 1592–7.

8 Devereux RB, Reichek N: Echocardiographic determination of left ventricular mass in man–anatomic validation of the method. *Circulation* 1977; **55**: 613–18.

9 Mosteller RD: Simplified calculation of body-surface area. *N Engl J Med* 1987; **317**: 1098 (abstract).

10 Levy D, Anderson KM, Savage DD et al: Echocardiographically detected left ventricular hypertrophy: prevalence and risk factors. *Ann Int Med* 1988; **108**: 7–13.

11 Devereux RB, Lutas EM, Casale PN et al: Standardisation of M-mode echocardiographic left ventricular anatomic measurements. *J Am Coll Cardiol* 1984; **4**: 1222–30.

12 Lauer MS, Larson MG, Levy D: Gender-specific reference M-mode values in adults: population-derived values with consideration of the impact of height. *J Am Coll Cardiol* 1995; **26**: 1039–46.

13 Levy D, Savage DD, Garrison RJ et al: Echocardiographic criteria for left ventricular hypertrophy: the Framingham heart study. *Am J Cardiol* 1987; **59**: 956–60.

14 Pellicia A, Maron BJ, Spataro A et al: The upper limit of physiologic cardiac hypertrophy in highly trained elite athletes. *N Engl J Med* 1991; **324**: 295–301.

15 Bland JM, Altman DG: Statistical methods for assessing agreement between two methods of clinical measurement. *Lancet* 1986; **1**: 307–10.

16 Popp RL, Filly K, Brown OR, Harrison DC. Effect of transducer placement on echocardiographic measurement of left ventricular dimensions. *Am J Cardiol* 1975; **35**: 537–40.

17 Stefadouros MA, Canedo MI: Reproducibility of echocardiographic estimates of left ventricular dimensions. *Br Heart J* 1977; **39**: 390–8.

18 Reichek N, Helak J, Plappert T et al: Anatomic validation of left ventricular mass estimates from clinical two-dimensional echocardiography; initial results. *Circulation* 1983; **67**: 348–52.

19 Collins HW, Kronenberg MW, Byrd III BF: Reproducibility of left ventricular mass measurements by two-dimensional and M-mode echocardiography. *J Am Coll Cardiol* 1996; **14**: 672–6.

20 Schiller NB, Shah PM, Crawford M et al: Recommendations for quantitation of the left ventricle by two-dimensional echocardiography. *J Am Soc Echocardiogr* 1989; **2**: 358–67.

21 Schiller NB: Two-dimensional echocardiographic determination of left ventricular volume, systolic function, and mass. Summary and discussion of the 1989 recommendations of the American Society of Echocardiography. *Circulation* 1991; **84**: I-280–7.

22 Devereux RB: Left ventricular geometry, pathophysiology and prognosis. *J Am Coll Cardiol* 1995; **25**: 885–7.

23 Helak JW, Reichek N: Quantitation of human left ventricular mass and volume by two-dimensional echocardiography: in vitro anatomic validation. *Circulation* 1981; **63**: 1398–407.

24 Schiller NB, Shah PM, Crawford M et al: Recommendations for quantitation of the left ventricle by two-dimensional echocardiography. American Society of Echocardiography Committee on Standards, Subcommittee on Quantitation of Two-Dimensional Echocardiograms. [Review]. *J Am Soc Echocardiogr* 1989; **2**: 358–67.

25 Gaasch WH: Left ventricular radius to wall thickness ratio. *Am J Cardiol* 1979; **42**: 1189–94.

26 St John Sutton M, Reichek N, Lovett J et al: Effects of age, body size, and blood pressure on the normal human left ventricle. Presentation at the American Heart Association, 53rd Scientific Session, Miami, Florida, November 1980. *Circulation* 1980; **62**: III–305 (abstract).

27 Reichek N, Devereux RB: Reliable estimation of peak left ventricular systolic pressure by M-mode echocardiographic determined end-diastolic relative wall thickness; identification of severe valvular aortic stenosis in adult patients. *Am Heart J* 1982; **103**: 202–3.

28 Gaasch WH, Andrias W, Levine HJ: Chronic aortic regurgitation: the effect of aortic valve replacement on left ventricular volume, mass, and function. *Circulation* 1980; **58**: 825–36.

29 Verdecchia P, Schillaci G, Borgioni C et al: Adverse prognostic significance of concentric remodelling of the left ventricle in hypertensive subjects with normal left ventricular mass. *J Am Coll Cardiol* 1995; **25**: 871–8.

30 Devereux RB, James GD, Pickering TG: What is normal blood pressure? Comparison of ambulatory pressure level and variability in patients with normal or abnormal left ventricular geometry. *Am J Hypertension* 1993; **6**: 211S–215S.

31 Ganau A, Devereux RB, Roman MJ et al: Patterns of left ventricular hypertrophy and geometric remodeling in essential hypertension [see comments]. *J Am Coll Cardiol* 1992; **19**: 1550–8.

32 Ganau A, Arru A, Saba PS et al: Stroke volume and left heart anatomy in relation to plasma volume in essential hypertension. *J Hypertension Supplement* 1991; **9**: S1504–11.

33 Linzbach AJ: Hypertrophy, hyperplasia, and structural dilatation of the human heart. *Adv Cardiol* 1976; **18**: 1–14.

34 Byrd III BF, Wahr D, Wang YS et al: Left ventricular mass and volume/mass ratio determined by two-dimensional echocardiography in normal adults. *J Am Coll Cardiol* 1985; **6**: 1021–5.

35 Pearlman JD, Triulzi MO, King ME et al: Left atrial dimensions in growth and development: normal limits for two-dimensional echocardiography. *J Am Coll Cardiol* 1990; **16**: 1168–74.

36 Kitzman DW, Sheikh KH, Beere PA et al: Age-related alterations of Doppler left ventricular filling indexes in normal subjects are independent of left ventricular mass, heart rate, contractility and loading conditions. *J Am Coll Cardiol* 1991; **18**: 1243–50.

37 Wahr DW, Wang YS, Schiller NB: Left ventricular volumes determined by two-dimensional echocardiography in a normal adult population. *J Am Coll Cardiol* 1983; **1**: 863–8.

38 Inuoye I, Massie B, Loge D et al: Abnormal left ventricular filling: an early finding in mild to moderate systemic hypertension. *Am J Cardiol* 1984; **53**: 120–6.

39 Cuocolo A, Sax FL, Brush JE et al: Left ventricular hypertrophy and impaired diastolic filling in essential hypertension. *Circulation* 1990; **81**: 978–86.

40 Fouad FM, Slominski M, Tarazi RC: Left ventricular diastolic function in hypertension: relation to left ventricular mass and systolic function. *J Am Coll Cardiol* 1984; **3**: 1500–6.

41 Hess OM, Villari B, Krayenbuhl HP: Diastolic dysfunction in aortic stenosis. *Circulation* 1993; **87**: IV-73–6.

42 Rossvoll O, Hatle LK: Pulmonary venous flow velocities recorded by transthoracic Doppler ultrasound: relation to left ventricular diastolic pressures. *J Am Coll Cardiol* 1993; **21**: 1687–96.

43 Tenenbaum A, Motro M, Hod H et al: Shortened Doppler-derived mitral A wave deceleration time: an important predictor of elevated left ventricular filling pressure. *J Am Coll Cardiol* 1996; **27**: 700–5.

44 Salustri A, Roelandt JRTC: Ultrasonic three-dimensional reconstruction of the heart. *Ultrasound Med Biol* 1995; **21**: 281–93.

45 von Ramm OT, Pavy HA, Smith SW, Kisslo J. Real-time three-dimensional echocardiography: the first human images. *Circulation* 1991; **84**: II-685 (abstract).

46 King DL, King Jr DL, Smith MD, Kwan OL: Three-dimensional spatial registration and interactive display of position and orientation of real-time ultrasound images. *J Am Coll Cardiol* 1992; **20**: 1238–45.

47 Handschumacher MD, Lethor J, Siu SC et al: A new integrated system for the three-dimensional echocardiographic reconstruction: development and validation for ventricular volume with application in human subjects. *J Am Coll Cardiol* 1993; **21**: 737–42.

48 Jiang L, Levine RA, Weyman AE, Handschumacher MD: Accuracy of three-dimensional echocardiographic reconstruction by electromagnetic positional location: a further step toward practical implementation of the technique. *J Am Coll Cardiol* 1994; **9**: 701–3.

49 Roelandt J, Salustri A, Bruining N: Precordial and transesophageal dynamic three-dimensional echocardiography with rotatable (multiplane) transducer systems. *Ultrasound Med Biol* 1994; **20**: S411–4 (abstract).

50 Sapin PM, Schroeder KD, Smith MD et al: Three-dimensional echocardiographic measurement of left ventricular volume in vitro: comparison with two-dimensional echocardiography and cineventriculography. *J Am Coll Cardiol* 1993; **22**: 1530–7.

51 Gopal AA, Keller AM, Shen Z et al: Three-dimensional echocardiography: in vitro and in vivo validation of let ventricular mass and comparison with conventional echocardiographic methods. *J Am Coll Cardiol* 1994; **24**: 504–13.

52 Diethelm L, Simonson JS, Dery R et al: Determination of left ventricular mass with ultrafast CT and two-dimensional echocardiography. *Radiology* 1989; **171**: 213–17.

53 Feiring AJ, Rumberger JA, Reiter SJ et al: Determination of left ventricular mass in dogs with rapid acquisition cardiac computed tomographic scanning. *Circulation* 1985; **72**: 1355–64.

54 Roig E, Geirgiou D, Chomka EV et al: Reproducibility of left ventricular myocardial volume and mass measurements by ultrafast computed tomography. *J Am Coll Cardiol* 1991; **18**: 990–6.

55 Katz J, Milliken MC, Stray-Gunderson J et al: Estimation of human myocardial mass with MR imaging. *Radiology* 1988; **169**: 495–8.

56 Allison JD, Flickenger FW, Wright JC et al: Measurement of left ventricular mass in hypertrophic cardiomyopathy using MRI: comparison with echocardiography. *Magn Res Imag* 1993; **11**: 329–34.

57 Keller AM, Peshock RM, Malloy CR et al: In vivo measurement of myocardial mass using nuclear magnetic resonance imaging. *J Am Coll Cardiol* 1986; **8**: 113–17.

58 Aurigemma G, Davidoff A, Silver K et al: Left ventricular mass quantitation using single-phase cardiac magnetic resonance imaging. *Am J Cardiol* 1992; **70**: 259–62.

59 Shapiro EP, Rogers WJ, Beyar R et al: Determination of left ventricular mass by magnetic resonance imaging in hearts deformed by acute infarction. *Circulation* 1989; **79**: 706–11.

60 Forbat SM, Karwatowski SP, Gatehouse PD et al: Technical note: rapid measurement of left ventricular mass by spin echo magnetic resonance imaging. *Br J Radiol* 1994; **67**: 86–90.

3

Imaging of the coronary artery in ischemic syndromes

Jon Resar

The spectrum of syndromes encompassing ischemic coronary artery disease includes stable angina, unstable angina, and acute myocardial infarction (both Q wave and non-Q wave). Although these entities have distinct criteria that help to categorize patients presenting with chest pain, there is in fact, considerable overlap in clinical presentation between these groups. Moreover, there are consistent data from pathologic, angiographic, and angioscopic studies showing a common pathophysiologic basis for these syndromes, namely, an atherosclerotic plaque with varying degrees of plaque disruption and superimposed thrombus.[1–3] The specific clinical presentation of one of these ischemic syndromes depends on the severity and duration of ischemia as modified by whether the obstruction is occlusive or nonocclusive, transient or persistent, or attenuated by collateral flow. The purpose of this chapter is to review the findings of various imaging modalities including angiography, angioscopy, and intravascular ultrasound in the setting of clinically apparent coronary artery disease with particular emphasis on unstable angina.

Angiography

Acute myocardial infarction

The demonstration by De Wood et al[4] of intracoronary thrombus in the early hours after acute transmural myocardial infarction was a seminal finding in acute coronary syndromes. Eighty-seven per cent of patients had total occlusion of the infarct-related artery within 4 h of the onset of symptoms. At 12–24 h, complete occlusion of the infarct-related artery was still present in nearly two-thirds of the patients studied. These results showing thrombus overlying a disruption in the fibrous cap of an atherosclerotic plaque as the cause of acute myocardial infarction had important therapeutic ramifications. The demonstration of thrombus formation in acute myocardial infarction ushered in the use of thrombolytic agents in the treatment of myocardial infarction. Depending on the regimen of the thrombolysis utilized, angiographic patency rates exceeding 80% can be achieved.[5,6]

Likewise, non-Q wave infarction which is defined as myocardial necrosis without the evolution of Q waves, is associated with total occlusion of the infarct-related vessel in 26% of patients studied within 24 h of symptoms and 42% of patients studied from 72 h to 7 days.[7] Thus, a marked increase in total coronary occlusion in the infarct-related vessel was observed over time, while the frequency of subtotal occlusion in this patient population declined. This is in contrast to that observed in Q wave myocardial infarctions in which the prevalence of total occlusion is high initially, but tends to decline with time after the infarction (Figs 3.1a, 3.1b, 3.2a, 3.2b).

Unstable angina

Unstable angina is defined as the:

- recent onset of chest pain at rest or with minimal exertion;
- rapid and marked progression of symptoms superimposed on a previously stable pattern of angina pectoris;
- recurrent episodes of angina at rest.

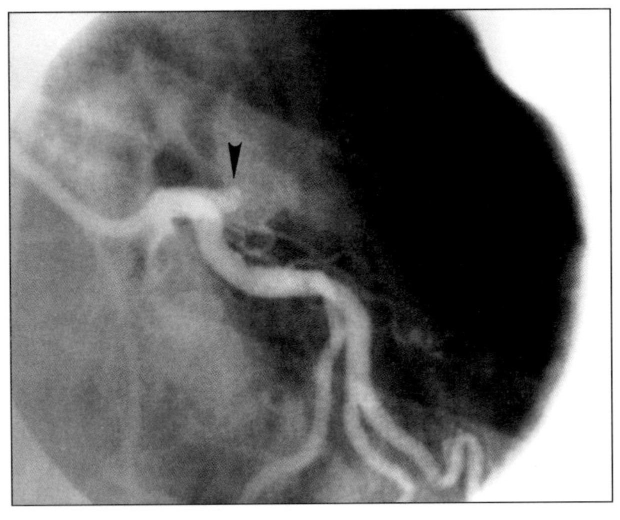
a

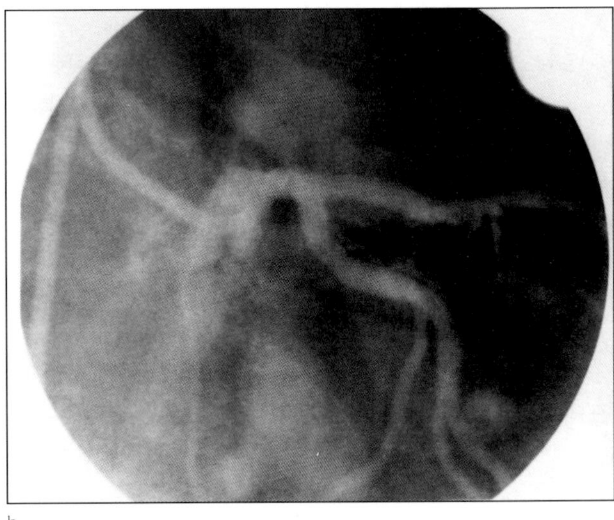
b

Figure 3.1
(a) Total thrombotic occlusion of the proximal left anterior descending coronary artery (arrow) 2 h after the onset of an acute anterior wall myocardial infarction. (b) Widely patent left anterior descending coronary artery following primary percutaneous transluminal angioplasty.

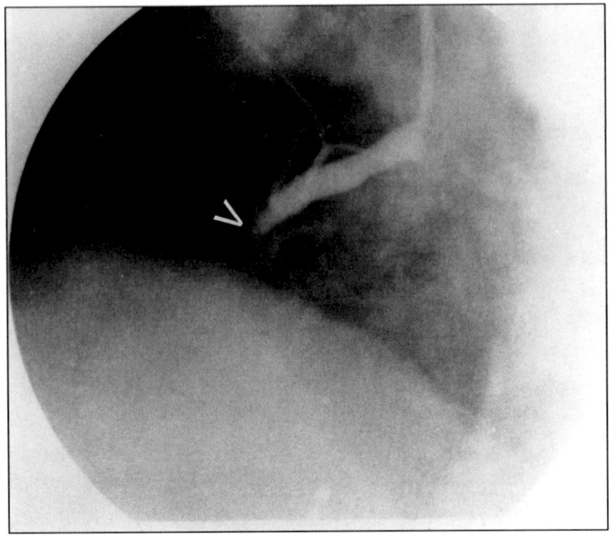
a

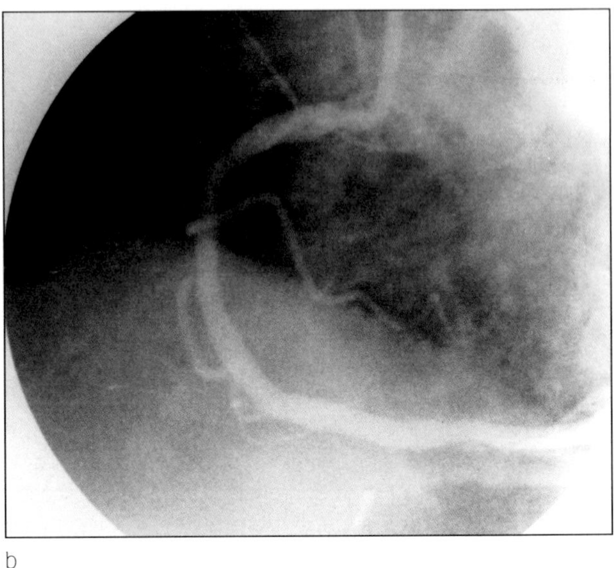
b

Figure 3.2
Total thrombotic occlusion of the proximal right coronary artery (arrow) 4 h after the onset of an acute inferior wall myocardial infarction. (b) Widely patent right coronary artery following primary percutaneous transluminal angioplasty.

Unstable angina and acute myocardial infarction can be considered a continuum as related to the process of coronary artery thrombosis. The distinction between acute myocardial infarction and unstable angina, namely whether myocardial necrosis occurs, relates to the duration and severity of the ischemic insult.

Early reports of angiography in the setting of unstable angina[8,9] highlighted the high incidence of severe coronary artery disease in selected patients undergoing coronary arteriography. Although no mention of angiographically evident thrombus was made in these papers, 83% of patients studied had at least one artery with greater than 70% stenosis. Morphologic features of lesions in patients progressing from stable to unstable angina include increased stenosis severity and eccentricity thought to represent plaque disruption or partially occlusive thrombus, or both.[10–13] Ambrose et al[10] observed angiographic features of complex coronary lesions including coronary thrombus and complex lesion morphology in 72% of patients with unstable angina undergoing early angiography.

The finding that angiographic stenosis complexity predicts subsequent in-hospital instability in patients with unstable angina has been confirmed by many[12,15] but not all[16] investigators. Furthermore, even in unstable angina patients who stabilize with medical management, subsequent short-term stenosis progression and coronary events are common.[17] Since patients presenting with unstable angina tend to be intervened on with percutaneous transluminal coronary angioplasty or coronary artery bypass surgery when significant coronary artery disease is identified, the natural history of unstable coronary lesions has not been well studied. Chen et al[17] performed repeat angiography on 84 patients 8 months after they had initially presented with unstable angina that had subsequently been stabilized on a standard medical regimen. At initial angiography, single-vessel disease was present in 61% and 39% had multivessel disease. Mean diameter stenosis severity of lesions causing ischemia was 67% by quantitative assessment. The lesions were judged complex (irregular borders, overhanging edges, or thrombus) in 64%. There were no differences in per cent stenosis or minimal stenosis diameter between complex ischemia-related stenoses and smooth ischemia-related stenoses at initial angiography. At restudy, 25% of ischemia-related stenoses and 7% of non-ischemia-related stenoses had progressed. Nearly 70% of ischemia-related stenoses that progressed were completely occluded at follow-up angiography. Both per cent stenosis and absolute stenosis diameter changed more significantly in complex ischemia-related stenoses compared with smooth ischemia-related lesions. Stenoses ≥50% progressed more frequently and showed a greater tendency toward total occlusion than mild stenoses. Clinical events were strongly correlated with disease progression as 72% of the patients with coronary events showed disease progression. The rapid progression of complex lesions in unstable angina confirmed work by previous investigators.[11,18] In addition, coronary artery disease progression was independent of conventional risk factors and of the actual extent of coronary disease.[17]

That coronary thrombosis plays an important role in unstable angina has been shown by angiography, angioscopy, autopsy and indirectly by biochemical methods.[13,19–26] The incidence of angiographically evident thrombus in patients presenting with unstable angina is likewise quite high. Angiographic findings thought to be characteristic of intracoronary thrombus include:

- total coronary artery occlusion with convex, irregular, or hazy distal margins and post-injection contrast retention or staining in the absence of adjacent branches to maintain run-off; or
- non-total occlusion with shaggy or irregular margins or a filling defect at or adjacent to a significant coronary stenosis seen in at least two projections.[27]

Of 67 patients with unstable angina, 36% had evidence of intra-arterial coronary thrombus, either proximal or distal to a significant stenosis.

The ability of angiography to identify intracoronary thrombus in unstable angina is dependent on the timing of angiographic study with respect to the last anginal attack. Freeman et al[28] randomized 78 patients admitted to the hospital for unstable angina to early (within 24 h) or late (5–6 days) angiography. The late angiography group was further subdivided into the patients who had elective or urgent cardiac catheterization. Cardiac events occurred more frequently in patients undergoing early angiography or urgent late angiography than in patients with late elective angiography. Coronary thrombus was detected in 43% of the early angiography patients compared to 21% in the late elective group. However, the frequency of coronary thrombus in the late angiography patients who required urgent study was 75%. Thrombus and multiple-vessel disease were the most powerful predictors of subsequent in-hospital cardiac events, while complex morphology alone was not predictive. Thus, intracoronary thrombus identified by coronary angiography was associated with a higher frequency of in-hospital cardiac events, including death, myocardial infarction, and urgent revascularization after an episode of unstable angina. When coronary angiography is performed more than 30 days after the last episode of chest pain, the incidence of thrombus is low (1–12%),[13,21,22,29,30] whereas within 2 weeks of angina, the incidence is considerably greater (52–85%).[27,31] Gotoh et al[20] studied 37 patients within 48 h of prolonged rest angina, not in the setting of acute infarction, and observed angiographic changes consistent with thrombus in 57%.

Although thrombus is likely to be present in more patients presenting with unstable angina, these data highlight the difficulties inherent to angiography in identifying thin-layered thrombus that may be indistinguishable from the underlying atherosclerotic plaque. Despite these limitations, the widespread use of angiography as a diagnostic tool in the assessment of coronary artery disease is likely to remain high. This may be especially true for issues relating to prognosis and percutaneous interventions (Figs 3.3–3.5).

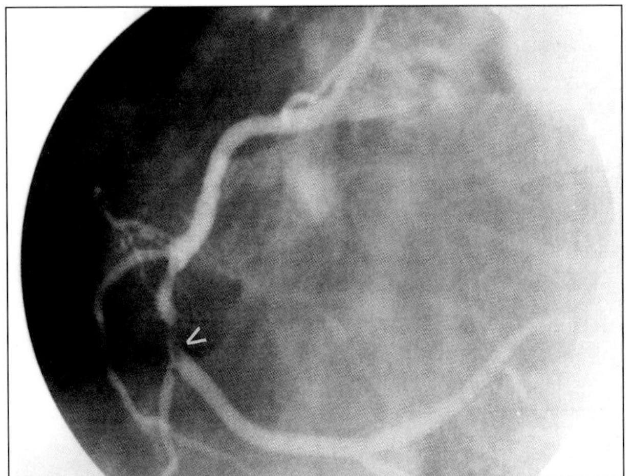

Figure 3.3
High grade stenosis with thrombus (arrow) in the mid right coronary artery following a non-Q wave inferior wall myocardial infarction.

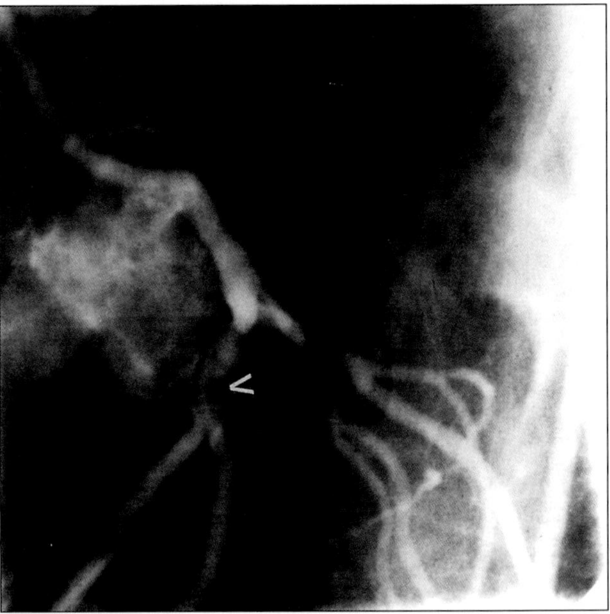

Figure 3.4
High grade stenosis with an ulcerative plaque (arrow) in the proximal left anterior descending coronary artery of a 49-year-old patient presenting with unstable angina.

Stable angina

Quantitative variables assessed angiographically such as the distribution of coronary lesions, number of diseased vessels, and the degree of coronary artery obstruction, have not been shown to be significantly different in patients with stable versus unstable angina.[9,10,19] However, there are important differences in the qualitative appearance of coronary lesions between the two syndromes.[10,32] Coronary lesions found in >71% of patients with unstable angina demonstrate marked eccentricity characterized by numerous irregularities or scalloped borders, whereas these findings are observed in only 16% of stable patients.[10] Conversely, concentric and minimally eccentric lesions were identified in the culprit arteries in 80% of patients with stable angina.[10] Numerous investigators have shown that stenoses with irregular borders often demonstrate plaque rupture or partially occlusive thrombi, thus accounting for the acute progression of coronary artery disease in these patients.[14]

Probably the most important angiographic difference between stable versus unstable patients is the incidence of intracoronary thrombus. Bresnahan et al[13] identified thrombus in only 2.5% of stable angina patients compared to 36% of patients with unstable symptoms. Furthermore, coronary artery thrombus was not found in patients who had stable angina without a prior myocardial infarction.

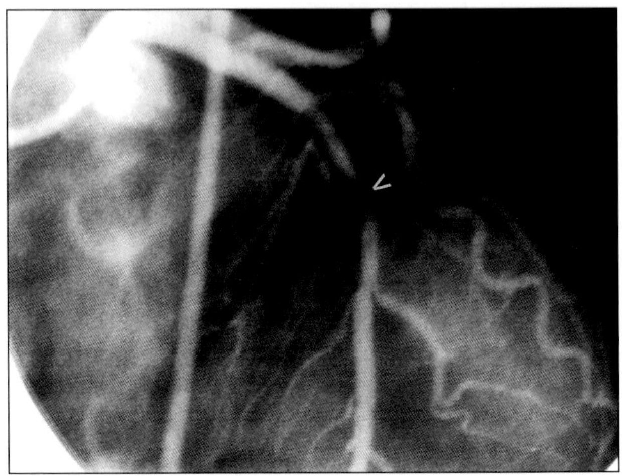

Figure 3.5
High grade stenosis in the mid left anterior descending coronary artery of a 38-year-old woman presenting with unstable angina.

Serial angiographic studies in patients with stable angina demonstrate progression in 40–50% of patients but, in contrast to unstable angina, the progression is generally of smaller magnitude and the occurrence of new occlusions occurs in less than 10% of patients.[33–35]

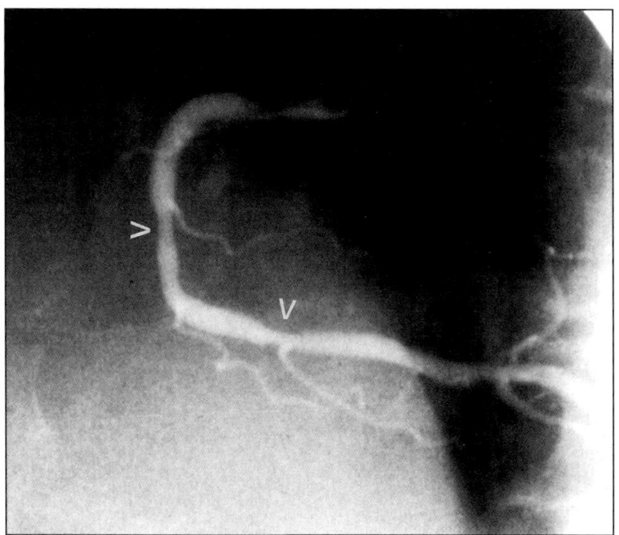

Figure 3.6
Multiple lesions of moderate severity (arrows) in the right coronary artery of a 60-year-old man with chronic, stable angina.

In the placebo group of a cholesterol lowering trial, Waters et al[34] documented a worsening of minimum lumen diameter by ≥ 0.4 mm of one or more lesions in 56% of stable angina patients, but only 9.6% exhibited a worsening of diameter stenosis by ≥15% and progression to a new total occlusion was seen in only 1.9%. Subsequent clinical follow-up of patients in such studies reveal that progression of disease assessed angiographically was as powerful a predictor of future coronary events as ejection fraction or number of diseased vessels, with a relative risk of 2.3 for death or nonfatal myocardial infarction in the ensuing 4 years[35] (Fig. 3.6).

Angioscopy

Percutaneous transluminal coronary angioscopy is a diagnostic imaging technique in which optic fibers are used to directly visualize the lumen of coronary arteries during cardiac catheterization. Angioscopy provides a full color, high resolution image of the intracoronary artery surface morphology. The main advantages of angioscopy are the ability to detect intraluminal thrombus and to identify surface features of the luminal surface. Angioscopy is highly sensitive at detecting even small thrombi on the endoluminal surface. Furthermore, qualitative features of thrombus such as color (red or white) can be readily ascertained.

Mizuno et al[23] studied 18 patients with unstable angina and 20 patients with acute myocardial infarction. Thrombi were defined as masses of red, of white or of both colors that adhered to the intima and protruded into the lumen. Angioscopy revealed coronary thrombi in all but two patients (one patient in each group) and this finding was not affected by whether angioscopy was performed early (<8 h) or late (>8 h) after the onset of pain at rest. Most important, the appearance of the thrombi differed between the two groups. In most unstable angina patients, grayish-white thrombi were observed, whereas in patients with acute myocardial infarction, reddish thrombi predominated. It was hypothesized that the differences in thrombus appearance between acute myocardial infarction and unstable angina were related to the dissimilar composition of the thrombus in the two clinical settings. Previous pathological studies have shown that white thrombi consist of a predominance of platelets, while red thrombi contain an abundance of fibrin mixed with erythrocytes.[36] Thrombi forming early in the course of rest angina are composed almost exclusively of platelets. These findings suggest that there may be subtle differences in thrombus formation between the two conditions, and these may account for the disparate results with thrombolytic therapy in acute myocardial infarction as compared to unstable angina.[37] Accordingly, the platelet-predominant thrombi observed in patients with unstable angina are more resistant to lysis by thrombolytic agents than the red thrombi commonly found in patients with acute myocardial infarction.

Angioscopy performed during coronary artery bypass surgery has demonstrated a high incidence of intracoronary thrombus in patients with a history of unstable angina. Sherman et al[38] demonstrated the superior sensitivity of angioscopy over angiography for the detection of thrombus and identification of complex plaque in a group of patients with unstable angina undergoing coronary artery bypass surgery. Angioscopy of the infarct-related artery following acute myocardial infarction nearly always demonstrates thrombus in those patients with post-infarction angina. Tabata et al[39] studied 51 patients following acute myocardial infarction (mean 13.9 days) and identified thrombus by angioscopy in 100% of patients with post-infarction angina but only in 15% of patients without post-infarction angina. There were no significant differences between groups for degree of stenosis in the infarct-related artery, number of vessels with significant stenosis, presence of collateral flow, type of therapy, or risk factors. Angiography was able to identify thrombus in only 35% of the patients in whom thrombus was identified by angioscopy. den Heijer et al[40] compared angioscopy to angiography and found that 48% of angioscopically observed thrombi remained undetected at angiography. Likewise, Ramee et al[41] demonstrated that lesion appearance, thrombus, and dissection can be identified more easily with angioscopy than angiography both before and

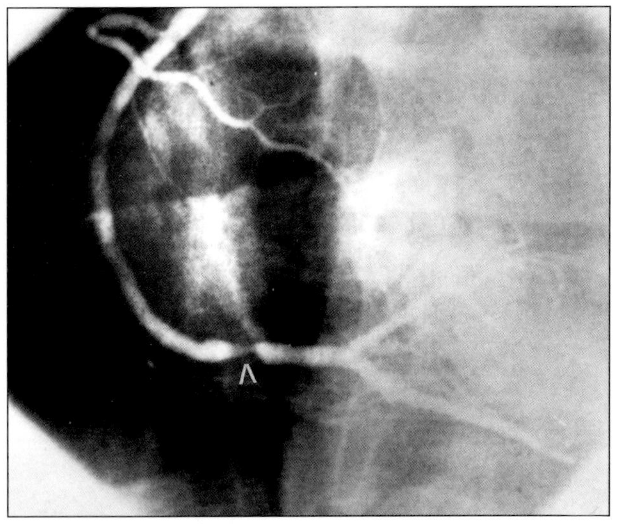

a

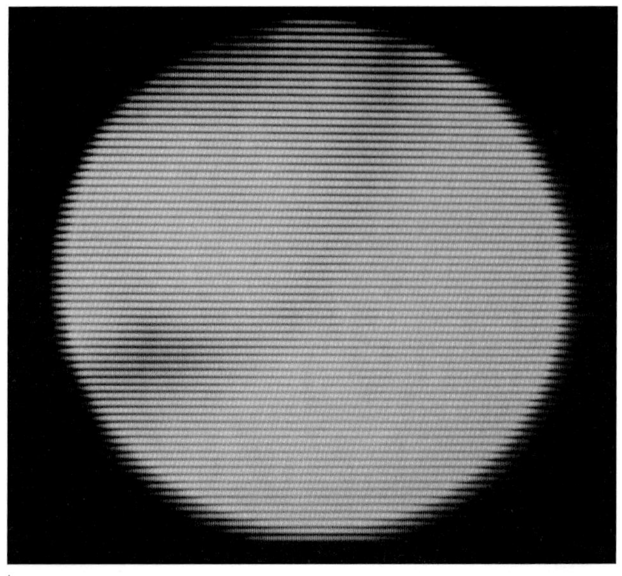

b

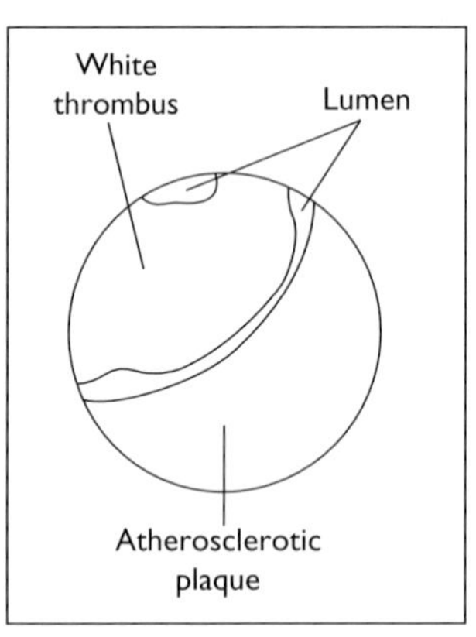

c

Figure 3.7
(a) Angiogram of the distal right coronary artery showing a hazy appearing focal stenosis in a 35-year-old man who presented with an inferior wall non-Q-wave myocardial infarction. (b) Angioscopy of the lesion showed a large, grayish-white fungating mass consistent with a platelet-rich intra-arterial thrombus in the upper left third of the image. (c) Schematic of the angioscopic image.

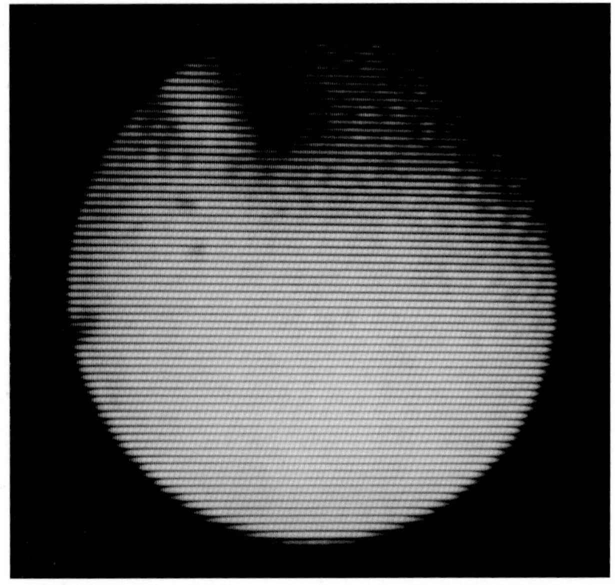

a

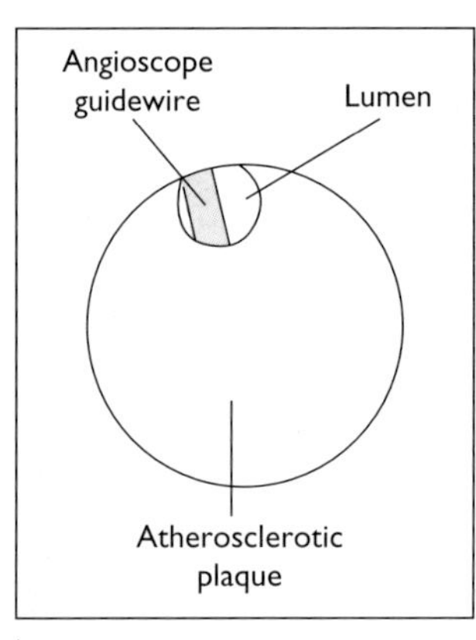

b

Figure 3.8
(a) Angioscopy of a smooth, glistening, concentric stenosis without ulceration or thrombus in a patient with stable angina. (b) Schematic of the angioscopic image.

after coronary angioplasty. The ability of angioscopy to delineate surface morphology including endothelial ulceration and partially occlusive thrombus is the major attribute of this imaging modality (Figs 3.7 and 3.8).

Intravascular ultrasound

Intravascular coronary ultrasound provides a unique approach to the assessment of coronary artery anatomy and lesion morphology. The tomographic orientation of ultrasound allows for imaging of the full 360° circumference of the vessel wall, not just the silhouette of the lumen as visualized by angiography. Thus, dimensional measurements such as diameter and cross-sectional area can be easily delineated. In addition, the ability of intravascular ultrasound to image vessel wall morphology facilitates the assessment of plaque composition, lesion morphology, extent of dissection, and overall plaque burden. In normal arteries, the ultrasound image reveals a smooth circular wall with a laminar appearance with a discrete linear reflectance at the acoustic interface between the lumen and intima.[42] Within the atheromatous plaque, ultrasound is able to distinguish certain characteristics such as fibrous tissue, calcification, and lipid or necrotic material.[43] Tobis et al[43] showed that intravascular ultrasound was more sensitive than angiography for demonstrating the presence and extent of atherosclerosis and arterial calcification. The correlation between angiographic and ultrasound measurements of coronary artery lumen in normal segments is quite variable (r = 0.26–0.92) depending on the investigator group.[42–44] Furthermore, extensive atheromatous involvement can be identified on the ultrasound images even in segments that appear normal on angiography. Mintz et al[45] found that only 6.8% of the angiographically normal coronary artery reference segments were found to be normal by intravascular ultrasound with the percent cross-sectional narrowing in these 'angiographically normal' vessels averaging 51 ± 13%.

Braden et al[46] compared lesion eccentricity by angiography to intravascular ultrasound and showed in that angiography was a poor predictor of lesion morphology in severe coronary stenoses in that only half of the lesions had concordant angiographic and ultrasound assessment.

Correlation of in vitro ultrasound images and histologic sections have been shown to be accurate in more than 90% of segments studied.[47,48] Hodgson et al[49] compared ultrasound characterization of plaque composition for patients with stable and unstable angina. No difference in angiographic percent area narrowing was seen between patients with unstable versus stable angina (90% versus 89%, respectively). Lesion composition was very different between the two groups, however, as patients with unstable angina had more soft lesions (74% versus 41%), fewer calcified and mixed plaques (fibrotic, soft or calcific components in one or more combinations) (25% versus 59%), and fewer intralesional calcium deposits (16% versus 45%) than patients with stable angina. Interestingly, morphologic plaque classification by ultrasound was closely correlated to the clinical angina pattern (stable versus unstable) but bore little relation to established angiographic morphologic

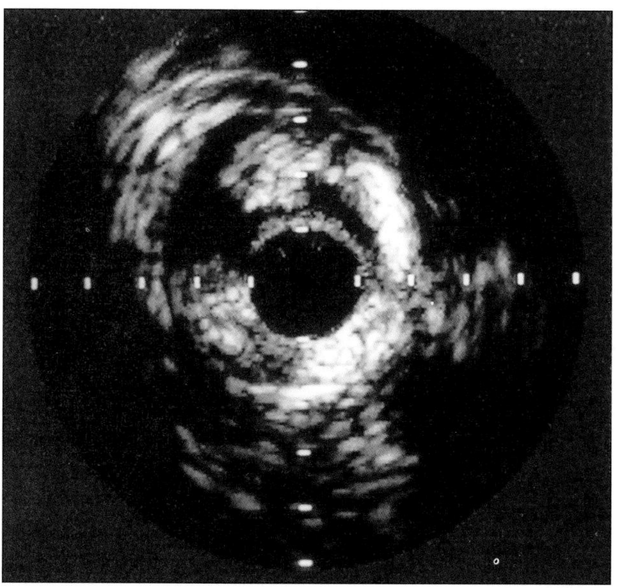

a

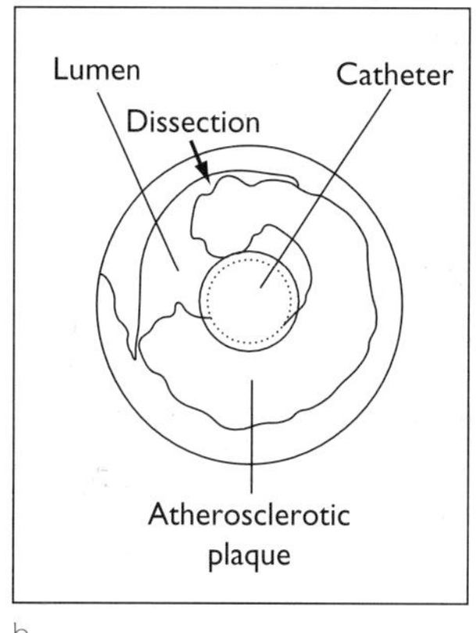

b

Figure 3.9
(a) Intravascular ultrasound of an ulcerative lesion demonstrating a severe atherosclerotic stenosis with plaque dissection. (b) Schematic of the ultrasound image.

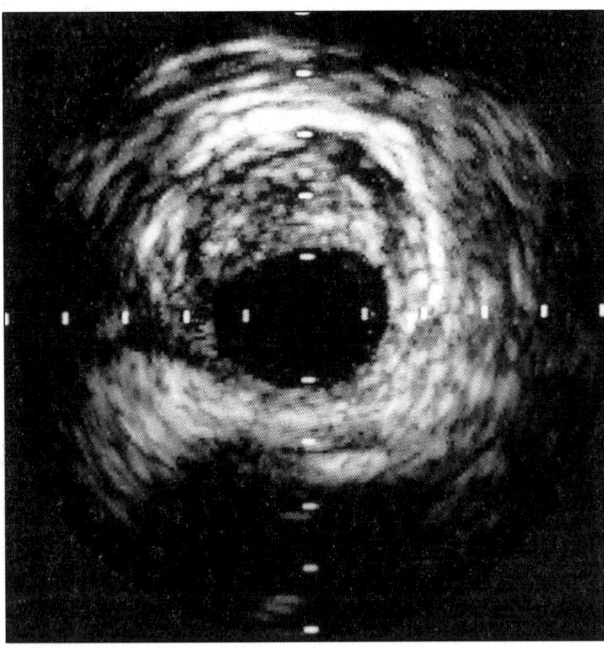

a

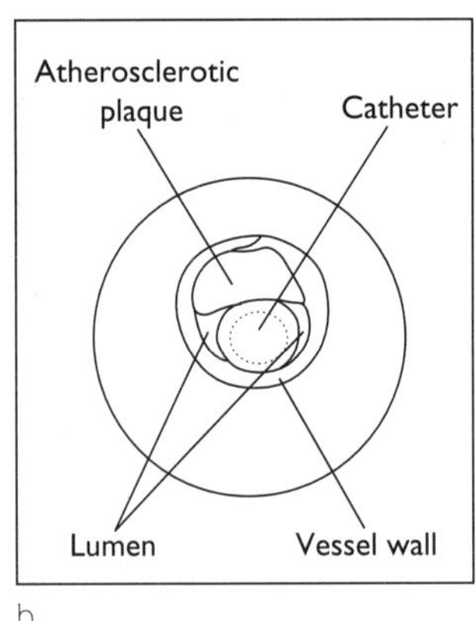

b

Figure 3.10
(a) Intravascular ultrasound of an eccentric atherosclerotic stenosis. (b) Schematic of the ultrasound image.

characteristics. This important study highlights the ability of intravascular ultrasound to characterize plaque composition and possibly to identify abnormal soft plaque regions that are the substrate for plaque rupture. Further study utilizing computer-assisted analysis of the backscattered ultrasound signal may further enhance the ability of ultrasound to characterize plaque composition in the future[50,51] (Figs 3.9–3.11).

Summary

This review has demonstrated that angiography, angioscopy, and intravascular ultrasound exhibit different imaging capabilities. What then is to be the reference or the 'gold standard' for the assessment of atherosclerotic coronary artery disease? Angiography is extremely well-suited at providing an overview or 'road-map' of the coronary artery network as a column of contrast outlining the lumen. The addition of computerized image analysis such as automatic edge detection and digital angiography improves angiographic reproducibility.[52,53] However, angiography is limited in its ability to detect early or minimal atherosclerotic disease, estimate severity of stenosis and vessel diameter, characterize plaque complexity and composition, and identify thrombus.[54] Although angioscopy is adept at characterizing intraluminal morphology such as thrombus formation and plaque rupture, it is limited by the requirement of a blood-free medium necessitating continuous flushing. Furthermore, it does not have the capacity to image beyond the intima. Angioscopic visualization is limited in tortuous segments of the coronary artery because of the lack of coaxial alignment of the angioscope. Intravascular ultrasound in addition to yielding information on intraluminal morphology is the only technique that is able to characterize intramural processes such as plaque area and wall thickness.

Thus, in an important sense, these imaging modalities provide complementary information that yields a more thorough delineation of the atherosclerotic process affecting the coronary arteries. In most instances, angiography is adequate for imaging the entire coronary arterial network and for defining significant coronary artery narrowings. If identification of thrombus is critical to the clinical setting, then angioscopy is the imaging modality of choice. If angiography cannot visualize certain arterial segments or additional information about the vascular wall is needed, then intravascular ultrasound may be required. Understanding the capabilities and limitations of these imaging modalities will enable the operator to utilize these techniques appropriately to provide information regarding the appearance of the luminal surface (in the case of angioscopy), or the structure and extent of atherosclerotic disease in the coronary artery wall (as by intravascular ultrasound).

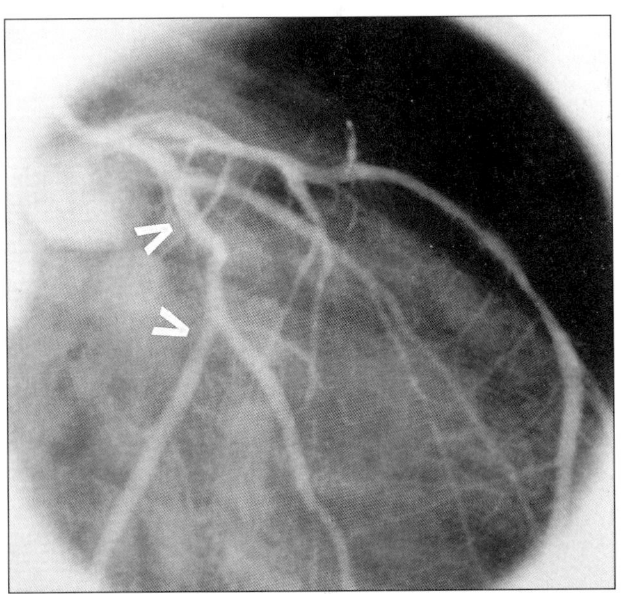

a

Figure 3.11

(a) Angiogram of the left coronary arteries show minimal disease of the left circumflex coronary artery. Arrows show location of areas imaged by intravascular ultrasound. (b) Intravascular ultrasound of the proximal left circumflex coronary artery showing moderate atherosclerotic burden in a region without angiographically evident disease. (c) Schematic of the ultrasound image. (d) Intravascular ultrasound of the mid left circumflex in a region of angiographic haziness showing an ulcerated atherosclerotic plaque of moderate severity. (e) Schematic of the ultrasound image.

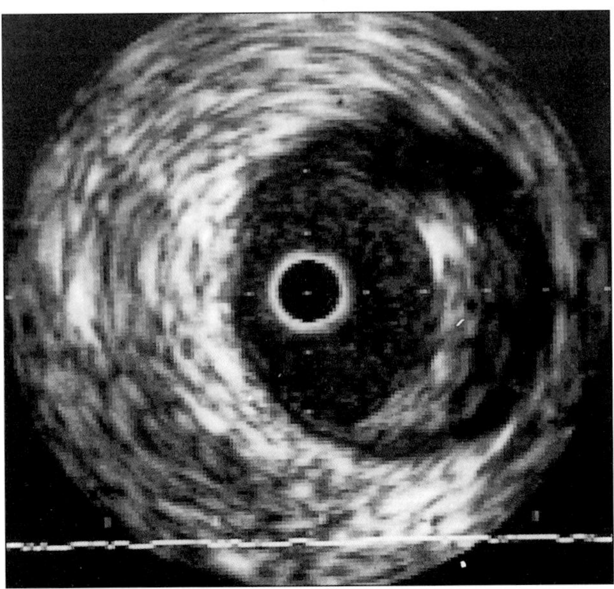

b

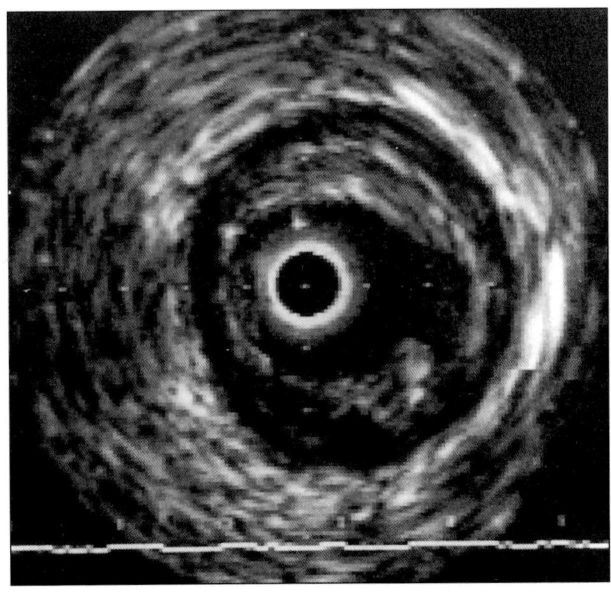

d

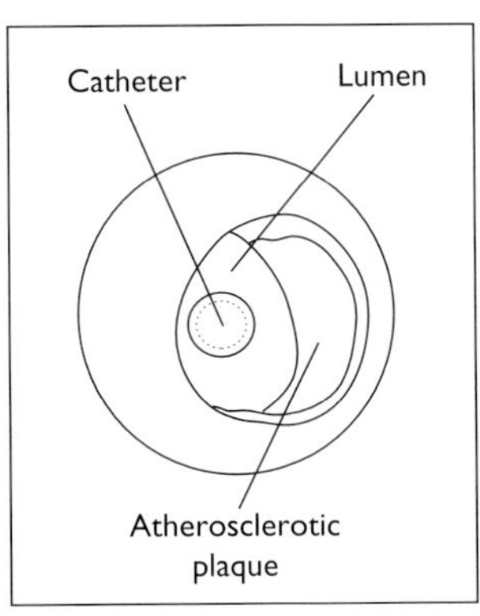

c

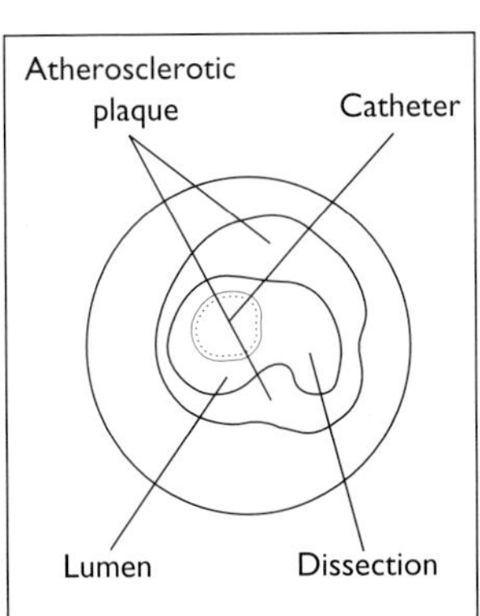

e

References

1 Fuster V, Badimon L, Cohen M et al: Insights into the pathogenesis of acute ischemic syndromes. *Circulation* 1988; **77**: 1213–20.

2 Forrester JS, Litvack F, Grunfest W et al: A perspective of coronary disease seen through the arteries of living man. *Circulation* 1987; **75**: 505–13.

3 Davies MJ, Thomas A: Thrombosis and acute coronary artery lesions in sudden cardiac ischemic death. *N Engl J Med* 1984; **310**: 1137–40.

4 DeWood MA, Spores J, Notshe RN et al: Prevalence of total coronary occlusion during the early hours of transmural myocardial infarction. *N Engl J Med* 1980; **303**: 897–902.

5 Neuhaus KL, Feuerer W, Jeep-Tebbe S, et al: Improved thrombolysis with a modified dose regimen of recombinant tissue-type plasminogen activator. *J Am Coll Cardiol* 1989; **14**: 1566–9.

6 Carney RJ, Murphy GA, Brandt TR et al: Randomized angiographic trial of recombinant tissue-type plasminogen activator (alteplase) in myocardial infarction. *J Am Coll Cardiol* 1992; **20**: 17–23.

7 DeWood MA, Stifter WF, Simpson CS et al: Coronary arteriographic findings soon after non-Q-wave myocardial infarction. *N Engl J Med* 1986; **315**: 417–23.

8 Conti CR, Brawley RK, Griffith LSC et al: Unstable angina pectoris: morbidity and mortality in 57 consecutive patients evaluated angiographically. *Am J Cardiol* 1973; **32**: 745–50.

9 Alison HW, Russell Jr RO, Mantle JA et al: Coronary anatomy and arteriography in patients with unstable angina pectoris. *Am J Cardiol* 1978; **41**: 204–9.

10 Ambrose JA, Winters SL, Stern A et al: Angiographic morphology and the pathogenesis of unstable angina pectoris. *J Am Coll Cardiol* 1985; **5**: 609–16.

11 Ambrose JA, Winters SL, Arora RR et al: Angiographic evolution of coronary artery morphology in unstable angina. *J Am Coll Cardiol* 1986; **7**: 472–8.

12 Williams AE, Freeman MR, Chisholm RJ et al: Angiographic morphology in unstable angina pectoris. *Am J Cardiol* 1988; **62**: 1024–7.

13 Bresnahan DR, Davis JL, Holmes DR et al: Angiographic occurrence and clinical correlates of intraluminal coronary artery thrombus: role of unstable angina. *J Am Coll Cardiol* 1985; **6**: 285–9.

14 Levin DC, Fallon JT: Significance of the angiographic morphology of localized coronary stenosis. Histopathologic correlations. *Circulation* 1982; **66**: 316–20.

15 Bugiardini R, Pozzati A, Borghi A et al: Angiographic morphology in unstable angina and its relation to transient myocardial ischemia and hospital outcome. *Am J Cardiol* 1991; **67**: 460–4.

16 Bar FW, Raynaud P, Renkin JP et al: Coronary angiographic findings do not predict clinical outcome in patients with unstable angina. *J Am Coll Cardiol* 1994; **24**: 1453–9.

17 Chen L, Chester MR, Redwood S et al: Angiographic stenosis progression and coronary events in patients with stabilized unstable angina. *Circulation* 1995; **91**: 2319–24.

18 Moise A, Theroux P, Taeymans Y et al: Unstable angina and progression of coronary atherosclerosis. *N Engl J Med* 1983; **309**: 685–9.

19 Fuster V, Frye RL, Connolly DC et al: Arteriographic patterns early in the onset of the coronary syndromes. *Br Heart J* 1975; **37**: 1250–5.

20 Gotoh K, Minamino T, Katoh O et al: The role of intracoronary thrombus in unstable angina: angiographic assessment and thrombolytic therapy during ongoing anginal attacks. *Circulation* 1988; **77**: 526–34.

21 Holmes Jr DR, Hartzler GO, Smith HC et al: Coronary artery thrombosis in patients with unstable angina. *Br Heart J* 1981; **45**: 411–16.

22 Vetrovec GW, Cowley MJ, Overton H et al: Intracoronary thrombus in syndromes of unstable myocardial ischemia. *Am Heart J* 1981; **102**: 1202–8.

23 Mizuno K, Satomura K, Miyamoto A et al: Angioscopic evaluation of coronary-artery thrombi in acute coronary syndromes. *N Engl J Med* 1992; **326**: 287–91.

24 Fitzgerald DJ: Platelet activation in the pathogenesis of unstable angina: importance in determining the response to plasminogen activators. *Am J Cardiol* 1991; **68**: 51B–57B.

25 Falk E: Unstable angina with fatal outcome: dynamic coronary thrombolysis leading to infarction and/or sudden death: autopsy evidence of recurrent mural thrombosis and peripheral embolization culminating in total vascular occlusion. *Circulation* 1985; **71**: 699–708.

26 Folts JD, Gallagher K, Rowe GG: Blood flow reductions in stenosed canine coronary arteries: vasospasm or platelet aggregation. *Circulation* 1982; **65**: 248–55.

27 Vetrovec GW, Leinbach RC, Gold HK et al: Intracoronary thrombolysis in syndromes of unstable ischemia: angiographic and clinical results. *Am Heart J* 1982; **104**: 946–52.

28 Freeman MR, Williams AE, Chisholm RJ et al: Intracoronary thrombus and complex morphology in unstable angina. *Circulation* 1989; **80**: 17–23.

29 Mandelkorn JB, Wolf NM, Singh S et al: Intracoronary thrombus in nontransmural myocardial infarction and in unstable angina pectoris. *Am J Cardiol* 1983; **52**: 1–6.

30 Zack PM, Ischinger T, Aker UT et al: The occurrence of angiographically detected intracoronary thrombus in patients with unstable angina pectoris. *Am Heart J* 1984; **108**: 1408–12.

31 Capone G, Wolf NM, Meyer B et al: Frequency of intracoronary filling defects by angiography in unstable angina pectoris at rest. *Am J Cardiol* 1985; **56**: 403–6.

32 Ambrose JA, Winters SI, Arora RR et al: Coronary angiographic morphology in myocardial infarction: a link between the pathogenesis of unstable angina and myocardial infarction. *J Am Coll Cardiol* 1985; **6**: 1233–8.

33 Singh AN: Progression of coronary atherosclerosis: clues to pathogenesis from serial coronary angiography, *Br Heart J* 1984; **52**: 451–61.

34 Waters D, Higginson L, Gladstone P: Effects of monotherapy with an HMG-CoA reductase inhibitor on the progression of coronary atherosclerosis as assessed by serial quantitative angiography: the Canadian Coronary Atherosclerosis Intervention Trial (CCAIT). *Circulation* 1994; **89**: 959–68.

35 Waters D, Lesperance J, Francetich M: A controlled clinical trial to assess the effect of a calcium channel blocker on the pregression of coronary atherosclerosis. *Circulation* 1990; **82**: 1940–53.

36 Miller RD, Burchell HB, Edwards JE: Myocardial infarction with and without acute coronary occlusion; a pathologic study. *Arch Intern Med* 1951; **88**: 597–604.

37 The TIMI IIIB Investigators: Effects of tissue plasminogen activator and a comparison of early invasive and conservative strategies in unstable angina and non-Q-wave myocardial infarction. *Circulation* 1994; **89**: 1545–56.

38 Sherman CT, Litvack F, Grunfest W et al: Coronary angioscopy in patients with unstable angina pectoris. *N Engl J Med* 1986; **315**: 913–19.

39 Tabata H, Mizuno Kyoichi, Arakawa K et al: Angioscopic identification of coronary thrombus in patients with postinfarction angina. *J Am Coll Cardiol* 1995; **25**: 1282–5.

40 den Heijer P, Foley DP, Escaned J et al: Angioscopic versus angiographic detection of intimal dissection and intracoronary thrombus. *J Am Coll Cardiol* 1994; **24**: 649–54.

41 Ramee SR, White CJ, Collins TJ et al: Percutaneous angioscopy during coronary angioplasty using a steerable microangioscope. *J Am Coll Cardiol* 1991; **17**: 100–5.

42 Nissen SE, Gurley JC, Grines CL et al: Intravascular ultrasound assessment of lumen size and wall morphology in normal subjects and coronary artery disease patients. *Circulation* 1991; **84**: 1087–99.

43 Tobis JM, Mallery J, Mahon D et al: Intravascular ultrasound imaging of human coronary arteries in vivo. *Circulation* 1991; **83**: 913–26.

44 Goar FGS, Pinto F, Alderman EL et al: Intravascular ultrasound imaging of angiographically normal coronary arteries: an in vivo comparison with quantitative angiography. *J Am Coll Cardiol* 1991; **18**: 952–8.

45 Mintz GS, Painter JA, Pichard AD et al: Atherosclerosis in angiographically normal coronary artery reference segments: an intravascular ultrasound study with clinical correlations. *J Am Coll Cardiol* 1995; **25**: 1479–85.

46 Braden GA, Herrington DM, Kerensky RA: Angiography poorly predicts actual lesion eccentricity in severe coronary stenoses: confirmation by intracoronary ultrasound. *J Am Coll Cardiol* 1994; **23**: 413A.

47 Hodgson JMcB, Graham SP, Sheehan H et al: Percutaneous intravascular ultrasound imaging: validation of a real time synthetic aperture array catheter. *Am J Card Imag* 1991; **5**: 65–71.

48 Bartorelli AL, Potkin BN, Almagor Y et al: Plaque characterization of atherosclerotic coronary arteries by intravascular ultrasound. *Echocardiography* 1990; **7**: 389–95.

49 Hodgson JMcB, Reddy KG, Suneja R et al: Intracoronary ultrasound imaging: correlation of plaque morphology with angiography, clinical syndrome, and procedural results in patients undergoing coronary angioplasty. *J Am Coll Cardiol* 1993; **21**: 35–44.

50 Barzilai B, Saffitz JE, Miller JG et al: Quantitative ultrasonic characterization of the nature of atherosclerotic plaques in human aorta. *Circ Res* 1987; **60**: 459–63.

51 Linker DT, Kleven A, Gronningsaether A et al: Tissue characterization with intra-arterial ultrasound: special promise and problems. *Int J Card Imaging* 1991; **6**: 255–63.

52 Spears JR, Sandor T, Als AV et al: Computerized image analysis for quantative measurement of vessel diameter from cineangiograms. *Circulation* 1983; **68**: 453–61.

53 Mancini GBJ, Simon SB, McGillem MJ et al: Automated quantitative coronary arteriography: morphologic and physiologic validation in vivo of a rapid digital angiographic method. *Circulation* 1987; **75**: 452–60.

54 Coy KM, Maurer G, Siegel RJ: Intravascular ultrasound imaging: a current perspective. *J Am Coll Cardiol* 1991; **18**: 1811–23.

4

Echocardiography in patients with acute myocardial infarction

Albert Andrew Burton and João A C Lima

Introduction

Echocardiography has become an important tool in the evaluation of patients with acute myocardial infarction. This imaging permits noninvasive assessment of the size and location of an infarction, facilitating early diagnosis and management. Echocardiography is comparable or superior to invasive methods in identifying many of the complications of acute myocardial infarction. In addition, rest and stress echocardiography provide prognostic information in survivors of infarction.

Regional function during myocardial ischemia and infarction

When blood flow to the myocardium is curtailed, ischemia or infarction develops causing systolic functional impairment of the affected ventricular segment.[1–3] These wall motion abnormalities develop almost immediately after a vessel is occluded, preceding electrocardiographic changes or chest pain. Systolic thinning or dyskinesis of the left ventricular wall is generally absent if ischemia involves only the subendocardial half of the wall segment (Fig. 4.1). As ischemia progresses across the entire thickness of the left ventricular wall, the injured segment becomes unable to generate tension during systole.[2] The ischemic segment is stretched passively at the onset of systole by contraction of the nonischemic portion of the left ventricle. Although the ischemic segment is compliant at the start of isovolemic contraction, it ultimately becomes stiff when fully stretched, allowing for intraventricular pressure increase, aortic valve opening, and ventricular emptying by further contraction of the nonischemic segments. Therefore, during transmural ischemia, the nonischemic portion of the left ventricle bears the burden of maintaining cardiac output while connected in series with ischemic tissue. This may result in increased thickening of regions distant from the ischemic border. At the same time, nonischemic segments adjacent to the ischemic area may thicken to a lesser degree or lack function entirely. The cross-sectional shape of the left ventricle during systole also changes significantly during transmural ischemia, assuming different configurations depending on depth and size of the ischemic area.[2]

If blood flow to a region of myocardium remains completely obstructed for several hours, the core of that region will undergo irreversible necrosis. The surrounding tissue may remain viable but ischemic. The final outcome of these regions around necrotic myocardium is determined by the presence of collateral flow or changes in myocardial oxygen demand. These border areas may recover if ischemia resolves (Fig. 4.2), or they may progress to myocardial death and necrosis if ischemia persists. Hearts that survive the first 2 weeks after myocardial infarction tend to show improved global left ventricular function, owing in part to the resolution of ischemia, but also because of stiffening of the infarcted tissue by fibrosis.[4] Distortion of the left ventricular architecture due to repeated bulging and stretching of the infarcted tissue may lead to infarct expansion, aneurysm formation, and cardiac dilatation. Return of perfusion to the myocardium may lead to partial or complete recovery of function in the ischemic region. Alternatively, reperfusion may cause edema or reperfusion injury in the region of ischemia, delaying recovery of function for days or weeks.[3] Histologically normal

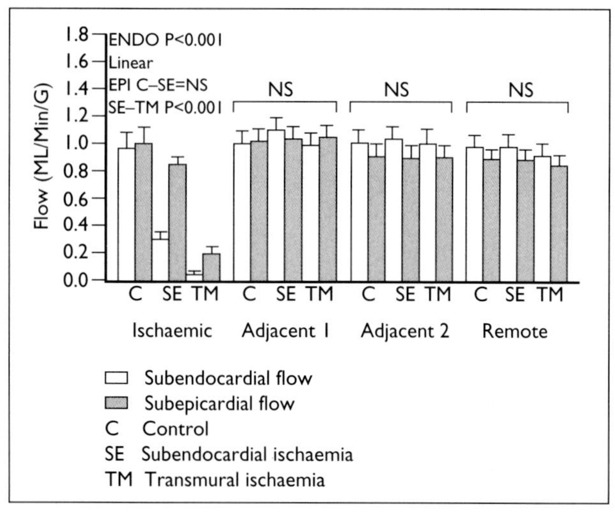

a

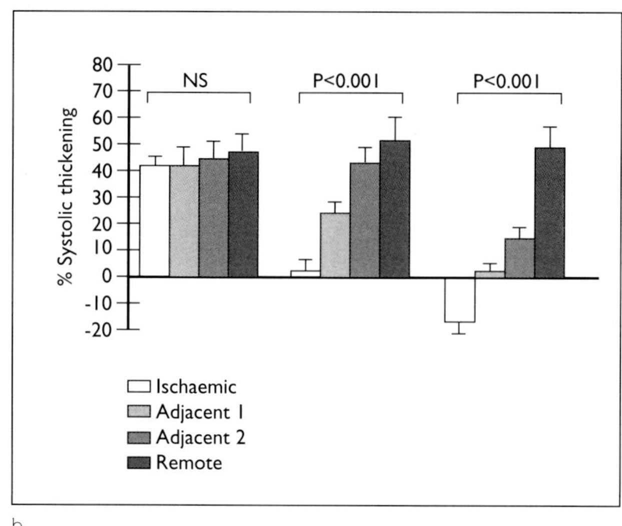

b

Figure 4.1
(a) Myocardial blood flow in four anatomic regions (defined on post-mortem examination as ischemic, adjacent 1, adjacent 2, and remote) at control and during subendocardial ischemia (SE) and transmural ischemia (TM). Flow changes were restricted to the subendocardial layer during critical stenosis (progressive decline in flow from control to transmural ischemia) but involved the entire left ventricular wall during transmural ischemia. (b) Per cent systolic thickening for the four anatomic regions (infarcted, adjacent 1, adjacent 2, and remote) at control and during subendocardial and transmural ischemia. In the ischemic region, systolic thickening was abolished during subendocardial ischemia and was replaced by thinning during transmural ischemia. In adjacent regions function was depressed during ischemia when compared to the remote regions, where function was unaltered during the entire experiment. (Reprinted with permission from Lima et al.[2]).

myocardium near the region of ischemia may be dysfunctional, behaving mechanically in much the same way as ischemic myocardium.[5] Further reduction in oxygen supply or increase in oxygen demand may extend the original infarcted region or create new areas of subendocardial or transmural necrosis. Thus, within the first 2 weeks or 3 weeks after myocardial infarction, hypofunctional segments of the left ventricle may be ischemic, infarcted, stunned or overloaded.[3] The variety of factors that contribute to abnormal wall motion in myocardial infarction may confound the relationship between regional ventricular function, blood flow and histology, having significant implications for the echocardiographic detection and quantitation of myocardial infarction.[3]

Echocardiography in the diagnosis and early management of myocardial infarction

Each year in the United States, 3.2 million people are evaluated in emergency departments because of chest pain.[6] In patients with classic symptoms and typical ECG findings, the diagnosis of acute myocardial infarction is straightforward. However, the classic clinical and electrocardiographic findings are present in only a minority of patients presenting with acute myocardial infarction. Fewer than one-third of patients presenting to the emergency department with chest pain have myocardial infarction and fewer than one-third of patients with an acute myocardial infarction have diagnostic ECG changes on presentation.[7] Because of the limitations of clinical findings and ECG, echocardiographic imaging is playing an increasing role in the early diagnosis and management of patients with chest pain. Echocardiography is more sensitive and specific than history and ECG findings in diagnosing myocardial infarction in patients presenting with chest pain. In several clinical series, left ventricular wall motion abnormalities were observed in 89–100% of patients with transmural infarction.[8–11] The sensitivity of echocardiography in detecting a nontransmural infarction is somewhat less and depends on the transmural thickness of the infarcted myocardial segment.[10] If available data are pooled, 82% of all patients eventually found to have an acute myocardial infarction had wall motion abnormalities detected on echocardiography at the time of the presentation. In addition, patients who had no echocardiographically detected wall motion abnormalities had smaller infarctions and fewer complications.[8–12]

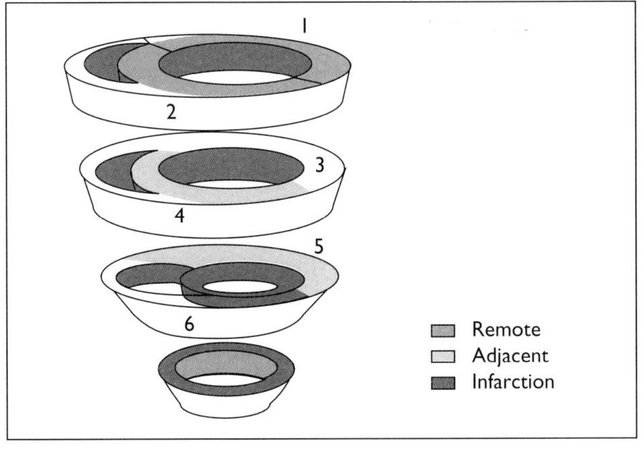

a

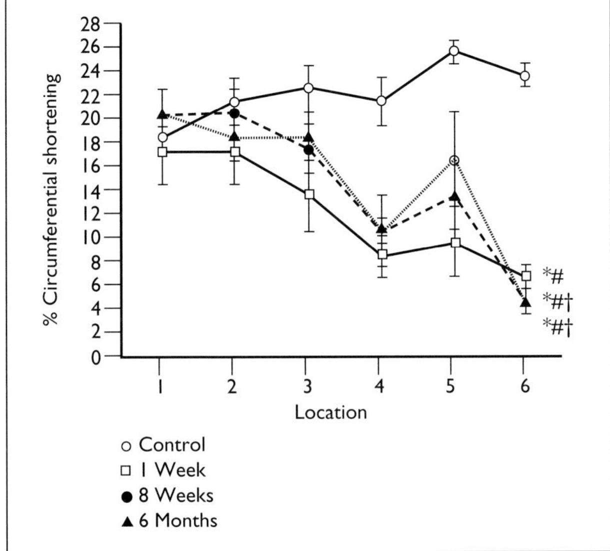

b

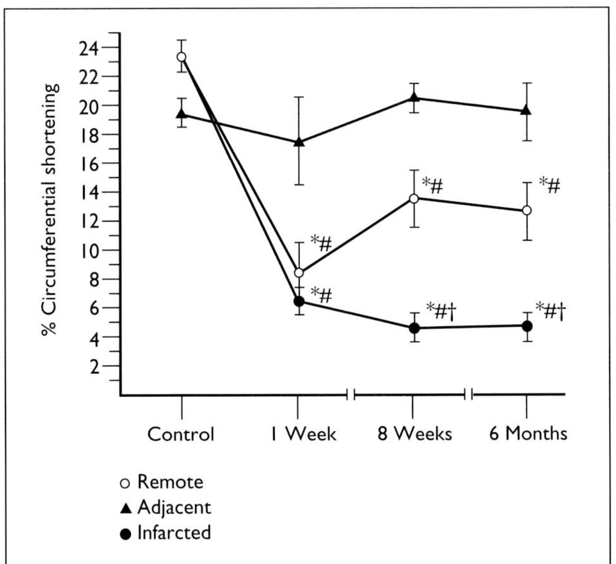

c

Figure 4.2
Schematic diagram of short-axis slices from a typical magnetic resonance imaging (MRI) study of an animal after anteroapical infarction. Regions 1 and 2 in the most basal slice are remote from the infarct. Region 6 is within the infarcted region. Regions 4 and 5 are immediately adjacent to the infarct. Region 3 is at an intermediate distance from the most remote and immediately adjacent segments and was left out of the analysis. (b) Graph showing per cent circumferential shortening in the subendocardium by regions; corresponding to the regions shown in (a) at control and at 1 week, 8 weeks, and 6 months after myocardial infarction. The statistical significance of differences between regions was calculated by repeated-measures ANOVA. During control, shortening increased from base to apex ($P<0.05$). At 1 week, after infarction, shortening decreased from base to apex $P<0.003$). This same decreasing gradient in function from base to apex was seen at 8 weeks and 6 months after infarction ($P<0.0001$ for both), but there was a trend toward improved function in regions 1 through 5 compared with that at 1 week. By Scheffé subtesting, *$P<0.05$ versus region 1, #$P<0.05$ versus region 2, and †$P<0.03$ versus region 3. Similar changes were seen for subepicardial shortening. (c) Graph depicting subendocardial per cent circumferential shortening for infarcted, adjacent, and remote regions over time. Segmental function in the remote region did not change over time (P = NS), whereas per cent shortening in the infarcted region fell at 1 week and remained depressed ($P<0.0001$). Adjacent region function fell at 1 week and improved in part from 1 to 8 weeks $P<0.0001$). The statistically significant differences between regions at each time point calculated by repeated-measures ANOVA were as follows: control, NS; 1 week, $P<0.05$; 8 weeks, $P<0.0001$; 6 months, $P<0.0002$. By Scheffé subtesting, *$P<0.05$ versus control, #$P<0.05$ versus remote, and †$P<0.05$ versus adjacent. Similar changes were seen in the subendocardium. (Reprinted with permission from Kramer et al.[1]).

Echocardiography is also useful in the diagnosis and management of chest pain due to causes other than myocardial infarction. Patients with chest pain due to myocardial ischemia usually have echocardiographically detectable wall motion abnormalities with pain, even in the absence of infarction. Other causes of chest pain including aortic dissection, hypertrophic cardiomyopathy, valvular heart disease, pericarditis, and pulmonary embolism can frequently be identified or suspected based on transthoracic echocardiography.

In addition to facilitating diagnosis, echocardiography early in the course of acute myocardial infarction provides information important in guiding early management and determining short-term prognosis. The location and size of wall motion abnormalities correlate well with the coronary artery involved in an infarction.[13] Infarction resulting from obstruction of the left anterior descending coronary artery usually causes abnormal function in the anterior, septal, and apical segments of the left ventricle (Figs 4.3 and 4.4). Akinesis of the basal anterior segment predicts occlusion of the left anterior descending coronary artery, proximal to the first septal perforator, a finding of prognostic significance. There is overlap in the areas of abnormal wall motion in myocardial infarcts involving the left circumflex and right coronary arteries. Occlusion of either vessel can cause abnormal motion in the middle and basilar segments of the posterior and inferior walls (Figs 4.5 and 4.6). Wall motion abnormalities confined to the posterior and lateral walls are usually caused by obstruction of the circumflex, while abnormalities confined to the inferior basal segment are characteristic of obstruction of the right coronary artery. Evidence of right ventricular infarction usually indicates that the proximal right coronary artery is occluded.[14] In patients with single-vessel coronary artery disease, the stress of myocardial infarction usually causes hyperkinesia of uninvolved segments. The absence of hyperkinesis or the presence of hypofunction in areas not adjacent to the infarcted zone suggests that significant multivessel disease is present.[12]

As previously discussed, a number of factors, including the presence of ischemia, stunning or overload, confound the relationship between the size of regional wall motion abnormalities and the amount of infarcted myocardium. When compared to pathological examination, echocardiography tends to overestimate the amount of necrosed myocardium early in the course of myocardial infarction.[3] Despite this limitation, echocardiographic estimation of the extent of myocardial infarction correlates well with infarct size as determined by peak creatine kinase, radionuclide imaging, and contrast ventriculography.[1–18] Echocardiographic evaluation of left ventricular function early in the course of myocardial infarction has been found to be a better predictor of in-hospital mortality than the prognostically strongest clinical parameters, including Killip class.[12,19–21] In several series, an echocardiographically determined ejection fraction of over 40% correlated with a low short-term mortality and could potentially be used to select low-risk patients for early discharge.[14,21] By contrast, a tall peaked E wave on Doppler evaluation of left ventricular filling has been correlated with elevated left ventricular end-diastolic pressure and worse prognosis.[24]

Echocardiography has been used to assess the efficacy of thrombolytic therapy. The time required for improvement of left ventricular function after reperfusion is related to the

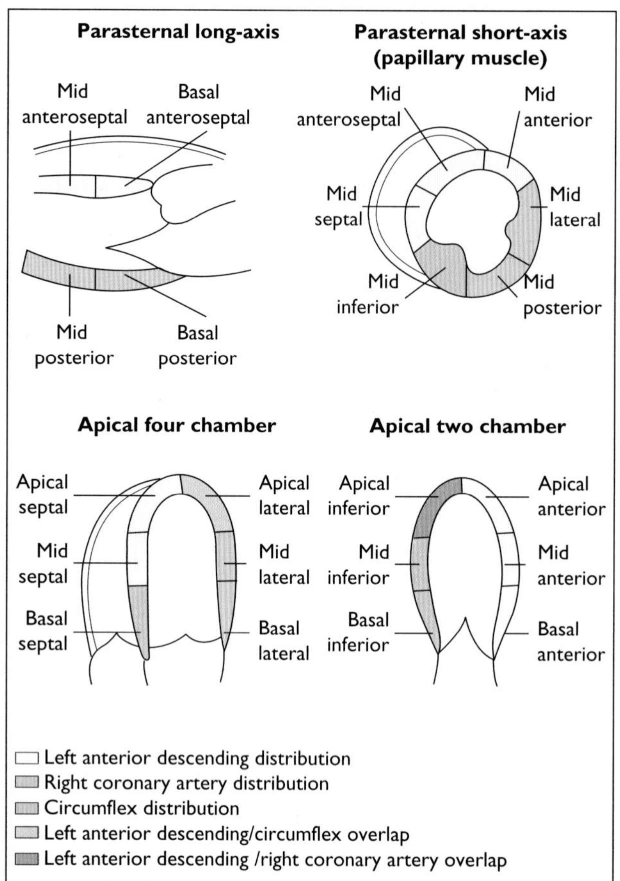

Figure 4.3
Four diagrams representing the four standard echocardiographic views (parasternal long-axis and short-axis, apical 4-chamber, and apical 2-chamber). Sixteen segments of the left ventricular wall are displayed according to coronary blood flow. The apical lateral segment can be perfused by either the left anterior descending or left circumflex coronary arteries. The apical inferior segment can be perfused by either the left anterior descending or right coronary arteries. (Reprinted with permission from Segar et al.[84]).

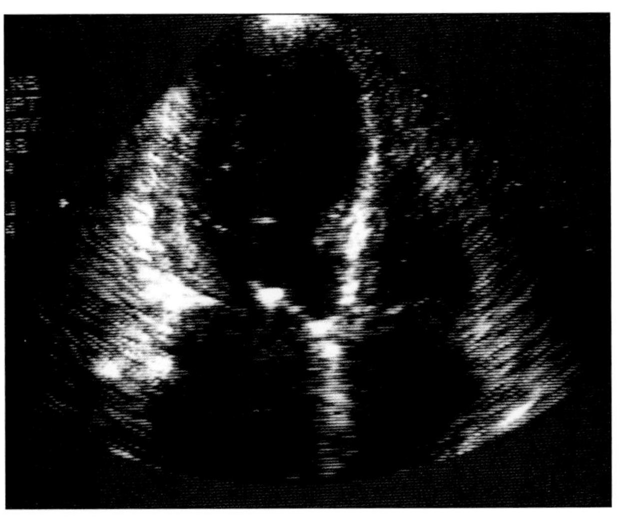

a

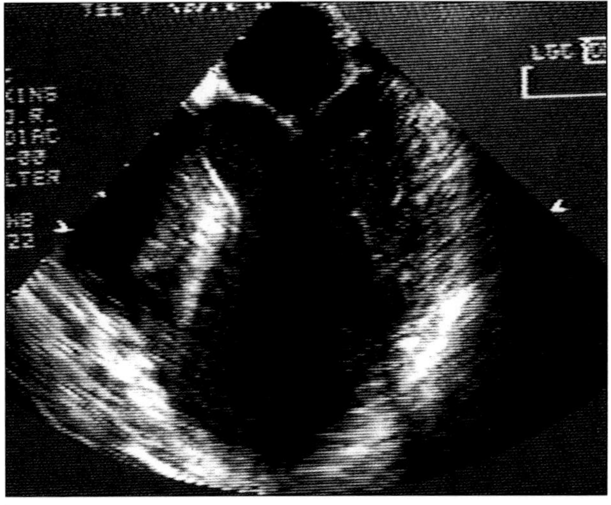

b

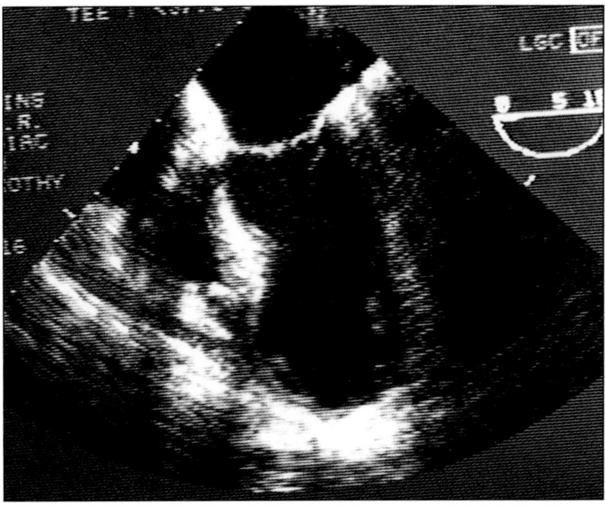

c

Figure 4.4
Echocardiographic 4-chamber view demonstrating anteroapical left ventricular infarction at end-diastole (a) and end-systole (b). Anteroapical segment corresponds to left anterior descending coronary artery occlusion.

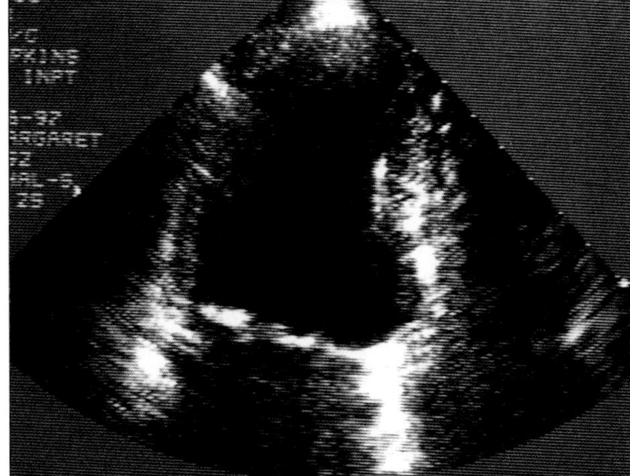

Figure 4.5
Left ventricular short-axis echocardiographic cross-section at end-systole demonstrating inferior wall thinning corresponding to inferior wall myocardial infarction caused by right coronary artery occlusion. Frequently, when the posterior descending artery is occluded, the inferoseptal segment underlying the posteromedial papillary muscle is involved and becomes scarred or dysfunctional.

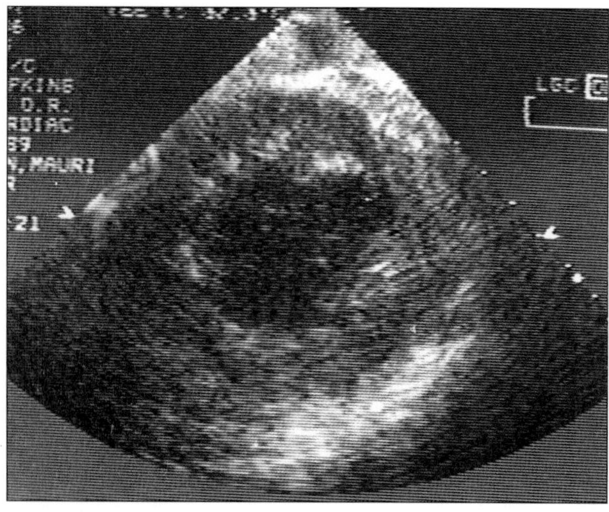
a

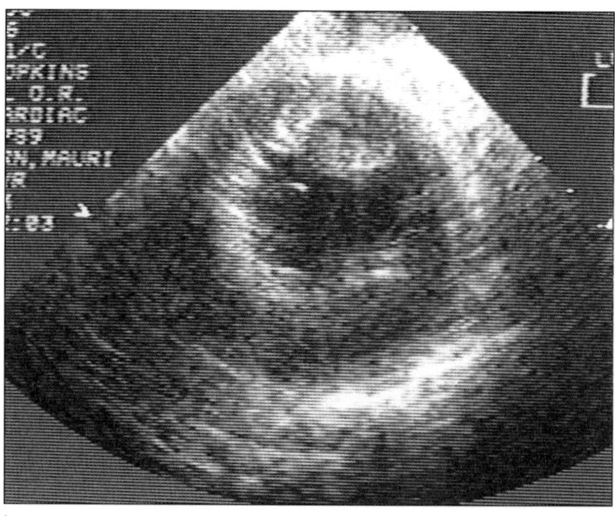
b

Figure 4.6
Left ventricular short-axis at end-systole showing inferolateral myocardial infarction caused by left circumflex occlusion.

duration of ischemia and size of the ischemic zone. In patients with successful reperfusion induced by thrombolytic agents or direct angioplasty, echocardiographically detectable improvement in contractility can occur in the first 24 h, with some improvement occurring as late as 10 days after reperfusion.[22] The delay in recovery of function, even after successful reperfusion, limits the utility of echocardiography in acutely assessing the success of thrombolytic therapy. Echocardiographic techniques using microbubble contrast to evaluate intramyocardial blood flow may eventually have a clinically significant role in assessing the success of reperfusion therapy.[23]

The widespread use of echocardiography early in the evaluation of myocardial infarction reflects the clinical utility, availability and safety of this technique. Echocardiography does have a number of potential shortcomings in the early diagnosis and management of acute myocardial infarction. The quality of echocardiographic images depends on the skill of the operator and the habitus of the patient. Images adequate for evaluation of wall motion could not be obtained in 5–15% of patients in clinical studies of myocardial infarction.[8–11] Abnormal wall motion can be present in patients with Wolfe–Parkinson–White syndrome, bundle branch block, right ventricular overload, and after cardiac surgery. However, in contrast to patients with myocardial infarction, in these patients wall thickening is usually preserved. On the other hand, myocarditis may cause regional loss of wall thickening and be indistinguishable from infarction by echocardiography.[25] In addition, it is sometimes difficult to differentiate new wall motion abnormalities from pre-existing ones by echocardiography.

Echocardiography in the assessment of complications after acute myocardial infarction

At present most in-hospital deaths of patients with acute myocardial infarction are due to cardiogenic shock or mechanical complications of infarction.[26] Echocardiography now plays a central role in the diagnosis and evaluation of patients with complicated myocardial infarction. Developments in echocardiography, including color flow imaging, Doppler and transesophageal echocardiography allow early identification of conditions that historically required invasive methods for diagnosis.

Infarct extension occurs in 10–20% of patients in the first 10 days after acute myocardial infarction.[27,28] This complication is more common after thrombolytic therapy and is seen in most patients with cardiogenic shock.[28,29] Infarct extension is recognized echocardiographically by the appearance of new areas of abnormal wall motion.[30] This is in contrast to infarct expansion, in which the infarcted region dilates, but additional wall motion abnormalities do not appear in previously uninvolved segments of myocardium.

Rupture of the free wall of the left ventricle is the cause of death in up to 10% of patients dying in the hospital from acute myocardial infarction. Ventricular free wall rupture usually rapidly leads to hemopericardium and death from pericardial tamponade. Occasionally, hemorrhage into the pericardial space is slow or repetitive, allowing survival for hours or days after rupture. Rarely, hemorrhage into the pericardial space may be confined by organizing thrombus, hematoma and/or pericardial adhesions leading to a pseudoaneurysm. Despite the frequently catastrophic presentation of free wall rupture, long-term survival is sometimes possible with early diagnosis and surgical intervention.[31]

Pericardial effusion can be detected in virtually all patients with free wall rupture, and the absence of a pericardial effusion and pseudoaneurysm on echocardiographic examination virtually excludes the possibility of cardiac rupture. However, pericardial effusions are frequently present in patients with myocardial infarction who do not have free wall rupture.[32–36] Echocardiographic images suggestive of thrombus within the pericardial space are frequently present after free wall rupture, although this finding can be present in other conditions, including fibrinous pericarditis.[32] Echocardiographic evidence of cardiac tamponade in patients with a recent myocardial infarction is strongly associated with free wall rupture.[32] The tear in the free wall may occasionally be directly visualized or identified by the presence of Doppler flow signal traversing the wall of the left ventricle.[32–36] However, these findings are present in only a few transthoracic echocardiograms from patients with free wall rupture. In a prospective study, the presence of hemopericardium was highly predictive of free wall rupture after infarction. Pericardiocentesis was recommended in patients with clinical and echocardiographic features suggestive of free wall rupture. If results of pericardiocentesis were consistent with hemopericardium, immediate surgical exploration for definitive diagnosis and repair of the ruptured wall segment was recommended.[32] Transesophageal echocardiography is frequently useful in identifying free wall rupture in cases in which transthoracic images are equivocal.[37]

Pseudoaneurysm formation is an uncommon late outcome of left ventricular free wall rupture. The wall of a pseudoaneurysm is composed of clot and pericardium, while the wall of a true aneurysm is derived from myocardium. Recognition of pseudoaneurysms is important because, in contrast to true left ventricular aneurysms, pseudoaneurysms are prone to spontaneous rupture.[38] Pseudoaneurysms generally communicate with the left ventricle through a narrow neck (Fig. 4.7). The portion of a pseudoaneurysm that communicates with the ventricular cavity is usually not as wide as the pseudoaneurysm at its greatest width, while the portion of a true aneurysm that communicates with the ventricle is usually the widest aspect of the aneurysm. There is usually an abrupt interruption of myocardium at the neck of pseudoaneurysms, while in true aneurysms (Fig. 4.8) the myocardium tapers

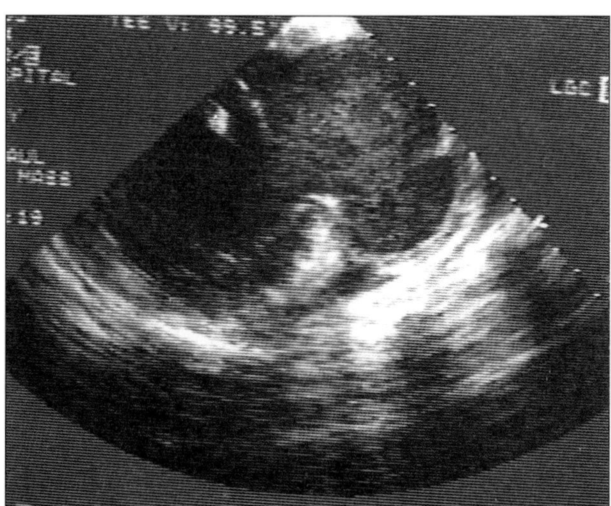

Figure 4.7
Inferior wall pseudoaneurysm reflecting prior rupture of the left ventricular wall with localized tamponade by intrapericardial thrombus formation.

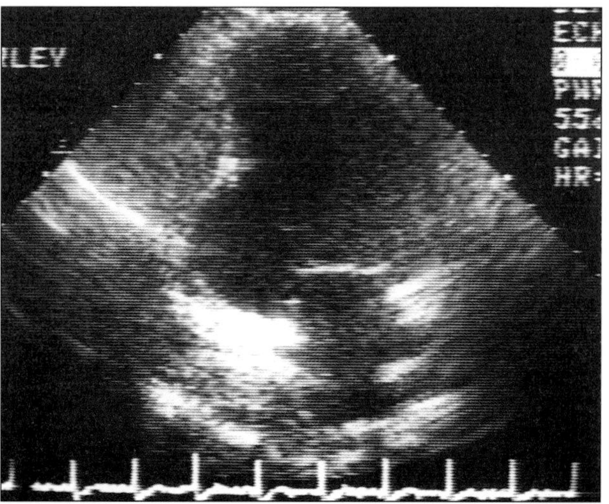

Figure 4.8
Inferior wall aneurysm with ventricular wall thinning. The larger diameter of the aneurysm's mouth relative to the diameter of its fundus indicates that the sacular structure is a true aneurysm as opposed to a ruptured infarct with pseudoaneurysmatic formation.

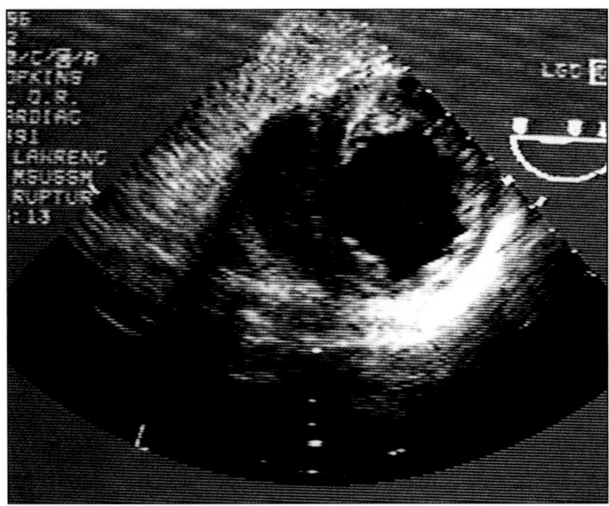

a

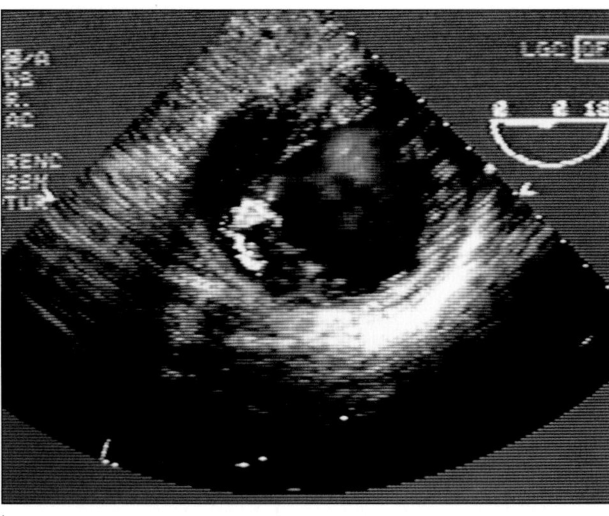

b

Figure 4.9
End-diastolic image of the left ventricle with interventricular septal rupture at the border of a large anterior myocardial infarction (a). Systolic high velocity jet is seen in (b) generating fast (mosaic like) color flow velocities in the right ventricular apex which strongly suggest the presence of a ventricular septal defect.

gradually to form the aneurysm wall.[38] The use of Doppler imaging to demonstrate blood flow in the pseudoaneurysm is useful in distinguishing localized pericardial effusions from pseudoaneurysms.[39] While these differences are generally helpful in differentiating true aneurysms from pseudoaneurysms, some true aneurysms, particularly those arising from the posterior and inferior walls, may have a narrow neck. It may be difficult to distinguish pseudoaneurysms and true aneurysms by echocardiography in these cases.[40,41]

Rupture of the ventricular septum is an infrequent but serious complication of acute myocardial infarction. Septal rupture occurs in 1–2% of infarcts, and accounts for approximately 5% of deaths in acute myocardial infarction.[42] Mortality in patients with rupture of the ventricular septum approaches 90% in patients treated medically.[43] Mortality is significantly reduced by surgical intervention, making early recognition of this condition important.[44] Ventricular septal rupture is more common in anterior than in inferior wall infarction. Septal rupture in anterior wall infarction is usually located near the apex of the left ventricle (Fig. 4.9), while in inferior wall infarction[45] rupture usually occurs in the basal septum (Fig. 4.10). The septal defect may be a direct through-and-through perforation or a complex serpiginous tract that dissects into regions remote from the primary site of the septal tear.[46]

Septal rupture characteristically presents with hemodynamic deterioration and a new murmur. This clinical presentation is similar to that of acute mitral regurgitation after myocardial infarction. Current echocardiographic techniques, including color flow imaging and transesophageal echocardiography, have simplified the diagnosis of ventricular septal rupture and generally eliminated the need for invasive confirmatory studies.[26] Segmental wall motion abnormalities consistent with infarction are invariably present in patients with this condition. An aneurysmal bulging of the septum into the right ventricular cavity is frequently present. Direct observation of the defect by echocardiography was reported in 60% (122/205) of cases described in recent series.[26,45–47] Rupture of the septum usually results in shunting of blood flow from the left ventricle to the right ventricle, creating a high velocity systolic jet within the right ventricle, which can be readily detected with Doppler imaging.[47] Doppler techniques, particularly color flow imaging, increase the sensitivity of echocardiography in identifying septal rupture. In several recent series, color flow Doppler identified septal rupture in 98% (119/122) of patients with confirmed rupture.[26,46–47] Color flow imaging is particularly useful in delineating the course of serpiginous ruptures. Echocardiographic contrast injected into a peripheral vein has been used in the past to identify

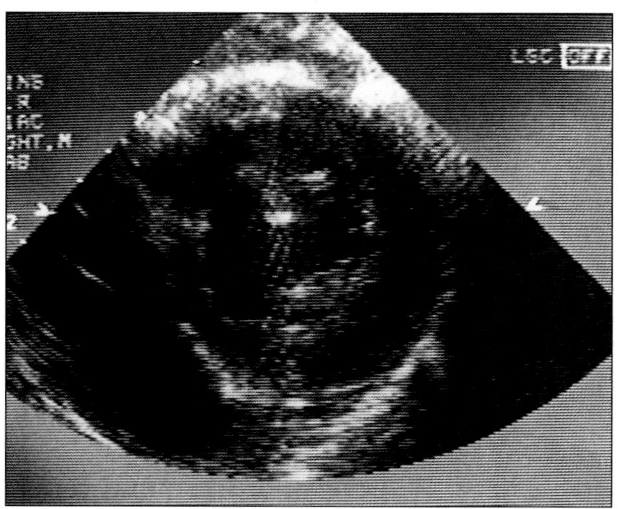
a

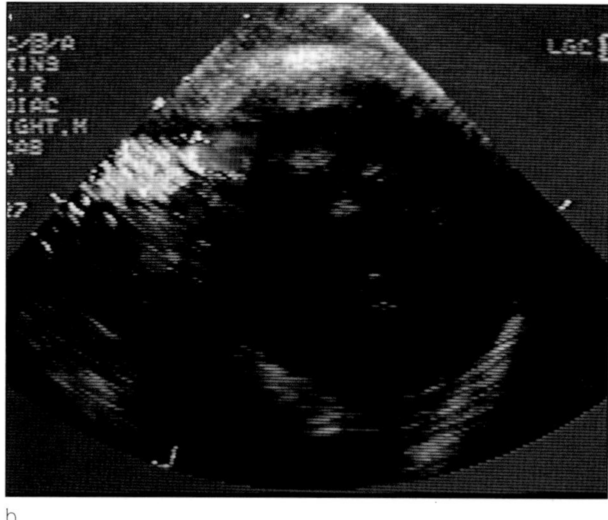
b

Figure 4.10
Ventricular septal defect caused by inferior wall myocardial infarction seen by transgastric echocardiogram. The septal defect is seen as a systolic jet between the left and right ventricles at the level of the border of the infarcted region.

septal rupture, but this approach has been largely supplanted by Doppler techniques.[46,47] As patients with rupture of the ventricular septum are frequently mechanically intubated, transthoracic echocardiographic images may be suboptimal. Transesophageal echocardiography reliably demonstrates the septal defect in this setting.[26,48]

Complete or partial rupture of a papillary muscle is a rare but frequently fatal complication of myocardial infarction, occurring in approximately 1% of infarctions.[49] The posteriomedial papillary muscle is supplied by a single artery, unlike the anterolateral papillary muscle which usually has a dual blood supply. Because of this difference, muscle rupture occurs more often in the posteriomedial than in the anterolateral papillary muscle, and is much more common after inferior than after anterior acute myocardial infarction.[49] Complete rupture of a papillary muscle is frequently fatal and rarely observed. Partial rupture usually involves one of the heads of the muscle. Patients with partial rupture of a papillary muscle usually develop pulmonary edema and severe hemodynamic compromise. Although in historical descriptions, papillary muscle rupture is associated with a new loud systolic murmur, the murmur may be soft or absent.[50,51] In patients with papillary muscle rupture, overall left ventricular function is often preserved and the long-term prognosis after surgical intervention is good if prompt intervention is made.[52] Without surgical treatment the mortality is 50% in the first 24 h and 90% in the first week.[49] Two-dimensional echocardiography has greatly simplified the diagnosis of papillary muscle rupture, facilitating early intervention (Fig. 4.11). Echocardiographic findings in partial papillary muscle rupture include direct visualization of the ruptured head, flail mitral leaflets, a mobile mass appearing in the left atrium during systole, and in the left ventricle during diastole, as well as new holosystolic prolapse of a mitral valve leaflet.[26,46,51] The partially ruptured muscle was directly observed using transthoracic echocardiography in 48% (23/48) of patients with confirmed partial rupture of a papillary muscle in recent series.[26,46] Indirect echocardiographic evidence of papillary muscle rupture was reported in almost all patients with confirmed partial papillary muscle rupture.[26,46–53] Evidence of mitral regurgitation on color flow imaging is present in almost all patients with this condition. However, when compared to angiography, color flow imaging may significantly underestimate the severity of mitral regurgitation, particularly if the regurgitant jet is eccentric or the left atrium is small and noncompliant.[26,46] In cases in which transthoracic images are nondiagnostic, transesophageal echocardiography can establish the diagnosis of partial rupture of the papillary muscle in virtually all cases.[26,46,52,53]

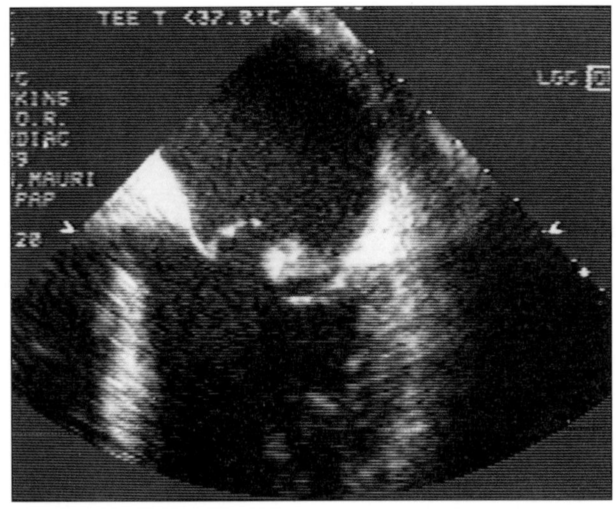

a

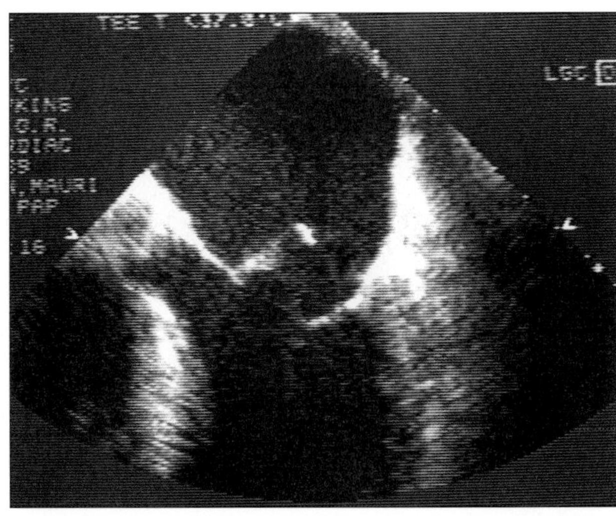

b

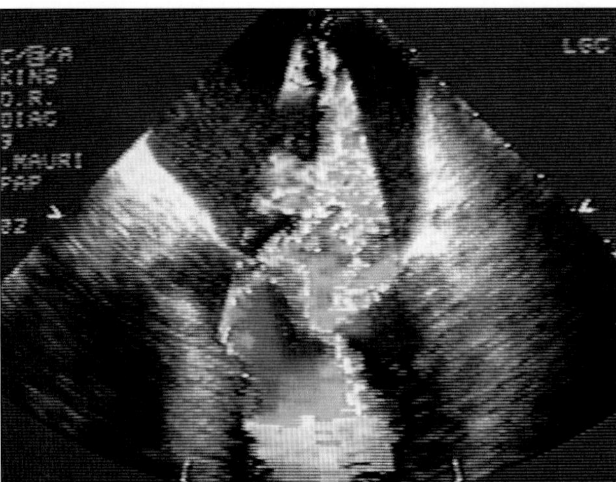

c

Figure 4.11
Papillary muscle rupture diagnosed by transesophageal echocardiography 2 days after myocardial infarction causing severe mitral regurgitation and pulmonary edema.

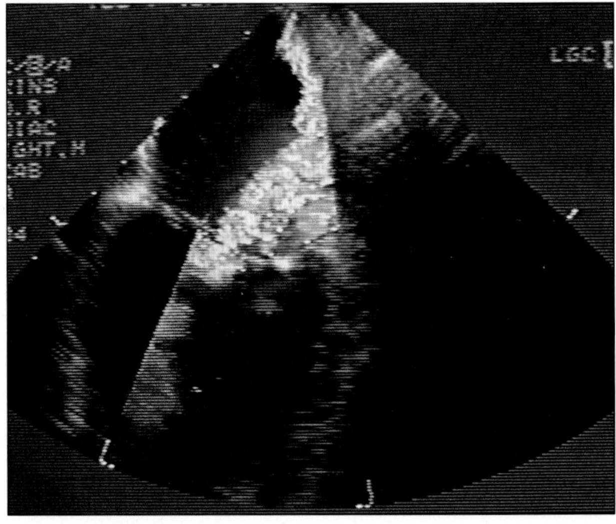

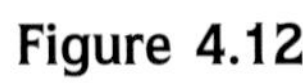

Figure 4.12
Moderate, or sometimes severe, mitral regurgitation may develop after inferior myocardial infarction if both papillary muscle infarction and ventricular dilatation develop after infarction. The time course for mitral valve failure to become clinically significant is generally measured in weeks (6–8) or months after acute myocardial infarction.

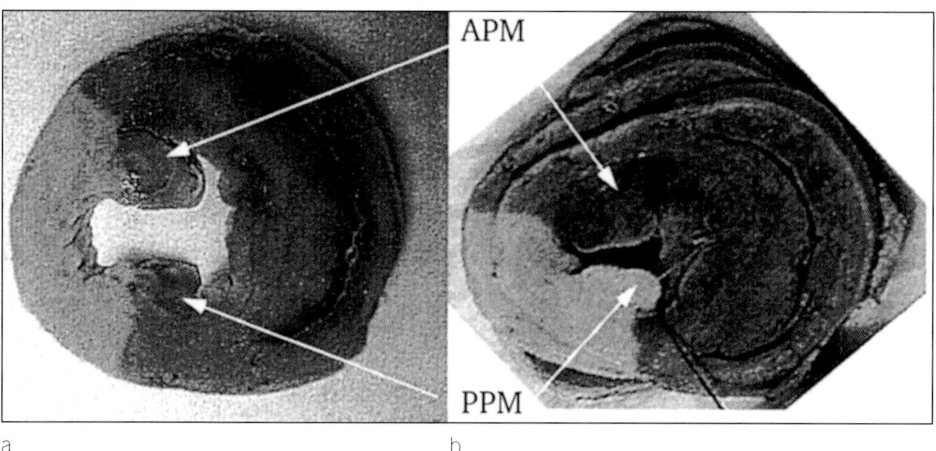

Figure 4.13
Left ventricular cross-sections (5-mm) from ovine hearts at post-mortem examination. Inferior wall myocardial infarction was produced sparing both papillary muscles in one group or animals (a) or involving at least one of them in a second group (b). Infarct size and left ventricular dilatation were similar in both groups of animals. However, only animals from group b developed significant chronic or subacute mitral regurgitation in the ensuing 6–8 weeks emphasizing the contribution of papillary muscle scarring and shortening in the pathophysiology of this condition (Reprinted with permission from Llanera et al.[54]).

More commonly, mitral regurgitation may develop after myocardial infarction in the absence of partial rupture of the papillary muscle. In these cases regurgitation develops after an infarction as a result of restriction of leaflet motion due to fibrosis of the papillary muscle combined with left ventricular dilatation (Fig. 4.12). In contrast to partial rupture of a papillary muscle, mitral regurgitation in this setting develops chronically over weeks or months,[54] and is also more common after inferior myocardial infarction, frequently accompanied by fibrosis of the posteriomedial papillary muscle (Fig. 4.13). However, mitral regurgitation immediately after myocardial infarction, but not caused by a ruptured papillary muscle, is more commonly due to acute left ventricular dilatation following extensive anterior myocardial infarction.

Mural thrombus is a common complication of myocardial infarction. Two-dimensional echocardiography is a reliable and noninvasive method for diagnosing this condition.[55] Thrombi most frequently occur in dyskinetic or aneurysmal regions of the left ventricle and are more common in the anterior wall and apex than in the inferior wall.[55,58] Thrombi may appear as protruding and mobile irregularly-shaped masses or as smooth masses layered on the ventricular wall (Fig. 4.14). Pooled data from studies of ventricular thrombosis suggest that the presence of echocardiographically demonstrated thrombus in the left ventricle is associated with increased risk of embolism and that this risk can be reduced with anticoagulation.[57–58] Protruding or mobile thrombi appear to be more likely to embolize, but anticoagulation also appears beneficial in patients without these high risk features.[57–58]. Various ventricular structures, including papillary muscles, chordae tendinae and muscle trabeculations, may be misidentified as mural thrombus. Spurious intracavitary echoes and reverberation artifact may also be mistaken for thrombus. However, ventricular thrombus almost never occurs in a region of normal ventricular wall motion, an important feature in identifying true intracavitary thrombus.[56]

Most left ventricular thrombi develop within 48 h of infarction. However, thrombi may develop as late as 8–10 days after infarction. Intracavitary spontaneous echocardiographic contrast has been observed to precede the formation of thrombus on an akinetic segment of the left ventricle.[59] In one study, abnormal pulse Doppler flow patterns in the left ventricle predicted the formation of left ventricular thrombus.[60] However this finding was not confirmed in a subsequent study.[61]

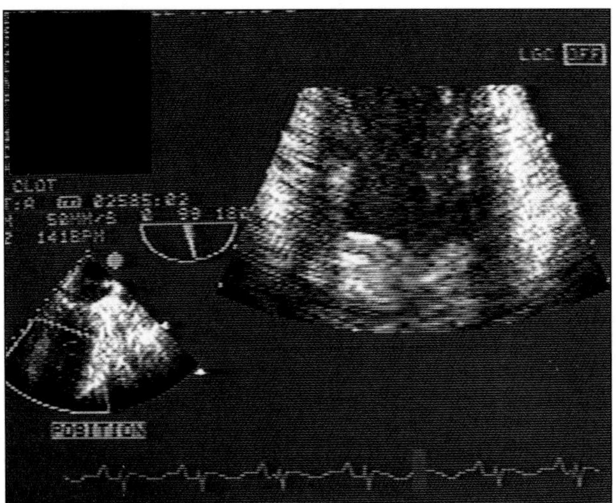

Figure 4.14
Transesophageal echocardiogram depicting the presence of a large apical thrombus in a patient with a recent anterior myocardial infarction. The thrombus is protuberant and particularly prone to embolization from the anatomic standpoint.

Infarction of the right ventricle complicates nearly half of all inferior myocardial infarctions. Right ventricular infarction can cause hypotension and hemodynamic decompensation in the absence of severe left ventricular compromise.[62] Because the medical management of right ventricular infarction differs significantly from that of left ventricular infarction, early and accurate diagnosis of right ventricular infarction is clinically important. Echocardiography is helpful in the diagnosis of this condition.[14,62–65]

Patients with right ventricular infarction usually show akinesis of the inferior and posterior walls of the left ventricle.[20,62–66] Wall motion abnormalities in the right ventricular wall are present in almost all patients with confirmed right ventricular infarction. Right ventricular dilatation is frequently present. Paradoxical motion of the interventricular septum during diastole is sometimes observed and is caused by changes in transeptal pressure gradient.[65] Right ventricular thrombus and tricuspid regurgitation may also be present.[20,62–66]

Bowing of the interatrial septum toward the left atrium, indicating increased right atrial pressure, is an important prognostic finding in right ventricular infarction. This finding was present in 25% of patients with right ventricular infarction in one large series and was associated with a higher incidence of hypotension, heart block and mortality.[66] Increased right atrial pressures in right ventricular infarction can lead to right-to-left shunting in patients with a patent foramen ovale, producing arterial hypoxemia,[67] cerebral or other peripheral embolic events. Contrast echocardiography, used with or without transesophageal echocardiography, can demonstrate right-to-left shunting through a patent foramen ovale in these patients.

Echocardiography in risk stratification after myocardial infarction

The prognosis in survivors of acute myocardial infarction depends on multiple factors which relate both to the acute event, including infarct size, location and transmurality, and factors preceding the infarction, such as age, sex, risk factors and a history of prior myocardial infarction. However, the single most important determinant of long-term outcome after myocardial infarction is the degree of left ventricular post-infarction dysfunction.[12,68–71] Several series have shown that infarct size and left ventricular function, as assessed by rest echocardiography, were more predictive of death following discharge after infarction than the prognostically strongest clinical parameters, including Killip class.[12,68–71] In the Survival and Ventricular Enlargement trial,[71] increased left ventricular area at the time of discharge from the hospital, and also at 1 year after discharge, strongly predicted adverse cardiovascular events, including death (see also Chapter 5). Therefore, two-dimensional echocardiography has been found to be comparable or superior to radionuclide imaging in post-infarction patients for:

- detecting wall motion abnormalities;
- evaluating global left ventricular dysfunction; and thus
- assessing the individual patient's prognosis after hospital discharge.

While rest echocardiography provides important prognostic information, this technique does not predict which patients are likely to have recurrent ischemia or infarction after discharge. Exercise echocardiography alone has several limitations, including relatively low diagnostic accuracy for predicting multivessel disease, low sensitivity in predicting clinical outcome, inability to localize ischemic regions, and dependency on the patient's ability to exercise.[72–74] The utility of predischarge stress testing after thrombolytic therapy has recently been questioned.[72] However, it appears that stress echocardiography provides useful information in some subsets of patients, although the paucity of long-term trials using stress echocardiography (Fig. 4.15) to determine prognosis in patients treated with thrombolytics is an important shortcoming.[72] At present, four types of stressors are widely used with echocardiography for evaluation of patients after myocardial infarction: exercise, dobutamine, dipyridamole, and atrial pacing.

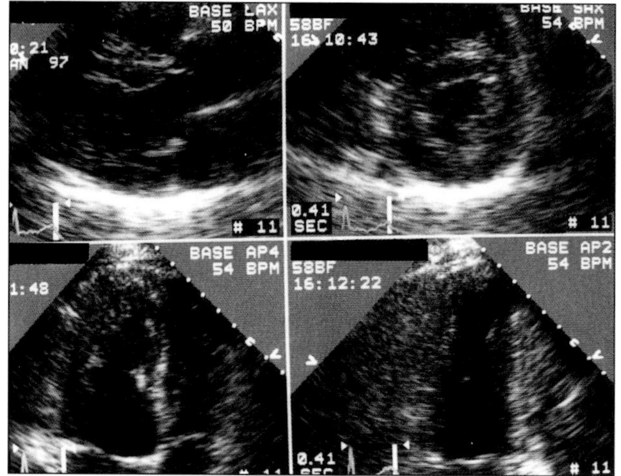

Figure 4.15
The introduction of digital technology to the echocardiographic laboratory facilitated the development of stress echocardiography. The standard views used in this modality are shown: parasternal long- and short-axis views are seen at the top (left and right, respectively) and apical 4- and 2-chamber views are seen in the bottom (left and right, respectively). Notice that, contrary to echocardiograms obtained in most institutions around the world, the left ventricle is displayed on the left in the 4-chamber view, and the inferior wall is displayed on the right in the 2-chamber view at the Johns Hopkins Hospital.

Exercise echocardiography (Fig. 4.16) adds to the accuracy of exercise treadmill testing in detecting patients with multivessel coronary artery disease after myocardial infarction. Three studies in post-infarction patients, performed before widespread use of thrombolytic therapy, found that exercise echocardiography was superior to exercise ECG alone in identifying patients at high risk for adverse events after discharge.[74–76] Meta-analysis of studies of exercise echocardiography in patients after infarction indicates that failure to increase ejection fraction by more than 5%, or the appearance of new wall motion abnormalities, were strongly associated with death or recurrent myocardial infarction.[74–76]

Exercise echocardiography is not useful in patients who cannot perform significant physical activity, and patients who cannot exercise after infarction are at higher risk for recurrent ischemic events.[72] Several studies suggest a role for dobutamine stress echocardiography for risk stratification in

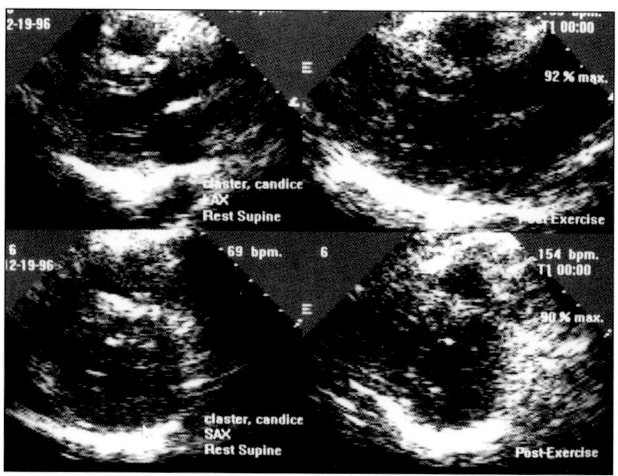

a

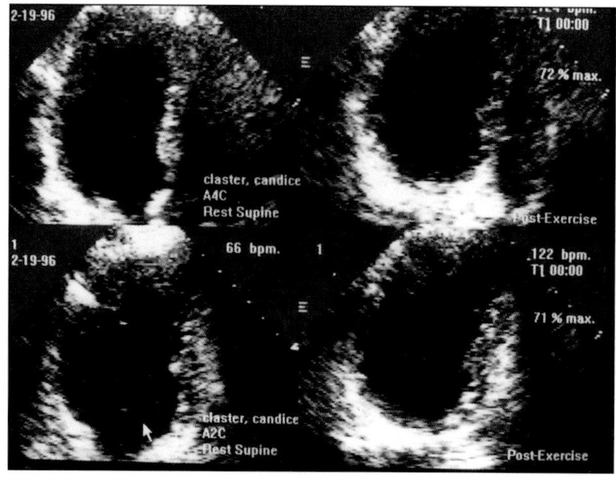

b

Figure 4.16
The protocol involved in exercise stress echocardiography involves the comparison of multiple frames (generally eight or more) obtained at the time of the R wave in the electrocardiogram and then at each 50 ms afterwards. Images obtained at rest on the left are compared with images obtained immediately after cessation of treadmill exercise on the right. The entire data set consists of parasternal views shown in (a) and apical views shown in (b).

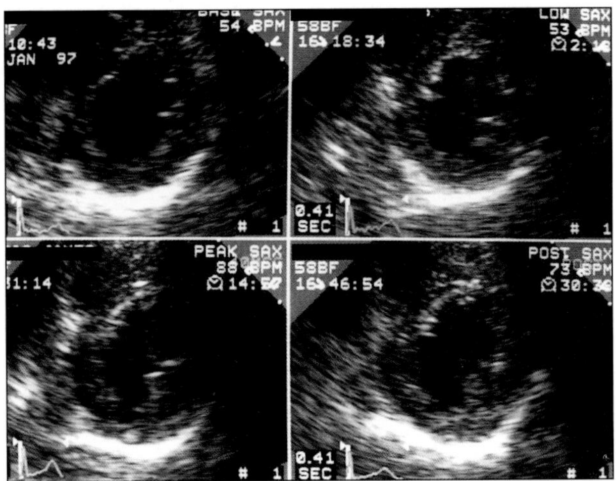

Figure 4.17
Dobutamine stress echocardiography is now commonly used to assess the presence of significant coronary artery disease and myocardial viability after infarction or in patients with heart failure. The most used protocols involve the display of images obtained at rest and low dose (5–10 μg/kg per min) dobutamine on top (left and right, respectively) and peak dose (40–50 μg/kg per min) and recovery on the bottom (left and right, respectively). However, modifications of such protocol are common particularly when atropine is routinely utilized to increase the heart rate at the peak of dobutamine stimulation.

patients who cannot perform significant physical activity after a myocardial infarction.[76–79] Dobutamine echocardiography (Fig. 4.17) has been used safely as early as 5 days after an infarction.[77] The presence of new wall motion abnormalities with dobutamine stress accurately predicted the presence of multivessel coronary artery disease after infarction in several studies. This technique has also been used to assess myocardial viability after infarction.[77–81] A biphasic response to dobutamine stress (improvement in wall motion abnormalities at low dose followed by deterioration at higher doses) identifies patients with viable but jeopardized myocardium who are at higher risk for further events.[81] Finally, dipyridamole has also been used as a pharmacological stressor after infarction.[82,83] This agent appears to be less likely to induce arrhythmias than dobutamine, and when combined with two-dimensional echocardiography, appears comparable to dobutamine echocardiography in identifying high-risk patients after myocardial infarction.[83]

Summary

The development of transthoracic echocardiography has revolutionized the management of patients with myocardial infarction. This noninvasive method, which can be easily performed at the bedside, yields important information on the extent of ischemic injury, and ultimately on the impact that such injury will have on the patient with infarction. Infarct size and location can be ascertained during or immediately after coronary occlusion in the emergency department or coronary care unit. The presence of several types of underlying cardiac diseases as well as the development of complications following myocardial infarction can be evaluated by echocardiography: infarct extension, infarct expansion, mitral regurgitation, and cardiac rupture can be diagnosed by echocardiography during the acute post-infarction period. Similarly, left ventricular thrombus formation and right ventricular infarction can be diagnosed by two-dimensional echocardiography, and have important implications for the management of patients with acute myocardial infarction.

While the ultrasound technology involved in the acquisition of real-time cardiac transthoracic images and Doppler signal has evolved markedly since the introduction of unidimensional techniques 30 years ago, several limitations are important relative to the patient with acute myocardial infarction. The hardware necessary for adequate Doppler echocardiographic studies is expensive, and a great deal of expertise is required, not only in the acquisition but also in the interpretation of images from patients with myocardial infarction. This has limited the widespread use of this technology in emergency departments and small hospitals or patient care units. Further technological improvement, including the development of three-dimensional real-time techniques may address some of the above mentioned limitations in the future.

The acquisition of echocardiographic images during diverse physiologic or pharmacological stimuli enhances the application of ultrasound to the study of cardiovascular function in patients with infarction. Exercise, pacing, dobutamine, adenosine, and dypiridamole have all been used to produce different types of controlled stressful interventions in post-infarction patients. These studies have been utilized to evaluate the presence of viable but stunned myocardium, the presence of blood flow limiting lesions in the infarct-related artery or elsewhere in the coronary arterial tree, and thus, to assess the prognosis of patients with myocardial infarction. Finally, the detailed assessment of cardiac structure and function as the heart remodels in response to myocardial loss by infarction represents another important application of echocardiography to the individual post-infarct patient, as well as a tool to elucidate the pathophysiology of cardiomyopathy and heart failure in ischemic heart disease.

References

1 Kramer CM, Lima JAC, Reichek N et al: Regional differences in function within noninfarcted myocardium during left ventricular remodeling. *Circulation* 1993; **88**: 1279–88.

2 Lima JAC, Becker LC, Melin JA et al: Impaired thickening of nonischemic myocardium during acute regional ischemia in the dog. *Circulation* 1985; **71**: 1048–59.

3 Lima JAC, Weiss JL: Use of echocardiographic regional contraction abnormalities for the estimation of infarct size. *Am J Card Imag* 1990; **4**: 23–32.

4 Lew WYW, Chen Z, Guth B et al: Mechanisms of augmented segment shortening in non ischemic areas during acute ischemia of the canine left ventricle. *Cir Res* 1985; **56**: 351–8.

5 Braunwald E, Kloner RA: The stunned myocardium: prolonged, post-ischemic ventricular dysfunction. *Circulation* 1981; **63**: 739–46.

6 Roberts R, Kleiman NS: Earlier diagnosis and treatment of acute myocardial infarction necessitates the need for a 'new diagnostic mind-set'. *Circulation* 1994; **89**: 872–81.

7 Lee TH, Rouan GW, Weisberg MC et al: Sensitivity of routine clinical criteria in diagnosing myocardial infarction within the first 24 hours of hospitalization. *Ann Int Med* 1987; **106**: 181–6.

8 Peels CH, Visser CA, Kupper AJ et al: Usefulness of two-dimensional echocardiography for immediate detection of ischemia in the emergency room. *Am J Cardiol* 1990; **65**: 687–91.

9 Sabia P, Afrooktch A, Touchstone DA et al: Value of regional wall motion abnormality in the emergency room diagnosis of acute myocardial infarction. *Circulation* 1991; **84**: I-85–I-92.

10 Loh IK, Charuzi Y, Beeder C et al: Early diagnosis of nontransmural infarction by two-dimensional echocardiography. *Am Heart J* 1982; **104**: 963–8.

11 Oh JK, Miller FA, Shub C et al: Evaluation of acute chest pain syndromes by two-dimensional echocardiography: its potential application in the selection of patients for acute reperfusion therapy. *Mayo Clin Proc* 1987; **62**: 59–66.

12 Launbjerg J, Berning J, Fouergaard P et al: Sensitivity and specificity of echocardiographic identification of patients eligible for safe early discharge after acute myocardial infarction. *Am Heart J* 19??; **124**: 846–53.

13 Stamm RB, Gibson RS, Biship HC et al: Echocardiographic detection of infarct-localized asynergy and remote asynergy during myocardial infarction: correlation with the extent of angiographic disease. *Circulation* 1983; **67**: 233–44.

14 D'Arcy B, Nanda NC: Two-dimensional echocardiographic features of right ventricular infarction. *Circulation* 1982; **65**: 167–73.

15 Nixon JV, Narahara KA, Smitherman TC: Estimation of myocardial involvement in patients with acute myocardial infarction by two dimensional echocardiography in acute myocardial infarction. *Circulation* 1980; **62**: 1248–55.

16 Kisslo JA, Robertson D, Gilbert BW et al: A comparison of real-time, two dimensional echocardiography and cineangiography in detecting left ventricular asynergy. *Circulation* 1977; **55**: 134–41.

17 Hect HS, Taylor R, Wong M, Shah PM: Comparative evaluation of segmental asynergy in remote myocardial infarction by radionuclide angiography, two dimensional echocardiography and contrast ventriculography. *Am Heart J* 1981; **101**: 740–7.

18 Heger JJ, Weyman AE, Wann LS et al: Cross-sectional echocardiography in acute myocardial infarction: detection and localization of regional left ventricular asynergy. *Circulation* 1979; **66**: 531–8.

19 Horowitz RS, Morganroth J: Immediate detection of early high-risk patients with acute myocardial infarction using two-dimensional echocardiographic evaluation of left ventricular regional wall motion abnormalities. *Am Heart J* 1982; **103**: 814–22.

20 Launbjerg J, Berning J, Fruergaard D et al: Risk stratification after acute myocardial infarction by means of echocardiographic wall motion scoring and Killip classification. *Cardiology* 1992; **80**: 375–81.

21 Berning J, Steensgaard-Hansen F: Early estimation of risk by echocardiographic determination of wall motion index in an unselected population with acute myocardial infarction. *Am J Cardiol* 1990; **65**: 567–76.

22 Topol E, Weiss JL, Brinker JA et al: Regional wall motion improvement after coronary thrombolysis with recombinant tissue plasminogen activator: importance of coronary angioplasty. *J Am Coll Cardiol* 1985; **6**: 426–33.

23 Sanjiv K: Myocardial contrast echocardiography in coronary artery disease: potential applications using venous injections of contrast. *Am J Cardiol* 1995; **75**: 61D.

24 Delemarre BJ, Visser CA, Bot H et al: Predicitive value of pulsed Doppler echocardiography in acute myocardial infarction. *J Am Soc Echocardiogr* 1989; **2**: 102–9.

25 Weyman AE: *Cross-sectional echocardiography* (Lea & Febinger, Philadelphia, 1982).

26 Buda AJ: The role of echocardiography in the evaluation of mechanical complications of acute myocardial infarction. *Circulation* 1991; **84**: I–109.

27 Muller JE, Rude RE, Braunwald E et al: Myocardial infarct extension: recurrence, outcome, and risk factors in the Multicenter Investigation of Infarct Size. *Ann Intern Med* 1988; **108**: 1–6.

28 Ellis SG, Topal EJ, George BS et al: Recurrent ischemia without warning. Analysis of risk factors for in-hospital ischemic events, following successful thrombolysis with intravenous tissue plasminogen activator. *Circulation* 1989; **80**: 1482–5.

29 Baker JT, Bramlet DA, Lester RM et al: Myocardial infarction extension: incidence and relationship to survival. *Circulation* 1982; **65**: 918–23.

30 Isaacsohn NJ, Earle MJ, Kember AJ, Parisi AF: Postmyocardial infarction pain and infarction pain and infarct extension in the coronary care unit: role of two-dimensional echocardiography. *J Am Coll Cardiol* 1988; **11**: 246–51.

31 Pastornak R, Braunwald E, Sobel B: Acute myocardial infarction. In: Branwauld E, ed., *Heart Disease: A Textbook of Cardiovascular Medicine*, 4th edn (WB Saunders, Philadelphia, PA, 1992).

32 Lopez-Sendon J, Gonzalez A, Lopez E et al: Diagnosis of subacute ventricular wall rupture after acute myocardial infarction: sensitivity and specificity of clinical, hemodynamic, and echocardiographic criteria. *J Am Coll Cardiol* 1992; **19**: 1145–53.

33 Oliva PB, Hammill SC, Edwards WD: Cardiac rupture, a clinically predictable complication of acute myocardial infarction: report of 70 cases with clinicopathologic correlations. *J Am Coll Cardiol* 1993; **22**: 720–6.

34 Raitt MH, Kraft CD, Gardner CJ et al: Subacute ventricular free wall rupture complicating myocardial infarction. *Am Heart J* 1993; **126**: 946–55.

35 Pollak H, Nobis H, Miczoch J: Frequency of left ventricular free wall rupture complicating acute myocardial infarction since the advent of thrombolysis. *Am J Cardiol* 1994; **74**: 184–6.

36 Pollak H, Dietz W, Speil R et al: Early diagnosis of subacute free wall rupture complicating acute myocardial infarction. *Eur Heart J* 1993; **14**: 640–8.

37 Stoddard MF, Dawkins PR, Longaker RA et al: Transesophageal echocardiography in the detection of left ventricular pseudoaneurysm. *Am Heart J* 1993; **125**: 534–9.

38 Nanda NC, Gatewood RD: Differentiation of left ventricular pseudoaneurysm from true aneurysms by two-dimensional echocardiography. *Circulation* 1979; **60**: II–144.

39 Sutherland GR, Smyllie JH, Roelandt JRT: Improved diagnosis and characterization of left ventricular pseudoaneurysm by Doppler color flow imaging. *Br Heart J* 1989; **61**: 59–66.

40 Reeves F, Drobinski G: Evidence of the inaccuracy of standard echocardiographic and angiographic criteria used for the recognition of true or 'false' left ventricular inferior aneurysm. *Br Heart J* 1988; **60**: 125–7.

41 Davies MJ: Ischaemic ventricular aneurysms: true or false? *Br Heart J* 1988; **60**: 95–7.

42 Radford MJ, Johnson RA, Dagett WM et al: Ventricular septal rupture: a review of clinical and pathological features and an analysis of survival. *Circulation* 1981; **64**: 545–53.

43 Sanders RJ, Kern WH, Blount SJ: Perforation of the interventricular septum in myocardial infarction. *Am Heart J* 1956; **51**: 736–42.

44 Montoya A, McKeever L, Scanlon PJ et al: Early repair of ventricular septal rupture after infarction. *Am J Cardiol* 1980; **45**: 345–8.

45 Topaz O, Taylor AL: Interventricular septal rupture complicating acute myocardial infarction: from pathophysiologic features to the role of invasive and noninvasive diagnostic modalities in current management. *Am J Med* 1992; **93**: 683–8.

46 Kishon Y, Iaqbal A, Oh JK et al: Evolution of echocardiographic modalities in detection of postmyocardial infarction ventricular septal defect and papillary muscle rupture: study of 62 patients. *Am Heart J* 1993; **126**: 667–75.

47 Smyllie JH, Sutherland GR, Geuskens R et al: Doppler color flow mapping in the diagnosis of ventricular septal rupture and acute mitral regurgitation after myocardial infarction. *Am J Cardiol* 1990; **15**: 1449–55.

48 Ballal R, Sanyal RS, Nanda NC, Mahan EF. Usefulness of transesophageal echocardiography in the diagnosis of ventricular septal rupture secondary to acute myocardial infarction. *Am J Cardiol* 1993; **71**: 367–70.

49 Clements SD, Story WE, Hurst JW et al: Ruptured papillary muscle a complication of myocardial infarction: clinical presentation, diagnosis and treatment. *Clin Cardiol* 1985; **8**: 93–103.

50 Efthimiou J, Pitcher M, Ormerod O et al: Severe 'silent' mitral regurgitation after myocardial infarction: a clinical conundrum. *Br Med J* 1992; **305**: 105–6.

51 Goldman AP, Glover MU, Mick W et al: Role of echocardiography/Doppler in cardiogenic shock: silent mitral regurgitation. *Ann Thoracic Surg* 1991; **52**: 296–9.

52 Stoddard MF, Keedy DL, Kuppersmith J: Transesophageal echocardiographic diagnosis of papillary muscle rupture complicating acute myocardial infarction. *Am Heart J* 1990; **120**: 690–2.

53 Zotz RJ, Dohmen G, Genth S et al: Diagnosis of papillary muscle rupture after acute myocardial infarction by transthoracic and transesophageal echocardiography. *Clin Cardiol* 1993; **16**: 665–70.

54 Llaneras MR, Nance ML, Streicher JT et al: Pathogenesis of ischemic mitral insufficiency. *J Thoracic Cardiovasc Surg* 1993; **105**: 439–43.

55 Asinger RW, Mikell FL, Elsperger J, Hodges M. Incidence of left-ventricular thrombosis after acute transmural myocardial infarction. *N Engl J Med* 1981; **305**: 297–302.

56 Asinger RW, Mikell FL, Sharma B, Morrison H. Observations on detecting left ventricular thrombus with two dimensional echocardiography: emphasis on avoidance of false positive diagnoses. *Am J Cardiol* 1981; **47**: 145–56.

57 Kontny F, Dale J, Nesvold A et al: Left ventricular thrombosis and arterial embolism in acute anterior myocardial infarction. *J Internal Med* 1993; **233**: 139–43.

58 Vecchio C, Chiarella F, Lupi G et al: Left ventricular thrombus in anterior acute myocardial infarction after thrombolysis. *Circulation* 1991; **84**: 512–19.

59 Glikson M, Agranat O, Ziskind Z et al: From swirling to a mobile pedunculated mass–the evolution of left ventricular thrombus despite full anticoagulation. *Chest* 1993; **103**: 281–3.

60 Delemarre BJ, Visser CA, Bot H, Dunning A: Prediction of apical thrombus formation in acute myocardial infarction based on left ventricular spatial flow pattern. *J Am Coll Cardiol* 1990; **15**: 355–60.

61 Bhatnagar SK, Al-Yusuf AR: Left ventricular blood flow analysis in patients with and without a thrombus after first Q wave anterior myocardial infarction: two-dimensional Doppler echocardiographic study. *Angiology* 1992; **3**: 188–94.

62 Kinch J, Ryan TJ: Right ventricular infarction. *N Engl J Med* 1994; **330**: 1211–17.

63 Jugdutt BI, Sussex BA, Sivaram CA, Rossall RE. Right ventricular infarction: two dimensional echocardiographic evaluation. *Am Heart J* 1984; **107**: 505–18.

64 Bellamy GR, Rasmussen HH, Nasser FN et al: Value of two-dimensional echocardiography, and clinical signs in detecting right ventricular infarction. *Am Heart J* 1986; **112**: 304–9.

65 Lopez-Sendon J, Garcia-Fernandez MA, Coma-Canella I et al: Segmental right ventricular function after acute myocardial infarction: two-dimensional echocardiographic study in 63 patients. *Am J Cardiol* 1983; **51**: 390–6.

66 Lopez-Sendon J, Lopez de Sa E, Fernandez de Soria R et al: Inversion of the normal interatrial septum convexity in acute myocardial infarction: incidence, clinical relevance and prognostic significance. *J Am Coll Cardiol* 1990; **15**: 806–7.

67 Manno BV, Beemis CE, Carver, Mintz GS: Right ventricular infarction complicated by right to left shunt. *J Am Coll Cardiol* 1983; **1**: 554–7.

68 Madsen BK, Egeblad H, Hojberg S et al: Prognostic value of echocardiography compared to other clinical findings. *Cardiology* 1995; **86**: 157–62.

69 Berning J, Steensgaard-Hansen F, Appleyard M: Relative prognostic value of clinical heart failure and early echocardiographic parameters in acute myocardial infarction. *Cardiology* 1991; **79**: 64–72.

70 Berning J, Steensgaard-Hansen F: Early estimation of risk by echocardiographic determination of wall motion index in an unselected population with acute myocardial infarction. *Am J Cardiol* 1990; **65**: 567–76.

71 Sutton MSJ, Pfeffer MA, Plappert T et al: Quantative two-dimensional echocardiographic measurements are major predictors of adverse cardiovascular events after myocardial infarction. *Circulation* 1994; **89**: 68–75.

72 Reeder S, Gibbons RJ: Acute myocardial infarction: risk stratification in the thrombolytic era. *Mayo Clin Proc* 1995; **70**: 87–94.

73 Armstrong WF. Stress echocardiography: clinical influence and future role. *Mayo Clin Proc* 1995; **70**: 5–15.

74 Ryan T, Armstrong WF, O'Donnell JA, Feigenbaum H: Risk stratification after acute myocardial infarction by means of exercise two-dimensional echocardiography. *Am Heart J* 1987; **114**: 1305–16.

75 Applegate RJ, Dell'Italia LJ, Crawford MH: Usefulness of two-dimensional echocardiography during low level exercise testing early after uncomplicated myocardial infarction. *Am J Cardiol* 1987; **60**: 10–14.

76 Roger VL, Pellikka PA, Oh JK et al: Stress echocardiography. Part I. Exercise echocardiography: techniques, implementation, clinical applications and correlations. *Mayo Clin Proc* 1995; **70**: 95–96.

77 Berthe C, Pierard LA, Hiernaux M et al: Predicting the extent and location in acute myocardial infarction by echocardiography during dobutamine infusion. *Am J Cardiol* 1986; **58**: 1167–72.

78 Smart SC, Sawada SG, Ryan T et al: Dobutamine echocardiography identifies restenosis and multivessel disease in myocardial infarction. *J Am Coll Cardiol* 1991; **17** (suppl 277a): (abstract).

79 Smart SC, Sawada SG, Ryan T et al: Low dose dobutamine echocardiography to assess prognosis after thrombolysis for M.I. *Circulation* 1991; **84** (suppl 2): 478 (abstract).

80 Shaw LJ, Peterson ED, Keesler KL, Califf RM: Are stress imaging modalities of value in post-myocardial infarction predischarge risk stratification? A meta-analysis of stress perfusion and ventricular function imaging studies. *J Am Coll Cardiol* 1996; **27** (suppl 1): 329a.

81 Previtali M, Poli A, Lazarina L et al: Dobutamine stress echocardiography for assessment of myocardial viability and ischemia and acute myocardial infarction treated with thrombolysis. *Am J Cardiol* 1993; **72**: 124–30.

82 Sclavo MG, Noussan P, Pallisco O, Presbitero P: Usefulness of dipyridamole–echocardiographic test to identify jeopardized myocardium after thrombolysis. *Eur Heart J* 1992; **13**: 1348–55.

83 Camerieri A, Picano E, Lendi P: Prognostic value of dipyridamole–echocardiography early after myocardial infarction in elderly patients. *J Am Coll Cardiol* 1993; **22**: 1809–15.

84 Segar et al: Dobutamine stress echocardiography: correlation with coronary lesion severity as determined by quantitative angiography. *J Am Coll Cardiol* 1992; **13**: 70–7.

5

Left ventricular post-infarct remodeling

João AC Lima

Natural history

Anterior myocardial infarction

The alterations of left ventricular structure and function developed in response to myocardial loss by infarction have been described as ventricular remodeling.[1–5] These alterations represent response mechanisms designed to maintain cardiac output in the face of significant myocardial loss. However, the magnitude of such response may be disproportional to the degree of myocyte loss and become detrimental to the patient with infarction. Thus, the increased rate of cardiac complications associated with greater post-infarct remodeling[6] are in part caused by an appropriate response to a large infarct, and in part secondary to an exaggerated compensatory response to a given degree of myocardial loss.

The process of ventricular remodeling after a non-reperfused anterior myocardial infarction commences with thinning and expansion of the infarcted segment in the first days which follow coronary occlusion.[1–8] Typically, most human anterior infarcts result from lesions situated in the left anterior descending coronary artery beyond the first septal perforator branch. In this case, the mid and distal portions of the interventricular septum and anterior wall are damaged and become akinetic while the left ventricular apex, which is commonly completely involved by infarction, become dyskinetic (Fig. 5.1). Initially, the remaining portions of the left ventricle maintain normal function or become hypercontractile,[9] obscuring the impact of infarction on global left ventricular function. In fact, the most common mistake in the evaluation of left ventricular function after acute myocardial infarction is the overestimation of global function and stroke volume because of non-infarcted tissue hyperfunction. Permanent or prolonged obstruction of the very proximal left anterior descending coronary artery results in marked ventricular dilatation and global dysfunction[10] leading to clinical signs and symptoms typical of patients with dilated cardiomyopathies (Fig. 5.2).

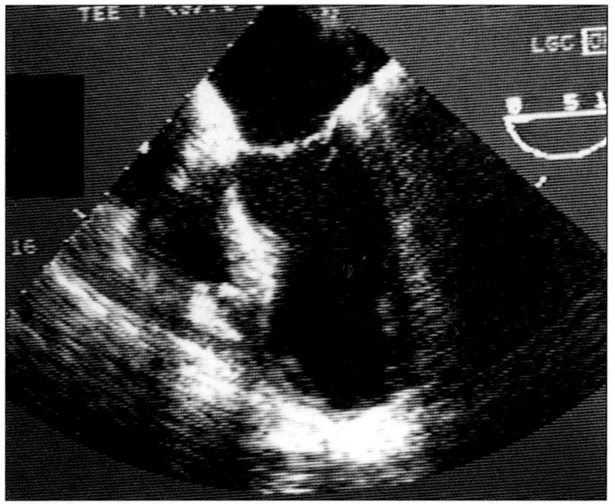

Figure 5.1
Cross-sectional apical image of the heart (4-chamber view) with the left ventricle displayed on the left. The echocardiogram was obtained from a patient who suffered an anterior myocardial infarction months prior to the echocardiographic study. The distal portion of the septum and apex is thin and akinetic reflecting aneurysm formation. Patients with such abnormalities are at increased risk of developing complications such as embolism and ventricular arrhythmias.

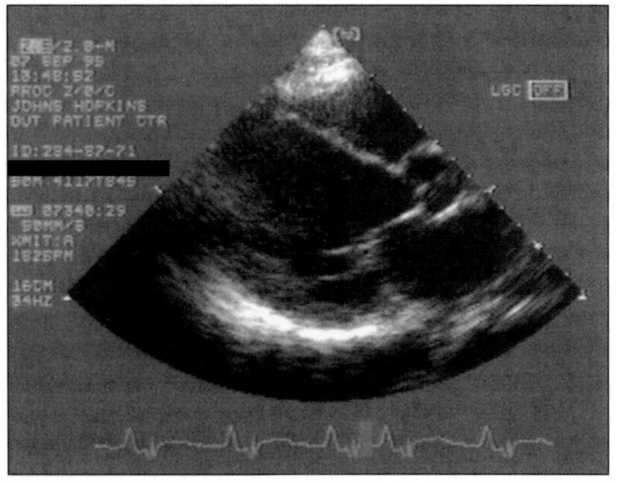

a

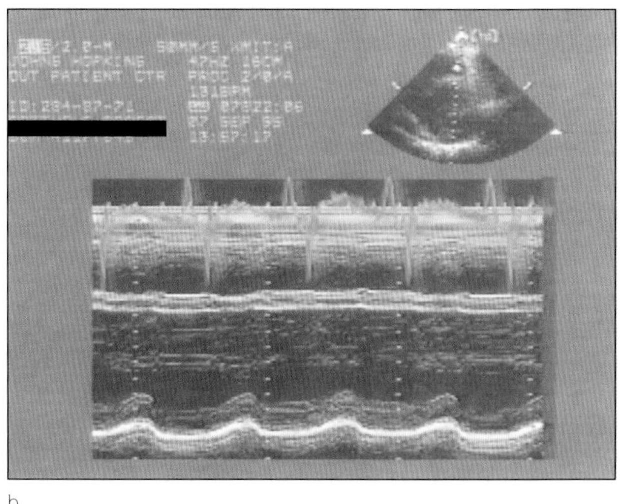

b

Figure 5.2

(a) Longitudinal cross-sectional image of the infarcted left ventricle (long-axis views) displaying region of septal thinning and akinesis compatible with healed myocardial infarction. The culprit lesion was located very proximally in the left anterior descending coronary artery with resultant post-infarction ventricular dilatation with poor global left ventricular function. (b) M-mode echocardiogram obtained at the level of the left ventricular equator in the same patient displaying akinetic septum and contractile inferior wall.

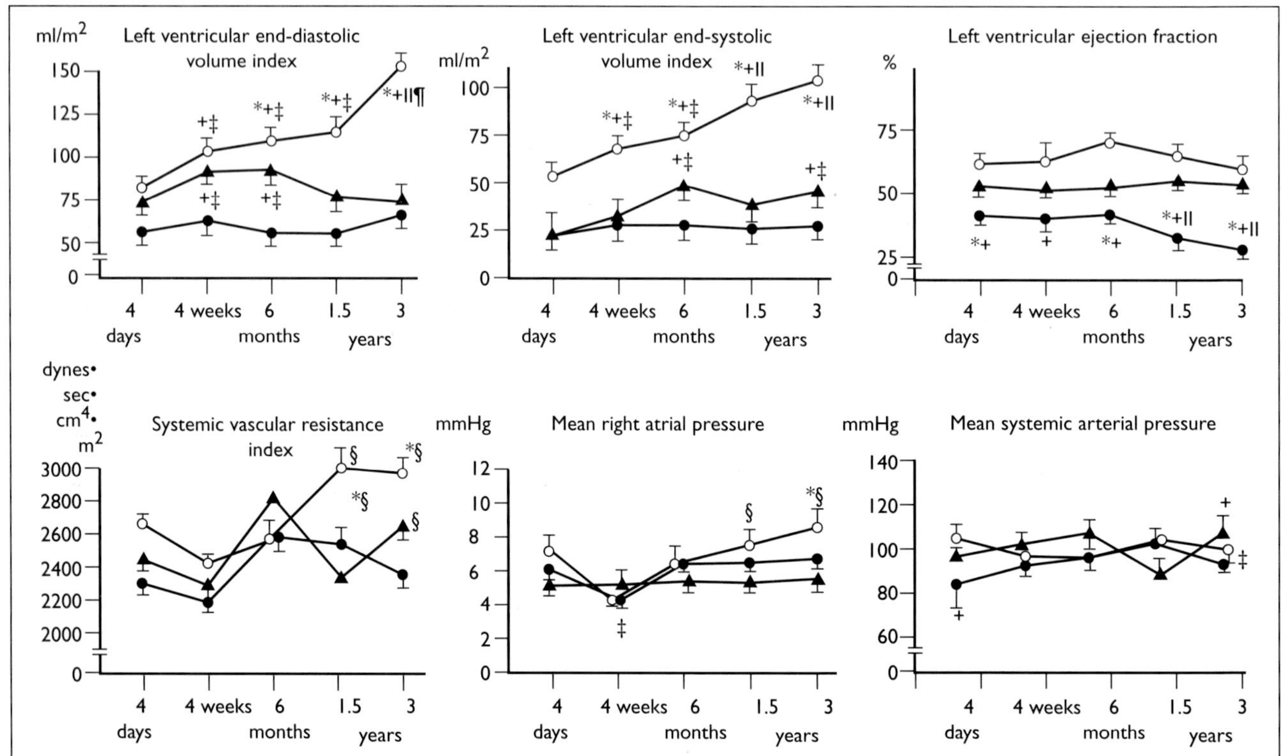

Figure 5.3

The time course of hemodynamic changes after myocardial infarction is depicted in six panels: top, left ventricular end-diastolic volume, end-systolic volume and ejection fraction; bottom, systemic vascular resistance index, mean right atrial pressure and mean systemic arterial pressure. Data are categorized by the magnitude of initial damage assessed as the extent regional left ventricular dysfunction. (Reprinted with permission from Gaudron et al.[5]).

The natural history of anterior myocardial infarcts managed before the advent of therapeutic reperfusion is well recognized. Infarct expansion and thinning which characterize the first few days after coronary occlusion[1,8] are followed by infarct healing, with the eventual formation of a fibrous scar 6–8 weeks after the acute episode.[7] However, the non-infarcted portion of the left ventricle undergoes marked changes during the same period of time. The left ventricle dilates and hypertrophies in response to the activation of the Frank–Starling mechanism.[4] This mechanism is activated by the sudden drop in chamber function caused by infarction, with insufficient compensatory response from non-infarcted myocardium. In cases of severe myocardial damage,[5] the left ventricle may continue to dilate up to at least 3 years following myocardial infarction (Fig. 5.3).

Left ventricular hypertrophy[4,11] and chamber distortion[1,8,12] accompany left ventricular dilatation after infarction. Left ventricular mass augmentation is well documented in both small[11] and large[4] animal models of myocardial infarction. This post-infarct hypertrophy is eccentric, i.e. the increase in left ventricular mass is not accompanied by an increase in wall thickness relative to the cavity diameter.[13] Therefore, the increase in volume is greater than the increase in mass leading to a progressive reduction in the volume/mass ratio.[4] Such remodeling of the left ventricular chamber is commonly associated with an increased end-diastolic pressure leading to dyspnea on effort and eventually congestive heart failure.[5,6] The stasis of blood in the left ventricular apex frequently causes thrombus formation and embolization resulting in stroke, peripheral embolization, and/or myocardial reinfarction.[3,10] Finally, the most feared outcome of large anterior infarctions is the development of malignant ventricular arrhythmias causing sudden death.[10,14]

Inferior myocardial infarction

Large inferior (Fig. 5.4) or lateral (Fig. 5.5) myocardial infarcts produce remodeling of the left ventricle of similar magnitude to anterior infarcts in terms of ventricular dilatation and hypertrophy. However, the importance of differences in ventricular shape and function after inferior versus anterior infarcts have not been well characterized, in part due to the lack of methods to accurately measure infarct size in humans. After large inferior or lateral infarcts, the ventricle becomes dilated particularly at the level of the equator, assuming a more globular shape.[15,16] Infarct thinning and expansion take place as in anterior infarcts but lead to aneurysm formation less frequently. In fact, the presence of an inferior wall aneurysm identified by imaging, should raise the possibility of a pseudoaneurysm caused by rupture of the left ventricular wall, tamponaded

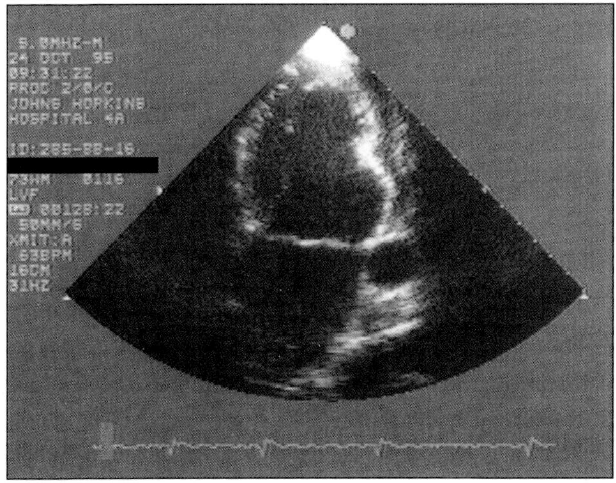

Figure 5.4
Echocardiographic apical image (2-chamber view) of infarcted left ventricle displaying inferior wall thinning and dyskinesis corresponding to large healed inferior infarction. The inferior wall aneurysm in this case can be differentiated from a pseudoaneurysm by its large neck relative to the fundus.

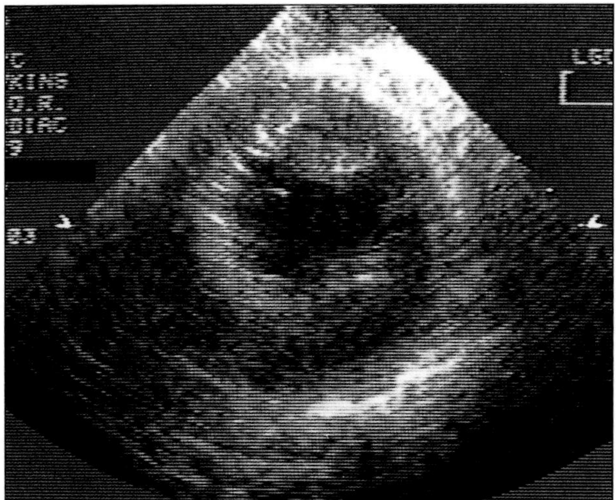

Figure 5.5
Left ventricular short-axis cross-section obtained from the transgastric approach to illustrate a lateral myocardial infarct in a patient with left circumflex coronary occlusion. The ventricular short-axis cross-section is displayed with inferior wall on top and anterior wall at the bottom, septum to the left and lateral wall to the right side of the reader. Myocardial infarcts caused by left circumflex occlusion are predominantly inferobasal or posterobasal in location and characterized by a paucity of ECG findings.

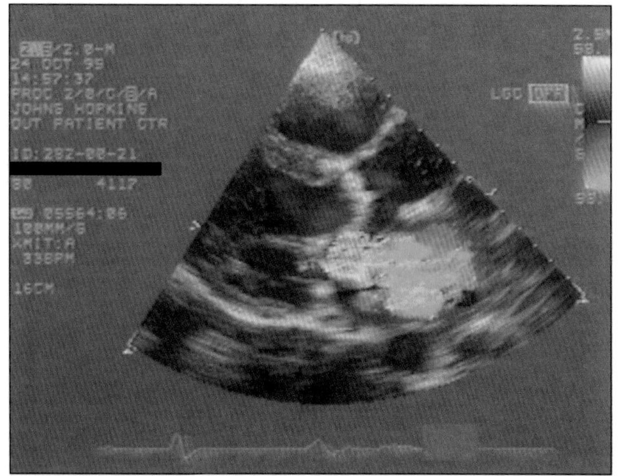

a

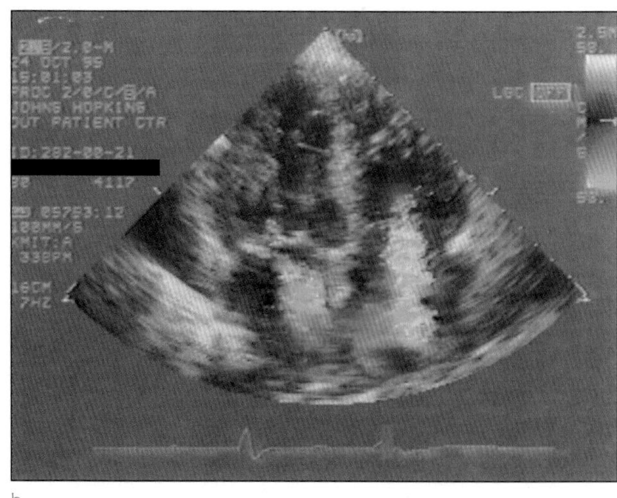

b

Figure 5.6
(a) Left ventricular long-axis image of another patient with inferior infarction to illustrate the presence of ischemic mitral regurgitation which is severe in this case. Leaflet apposition becomes impaired by chordae scarring superimposed to inferior wall akinesis and ventricular dilatation, which is more prominent at the level of the left ventricular base in cases of inferior wall infarction.
(b) Four-chamber view from the same patient to confirm the severity of mitral regurgitation and illustrate the presence of tricuspid regurgitation as a consequence of left ventricular dysfunction and pulmonary hypertension.

by pericardial thrombus formation (Fig. 5.4). Left ventricular remodeling caused by large inferior or lateral infarcts, although not as well characterized as remodeling caused by anterior infarcts, also includes the frequent development of ventricular arrhythmias, congestive heart failure, and occasionally thromboembolism.[3,5,14]

Mitral regurgitation is a common complication of inferior myocardial infarction (Fig. 5.6). Intrinsic papillary muscle damage, combined with asynergy of the left ventricular wall segment to which papillary muscles attach, may result in shortened chordae and incomplete aposition of mitral valve leaflets with regurgitation of blood into the left atrium during systole.[17,18] This process usually takes weeks to mature, generally causing mitral insufficiency 6–8 weeks after acute myocardial infarction (Fig. 5.6). It is different than the processes which lead to acute mitral regurgitation after myocardial infarction which include: rupture of a papillary muscle, papillary muscle dysfunction due to ischemia, or acute left ventricular dilatation secondary to marked myocardial loss.

The natural history of small inferior infarcts is significantly different to that of anterior infarcts. Most small inferior infarcts lead to limited ventricular post-infarct remodeling, frequently resulting in little or no dilatation and mild global dysfunction. In many cases, the substitution of necrotic tissue by fibrous scar results in infarct size reduction by imaging methods performed serially after coronary occlusion.[16] Frequently, inferior or lateral infarcts are not transmural, and their relative transmural extent may decrease as the epicardial rim of surviving myocardium hypertrophies. This may lead to the disappearance of electrocardiographic Q waves and varying reduction in the magnitude of the corresponding wall motion abnormality which may ultimately become imperceptible to the naked eye.

Pathophysiology of post-infarct left ventricular remodeling

Infarct expansion

Transmural non-reperfused myocardial infarcts expand in the first 24–48 h after coronary occlusion.[8] This expansion (Fig. 5.7) is caused by passive wall stress secondary to forces imposed on the necrotic segment by contraction of non-infarcted myocardium.[9] In addition, the outward forces

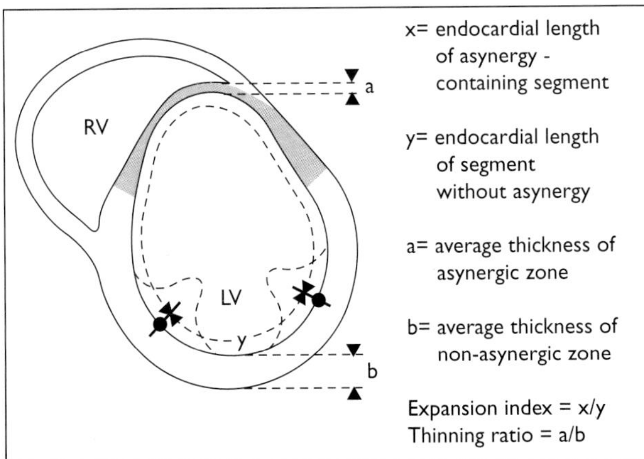

Figure 5.7
Short-axis left ventricular cross-section at the level of the ventricular equator illustrating a geometric method of quantifying the magnitude of infarct expansion early after infarction, as the ratio of thinning of infarcted to non-infarcted wall segments. (Reprinted with permission from Jugdutt and Michorowski[57]).

generated by the rise in the intracavitary pressure during each systole leads to progressive bulging of the stretched infarcted segment with the ultimate formation of an aneurysm.[10] As mentioned above, anterior infarcts are more susceptible than inferior infarcts to undergo infarct expansion and aneurysm formation. Topographic location and the shape of the infarcted territory may represent important determinants of such predisposition in patients with anterior myocardial infarction.[15,16]

Infarct expansion results from mechanical slippage and stretch of necrotic fibers in the hours which follow coronary occlusion.[19] Disrupted fibers are slowly substituted by fibrous tissue in a process frequently referred to as infarct healing.[7] Corticosteroids unfavorably influence this process increasing the chances of ventricular rupture and mortality after myocardial infarction.[20] Similarly, increases in ventricular afterload lead to increased infarct expansion and wall thinning experimentally, resulting in larger aneurysms after myocardial infarction.[21] Previous pharmacologic attempts to alter infarct healing directly have been ineffective or produced marginal benefits in terms of ventricular remodeling and mortality after myocardial infarction.[7,20]

Myocardial reperfusion may totally or partially prevent infarct expansion after infarction, depending on its timing relative to the onset of coronary occlusion and tissue oxygen deprivation.[22,23] The beneficial influence of myocardial reperfusion on infarct expansion when myocardial salvage is no longer feasible[24] forms the basis for the open artery hypothesis and the rationale for therapeutic intervention in patients who are no longer candidates for direct myocardial salvage after acute myocardial infarction. The mechanisms by which reperfusion alters infarct expansion are not entirely clarified. Marked edema formation by reflow through the infarct-related artery may alter the material properties of infarcted tissue after reperfusion. This increased stiffness may in turn provide mechanical resistance to longitudinal, circumferential, and shear forces produced by contraction of the remaining non-infarcted myocardium. In addition, the increased thickness of reperfused segments in comparison to non-reperfused infarcts may also play an important role in preventing the outward systolic bulge of expanded segments which ultimately results in aneurysm formation. However, further studies are necessary to characterize more clearly the beneficial effects of reperfusion on left ventricular post-infarct remodeling.

Mechanisms of post-infarct left ventricular remodeling

The process of post-infarct ventricular remodeling is driven mainly by increased intraventricular diastolic pressures, resulting from the activation of the Frank–Starling mechanism.[2,4,5,11] This increased pressure leads to cell slippage[19] and myocyte elongation[25] in the non-infarcted portion of the left ventricle which dilates progressively to accommodate increasingly large end-diastolic volumes. However, the distribution of stresses in the non-infarcted portion of the infarcted heart is not homogeneous.[12,26–28] Evidence from studies using geometric models to estimate wall stress in the human heart after infarction[26] confirmed earlier predictions obtained from mathematical models of the infarcted left ventricle which found elevated stresses in non-infarcted regions located adjacent to the infarct scar.[27] Similarly, numerous previous studies[4,28–30] have characterized differences in segmental function after myocardial infarction with greater dysfunction in the adjacent non-infarcted regions (Fig. 5.8). These findings support the concept that increased systolic wall stresses in adjacent non-infarcted regions after myocardial infarction may contribute to the post-infarct remodeling process, in addition to the augmentation of end-diastolic volumes generated via the renin–angiotensin mechanism.[31]

The concept that adjacent region dysfunction is related to local mechanical overload is further supported by cellular studies which have demonstrated greater hypertrophy in adjacent regions compared to regions remote from the

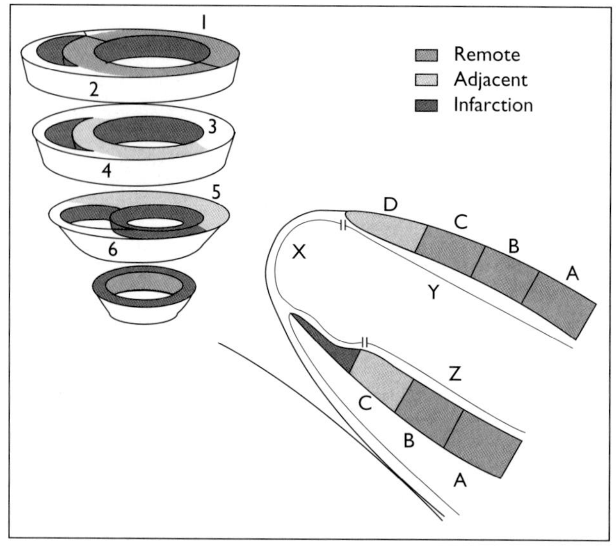

a

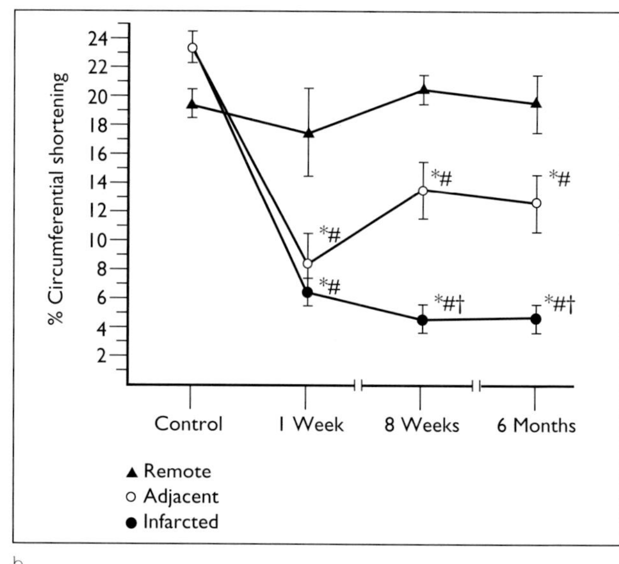

b

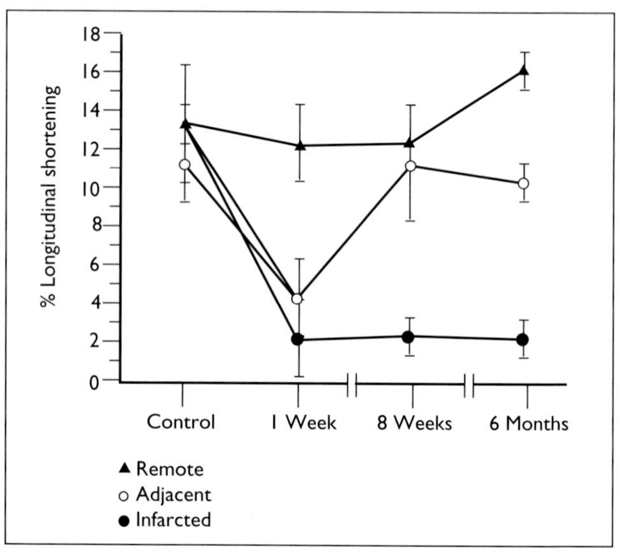

c

Figure 5.8

(a) Top: schematic diagram of short-axis slices from a typical magnetic resonance imaging (MRI) study of an animal after anteroapical infarction. Regions 1 and 2 in the most basal slice are remote from the infarct. Region 6 is within the infarcted area. Regions 4 and 5 are immediately adjacent to the infarct. Region 3 is at an intermediate distance from the most remote and immediately adjacent segments and was left out of the analysis. The regional analysis of circumferential shortening was based on this classification scheme. Bottom: schematic diagram of a long-axis image from MRI study of an animal after anteroapical infarction. To distinguish between the analysis of longitudinal and circumferential shortening, letters were used in lieu of numbers to label regions in the long-axis orientation. Regions A and B in both the septum and lateral free wall are remote from the infarction. Region D in the septum encompasses thinned infarcted tissue. Regions C in the septum and D in the lateral wall are defined as adjacent because of their proximity to infarcted myocardium. Region C in the lateral wall is at an intermediate distance from the most remote regions and immediately adjacent regions and was left out of the analysis. Regional analysis of longitudinal shortening was based on this classification scheme. The segment labeled X represents the thinned infarcted region and segments Y and Z, the non-infarcted lateral free wall and septum, respectively. (b) Graph showing per cent circumferential shortening (measured as systolic changes in intertag distances) in the subendocardium of infarcted, adjacent and remote regions as depicted in (a), up to 6 months after myocardial infarction in the ovine model of myocardial infarction. (c) Graph depicting subendocardial per cent longitudinal shortening in infarcted, adjacent and remote regions as shown in (a) up to 6 months after myocardial infarction in the same animals represented in (b). (Reprinted with permission from Kramer et al.[4]).

infarct scar.[32–34] In recent studies, adjacent region dysfunction has been associated with local cell hypertrophy as early as 2 weeks after coronary occlusion in experimental models.[32] Conversely, the possibility that humoral factors released by cells adjacent to the infarct border influence the degree of cellular remodeling in adjacent regions cannot be excluded.[32] In any case, these cellular alterations relate to evidence from other studies which have demonstrated differences in autonomic innervation,[35] local metabolism,[36] and propensity for arrhythmias[37] in non-infarcted myocardium adjacent to infarct scars. In fact, previous studies which have attempted to localize the origin of malignant ventricular tachycardia in patients who were rescued from sudden death have identified the adjacent regions as the common focus of abnormal re-entrant electric activity. Given the fact that sudden death is the most common mechanism of mortality in patients exhibiting severe post-infarct remodeling, further studies designed to elucidate the cellular mechanisms involved in the remodeling process are needed for the development of therapies specifically targeted to alter the remodeling process.

Clinical trials

The notion that post-infarct ventricular remodeling can be modified by therapy to prevent or diminish the incidence of its associated complications is gaining increasing attention.[38] However, the first concern regarding these patients should obviously be directed towards preventing reinfarction or further episodes of myocardial ischemia. In this regard, risk stratification to identify patients with myocardial ischemia or large territories at risk, and intervention to optimize myocardial vascularization and diminish the chances of coronary reocclusion (aspirin), are paramount in the care of patients with acute myocardial infarction.[39,40] Chronically, the importance of risk factor control and aspirin used to alter coronary atherosclerosis and/or prevent reinfarction cannot be overestimated. They represent the cornerstones of post-myocardial infarction patient care along with therapeutic strategies designed to alter the remodeling process itself.

Previous attempts to influence infarct healing were unsuccessful as were attempts to unload the left ventricle immediately after myocardial infarction with vasodilator therapy. However, experimental studies demonstrating the protective effects of the angiotensin converting enzyme (ACE) inhibitor captopril[41] were followed by imaging studies which demonstrated the beneficial effects of chronic ACE inhibition on post-infarct left ventricular dilatation in humans.[42,43] These studies formed the rationale for multicenter clinical trials which tested the hypothesis that chronic ACE inhibition could limit left ventricular post-infarct remodeling and the cardiac complications typically associated with that process.[38]

The SAVE trial

The Survival and Ventricular Enlargement (SAVE) trial enrolled 2231 patients with left ventricular ejection fraction below 40% as assessed by radionuclide ventriculography.[44] Patients were randomized to captopril (target dose of 50 mg t.i.d.) or placebo (*n* = 1116) and followed for 42±10 months. Fifty-five per cent of the infarcts were anterior, 17.5% were inferior and 11.5% of all patients had combined anterior and inferior myocardial infarcts. Thirty-five per cent of patients had had previous infarctions at the time of randomization and only one-third of patients in both groups received thrombolytics before treatment. Treatment was started 11 days on average after infarction in patients of both groups.

Cardiovascular mortality was greater in patients taking placebo (*n* = 234) than in those taking captopril (*n* = 188, 21% risk reduction, 95% confidence interval = 5–35%, *P* = 0.014, Fig. 5.9). There was also a marked reduction in mortality secondary to congestive heart failure in the treatment group as compared with the placebo group (38 versus 58 deaths, respectively). There were no differences between the two groups with respect to deaths from non-cardiac causes (41 versus 40, NS in the placebo and captopril groups, respectively). Similarly, cardiovascular morbidity was significantly reduced by treatment with captopril after

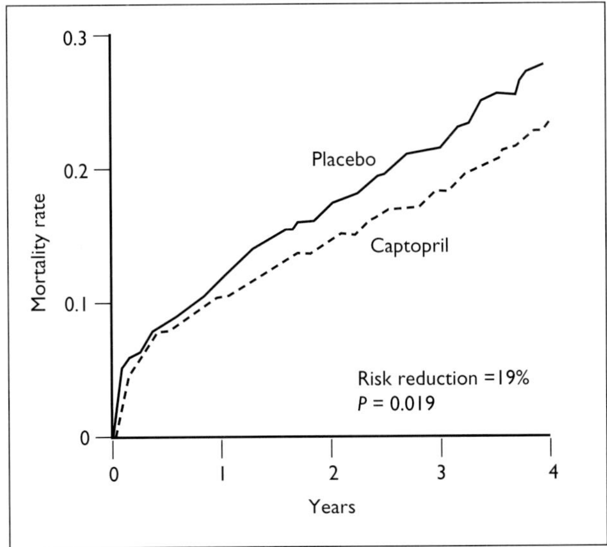

Figure 5.9
Cumulative mortality from all causes in post-infarct patients taking captopril and placebo. (Reprinted with permission from Pfeffer et al.[44]).

myocardial infarction. Patients in the treatment arm of the trial had less congestive heart failure requiring open label treatment with ACE inhibitors, less failure requiring hospitalization, and less recurrent myocardial infarction which was in some ways surprising, since this class of agents was not thought to protect for recurrent coronary occlusion. The mechanisms by which captopril reduced the risk of cardiovascular death and congestive heart failure in post-infarction patients are mediated mainly by reductions in post-infarction remodeling.[45]

Two-dimensional echocardiograms were obtained in 512 patients enrolled in the SAVE study and repeated at 1 year in 420 survivors.[45] Parameters of left ventricular size and function were related to the incidence of adverse cardiovascular events including death, heart failure requiring hospitalization, or open label ACE inhibition, and recurrent infarction, for a follow-up period averaging 3.0±0.6 years. Left ventricular end-systolic area and the fractional change in cavity area during systole (i.e. two-dimensional ejection fraction) were strongly related to cardiovascular mortality and morbidity irrespective of treatment assignment. In addition, left ventricular end-diastolic and end-systolic areas were larger in the placebo than in the captopril group, while the fractional change in cavity area was lower in the placebo than in the captopril group.

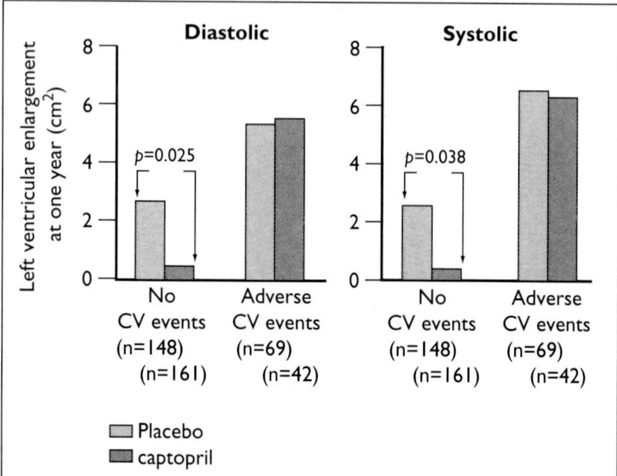

Figure 5.10
Bar graphs showing changes in left ventricular area between baseline and 1 year in patients who did, versus those who did not, experience an adverse cardiovascular (CV) event according to whether they were assigned to placebo or captopril therapy. (Reprinted with permission from St John Sutton et al.[45]).

About one-quarter of the 1-year survivors (26.4%) experienced a major adverse cardiovascular event during the follow-up period. These patients had greater ventricular size than patients who did not experience cardiovascular events (Fig. 5.10). This analysis in a subset of patients enrolled in the SAVE study demonstrates the link between attenuation of left ventricular remodeling by captopril after infarction and improved clinical outcome.

Other clinical trials involving ACE inhibition after myocardial infarction

The benefits of ACE inhibition on post-infarct ventricular remodeling have been evaluated in another trial of similar size to the SAVE trial. The Acute Infarction Ramipril Efficacy (AIRE) study enrolled 2006 patients on average 5 days after infarction and randomized them to placebo or ramipril with a mean follow-up of 15 months.[46] The study demonstrated a reduced overall mortality of 27% in patients taking ramipril and a reduction in resistant congestive heart failure of 19% compared with placebo. Interestingly, while mortality differences in the SAVE trial became significant only after 1 year of post-infarct follow-up, the benefit of ramipril on mortality became apparent as early as 30 days after the acute myocardial infarction event. Similarly, the effects of early ACE inhibition with zofenopril on the prevention of severe congestive heart failure were assessed in 1556 patients with an acute anterior wall myocardial infarction.[47] The Survival of Myocardial Infarction Long-Term Evaluation (SMILE) trial involved careful drug titration in the acute phase of anterior myocardial infarction to avoid hypotension. During the 6 weeks of double-blind treatment, 32 patients (4.1%) developed severe congestive heart failure in the placebo group while only 17 (2.2%) developed failure in the zofenopril treated group. The risk reduction afforded by the ACE inhibitor was 46% ($P<0.018$). Most importantly, there was a trend towards less mortality in the zofenopril group (38 deaths) versus the placebo group (51 deaths) with a risk reduction of 25% (95% confidence interval = 11–60%, $P = 0.19$). However, the 1-year mortality rate for patients who received zofenopril for 6 weeks after infarction was less than for those who received placebo (10 versus 14%, $P = 0.011$, Fig. 5.11). Although the drug was started early after the onset of acute infarction, discontinuation of the study drug due to hypotension was not greater in the zofenopril versus the placebo groups (3.8% versus 2.7%, NS).

Two other large trials have investigated the influence of ACE inhibition on survival after myocardial infarction.[48,49] The Gruppo Italiano per lo Studio della Sopravvivenza nell'Infarto Miocardico (GISSI-3) trial treated patients with

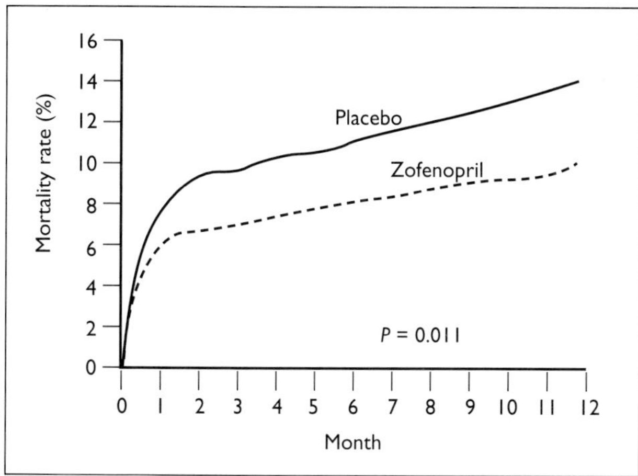

Figure 5.11
Cumulative mortality during 1 year of follow-up among patients with acute myocardial infarction treated for 6 weeks with zofenopril or placebo. (Reprinted with permission from Ambrosioni et al.[47]).

acute myocardial infarction in Killip class I or 2 within 24 h of symptoms of chest pain with lisinopril.[48] Follow-up was limited to 6 weeks, but patients treated with ACE inhibitors had a lower mortality rate than those treated with placebo (6.3% versus 7.1%, $P<0.03$). Similarly, the Collaborative Group Fourth International Study of Infarct Survival (ISIS-4) also found a lower mortality rate at 35 days in patients with acute myocardial infarction[49] treated with captopril relative to patients treated with placebo (7.1% versus 7.6%, $P<0.02$). These preliminary results are in agreement with the results from the SAVE, AIRE, SMILE and GISSI-3 trials. By contrast, the Cooperative New Scandinavian Enalapril Study (CONSENSUS-2) was interrupted after 6 months' follow-up by the Safety Committee because of concerns about the possible adverse effects of enalapril in elderly patients with early hypotension possibly caused by intravenous enalapril use.[50] The trial was originally designed to test the hypothesis that enalapril started immediately after thrombolysis was beneficial in diminishing mortality in patients with myocardial infarction. However, the analysis of data available at the time the trial was interrupted revealed no benefit in terms of mortality, even in the subgroups with a history of congestive heart failure, pulmonary edema or heart failure on admission to the coronary care unit.

The different results between CONSENSUS-2 and the other trials can be explained by the use of an intravenous vasodilator which not only lowers mean arterial pressure but also lowers ventricular filling pressures, narrowing myocardial perfusion pressure, and potentially causing additional ischemia. These results are in agreement with other failed attempts to lower ventricular afterload with intravenous vasodilators during the acute phase of acute myocardial infarction. In addition, the follow-up for the CONSENSUS-2 trial was aborted, and it is theoretically possible that a longer follow-up would reveal a benefit of enalapril therapy over and above the potentially harmful effects of the early intravenous administration of the agent. By contrast, in the SMILE trial the ACE inhibitor was administered early by mouth with careful monitoring of blood pressure reduction in the acute post-infarct period.

Indications for ACE inhibition after myocardial infarction

The results of large clinical trials strongly support the use of ACE inhibitors in patients who have suffered myocardial infarction.[38] The benefits are clearly greater in patients with large infarctions: patients with anterior wall infarctions, significant left ventricular dysfunction and signs or symptoms of heart failure early after coronary thrombosis should receive ACE inhibition by mouth as soon as they are considered stable hemodynamically. The starting dose should correspond to 6.25 mg of captopril with progressive increments in the following days or weeks to a dose corresponding to 25–75 mg of captopril three times a day. Particular attention should be paid to the possibility of hypotension in these patients (systolic blood pressure should be kept above 95 mmHg during the acute post-infarction period). In patients with small inferior infarctions, the benefits of such agents are reduced by the absence of left ventricular dilatation and limited dysfunction as a consequence of the initial insult. The value of these agents in preventing reinfarction[44,51] over and above its effect on ventricular remodeling has not been established empirically, but is currently the object of intense investigation.

Future trends

Ventricular remodeling after myocardial infarction refers to the architectural and functional alterations which occur in response to myocardial loss caused by sudden oxygen deprivation.[2–4] During post-infarct remodeling the left ventricle dilates and becomes distorted assuming complex shapes depending on the size and location of the infarcted

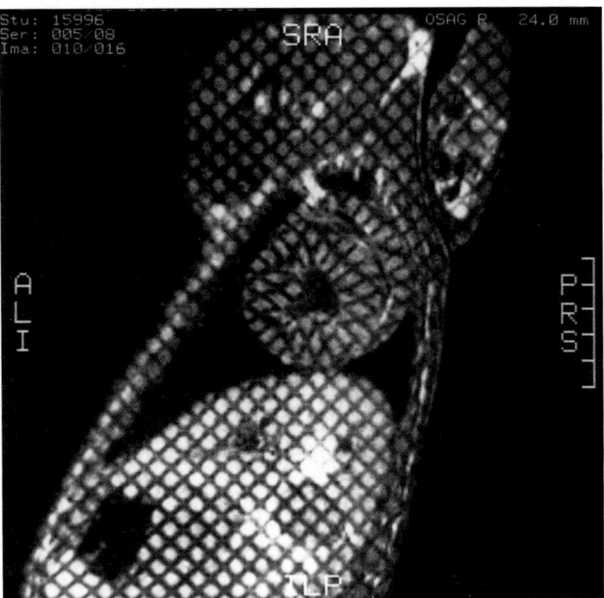

Figure 5.12
Left ventricular cross-section of canine ventricle at mid-systole. Myocardial tags placed at end-diastole in a grid pattern (Spatial Modulation of Magnetization)[4,53,54] are not deformed in the liver but have deformed in the myocardium reflecting muscle contraction during systole.

region.[1,12,15] The possibility of multiple infarcted segments further complicates the ventricular anatomical response to myocardial loss by disrupting the intricate balance of mechanical forces which produce normal left ventricular systolic emptying and diastolic filling. For these reasons, methods which allow a detailed assessment of segmental architecture and function are necessary for a better understanding of the remodeling process.

Magnetic resonance imaging has the potential to fill this gap[4,52,53] by providing a three-dimensional assessment of ventricular architecture coupled with myocardial tagging (Fig. 5.12). This method consists of exciting a plane of myocardial protons at end-diastole, in an orientation which is perfectly perpendicular to the plane of imaging.[52] Such alteration in the state of magnetization will persist for typically 500 s in spin-echo imaging, resulting in stripes which accurately index myocardial motion during a given time interval, typically during systole or diastole. This methodology permits a precise characterization of segmental myocardial motion and deformation[54] which can be repeated serially to study the remodeling process in evolution (Fig. 5.13). Initial studies in experimental models[4] have led to ongoing clinical studies (Fig. 5.14) which may contribute significantly to our understanding of the remodeling process.

Similarly, the characterization of myocardial remodeling at the cellular level is crucial to a better understanding of ventricular post-infarct architectural and functional alterations. Myocyte slippage[19] and elongation,[25,32–34] (Fig. 5.15) take place in the hours or days which immediately follow myocardial infarction. However, the intracellular signals which trigger protein production, sarcomere assembly, and cellular elongation are still unknown. The possibility that such processes occur at different rates in different regions of the left ventricle is underscored by recent studies which have emphasized regional differences in myocyte hypertrophy and dysfunction in the remodeled ventricle.[32–34] Cellular alterations appear to be greater in the regions adjacent to the infarct scar relative to those located far from the infarcted region. Moreover, myocyte elongation appears to result from a cascade of intracellular processes which involve the tyrosine kinase pathway at the membrane level.[32] This pathway may be activated by the angiotensin II receptor, which appears to play an important role as the transducer of mechanical and/or humoral stimuli which instruct the surviving myocyte to hypertrophy.[55] After myocardial infarction, this cascade of intracellular processes could be triggered in response to the augmented stress caused by the burden of maintaining the circulation with fewer contractile units. The elucidation of intracellular mechanisms responsible for myocyte hypertrophy and failure may provide future avenues for controlling the response to infarction by specific modulation of myocardial post-infarct remodeling.

Summary

Left ventricular post-infarct remodeling represents in part an adaptive response to significant myocardial loss after coronary occlusion, and in part a malignant process leading to greater chamber dysfunction and heart failure. The process consists of left ventricular cavity enlargement, left ventricular eccentric hypertrophy, and infarct healing which is more intense in the subacute post-infarct period, but persists for weeks after infarction. Moreover, cavity dilatation continues beyond infarct healing in patients with large infarcts with progressive decline in global left ventricular function. ACE inhibitors can reduce the magnitude of post-infarct remodeling and at the same time decrease the risk of untoward complications after acute myocardial infarction.

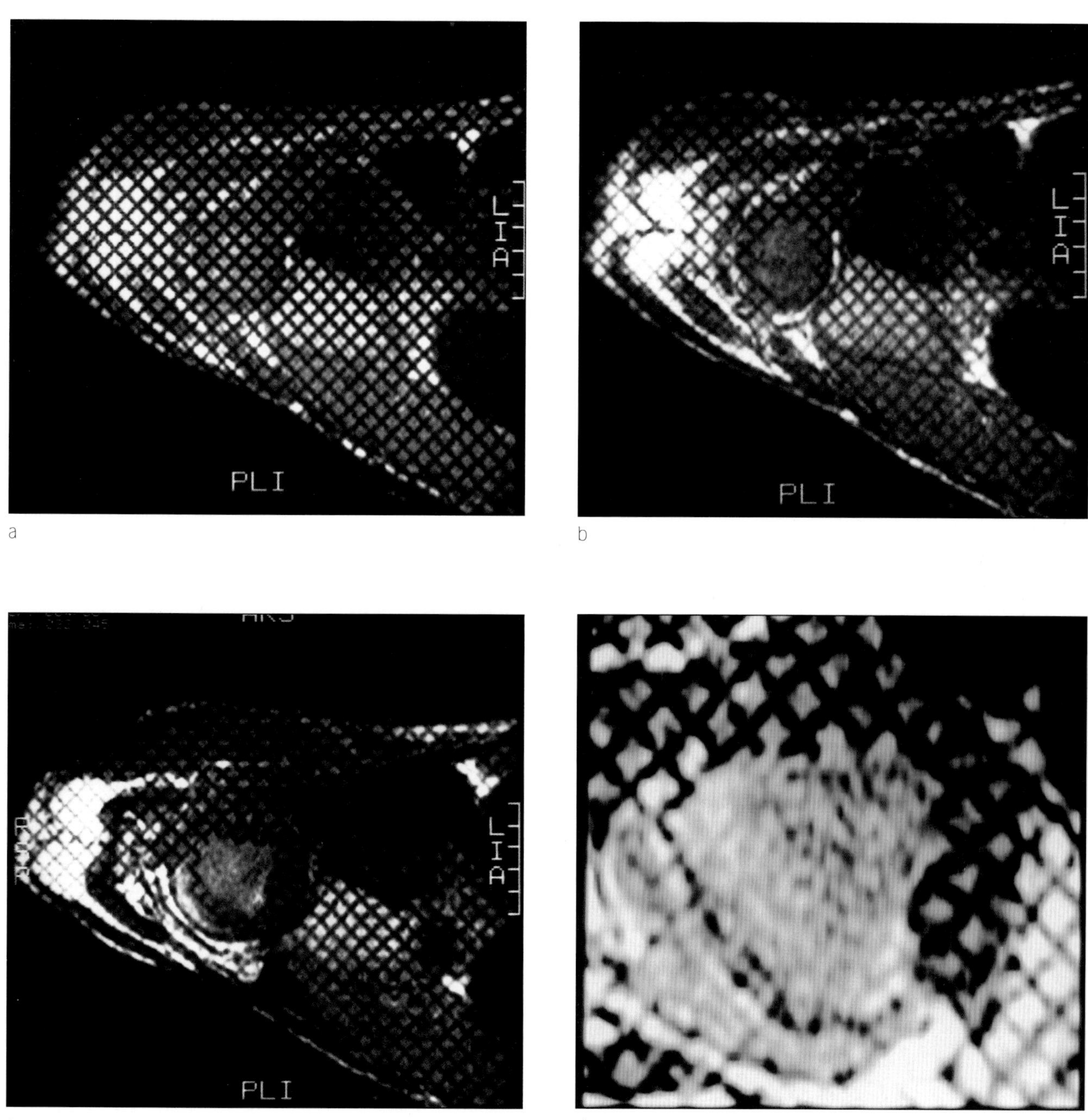

Figure 5.13
The same method illustrated in Figure 5.12 was used to study left ventricular cross-section of infarcted ovine hearts 8 weeks after coronary occlusion. (a) At end-diastole, because all cardiac and surrounding structures are marked by tagging, it is difficult to discern cardiac structures from intracavitary blood. (b) At end-systole, tags within both ventricles have vanished and those in non-infarcted myocardium are deformed by systolic myocardial contraction. The infarcted septum appears thin secondary to the infarct scar. (c) Left ventricular cross-section at mid-systole but at a more basal plane than previous panels. Myocardial tags have undergone significant deformation, particularly in non-infarcted regions like the left ventricular free wall. (d) Left ventricular cross-section of a different animal obtained at end-systole. The infarcted septum appears thin secondary to infarct scar. Myocardial tags in non-infarcted regions are deformed by systolic contraction.

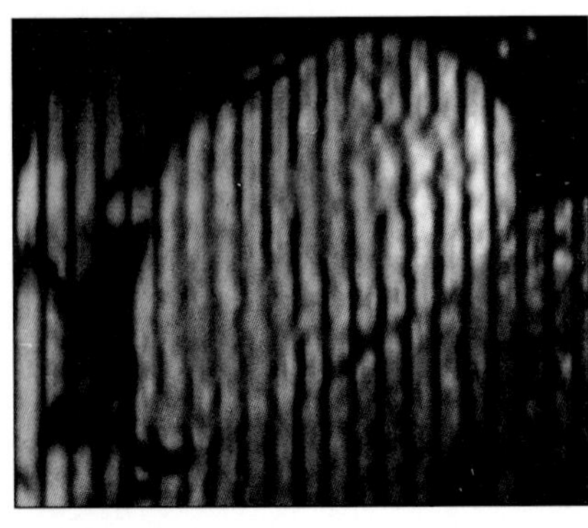
a

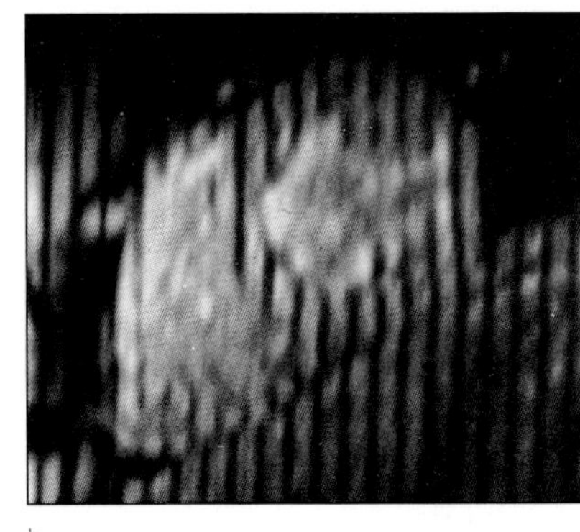
b

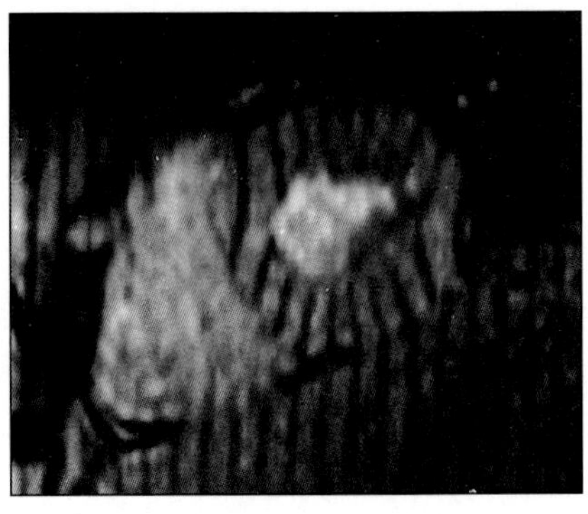
c

Figure 5.14
Left ventricular cross-section of a patient with a large inferior wall infarction 6 months after coronary occlusion. Myocardial tags placed in a striped pattern were applied using a modified spoiled GRASS pulse sequence which allows fast imaging by magnetic resonance imaging. (a) At end-diastole, similar to Figure 5.13a, magnetic tags involve intracavitary blood and myocardium. (b) Early in systole tags no longer present within the cavity but show some degree of systolic deformation in the myocardium. (c) At end-systole, myocardial tags reflect systolic myocardial deformation.

References

1 Bulkley B, Hutchins G, Bulkley BH: Infarct expansion versus extension: two different complications of acute myocardial infarction. *Am J Cardiol* 1978; **41**: 1127–32.

2 McKay RG, Pfeffer MA, Pasternak RC et al: Left ventricular remodeling following myocardial infarction; a corollary to infarct expansion. *Circulation* 1986; **74**: 693–702.

3 Pfeffer MA, Braunwald E: Ventricular remodeling after myocardial infarction. *Circulation* 1990; **81**: 1161–72.

4 Kramer CM, Lima JAC, Reichek N et al: Regional differences in function within noninfarcted myocardium during left ventricular remodeling. *Circulation* 1993; **88**: 1279–88.

5 Gaudron P, Eilles C, Kugler I, Ertl G: Progressive left ventricular dysfunction and remodeling after myocardial infarction. Potential mechanisms and early predictors. *Circulation* 1993; **87**: 755–63.

6 Erlebacher JA, Weiss JL, Eaton LW et al: Late effects of acute infarct dilatation on heart size: a two dimensional echocardiographic study. *Am J Cardiol* 1982; **49**: 1120–6.

7 Jugdutt BI, Amy RWN: Healing after myocardial infarction in the dog; changes in infarct hydroxyproline and topography. *J Am Coll Cardiol* 1986; **7**: 91–102.

8 Eaton LW, Weiss JL, Bulkley BH et al: Regional cardiac dilatation after acute myocardial infarction. *N Engl J Med* 1979; **300**: 57–62.

9 Goto Y, Igarashi Y, Yamada O et al: Hyperkinesis without the Frank–Starling mechanism in a nonischemic region of acutely ischemic excised canine heart. *Circulation* 1988; **77**: 468–77.

10 Meizlish JL, Berger HJ, Plankey M et al: Functional left ventricular aneurysm formation after acute anterior transmural myocardial infarction: incidence, natural history and prognostic implications. *N Engl J Med* 1984; **311**: 1001–6.

11 Pfeffer MA, Pfeffer JM, Fishbein MC et al: Myocardial infarct size and ventricular function in rats. *Circ Res* 1979; **44**: 503–12.

12 Mitchel GF, Lamas GA, Vaughan ED, Pfeffer MA: Left ventricular remodeling in the year after first anterior myocardial infarction: a quantitative analysis of contractile segment lengths and ventricular shape. *J Am Coll Cardiol* 1992; **19**: 1136–44.

13 Grossman W, Jones D, McLaurin LP: Wall stress patterns of hypertrophy in the human left ventricle. *J Clin Invest* 1975; **56**: 56–64.

14 Bigger JT, Fleiss JL, Kleiger R et al: The relationships among ventricular arrhythmias, left ventricular dysfunction, and mortality in the 2 years after myocardial infarction. *Circulation* 1984; **69**: 250–60.

15 Marino P, Kass D, Lima JAC et al: Influence of site of regional ischemia on LV cavity shape change in dogs. *Am J Physiol* 1988; **254**: H547–H557.

16 Picard MH, Wilkins GT, Ray PA, Weyman AE: Natural history of left ventricular size and function after acute

myocardial infarction. Assessment and prediction by echocardiographic endocardial surface mapping. *Circulation* 1990; **82**: 484–94.

17 Izumi S, Miyatake K, Beppu S et al: Mechanism of mitral regurgitation in patients with myocardial infarction: a study using real-time two-dimensional Doppler flow imaging and echocardiography. *Circulation* 1987; **76**: 777–85.

18 Llaneras MR, Nance ML, Streicher JT et al: Pathogenesis of ischemic mitral insufficiency. *J Thorac Cardiovasc Surg* 1993; **105**: 439–43.

19 Weissman HF, Bush DE, Mannisi JA et al: Cellular mechanisms of myocardial infarct expansion. *Circulation* 1988; **76**: 186–201.

20 Jugdutt BI, Basualdo CA: Myocardial infarct expansion during indomethacin or ibuprofen therapy for symptomatic post-infarction pericarditis: influence of other pharmacologic agents during remodeling. *Can J Cardiol* 1989; **5**: 211–21.

21 Nolan SE, Mannisi JA, Bush DE et al: Increased afterload aggravates infarct expansion after acute myocardial infarction. *J Am Coll Cardiol* 1988; **12**: 1318–25.

22 Marino P, Zanolla L, Zardini P on behalf of GISSI: Effect of streptokinase on left ventricular modeling and function after myocardial infarction: the GISSI (Greppo Italiano per lo studio della Streptochinaisi nell'Infarto Miocardico) trial. *J Am Coll Cardiol* 1989; **14**: 1149–58.

23 Koren GT, Hasin Y, Appelbaum D et al: Prevention of myocardial damage in acute myocardial ischemia by early treatment with intravenous streptokinase. *N Engl J Med* 1985; **313**: 1384–9.

24 Hochman JS, Choo H: Limitation of myocardial infarct expansion by reperfusion independent of myocardial salvage. *Circulation* 1987; **75**: 299–306.

25 Anversa P, Laoud AV, Levicky V, Guilderi G. Left ventricular failure induced by myocardial infarction. I. Myocyte hypertrophy. *Am J Physiol* 1985; **248**: H876–H882.

26 Lessick J, Sideman S, Azhari H et al: Regional three-dimensional geometry and function of left ventricles with fibrous aneurysm. *Circulation* 1991; **84**: 1071–86.

27 Bogen DK, Rabinowitz SA, Needleman A et al: An analysis of the mechanical disadvantage of myocardial infarction in the canine left ventricle. *Circ Res* 1980; **47**: 728–41.

28 Lima JAC, Becker LC, Melin JA et al: Impaired thickening of nonischemic myocardium during acute regional ischemia in the dog. *Circulation* 1985; **71**: 1048–59.

29 Gallagher KP, Gerren RA, Starling MC et al: The distribution of functional impairment across the lateral border of acutely ischemic myocardium. *Circ Res* 1986; **58**: 570–83.

30 Force T, Kemper A, Perkins L et al: Overestimation of infarct size by quantitative two-dimensional echocardiography: the role of tethering and of analytic procedures. *Circulation* 1986; **73**: 1360–8.

31 Swedberg K, Eneroth P, Kjekshus J, Wilhelmsen L: Hormones regulating cardiovascular function in patients with severe congestive heart failure and their relation to mortality. CONSENSUS trial Study Group. *Circulation* 1990; **82**: 1730–6.

32 Melillo G, Lima JAC, Judd RM et al: Intrinsic myocyte dysfunction and tyrosine kinase pathway activation underlie the impaired wall thickening of adjacent regions during post-infarct left ventricular remodeling. *Circulation* April, 1995.

33 Olivetti G, Capasse JM, Meggs LG et al: Cellular basis of chronic ventricular remodeling after myocardial infarction in rats. *Circ Res* 1991; **68**: 856–69.

34 Kozlovskis PL, Silver JD, Rubin RW et al: Regional variations in myosin heavy chain concentration after healing of experimental myocardial infarction in cats. *J Mol Cell Cardiol* 1984; **16**: 559–66.

35 Barber MJ, Mueller TM, Henry DP et al: Transmural myocardial infarction in the dog produces sympathectomy in non-infarcted myocardium. *Circulation* 1983; **67**: 787–96.

36 Liedke AJ, Nellis SH, Whetesell LF: Effects of regional ischemia on metabolic function in adjacent aerobic myocardium. *J Mol Cell Cardiol* 1982; **14**: 195–205.

37 Gough WB, Mehra R, Restivo M et al: Reentrant ventricular arrhythmias in the late myocardial infarction period in the dog. 13. Correlation of activation and refractory maps. *Circ Res* 1985; **57**: 432–42.

38 Ball SG, Hall AS, Murray GD: Angiotensin-converting enzyme inhibitors after myocardial infarction: indications and timing. *J Am Coll Cardiol* 1995; **25**(suppl):42S–46S.

39 Chesebro JH, Knatterud G, Roberts R et al: Thrombolysis in myocardial infarction (TIMI) trial, Phase I: a comparison between intravenous tissue plasminogen activator and intravenous streptokinase. *Circulation* 1987; **76**: 142–54.

40 ISIS-3 (Third International Study of Infarct Survival) Collaborative Group: ISIS-3: a randomized comparison of streptokinase vs. tissue plasminogen activator vs. anistreplase and of aspirin plus heparin vs. aspirin alone among 41,229 cases of suspected acute myocardial infarction. *Lancet* 1992; **339**: 753–70.

41 Pfeffer JM, Pfeffer MA, Braunwald E: Influence of chronic captopril therapy on the infarcted left ventricle of the rat. *Circ Res* 1985; **57**: 84–95.

42 Pfeffer M, Lamas G, Vaughan D et al: Effect of captopril on progressive ventricular dilatation after anterior myocardial infarction. *N Engl J Med* 1988; **319**: 80–6.

43 Sharpe N, Smith H, Murphy J, Hannan SP: Treatment of patients with symptomless left ventricular dysfunction after myocardial infarction. *Lancet* 1988; **1**: 255–9.

44 Pfeffer MA, Braunwald E, Moye LA et al: Effect of captopril on mortality and morbidity in patients with left ventricular dysfunction after myocardial infarction. Results of the Survival and Ventricular Enlargement Trial. *N Engl J Med* 1992; **327**: 669–77.

45 St John Sutton M, Pfeffer MA, Plappert T et al: Quantitative two-dimensional echocardiographic measurements are major predictors of adverse cardiovascular events after acute myocardial infarction: the protective effects of captopril. *Circulation* 1994; **89**: 68–75.

46 The Acute Infarction Ramipril Efficacy (AIRE) Study Investigators: Effect of ramipril on mortality and morbidity of survivors of acute myocardial infarction with clinical evidence of heart failure. *Lancet* 1993; **342**: 821–8.

47 Ambrosioni E, Borghi C, Magnani B on behalf of the SMILE Study Investigators: Effects of the early administration of zofenopril on mortality and morbidity in patients with anterior myocardial infarction. Results of the Survival of Myocardial Infarction Long-Term Evaluation Trial. *N Engl J Med* 1995; **332**: 80–5.

48 Gruppo Italiano per lo Studio della Sopravvivenza nell'Infarto Miocardico: GISSI-3: effects of lisinopril and transdermal glyceryl trinitrate singly and together on 6-week mortality and ventricular function after acute myocardial infarction. *Lancet* 1994; **343**: 1115–22.

49 ISIS 4 Collaborative Group: Fourth International Study of Infarct Survival: protocol for a large simple study of the effects of oral mononitrate, of oral captopril and of intravenous magnesium. *Am J Cardiol* 1991; **68**: 87D–100D.

50 Swedberg K, Held P, Kjekshus J et al: Effects of the early administration of enalapril on mortality in patients with acute myocardial infarction. Results of the Cooperative New Scandinavian Enalapril Survival Study II (CONSENSUS II). *N Eng J Med* 1992; **327**: 678–84.

51 Yusef S, Pepine C, Garces C et al: Effect of enalapril on myocardial infarction and unstable angina in patients with low ejection fraction. *Lancet* 1992; **340**: 1173–8.

52 Zerhouni E, Parish D, Rogers WJ et al: Human heart: tagging with MR imaging—a method for noninvasive measurement of myocardial motion. *Radiology* 1988; **169**: 59–64.

53 Clark N, Reichek N, Bergey P et al: Normal segmental myocardial function: assessment by magnetic resonance imaging using spatial modulation of magnetization. *Circulation* 1991; **84**: 67–74.

54 Lima JAC, Ferrari VA, Reichek N et al: Segmental motion and deformation of transmurally infarcted myocardium in acute postinfarct period. *Am J Physiol* 1995; **268**: H1304–H1312.

55 Sadoshima J, Qiu Z, Morgan JP, Izumo S. Angiotensin II and other hypertrophic stimuli mediated by G protein-coupled receptors activate tyrosine kinase, mitogen activated protein kinase, and 90-kD S6 kinase in cardiac myocytes. The critical role of calcium-dependent signaling. *Circ Res* 1995; **76**: 1–15.

56 Jugdutt BI, Michorowski BL: Role of infarct expansion in rupture of the ventricular septum after acute myocardial infarction: a two-dimensional echocardiographic study. *Clin Cardiol* 1987; **10**: 641–52.

6

Mitral regurgitation

Jennifer W Tanio and Nicholas J Fortuin

One can recognize the presence of mitral regurgitation readily by auscultation. Imaging techniques are employed to answer the following questions:

1. What is the etiology of the valvular lesion?
2. What is its severity?
3. What is the natural history likely to be?
4. What are the effects of the lesion on other cardiac structures, such as the left ventricular myocardium and the pulmonary vasculature?

The answers to these questions permit physicians to plan appropriate management and correctly time surgical intervention.

The mitral valve apparatus is composed of a fibrous annulus, two major leaflets (anterior and posterior), two (or three) papillary muscles, and multiple chordae tendineae which interconnect the papillary muscles and the leaflets. The anterior leaflet, which is adjacent to the aortic valve, is larger and semicircular in shape. The posterior leaflet is tripartite, with anterolateral, posteromedial, and middle scallops. Each leaflet is connected to both papillary muscles by multiple branching chordae tendineae. The anterolateral papillary muscle generally receives blood supply from both the left anterior descending and the left circumflex coronary arteries, while the posteromedial papillary muscle is only supplied by the posterior descending coronary artery. In the adult, the normal mitral valve cross-sectional area is 4–6 cm^2.

Mitral regurgitation may result from alterations in any part of the apparatus, as well as abnormalities in left ventricular wall motion in areas adjacent to the insertion of the papillary muscles. Numerous disease processes may impair the function of each component of the mitral apparatus. Imaging techniques allow easy recognition of mitral regurgitation and, more importantly, a determination of the etiology and (within limits) the severity of this condition. In addition, imaging techniques can provide information about the size and function of various cardiac chambers and the pulmonary artery pressure.

Imaging and mitral regurgitation

Echocardiography has proven to be the most useful imaging modality in the evaluation of mitral regurgitation. Two-dimensional and to a lesser extent M-mode echocardiography can detect abnormalities in valve structure such as congenital defects, rheumatic scarring, myxomatous disease, mitral valve vegetations, and chordal/papillary muscle rupture. These modalities provide information about chamber sizes and left ventricular function. This can help to estimate chronicity and severity, and to suggest the appropriate timing and risk of surgery.[1–4]

Doppler techniques (both color flow and pulsed/continuous wave) are used to demonstrate the regurgitant jet of mitral regurgitation and to map its location in the left atrium (Fig. 6.1). This may be useful in assessing severity (vide infra). Pulsed Doppler detects mitral regurgitation with a sensitivity and specificity of ≥90% and ≥95%, respectively.[5] Color flow Doppler, which is slightly more sensitive than pulsed or continuous wave Doppler, is sometimes used to ascertain the mechanism of regurgitation. For example, an extremely eccentric anteriorly directed jet suggests posterior leaflet prolapse, due to myxomatous degeneration or papillary muscle dysfunction. It is important to note that nearly half of normal subjects aged 6–49

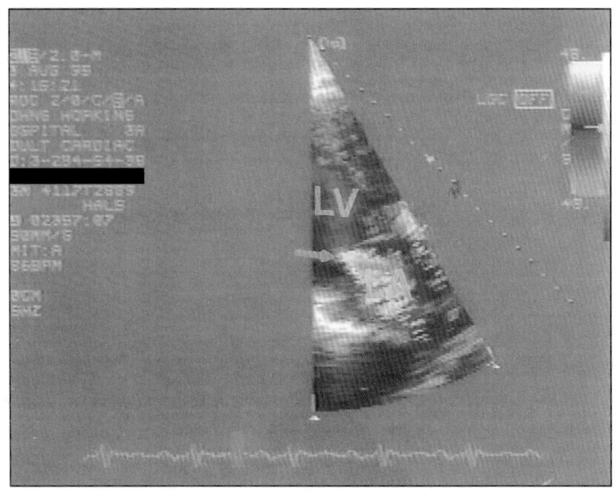

a

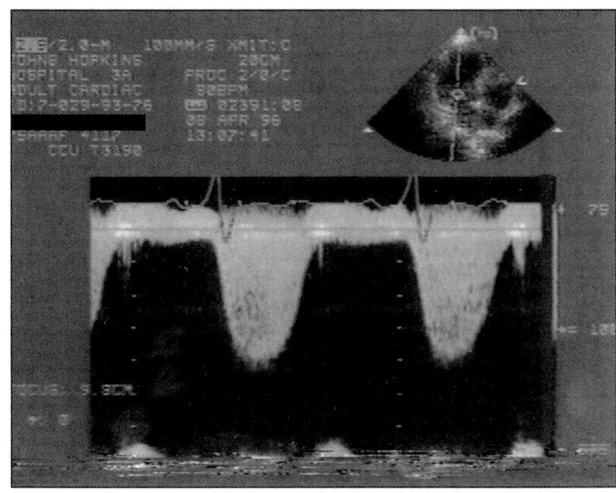

b

Figure 6.1 (a) Color mosaic (arrow) seen in the left atrium represents the jet of mitral regurgitation (LA: left atrium, LV: left ventricle). (b) Continuous wave Doppler interrogation demonstrates retrograde flow into the left atrium during systole consistent with mitral regurgitation.

years have some degree of mitral regurgitation on echocardiographic examination.[6] Echo-demonstrated mild mitral regurgitation occurring in a structurally normal heart without an audible murmur is unlikely to be of clinical significance.

Continuous wave Doppler can measure the peak velocity of a tricuspid regurgitation jet and estimate the right ventricular systolic pressure by the equation:

$$P = 4v^2 + 10$$

where v is the maximal regurgitant velocity (Fig. 6.2).

Assuming a normal pulmonic valve, this is an approximation of the pulmonary artery systolic pressure. Contrast echocardiography has been used to measure mitral regurgitation, but this technique is not yet in widespread clinical use.

Because of the superior image quality provided by the transesophageal approach, transesophageal echocardiography (TEE) often provides more information than transthoracic echocardiography (TTE) in certain clinical situations, including papillary muscle and chordal rupture, left atrial masses, leaflet perforation, and mechanical prosthetic mitral valve regurgitation.[7–9] TEE can interrogate the pulmonary veins, which are usually poorly seen in adults by TTE. Additionally, TEE is valuable in the intraoperative assessment of mitral regurgitation as it does not interfere with the sterile field. It must be noted, however, that TEE regurgitant jets are generally larger than those seen on TTE. Therefore, at least some of the criteria currently in use for the echocardiographic grading of severity of mitral regurgitation may need to be re-examined for TEE.[10,11]

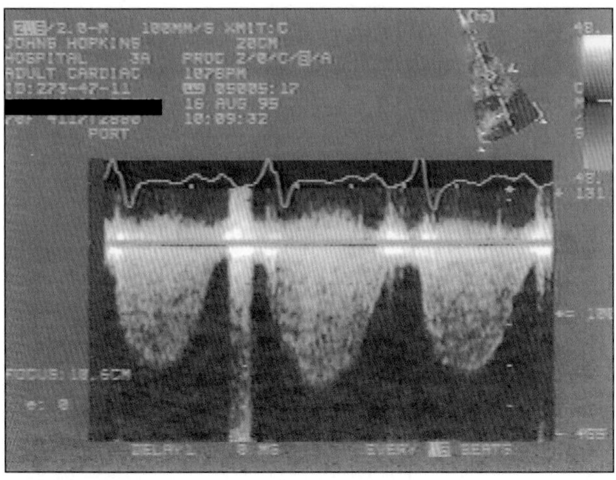

Figure 6.2
The velocity spectrum of tricuspid regurgitation is shown by continuous wave Doppler. Maximum velocity is approximately 3 m/s, consistent with a pulmonary artery systolic pressure of 36 mmHg plus right atrial pressure.

Evaluation of severity of mitral regurgitation

There is controversy regarding the optimal echocardiographic method for evaluating the degree of mitral regurgitation. Left atrial and left ventricular size are correlates of the severity of mitral regurgitation and are useful in assessing severity in chronic regurgitation. Generally, mild regurgitation is indicated by a left ventricular end diastolic cavity dimension of below 6 cm, moderate by 6–7 cm, and severe by greater than 7 cm. However, these values are less useful if chambers are normal sized, mitral regurgitation is of acute onset, or if left ventricular dysfunction or other valve disease is present.[12] Characteristics of the continuous wave Doppler signal which have been used for qualitative description of mitral regurgitation include signal strength and the presence of a late systolic 'shoulder' on the velocity curve.[5] Various properties of the jet seen on color flow Doppler may correlate with mitral regurgitation severity as determined by angiography (usually considered to be the 'gold standard') including the area of the maximum regurgitant jet, the depth of penetration of the jet retrograde into the left atrium, and the ratio of jet area to left atrial area.[13–15] There are numerous limitations to the accuracy of these techniques, since the size and depth of the jet depends on such technical factors as changes in transducer frequency and gain setting, echo factors such as jet eccentricity (the Coanda phenomenon), and clinical factors such as left atrial size and compliance, and preload and afterload.[16] It has been our experience that with color flow imaging, mitral regurgitation is overestimated in low output states, such as dilated cardiomyopathy, and underestimated in patients with eccentric jets. As a result, we cannot support the common practice of using this technique to make definitive statements about the severity of regurgitation.

There are several quantitative methods used to assess severity from Doppler data. Regurgitant fraction (RF) derived by echo is determined as follows:

$$RF = (LVI - LVO)/LVI$$

where LVI = left ventricular inflow = mitral valve orifice (the distance between the bases of the mitral leaflets in the apical four chamber view) × the integral of the transmitral flow velocity during diastole; and

LVO = left ventricular outflow = aortic valve orifice × the integral of the transaortic flow velocity during systole.

This calculation is confounded by coexisting mitral stenosis or atrial fibrillation, however.

Another way to assess the severity of mitral regurgitation involves the interrogation of pulmonary vein flow velocity. In normal subjects, there is phasic forward flow in the pulmonary veins during systole and early diastole, and retrograde flow in late diastole during atrial contraction. Forward flow during systole decreases with mitral regurgitation, and can even reverse direction with severe disease (Fig. 6.3).[17] However, decreased forward flow in systole can also occur due to other causes of elevated left atrial pressure, such as occurs in left ventricular dysfunction.

One of the newest and most promising techniques for echocardiographic quantification of mitral regurgitation,

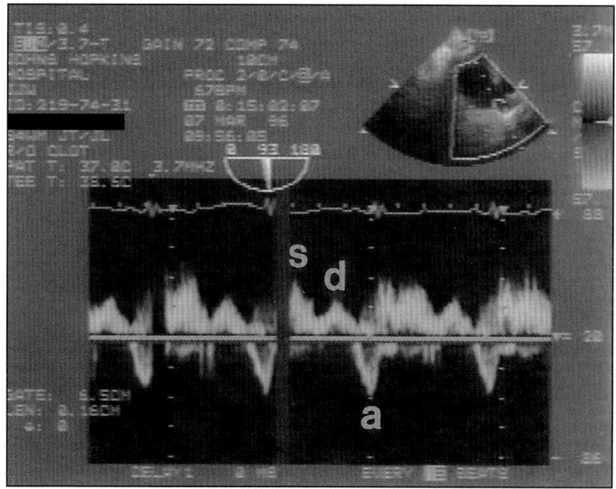

a

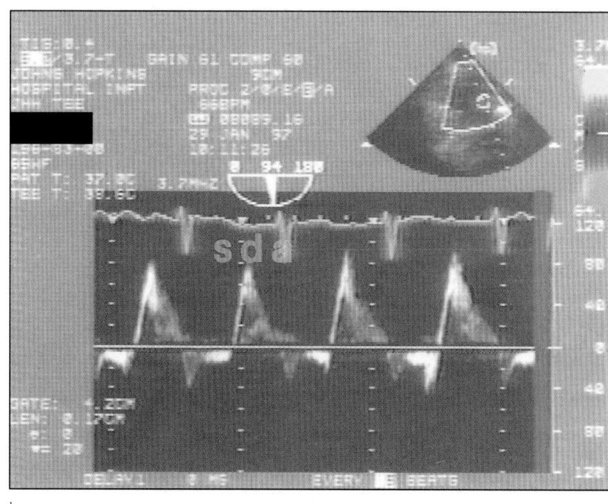

b

Figure 6.3 (a) Normal pulmonary vein flow, consisting of antegrade flow in systole (s) and early diastole [d], and retrograde flow with atrial systole [a]. (b) Abnormal pulmonary vein flow in a patient with severe mitral regurgitation; note that there is retrograde flow during systole.

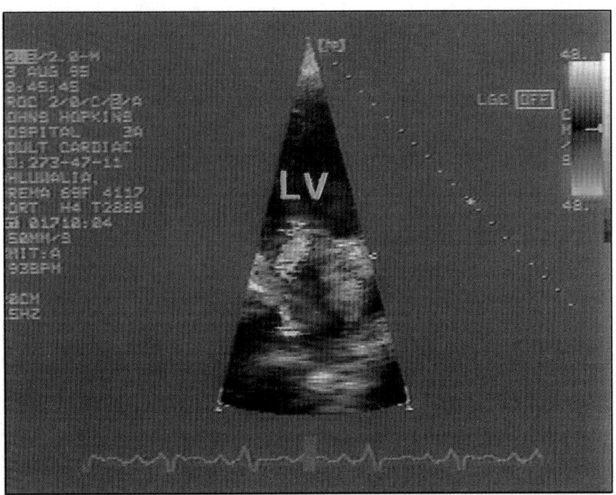

Figure 6.4
The hemispheric flow convergence region (FCR) is seen on the left ventricular side of the mitral valve during systole (see text).

known as the proximal isovelocity surface area (PISA) method, is based on the phenomenon of flow acceleration proximal to a regurgitant orifice.[18] Flow in this region gradually increases in velocity such that a series of hemispheric isovelocity surfaces is formed. These three-dimensional shells converge on the valve orifice, which is at their center. With mitral regurgitation, this is seen on color flow Doppler imaging as a rainbow of color on the ventricular side of the mitral valve (Fig. 6.4). This area is referred to as the flow convergence region (FCR).[19] Each 'color' in the rainbow represents an isovelocity shell. By the continuity principle, the flow crossing each of the isovelocity shells must be equal and must also equal the flow through the regurgitant orifice, and therefore:

$$\text{regurgitant flow rate} = 2\pi r^2 \times Vr$$

when r = radius of the measured shell;
$2\pi r^2$ = the surface area of that shell;
Vr = velocity of that shell.[20]

Peak flow rates of >500 ml/s generally correlate with several mitral regurgitations, and the absence of the FCR usually indicates mild regurgitation.[19] Regurgitant area (RA) is calculated as follows:

$$\text{RA} = \text{regurgitant flow/regurgitant velocity}$$

Regurgitant velocity is measured using continuous wave Doppler.

This can then be used to calculate the regurgitant stroke volume by integrating over a cardiac cycle:

$$\text{regurgitant stroke volume} = \text{regurgitant velocity time integral} \times \text{RA}$$

There are limitations to this technique as well, most significantly operator skill. However, unlike most of the methods above, it is not affected by factors which alter the distal regurgitant jet size.[19]

Contrast cardiac angiography is often used to assess the severity of mitral regurgitation. The extent of retrograde penetration of dye into the left atrium following left ventricular injection is used to grade the degree of regurgitation as follows:

- 0—none;
- 1+ (mild)—incomplete opacification of the left atrium, contrast clears with each beat;
- 2+ (moderate)—incomplete opacification of the left atrium less than that of the left ventricle after several beats, contrast does not clear with each beat;
- 3+ (moderately severe)—almost complete opacification of left atrium, intensity equal to that of the left ventricle;
- 4+ (severe)—almost complete opacification of the left atrium after the first beat, degree equal to that of the left ventricle, contrast may reflux into the pulmonary veins during systole.[9]

Regurgitant fraction can also be measured using ventricular angiography to measure total left ventricular stroke volume (SV_{total}) in an analogous fashion to that described above:

$$\text{regurgitant volume} = SV_{total} - SV_{forward}$$
$$\text{RF} = \text{regurgitant volume}/SV_{total}$$

A regurgitant fraction of >60% indicates severe, 40–60% moderate, and <40% mild mitral regurgitation.[21]

Left ventricular angiography is often considered to be the 'gold standard' for measuring the severity of mitral regurgitation. However, this scoring system is imprecise and subject to error from such factors as catheter position, chamber sizes, quantity and rate of injection of contrast, and dysrhythmias.[22]

Left ventricular function and mitral regurgitation

Another controversial issue is the assessment of left ventricular function in the patient with mitral regurgitation. Making the decision to proceed with surgery involves the consideration of many factors, but evaluation of systolic function can help the clinician to time and predict correctly the outcome of operative intervention. Diminished preoperative left ventricular contractile function is associated with postoperative left ventricular dysfunction and decreased postoperative survival.[1,3] Unfortunately, true myocardial function is notoriously difficult to assess in the patient with mitral regurgitation. Ejection fraction and left ventricular fractional shortening are easily obtained by echocardiography. However, increased preload and decreased afterload due to a low impedance pathway into the left atrium tend to lead to an increase in these indices of left ventricular contraction.[9] Indeed, patients with ejection fractions in the 'normal' range may already have some degree of left ventricular dysfunction.[23] Preload independent parameters such as left ventricular end-systolic volume and end-systolic volume index have been used to detect patients with early myocardial dysfunction, before ejection fraction falls.[9] The end-systolic wall stress to end-systolic volume index ratio, preload and afterload independent, has been shown to be an excellent predictor of postoperative outcome.[24] In general, complex measurements of left ventricular function are most useful in planning the timing of surgery in the asymptomatic patient with mitral regurgitation and a 'borderline' ejection fraction in the 55–60% range.[2] Simply derived ejection fraction remains a powerful predictor of postoperative outcome.[3,4]

Left ventricular angiography is a reliable way to study left ventricular function and end-systolic volume in patients with mitral regurgitation, but it offers no advantages over echocardiography for estimating postoperative prognosis.[4]

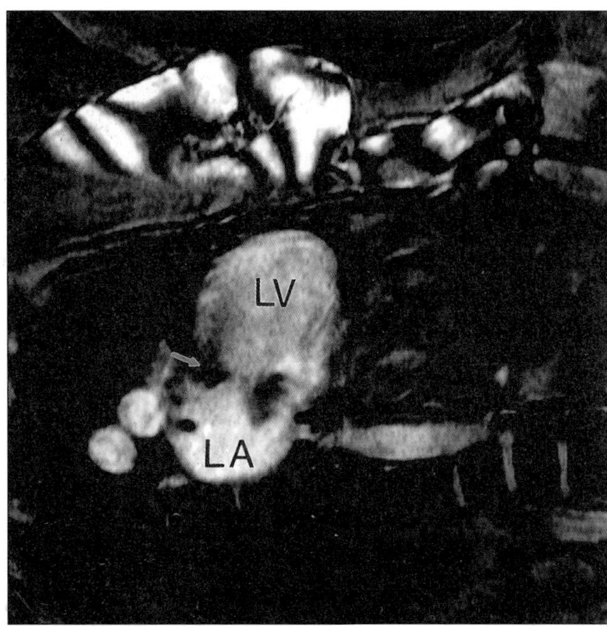

Figure 6.5
Demonstration of mitral regurgitation with magnetic resonance imaging. The arrow marks the 'flow void', which represents the regurgitant jet.

Additional methods for evaluating mitral regurgitation

Right heart catheterization with measurement of the pulmonary capillary wedge pressure may provide useful information in the management of patients with mitral regurgitation. The V wave normally occurs when blood fills the relaxing left atrium, peaking while the mitral valve is still closed during isovolumic relaxation of the left ventricle. Early appearance and increased size of the V wave may be seen with mitral regurgitation. However, V waves can also be present with mitral stenosis, congestive heart failure, and acute ventricular septal defects, and may be small with chronic mitral regurgitation due to increased left atrial compliance.[9,21] Invasive hemodynamic monitoring has been found to be of little use in the differential diagnosis or evaluation of mitral regurgitation in the acute setting.[25]

Radionuclide angiography is infrequently used to evaluate patients with mitral regurgitation. End-systolic left ventricular volume, an excellent predictor of postoperative outcome, is easily assessed by multigated acquisition radionuclide ventriculography (MUGA). The difference between right and left ventricular stroke volumes can be used to estimate the severity of mitral regurgitation. However, this is of little use in the setting of multivalvular disease.

Magnetic resonance imaging (MRI) has been used to study patients with valvular heart disease (Fig. 6.5). Currently available spin echo technology is suboptimal at visualizing the mitral valve structure compared to two-dimensional echo. Cine gradient echo imaging (GRE) can accurately detect endocardial/blood borders, and thus can be used to measure ventricular volumes.[27] The ratio of the size of the flow void seen with GRE to the left atrial area correlates well with Doppler derived measures of mitral regurgitation severity.[28] Cine MRI can provide images of the jet in three dimensions, so total jet volume can be calculated. However, like the measurements derived from color Doppler studies of the regurgitant jet, the size of the flow void is dependent on technical and hemodynamic factors, raising the question of whether this method offers any advantage over Doppler echocardiography. As with radionuclide angiography, regurgitant fraction can be calculated with MRI using differences between right and left ventricular stroke volumes. Velocity encoded cine GRE (VEC) can be used to quantify the actual regurgitant volume.

Mitral valve replacement and mitral valve repair

A major development in the management of the patient with mitral regurgitation has occurred in the past 10–15 years with the advent of excellent surgical techniques for mitral valve repair. It has long been known that patients who undergo mitral valve replacement often suffer a decline in left ventricular contractile function.[2] Initially this was thought to be due to the removal of the low pressure runoff into the left atrium when the valve is made competent. However, many studies have shown that patients who have mitral valve repair rather than mitral valve replacement are more likely to maintain normal ventricular function.[29,30] This may be explained by unfavorable changes in left ventricular geometry caused by interruption of the papillary muscle–valve continuity during mitral valve replacement.[31–33] Interestingly, at least in some groups of patients, leaving the chordopapillary support intact when the mitral valve is replaced is associated with improved survival compared to conventional mitral valve replacement.[34] Since its initial application in patients with mitral regurgitation resulting from myxomatous disease, mitral valve repair has been used in patients with rheumatic,[35] ischemic,[36] and infectious[37] mitral regurgitation.

In addition to its advantages in preserving left ventricular function, mitral valve repair is associated with a decreased risk of stroke and endocarditis compared to mitral valve replacement.[38] Patients who have undergone mitral valve repair do not need long-term anticoagulation if sinus rhythm is maintained. Mitral valve repair has also been shown to have lower operative and postoperative mortality rates, at least in certain patient groups.[36,39] Some studies show evidence of increased long-term survival as well.[40]

Unfortunately, not all patients with mitral regurgitation have valve anatomy that is amenable to repair. Even when repair is done, it is important to evaluate valve function prior to closing the chest so that re-repair or replacement can be performed if necessary. Echocardiography can address both of these concerns. Preoperative echocardiographic studies can determine whether repair is feasible. Myxomatous valves with predominant posterior leaflet prolapse or chordal rupture are best suited to repair. Two-dimensional and Doppler echocardiography have also been used intraoperatively to assess the mechanism of mitral regurgitation so the surgeon can select the optimal repair techniques.[41] Depending on the problem, diverse techniques such as chordal shortening, leaflet resection, chordal resuspension, and annuloplasty can be performed. Artificial chordal implantation has even been performed.[42] Although anterior leaflet procedures were previously less successful than posterior leaflet ones, recent data suggest equivalent short- and long-term results.[43] Intraoperative echocardiography has also been used to look for evidence of residual regurgitation following a repair procedure.[44] Although some investigators have used epicardial echocardiography, TEE is the most widely used approach in this setting.[44]

Specific conditions

Special case—acute mitral regurgitation

Acute mitral regurgitation differs from chronic mitral regurgitation with respect to pathophysiology, clinical presentation, and appropriate management. It can be caused by endocarditis, acute ischemia or myocardial infarction, prosthetic valve failure, chordal rupture due to myxomatous mitral disease, endocarditis or trauma, or rarely acute rheumatic fever. The left atrium and ventricle are not accustomed to the increased volume load, and therefore left ventricular filling pressure and left atrial pressure elevate dramatically, often leading to frank pulmonary edema. A significant amount of the cardiac output is directed backward into the left atrium, and therefore systemic vascular resistance goes up to maintain blood pressure. This leads to a vicious cycle of increasing regurgitant fraction, increased myocardial dilatation, increased myocardial workload, myocardial hypoxemia, and eventual pump failure.

Several echocardiographic findings may be seen with acute mitral regurgitation. The 'snake tongue' sign is the appearance of the high frequency fluttering of a ruptured chord in the left atrium. With papillary muscle rupture, the involved tip may be disconnected from the body of the muscle. The direction of the mitral regurgitant jet distinguishes anterior from posterior flail leaflet; with anterior flail the jet is directed posteriorly, and vice versa. TEE appears to be better at assessing the cause and severity of acute mitral insufficiency than TTE.[10]

Although many of the causes of acute mitral regurgitation are compatible with valve repair procedures, emergent surgery for acute mitral insufficiency is associated with a higher mortality than that for chronic disease.

Myxomatous valvular disease

Myxomatous mitral valve disease is the most common cause of mitral valve prolapse, and is the most common etiology of mitral regurgitation.[45] Indeed, mitral valve prolapse is the most common valvular heart disease, and it is seen in about 4% of the population.[46] Mitral valve prolapse may be familial or sporadic in occurrence. It is seen with diseases such as Marfan's syndrome, Ehlers–Danlos syndrome, pseudoxanthoma elasticum, and osteogenesis imperfecta. As it is commonly associated with bony abnormalities, it has been postulated that it may be part of a generalized connective tissue disorder.[47]

Myxomatous degeneration can affect the aortic, tricuspid, and even pulmonic valves, but most commonly affects the mitral valve. The posterior leaflet is often more severely affected than the anterior leaflet. The leaflets appear redundant and thickened, with an increased surface area. Microscopically, there is proliferation of the spongiosa layer with replacement of the normal dense collagen of the fibrosa layer.[48] The chordae tendineae may become elongated and thinned, and are more subject to spontaneous rupture. Fibrous deposits on the left ventricular surface of the leaflets and friction lesions on the left ventricular endocardium may be seen. It is important to note that mitral prolapse can occur whenever there is a sufficient size disproportion between the mitral leaflets and the left ventricular cavity. Thus, as large and floppy leaflets with a normal cavity lead to prolapse, so will normal-sized leaflets with an unusually small cavity. In the latter case, myxomatous change of the leaflets may be absent.

With myxomatous mitral valve disease, the oversized leaflets billow back into the left atrium during systole. This may lead to failure of leaflet coaptation and mitral regurgitation. Progressively severe mitral regurgitation may be due to annular dilatation, chordal rupture, or the development of endocarditis. Acute mitral regurgitation is caused by spontaneous or traumatic chordal rupture.

Echocardiography is the most useful imaging modality to evaluate myxomatous mitral valve disease. Two-dimensional examination may demonstrate thickened and redundant leaflets. There has been some debate as to the most accurate criteria for diagnosis of mitral valve prolapse. M-mode was originally used to visualize mitral valve prolapse, and typically shows late systolic posterior displacement of the mitral valve. This criterion is generally reliable, with few exceptions, including the presence of a sizable pericardial effusion with posterior swinging of the heart during systole (Fig. 6.6).[49] Other less specific signs include holosystolic hammocking of the valve leaflets and anterior motion of the leaflets in early systole. The most commonly used two-dimensional standard for prolapse is retrograde displacement of the mitral valve leaflets behind the plane of the valve annulus in systole. This is best evaluated in the parasternal long-axis view. Because of the saddle shape of the mitral annulus, using the apical 4-chamber view leads to an increased false positive rate of diagnosis.[50] Of note, this posterior displacement can be affected by changes in left ventricular size, such as occur with dehydration. Color flow Doppler is used to demonstrate mitral regurgitation, which is not always associated with a murmur on physical examination. The relationship between the physical examination

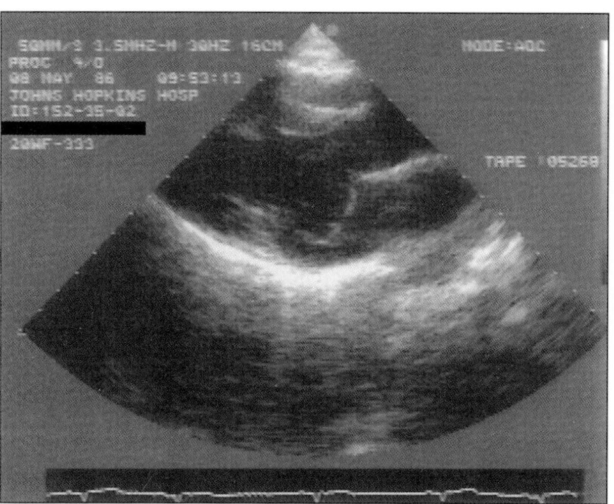

Figure 6.6
Mitral valve prolapse is evident on this 2-D view. Note the posterior displacement of the mitral valve leaflets into the left atrium.

findings of mitral valve prolapse and the typical echocardiographic appearance is not perfect, as some patients may have a consistent physical examination with a normal echo, and vice versa. Echocardiographic examination may also show other intracardiac anomalies known to be associated with myxomatous mitral valve disease, such as fossa ovalis aneurysm, Ebstein's anomaly, and ostium secundum atrial septal defect.

Contrast ventriculography can detect mitral valve prolapse with associated mitral regurgitation. Even in the absence of coronary artery disease, patients with severe mitral valve prolapse may have a peculiar abnormality of mid-ventricular wall motion on ventriculography which can disappear after operative correction.[50]

Patients with mitral valve prolapse may be referred for myocardial stress scintigraphy studies to differentiate chest pain associated with the mitral prolapse syndrome from that due to coronary artery disease. Unfortunately, such patients frequently have fixed or reversible myocardial perfusion defects in the absence of atherosclerotic coronary disease.[51]

Although uncomplicated mitral valve prolapse has a generally benign prognosis, a few patients will develop mitral regurgitation which is severe enough to warrant surgical intervention. Most prolapse-related mitral regurgitation is amenable to mitral valve repair, with its advantages as noted above. However, most centers have significantly more success and experience with posterior leaflet repair as opposed to anterior leaflet repair. Imaging techniques help to suggest the proper timing of surgery, which is often recommended at an earlier stage if repair appears feasible.

There has been some question as to whether all patients with suspected mitral prolapse on the basis of physical examination need an echocardiogram to assess the need for antibiotic prophylaxis. It is our opinion that only those patients with with audible mitral regurgitation on physical examination are at an increased risk for endocarditis.

Rheumatic valvular disease

Rheumatic disease is a rare cause of mitral regurgitation in the USA, although it remains frequent in underdeveloped nations. Rheumatic disease may cause acute or chronic mitral regurgitation. The mitral valve is the most common site of rheumatic valvular involvement, and mitral disease is abut three times as common as aortic valve disease.

Rheumatic carditis leads chronically to scarring and contraction of the chordae and the leaflets, the commissures may fuse, and the mitral valve orifice may become funnel shaped. The leaflets eventually become calcified. The mechanisms of mitral regurgitation due to rheumatic disease include unilateral commissural fusion and calcification which produces a teardrop-shaped orifice, and concentric calcification and fusion which produces a ring-shaped orifice.[47] Mitral regurgitation worsens as the left atrium dilates and distorts the shape of the mitral annulus, thus: 'mitral regurgitation begets more mitral regurgitation'. Interestingly, most patients with rheumatic mitral disease have some combination of mitral regurgitation and mitral stenosis, with an average mitral orifice of about 2 cm^2.[52]

Echocardiographic examination of a mitral valve affected by rheumatic heart disease typically shows thickened leaflets (Fig. 6.7). Areas of incomplete coaptation may be seen in the short-axis view. If some degree of mitral stenosis is present, there may be diastolic doming of the mitral valve, failure of mid-diastolic valve closure, and anterior motion of the posterior mitral leaflet in diastole. Echocardiography can also be used to study the subvalvular structures often affected by rheumatic disease; TEE is superior to TTE. Echocardiographic techniques can demonstrate the posterolaterally directed mitral regurgitant jet typically seen with acute rheumatic fever.[53]

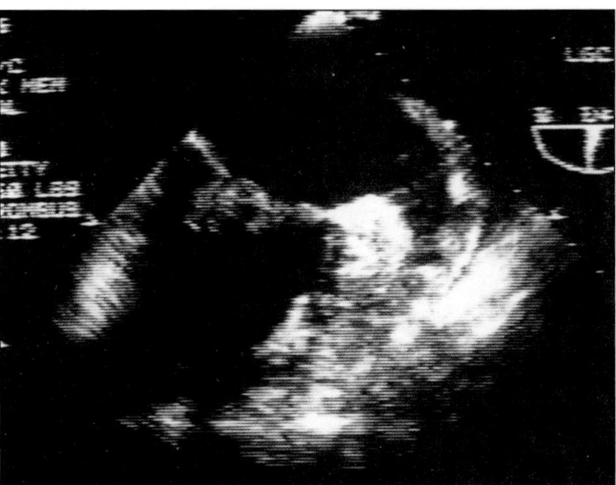

Figure 6.7
Transesophageal echocardiogram showing extensive rheumatic involvement of both leaflets of the mitral valve.

Ischemic heart disease

Mitral regurgitation is present in up to one-third of patients with ischemic heart disease, and the severity is inversely correlated with survival.[54] There are several mechanisms for ischemic mitral regurgitation, which can present in a chronic or acute manner. These include:

- papillary muscle dysfunction with diminished contraction and consequent leaflet prolapse;
- posterior infarction with scarring and shortening of the papillary muscle or abnormality of posterior wall motion causing apical leaflet displacement and failure of coaptation;
- mitral annular dilatation;
- papillary muscle rupture.

The most common mechanism is probably apical leaflet displacement due to ischemia or infarction. The most ominous type of ischemic mitral regurgitation is papillary muscle rupture (Fig. 6.8). This tends to occur about 2–7 days after acute myocardial infarction, and is associated with up to 5% of all deaths due to acute infarction.[55] Rupture of an entire papillary muscle generally results in immediate death, but fortunately, rupture usually affects one of several tips rather than the whole body. The posteromedial papillary muscle is more frequently affected because of its single blood supply.

In most patients with ischemic mitral regurgitation, the lesion is mild and the echocardiogram shows no abnormalities except for regional myocardial dysfunction. In some

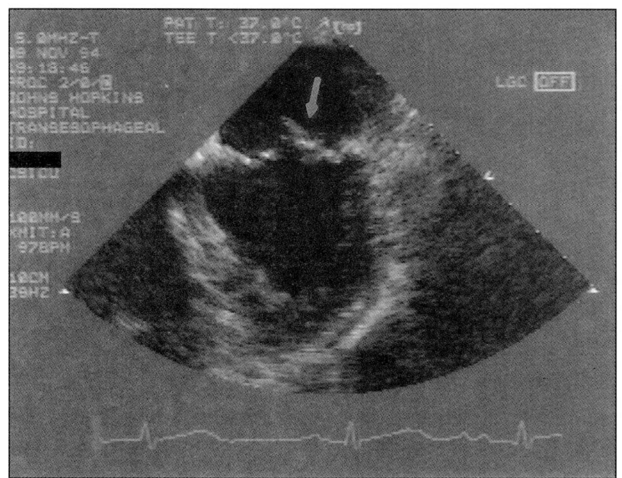

Figure 6.8
Papillary muscle rupture. Transesophageal echocardiogram demonstrates abnormal flailing motion of the mitral valve/subvalvular apparatus (arrow) posteriorly into the left atrium.

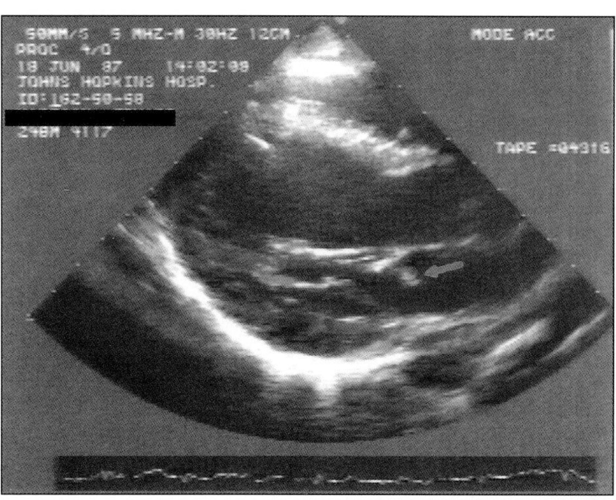

Figure 6.9
A large vegetation is present on the left atrial side of the anterior leaflet of the mitral valve (arrow).

more severe cases, echocardiographic examination shows severe prolapse, chaotic movements of parts of the mitral valve apparatus, or frank papillary muscle rupture, best seen by TEE.[7,25] In patients with mitral regurgitation who undergo surgery for ischemic heart disease, intraoperative TEE may demonstrate more severe mitral regurgitation than was appreciated by preoperative angiography. Up to 10% of those who undergo a pre-bypass TEE will have a change in operative plan.[54]

Infective endocarditis

About 75% of non-intravenous drug-using patients who develop endocarditis on a native mitral valve have a pre-existing valve abnormality, such as myxomatous mitral disease (most common), degenerative mitral disease (such as mitral annular calcification), rheumatic valvular disease, or congenital heart disease.

Endocarditis can cause mitral regurgitation due to leaflet perforation, interference with leaflet coaptation by vegetations, chordal rupture, or papillary muscle dysfunction due to abscess formation. Leaflet damage with chronic scarring and contraction can lead to mitral regurgitation which persists long after the acute infection has been successfully treated.

Currently available imaging technology allows visualization of several important abnormalities seen with mitral regurgitation due to mitral valve endocarditis. The most common of these are mitral valve vegetations (Fig. 6.9). The sensitivity for detection of vegetations by echocardiography varies from 30% to 90%; TEE is most sensitive while M-mode (vegetations appear as 'fluttering' echoes on the valve leaflet) is relatively insensitive.[56] Tiny vegetations are missed, as the lower size limit for detection is about 3 mm. Specificity for the detection of vegetations is not perfect; valve thickening and non-infectious valve nodules may be incorrectly identified. Echocardiography can demonstrate not only vegetations, but also the complications of mitral endocarditis, such as perivalvular abscesses, leaflet perforation, and chordal rupture. Abscesses are much more easily seen with TEE.[57] Echocardiographic examination can show whether other valves or cardiac structures are involved. In addition, the degree of mitral regurgitation can be determined. Mitral valve endocarditis associated with minimal mitral regurgitation has a significantly better prognosis.[58]

Echocardiography has become increasingly important in the management of the patient with mitral regurgitation due to mitral valve endocarditis. Traditionally, the diagnosis was made by clinical and laboratory factors such as positive blood cultures and a new murmur, without regard to echo findings.[59] In fact, early studies indicated that disease associated with visualizable vegetations was far advanced.[60,61]

However, many of these studies were done using insensitive M-mode techniques. A recent study has shown the superiority of a diagnostic strategy which utilizes two-dimensional echocardiographic data.[62] According to the current standard of practice, all patients with suspected endocarditis should have an echocardiogram. TTE is generally done first, with a subsequent TEE in the following situations:

- endocarditis strongly suspected, TTE equivocal or inadequate;
- high clinical suspicion of perivalvular abscess.

Echocardiographic criteria have been used to predict the likelihood of complications of infective endocarditis as well as the overall prognosis.[63] In some studies, the presence of large (≥10 mm) vegetations has been associated with a worse outcome.[56,63] However, the presence of large vegetations alone is not generally felt to be a sufficient indication for surgery. Echocardiographic evidence of vegetations may persist long after adequate antibiotic treatment. Although it has been difficult to differentiate 'active' vegetations from 'chronic' ones, a recent study successfully used digital image processing techniques to make this distinction.[64]

Nuclear scintigraphic imaging of the heart using radiolabeled white blood cells has been used to detect vegetations and valve abscesses; however, this technique has a poor sensitivity.

Prosthetic valve dysfunction

Mitral regurgitation is a common outcome of mitral prosthetic valve failure. This can occur by numerous mechanisms, the most common of which is the tissue degeneration seen with bioprostheses. These bioprosthetic leaflets are nonviable; with time they are prone to become thickened and stiff. Microscopically, there is deposition of calcium and disruption of collagen fibers. Linear tears can develop, especially near the leaflet base. After 10 years in place, failure due to this cause happens at a rate of 5% per year.[65] With the exception of severe leaflet dehiscence, this problem is usually gradual in onset, rather than acute. Another etiology of prosthetic valve failure which can lead to mitral regurgitation is paravalvular leak. This is equally common in bio- and mechanoprostheses. Although some degree of paravalvular leak is probably normal immediately after surgery,[66] leak that appears suddenly later on raises the concern of suture line failure (days to weeks) or an abscess due to endocarditis (weeks to years). Endocarditis can also lead to mitral regurgitation by the direct interference of vegetations with normal valve function. Another potential etiology of mitral regurgitation in a patient with a prosthetic mitral valve is valve thrombosis, usually in a patient with a mechanoprosthesis who has been inadequately anticoagulated. Thrombotic mitral valve occlusion can cause mitral regurgitation or mitral stenosis, depending on what position the orifice occluder is stuck in. Cage fracture (such as is infrequently seen with the Bjork Shiley device), and mechanical failure of the orifice occluder have become rare causes of mechanoprosthetic valve failure leading to mitral regurgitation. The clinical presentation of mitral prosthetic failure with mitral regurgitation can be chronic or acute, depending on the mechanism.

Echocardiography is an indispensable tool for assessing the patient with suspected mitral regurgitation due to prosthetic valve failure. However, because of the acoustic shadowing from the nonbiological materials common to all prosthetic valves, it can be difficult to diagnose mitral regurgitation by the usual criteria. When the valve is between the transducer and the regurgitant jet, as is the case with many common TTE views, the jet may be difficult to visualize. In addition, the structure of the valve itself may be lost in a blur of artifact. This is somewhat less of a problem with bioprostheses. The fluttering of a fractured porcine mitral leaflet produces a jet with a pathognomonic series of oscillating velocities that appear on pulsed Doppler as horizontal stripes.[49] When a jet cannot be well seen, but mitral regurgitation is suspected, PISA techniques can be used as described above. TEE, in which the left atrium (and thus the jet) is always between the transducer and the valve, is much less prone to shadow artifact. Because of the superior resolution of TEE, the prosthesis itself is also better seen, which permits the visualization of vegetations, clot, and perivalvular abscesses. For this reason, suspected mitral prosthetic failure with mitral regurgitation is an indication for TEE without preceding TTE.

It is important to distinguish the appearance of pathologic mitral regurgitation from the normal echocardiographic appearance of a prosthetic mitral valve. Small mitral regurgitant jets are seen on color Doppler in virtually all patients with mechanoprostheses, and up to 10% of patients with bioprostheses.[67] This is believed to be largely a result of valve design. These 'physiologic' mitral regurgitation jets originate inside the perimeter of the valve ring, and are often centrally oriented (Fig. 6.10). If they originate peripherally, such as the jets seen with St Jude prostheses, they are directed centrally. Physiologic jets also tend to be narrow-based and high velocity. Paraprosthetic jets tend to point toward and hug the left atrial wall (Fig. 6.11). For this reason, and due to the Coanda effect, the extent of these jets is usually difficult to determine.

As noted above, echocardiographic techniques, especially TEE, can also demonstrate vegetations, although with less sensitivity than with native valve endocarditis. It is also not uncommon for clot or prosthetic material such as the valve ring suture line to be incorrectly identified as a vegetation. In severe cases of suture line failure, valve instability may

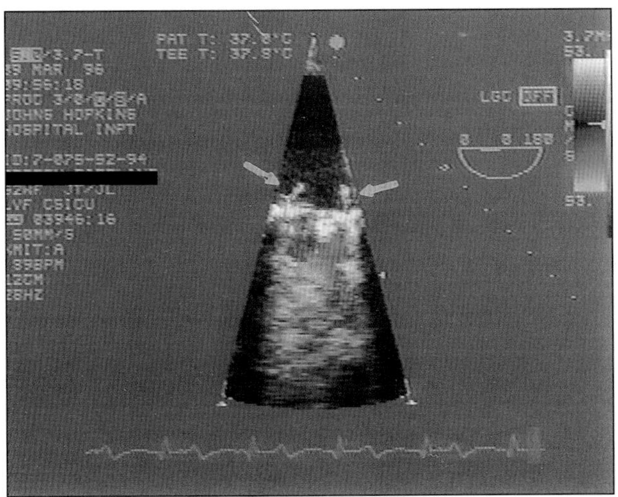

Figure 6.10
Transesophageal echocardiogram demonstrating normal mitral regurgitant jets seen with a St Jude mitral valve prosthesis (arrows).

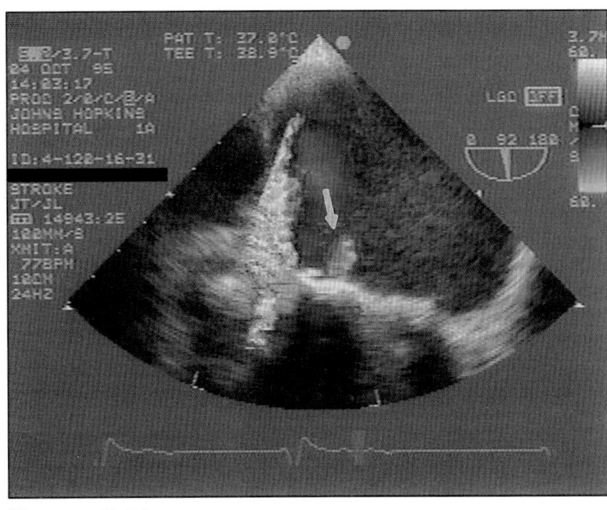

Figure 6.11
Pathologic mitral regurgitation (arrow) in a patient with a prosthetic mitral valve, most likely representing a periprosthetic leak. Note the high velocity and eccentric direction of the jet.

appear on echocardiogram as a rocking of the valve synchronized with the cardiac cycle.

Fluoroscopy is useful for detecting valve instability with abnormal valve motion. With mechanoprostheses, fluoroscopy can also demonstrate failure of one or both discs to open or close properly, which can be caused by vegetation or thrombosis. MRI of patients with prosthetic heart valves is safe, except for patients with early Star Edwards models. However, signal loss due to metal components renders it useless for the evaluation of prosthetic valve function.[68]

Cardiomyopathy

More than half of patients with dilated cardiomyopathy have some degree of mitral regurgitation.[69,70] Potential mechanisms for mitral regurgitation in these patients include:

- failure of the normal constriction of the mitral annulus during ventricular systole due to dysfunction of surrounding ventricular myocardium;
- papillary muscle displacement due to changes in left ventricular geometry, leading to coaptation failure (there is some debate as to whether or not annular dilatation is a salient part of this process).[71,72]

Echocardiographic evaluation in patients with this type of mitral regurgitation demonstrates impaired left ventricular systolic function which may be global or segmental, and left ventricular dilatation. The mitral valve may be free from pathology, although many of these patients have some degree of contributory intrinsic mitral valve disease. Regurgitant jets in these patients tend to be central in origin and direction. The severity of mitral regurgitation due to dilated cardiomyopathy is quite variable, and can be altered by hemodynamic changes in left ventricular mechanics such as those that occur during vasodilator therapy.[73] In addition, color flow mapping often overestimates the severity of mitral regurgitation.

Patients with hypertrophic cardiomyopathy also commonly have mitral regurgitation. Mechanisms of mitral regurgitation in these patients include abnormal anterior motion of the mitral valve during systole, myxomatous mitral valve disease with mitral prolapse, and chordal rupture.[74] Mitral regurgitation in these patients may be detected by pulsed or continuous wave Doppler, but it is important to differentiate the mitral regurgitant jet from high-frequency left ventricular outflow. The mitral regurgitant jet can usually be identified by the shape of the velocity curve; mitral regurgitation begins earlier in systole, whereas the left ventricular outflow velocity curve peaks late in systole and has the characteristic ski-slope appearance.

Congenital heart disease

Many congenital defects can be associated with abnormalities of various parts of the mitral apparatus which cause mitral regurgitation. These include several types of endocardial cushion defect, which can occur with cleft mitral valve, double orifice mitral valve, or a common atrioventricular valve with bridging anterior and posterior leaflets.[75] Cleft mitral valve can also appear as an isolated abnormality.[9] L-transposition, also known as corrected transposition, commonly involves abnormalities of the left-sided tricuspid valve, such as apical displacement of leaflet insertion. This leads to mitral regurgitation, which often presents later in life. An unusual congenital cause of mitral regurgitation is the anomalous origin of the left coronary artery from the pulmonary artery.[76] In this situation, mitral regurgitation is ischemic in etiology and develops progressively in childhood.

Echocardiography is the best imaging modality used to evaluate the patient with suspected congenital mitral disease. Especially in infants, high-frequency transducers can be used to produce two-dimensional images with exquisite anatomic detail. As patients with congenital mitral regurgitation commonly have other associated cardiac abnormalities, precise definition of cardiac anatomy is essential to proper management. Echocardiographic examination can be used to determine whether or not surgical correction is possible, for example, in patients with common atrioventricular canal. Cardiac catheterization may be necessary in patients with significant left-to-right shunt to evaluate pulmonary vascular resistance prior to operative repair. However, in infants, coronary anatomy can usually be defined noninvasively using echocardiographic techniques.

Summary

Mitral regurgitation is a common clinical problem with many potential etiologies. Currently available imaging modalities, especially echocardiography, provide the clinician with the means to make the diagnosis, define the cause, predict the natural history, and appropriately plan surgical intervention.

References

1. Reed D, Abbott RD, Smucker ML, Kaul S: Prediction of outcome after mitral valve replacement in patients with symptomatic chronic mitral regurgitation. *Circulation* 1991; **84**: 23–34.
2. Shahed MS, Tajik AJ: Echocardiography in valvular heart disease. In: Zaibag MA, Duran CG, eds. *Valvular Heart Disease* (Marcel Dekker, Inc.: New York, 1994) 65–130.
3. Enriquez-Sarano M, Tajik JL, Schaff HV et al: Echocardiographic prediction of left ventricular function after correction of mitral regurgitation: results and clinical implications. *J Am Coll Cardiol* 1994; **24**: 1536.
4. Enriquez-Sarano M, Tajik AJ, Schaff HV et al: Echocardiographic prediction of survival after surgical correction of organic mitral regurgitation. *Circulation* 1994; **90**: 830–43.
5. Weyman AE: *Principles and Practice of Echocardiography.* (Philadelphia: Lea and Febiger, 1994); 428–59.
6. Pollick C: What do echocardiographic reports of valvular regurgitation mean? *Cardiol Rev* 1994; **2**: 324–9.
7. Kranidis A, Koulouris S, Filippatos G et al: Mitral regurgitation from papillary muscle rupture: role of transesophageal echocardiography. *J Heart Valve Dis* 1993; **2**: 529–32.
8. Shyu K-G, Lei M-H, Hwang J-J et al: Morphologic characterization and quantitative assessment of mitral regurgitation with ruptured chordae tendineae by transesophageal echocardiography. *Am J Cardiol* 1992; **70**: 1152–6.
9. Fenster MS, Feldman MD: Mitral regurgitation: an overview. *Curr Prob Cardiol* 1995; **20**: 193–280.
10. Smith MD, Cassidy JM, Gurley JC et al: Echo Doppler evaluation of patients with acute mitral regurgitation: superiority of transesophageal echocardiography with color flow imaging. *Am Heart J* 1995; **129**: 967–74.
11. Castello R, Lenzen P, Aguirre F et al: Variability in the quantitation of mitral regurgitation by Doppler color flow mappings: comparison of transthoracic and transesophageal studies. *J Am Coll Cardiol* 1992; **20**: 433–8.
12. Burwash IG, Blackmore GL, Koilpillai CJ: Usefulness of left atrial and left ventricular chamber sizes as predictors of the severity of mitral regurgitation. *Am J Cardiol* 1992; **70**: 774–9.
13. Cujec B, Sullivan H, Willansky S et al: Color flow imaging in severe mitral and aortic regurgitation. *Can J Cardiol* 1988; **4**: 341–6.
14. Miyatake K, Izume S, Okamoto M et al: Semiquantitative grading of severity of mitral regurgitation by real-time two-dimensional Doppler flow imaging. *J Am Coll Cardiol* 1986; **7**: 82–8.
15. Cooper JW, Nanda NC, Philpot EF, Fan P: Evaluation of valvular regurgitation by color Doppler. *J Am Soc Echo* 1989; **2**: 56–66.
16. Salcado EE, Stewart WJ: Dependence of Doppler color flow spatial distribution on instrument settings. *Echocardiography* 1991; **8**: 319–22.
17. Klein AL, Obarski TP, Stewart WJ et al: Transesophageal Doppler echocardiography of pulmonary vein flow: a new

marker of mitral regurgitation severity. *J Am Coll Cardiol* 1991; **18**: 518–26.

18 Rodriguez L, Anconina J, Flachskampf FA et al: Impact of finite orifice size on proximal flow convergence: implications for Doppler quantification of valvular regurgitation. *Circ Res* 1992; **70**: 923–30.

19 Lewis JF: How to evaluate the severity of mitral regurgitation using conventional and newer methods such as 'PISA'. *Learning Center Highlights* 1995; **10**: 1–7.

20 Bargiggia GS, Tronconi L, Sahn DJ et al: A new method of quantitation of mitral regurgitation based on color flow Doppler imaging of flow convergence proximal to the regurgitant orifice. *Circulation* 1991; **84**: 1481–9.

21 Kern MJ: *The Cardiac Catheterization Handbook*. (Mosby: St Louis, 1991); 158–68.

22 Van den Brink RBA, Verneul HA, Hoedemaker G et al: The value of Doppler echocardiography in the management of patients with valvular heart disease: analysis of one year of clinical practice. *J Am Soc Echo* 1991; **4**: 109–20.

23 Schuler G, Peterson KL, Johnson A: Temporal response of left ventricular performance to mitral valve surgery. *Circulation* 1979; **59**: 1218–31.

24 Carabello B, Nolan SP, McGuire LB: Assessment of preoperative left ventricular function in patients with mitral regurgitation: value of end-systolic wall stress–end-systolic volume ratio. *Circulation* 1981; **64**: 1212–17.

25 Horstkotte D, Schulte HD, Niehues R et al: Diagnostic and therapeutic considerations in acute, severe mitral regurgitation: experience in 42 consecutive patients entering the intensive care unit with pulmonary edema. *J Heart Valve Dis* 1993; **2**: 512–22.

26 Globits S, Higgins CB: Assessment of valvular heart disease by magnetic resonance imaging. *Am Heart J* 1995; **129**: 369–81.

27 Semelka RC, Tomei E, Wagner S et al: Normal left ventricular dimensions and function: interstudy reproducibility of measurements with cine MR imaging. *Radiology* 1990; **174**: 763–8.

28 Aurigemma G, Reichek N, Schiebler M, Axel L: Evaluation of mitral regurgitation by cine MRI. *Am J Cardiol* 1990; **66**: 621–5.

29 Corin WJ, Sutsch G, Murakami T et al: Left ventricular function in chronic mitral regurgitation: preoperative and postoperative comparison. *J Am Coll Cardiol* 1995; **25**: 113–21.

30 Tischler MD, Cooper KA, Rowen M, LeWinter MM: Mitral valve replacement versus mitral valve repair: a Doppler and quantitative stress echocardiographic study. *Circulation* 1994; **89**: 132–7.

31 David TE, Uden DE, Strauss HD: The importance of the mitral apparatus in left ventricular function after correction of mitral regurgitation. *Circulation* 1983; **68**: II-76.

32 Hansen DE, Cahill PD, DeCompli WM et al: Valvular–ventricular interaction: importance of the mitral apparatus in canine left ventricular systolic performance. *Circulation* 1986; **73**: 1310–20.

33 Zile MR: Chronic aortic and mitral regurgitation: choosing the optimal time for surgical correction. *Cardiol Clin* 1991; **9**: 239–53.

34 Kaul TK, Ramsdale DR, Meek D, Mercer JL: Mitral valve replacement in patients with severe mitral regurgitation and impaired left ventricular function. *Int J Cardiol* 1992; **35**: 169–79.

35 Bernal JM, Rabasa JM, Vilchez FG et al: Mitral valve repair in rheumatic disease: the flexible solution. *Circulation* 1993; **88**: 1746–53.

36 Akins CW, Hilgenberg AD, Buckley MJ et al: Mitral valve reconstruction versus replacement for degenerative or ischemic mitral regurgitation. *Ann Thorac Surg* 1994; **58**: 668–76.

37 Michel PL, Iung B, Blanchard B et al: Long-term results of mitral valve repair for nonischaemic mitral regurgitation. *Eur Heart J* 1991; **12**(suppl B): 39–43.

38 Devlin WH, Starling MR: Mitral regurgitation: current concepts and future perspectives. *Cardiol Rev* 1994; **3**: 16–25.

39 Cosgrove DM, Stewart WJ: Mitral valvuloplasty. *Curr Prob Cardiol* 1989; **14**: 355–415.

40 Cohn LH: Surgery for mitral regurgitation. *JAMA* 1988; **260**: 2883–7.

41 Stewart WJ, Currie PJ, Salcedo EE: Evaluation of mitral leaflet motion by echocardiography and jet direction by Doppler color flow mapping to determine the mechanism of mitral regurgitation. *J Am Coll Cardiol* 1992; **20**: 1353–61.

42 Chachques JC, Pellerin M: Current status of valvular surgery. *Curr Opinion Cardiol* 1994; **9**: 186–90.

43 Grossi EA, Galloway AC, Le Boutillier M et al: Anterior leaflet procedures during mitral valve repair do not adversely influence long term outcome. *J Am Coll Cardiol* 1995; **25**: 134–6.

44 Stewart WJ, Currie PJ, Salcedo EE et al: Intraoperative Doppler color flow mapping for decision-making in valve repair for mitral regurgitation. *Circulation* 1990; **81**: 556–66.

45 Rosen SE, Borer JS, Hochreiter C et al: Natural history of the asymptomatic/minimally symptomatic patient with severe mitral regurgitation secondary to mitral valve prolapse and normal right and left ventricular performance. *Am J Cardiol* 1994; **74**: 374–9.

46 Perloff JC, Edwards JE: New guidelines for the clinical diagnosis of mitral valve prolapse. *Am J Cardiol* 1986; **57**: 1124–9.

47 Gaasch WH, Cohn LH, O'Rourke RA, Rackley CE: Mitral valve disease. In: Schlant RC, Alexander RW, eds, *The Heart* (McGraw-Hill: New York, 1994); 1483–518.

48 McAllister HA, Buja LM, Ferrans VJ: Valvular heart disease: anatomic abnormalities. In: Willerson JT, Cohn JN, eds, *Cardiovascular Medicine* (Churchill Livingstone: New York, 1995); 173–86.

49 Feigenbaum H: *Echocardiography* (Lea and Febiger: Philadelphia, 1994); 239–349.

50 Crawford MH, O'Rourke RA: Mitral valve prolapse: a cardiomyopathic state? *Prog Cardiovasc Dis* 1984; **27**: 133–9.

51 Butman S, Chandraratna PAN, Milne N et al: Stress myocardial imaging in patients with mitral valve prolapse: evidence of a perfusion abnormality. *Cathet Cardiovasc Diag* 1982; **8**: 243–52.

52 Rapaport E: Natural history of aortic and mitral valve disease. *Am J Cardiol* 1975; **35**: 221–7.

53 Zucker N, Goldfarb BL, Zalzstein E: A common color flow Doppler finding in the mitral regurgitation of acute rheumatic fever. *Echocardiography* 1991; **8**: 627–31.

54 Sheikh KH, Bengtson JR, Rankin JS et al: Intraoperative transesophageal Doppler color flow imaging used to guide patient selection and operative treatment of ischemic mitral regurgitation. *Circulation* 1991; **84**: 594–604.

55 Wei JY, Hutchins GM, Bulkley BH: Papillary muscle rupture in fatal acute myocardial infarction: a potentially treatable form of cardiogenic shock. *Ann Intern Med* 1979; **90**: 149–53.

56 Mugge A, Daniel WG, Frank G, Lichtlen PR: Echocardiography in infective endocarditis: reassessment of prognostic implications of vegetation size determined by the transthoracic and transesophageal approach. *J Am Coll Cardiol* 1989; **14**: 631–8.

57 Daniel WG, Mügge A, Martin RP et al: Improvement in the diagnosis of abscesses associated with endocarditis by transesophageal echocardiography. *N Engl J Med* 1991; **324**: 795–800.

58 Jaffe WM, Morgan DE, Pearlman AS, Otto CM: Infective endocarditis, 1983–1988: echocardiographic findings and factors influencing morbidity and mortality. *J Am Coll Cardiol* 1990; **15:** 1227–33.

59 von Reyn CF, Levy BS, Arbeit RD et al: Infective endocarditis: an analysis based on strict case definitions. *Ann Intern Med* 1981; **94**: 505–18.

60 Wann LS, Dillon JC, Weyman AE, Feigenbaum H: Echocardiography in bacterial endocarditis. *N Engl J Med* 1976; **295**: 135–9.

61 Hickey AJ, Wolfers J, Wilcken DEL: Reliability and clinical relevance of detection of vegetations by echocardiography in bacterial endocarditis. *Br Heart J* 1981; **46**: 624–8.

62 Durack DT, Lukes AS, Bright DK: New criteria for diagnosis of infective endocarditis: utilization of specific echocardiographic findings. *Am J Med* 1994; **96**: 200–9.

63 Sanfilippo AJ, Picard MH, Newell JB et al: Echocardiographic assessment of patients with infectious endocarditis: prediction of risk for complications. *J Am Coll Cardiol* 1991; **18**: 1191–9.

64 Tak T, Rahimtoola SH, Kumar A et al: Value of digital image processing of two-dimensional echocardiograms in differentiating active from chronic vegetations of infective endocarditis. *Circulation* 1988; **78**: 116–23.

65 Jamieson WRE, Janusz MT, Miyagishima RT et al: The Carpentier–Edwards standard porcine bioprosthesis: long-term evaluation of the high pressure glutaraldehyde fixed prosthesis. *J Cardiac Surg* 1988; **3**(suppl 3): 321–36.

66 Chambers J, Monaghan M, Jackson G: Colour flow Doppler mapping in the assessment of prosthetic valve regurgitation. *Br Heart J* 1989; **62**: 1–8.

67 Wilkins GT, Flachskampf FA, Weyman AE: Echo-Doppler assessment of prosthetic heart valves. In: Weyman AE, ed., *Principles and Practice of Echocardiography* (Lea and Febiger: Philadelphia, 1994); 1198–230.

68 Malloy CR, Peshock RM: Magnetic resonance. In: Willerson JT, Cohn JN, eds, *Cardiovascular Medicine* (Churchill Livingstone: New York, 1995); 1766–80.

69 Junker A, Thayssen P, Nielsen B, Andersen PE: The hemodynamic and prognostic significance of echo-Doppler-proven mitral regurgitation in patients with dilated cardiomyopathy. *Cardiology* 1993; **83**: 14–20.

70 Blondheim DS, Jacobs LE, Kotler MN et al: Dilated cardiomyopathy with mitral regurgitation: decreased survival despite a low frequency of left ventricular thrombus. *Am Heart J* 1991; **122**: 763–71.

71 Ballester M, Jajoo J, Rees S et al: The mechanism of mitral regurgitation in dilated left ventricle. *Clin Cardiol* 1983; **6**: 333–8.

72 Boltwood CM, Tei C, Wong M, Shah PM: Quantitative echocardiography of the mitral complex in dilated cardiomyopathy; the mechanism of functional mitral regurgitation. *Circulation* 1983; **68**: 498–508.

73 Seneviratne B, Moore GA, West PD: Effect of captopril on functional mitral regurgitation in dilated heart failure: a randomised double blind placebo controlled trial. *Br Heart J* 1994; **72**: 63–8.

74 Zhu W, Oh JK, Kopecky SL et al: Mitral regurgitation due to ruptured chordae tendineae in patients with hypertrophic obstructive cardiomyopathy. *J Am Coll Cardiol* 1992; **20**: 242–7.

75 Fyler DC: Endocardial cushion defects. In: Fyler DC, ed., *Nadas' Pediatric Cardiology* (Hanley and Belfus: Philadelphia, 1992); 577–87.

76 Roberts WC: Valvular heart disease of congenital origin in valvular heart disease: comprehensive evaluation and treatment. In: Frankl WS, Brest AN, eds, *Cardiovascular Clinics* (FA Davis: Philadelphia, 1993); 25–34.

7

Mitral stenosis and the role of echocardiography in mitral commissurotomy

James W Roberts and João AC Lima

There are well-defined roles for echocardiography in the evaluation of patients with mitral stenosis, particularly in those being considered for percutaneous transvenous mitral commissurotomy or surgical valve replacement. Echocardiography is used to assess mitral valve morphology with particular attention to commissural fusion and valve leaflet calcification, the two most important determinants of the severity of mitral stenosis. This assessment has proven to be useful in patient selection for surgical or catheter based commissurotomy, as immediate and long-term outcome can be predicted from echocardiographic grading scores. Transesophageal echocardiography aids the detection of left atrial thrombi and may be useful in guiding transseptal puncture and in predicting clinical outcomes. The degree of mitral regurgitation can also be assessed and this has influence on outcome after transvenous mitral valvuloplasty. Future imaging applications in this ever-expanding field may ultimately include the use of dobutamine stress echocardiography and intravascular ultrasound catheters. Therefore, the echocardiographic assessment of mitral stenosis plays a crucial role not only in the diagnosis and clinical staging of the rheumatic process, but also in defining the best therapeutic strategy for these patients.

Introduction

The clinical manifestations of mitral stenosis frequently prompt the use of cardiac imaging by ultrasound to confirm the clinical suspicion of valvular heart disease in patients with suggestive signs and symptoms of mitral stenosis. However, even in those with atypical clinical presentations such as new onset atrial fibrillation, a cerebral ischemic episode, or other peripheral embolic events, echocardiograms are often obtained to assess the presence of a potential cardiac source of embolus. Mitral stenosis is not infrequently diagnosed by echocardiography which is also routinely used in the follow-up of patients with established disease. The choice between different modalities of treatment is also made based mainly on valvular structural abnormalities determined by echocardiography. In this regard, one of the first considerations in patients with this condition who progress despite medical therapy, is the possibility of valvuloplasty by catheter based techniques.

Percutaneous transvenous mitral commissurotomy has rapidly become an acceptable alternative to surgical commissurotomy in the treatment of patients with mitral stenosis.[1–8] As the procedure has gained acceptance, well-defined roles for transthoracic echocardiography (TTE) have evolved. Experience has made it clear that outcomes are partially related to the valvular morphology.[2,7–11] This can be assessed with M-mode and two-dimensional echocardiography and graded by means of a standardized scoring system prior to the procedure. Doppler echocardiography can also be used to assess the presence or subsequent development of mitral regurgitation, another important determinant of outcome.[12] Transesophageal echocardiography (TEE) has a major role in the assessment of atrial thrombus, and may ultimately enjoy an expanded role in the prediction of clinical outcomes.

Pathology of mitral stenosis

Rusted and colleagues[13] described significant heterogeneity in the changes seen among various components of the mitral valve in hearts with mitral stenosis. The stenoses depended on changes in the chordae, the valvular leaflets, the commissures, or in combinations of all three components of the valve. They described four types of mitral stenosis in their series of 70 hearts: (1) commissural, (2) cuspal, (3) chordal, and (4) combined. The relative frequency of each of these was 31.4%, 15.7%, 8.6%, and 44.3%, respectively.

The first type of mitral stenosis has its most severe changes in the commissures, as the name implies. Different subtypes exist. One subtype has increased valve leaflet thickness and loss of pliability despite normal depth of the commissure. A second subtype is notable for fusion of the valvular leaflets in the vicinity of the commissures, leading to increased depth.

The cuspal type is marked by increased rigidity of the mitral leaflets. These cusps often become leathery in appearance. The anterior leaflet is usually more involved than the posterior leaflet. The greatest amount of fibrous thickening extends inward from the free edge of the leaflet for 1 cm or more and is usually more pronounced at the line of closure.

In the chordal type of mitral stenosis, the main pathology is thickening, shortening, and fusion of the chordae. It should be remembered that chordal shortening may lead to a pronounced reduction of leaflet mobility because each leaflet is attached to both the anterolateral and posteromedial sets of chordae. Shortening is often accompanied by chordal fusion, which leads to the formation of a new membrane, continuous with the commissural tissue. This, in turn, may ultimately distort the leaflets, leading to a funnel-shaped structure which sometimes causes greater obstruction to flow below, rather than at the level of the mitral leaflets.

The combined defects are most common, and variations on the above themes abound. There may be changes in commissural and leaflet thickening without changes in commissural depth. Another common scenario is the combination of leaflet and chordal fusion with commissural elongation. It is important to note that most hearts (75.7%) in Rusted's series fell into the commissural or the combined types, with significant changes seen at one or both of the commissures. This has important implications for percutaneous balloon corrective techniques, which rely on commissural splitting to achieve a satisfactory result.

The authors also described calcification as a common finding (31 of 50 hearts). Gross deposition was found in more than one location in a given valve and could be characterized as thin and superficial or thick and bulky. Calcification was most common in the valvular leaflets as opposed to the commissural junctions. The degree of calcification, in fact, is most important in considering surgical commissurotomy or valvuloplasty as a potential treatment for mitral stenosis.[2,9,14,15]

Echocardiographic assessment of mitral stenosis

There may be many effects of acquired rheumatic heart disease on the cardiovascular system, thus, the echocardiographic evaluation of patients with mitral stenosis is necessary not only to define the structure and function of the mitral valve per se, but also to detect the presence of other possible valvular conditions such as mitral, tricuspid or aortic regurgitation, as well as aortic or tricuspid stenosis. It is also used to assess the severity of pulmonary hypertension, and to evaluate the function of the left and right ventricular chambers. Knowing that valvular function and morphology are a major determinant of clinical outcomes after any form of invasive treatment for mitral stenosis, it is easy to understand the many applications of echocardiography in the assessment of patients with this disease. Currently, there are specific roles for several echocardiographic modalities including transthoracic M-mode and two-dimensional echocardiography, continuous wave and color flow Doppler, as well as transesophageal echocardiography.

M-mode echocardiography

Echocardiography was first used to detect mitral stenosis in 1956, as reported by Edler.[16] Currently, M-mode echocardiography allows a sensitive measure of valve leaflet thickness and motion. The normal mitral valve has an 'M'-shape configuration during diastole. The first peak represents early rapid filling, followed by a trough due to valve closure in mid-diastole. The valve then re-opens in late diastole, due to atrial contraction (Fig. 7.1a). The M-mode echocardiographic hallmark of mitral stenosis is the loss of this 'M'-shape configuration (Fig. 7.1b). The holodiastolic pressure gradient does not allow closure in mid-diastole, and hence there is limited or no valve reopening in late diastole. This flat diastolic E–F slope is characteristic of, but not specific for, mitral stenosis. Other conditions that may flatten the diastolic slope of mitral valve motion are those associated with decreased left ventricular compliance. However, when reduced diastolic slope is seen with increased thickness and anterior motion of the posterior leaflet, the M-mode provides a sensitive and accurate diagnosis of mitral stenosis.[17]

Nanda and colleagues[15] published data in 1975 that emphasized the importance of the degree of leaflet mobility and calcification on the M-mode echo in the management of symptomatic mitral stenosis patients. Mobility was graded as normal (>20 mm), restricted (16–19 mm) or poor (<15 mm). Calcification was graded as heavy (thick, conglomerate echoes), light (multiple, discrete linear echoes), or absent (thin single or duplicate signals).

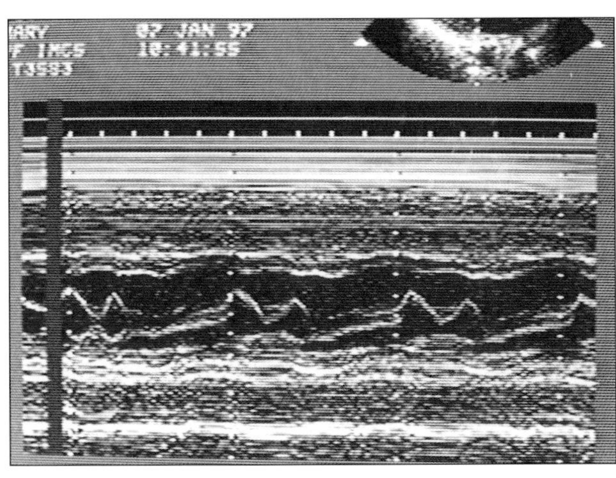

a

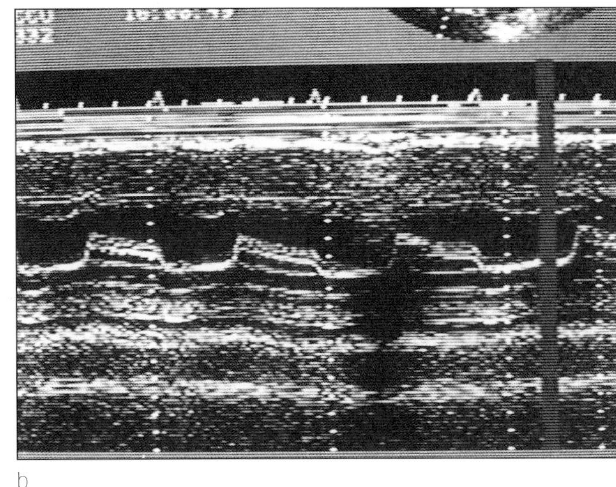

b

Figure 7.1
(a) An M-mode echocardiographic recording from a normal mitral valve with anterior displacement of the anterior leaflet in early diastole followed by partial leaflet closure and late reopening caused by atrial contraction. This normal (M) pattern can be contrasted with (b), from a patient with mitral stenosis. Both the anterior and posterior leaflets move anteriorly in diastole reflecting commissural fusion. In addition, leaflets are thickened and the anterior leaflet remains open throughout diastole, reflecting the transmitral gradient which characterizes mitral stenosis.

Eighteen of 19 patients without calcification on echo were treated with surgical commissurotomy. Eleven of 11 patients with heavy calcification and 11 of 11 patients with poor cusp mobility received valve replacement. Eight of the 11 patients with poor mobility also had heavy calcification. Thus heavy calcification and incipient poor leaflet mobility by echocardiography precluded surgical commissurotomy and resulted in valve replacement, whereas the absence of calcification indicated that commissurotomy could be performed. Therefore, in this series from 1975, 65% of patients were correctly triaged with relatively crude M-mode echocardiography simply on the basis of presence or absence of impaired leaflet mobility and heavy calcification. The two-dimensional echocardiography criteria used today represent an extension of the same principles identified by M-mode echocardiography nearly 20 years ago.

Two-dimensional echocardiography

Two-dimensional echocardiography can provide valuable morphologic information in patients with mitral stenosis, a fact that is underscored by the reliance on this modality to calculate echocardiographic scores. When valve leaflets are fibrotic and calcified, they produce a greater number of echoes due to increased thickness. Because of fusion, the anterior and posterior mitral leaflets do not separate properly during diastole and may appear to move in the same direction. When two-dimensional echocardiography is applied, the classic diagnostic features of mitral stenosis are thickened, domed leaflets with thickened tips and restricted motion near the commissures, giving a characteristic 'hockey stick' appearance in the long-axis view (Fig. 7.2). The ventricle fills slowly, the left atrial size is often markedly enlarged, and pulmonary hypertension may lead to right ventricular enlargement and hypertrophy (Fig. 7.3). The most useful application of two-dimensional echocardiography is in the assessment of leaflet mobility, leaflet thickening, subvalvular thickening and calcification which determine the severity of the rheumatic process. The stenotic orifice may be visualized directly and estimated accurately in the parasternal short-axis view. However, Doppler echocardiographic measurements allow a better hemodynamic assessment as summarized below.

Doppler echocardiography

The severity of mitral stenosis is frequently defined by the pressure gradient required to fill the left ventricle in

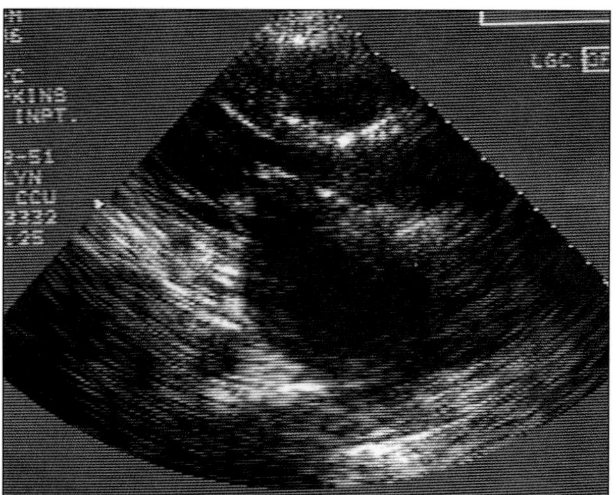

Figure 7.2
Two-dimensional echocardiographic long-axis view of the heart from a patient with mitral stenosis. Anterior mitral leaflet thickening and chordal shortening produces the typical 'hockey stick' pattern. The left atrium is significantly dilated. The left ventricle is typically of normal size and function when combined mitral regurgitation is either absent or mild, as in this patient with rheumatic mitral valve stenosis.

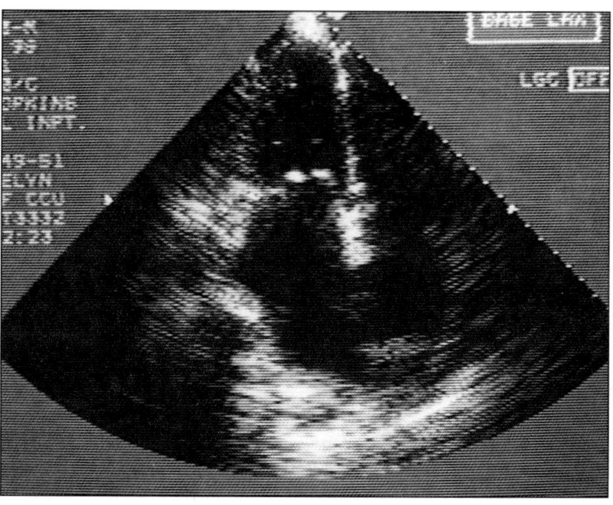

Figure 7.3
Two-dimensional echocardiographic four-chamber view of a patient with rheumatic mitral stenosis with the left ventricle and left atrium represented in the left side of the photograph. The left atrium is severely dilated and the mitral valve thickened. The right atrium is also dilated in this patient with mitral stenosis.

diastole, by forcing blood across the stenotic valve orifice. Such gradient can be measured directly by catheters placed in the left ventricle and left atrium after transseptal puncture of the interatrial septum. They can also be measured by Swan–Ganz catheterization of the pulmonary artery utilizing balloon occlusion of small pulmonary arterioles to assess pulmonary venous pressure which indirectly reflects left atrial pressure. These measurements can be contrasted with simultaneous measurements obtained inside the left ventricle permitting determination of the transvalvular gradient during diastole. Non-invasively however, the pressure gradient across the mitral valve can be accurately assessed by Doppler echocardiography. It is important to notice however, that despite the undisputed utility of quantitative measures of pressure gradients derived by Doppler or cardiac catheterization, the morphologic assessment obtained by M-mode and two-dimensional echocardiography described previously are equally important in the overall assessment of rheumatic mitral valve severity and disease progression.

Continuous wave Doppler echocardiography allows quantification of the severity of mitral valve stenosis.[18–21] Once the jet is identified, recording can be made from the apex with continuous wave Doppler to find the greatest velocities across the valve for best alignment of the beam (Fig. 7.4). Peak blood velocity can then be used to calculate the peak diastolic gradient by the modified Bernoulli equation:

$$\text{Pressure gradient} = 4V^2$$

Peak gradients are typically measured early in diastole and should not exceed 50–75 cm/s. However, it is difficult to distinguish stenotic from normal valves based on peak gradients alone because other conditions such as mitral regurgitation and atrial septal defects can produce increased peak gradients in the absence of mitral stenosis. Mean gradients are more reliable and should be calculated by averaging gradients from as many sampling points as possible during the diastolic period. While mean pressure gradients measured by continuous wave Doppler correlate well with mean pressure gradients directly measured at cardiac catheterization, the fact that the difference between abnormal (above 12 mmHg) and normal (below 12 mmHg) mean gradients is frequently not much larger than the standard error of the method (6–8 mmHg) diminishes the practical utility of this technique in the assessment of mitral stenosis severity.

In patients with mitral stenosis, the peak velocity of blood inflow across the mitral valve is increased as

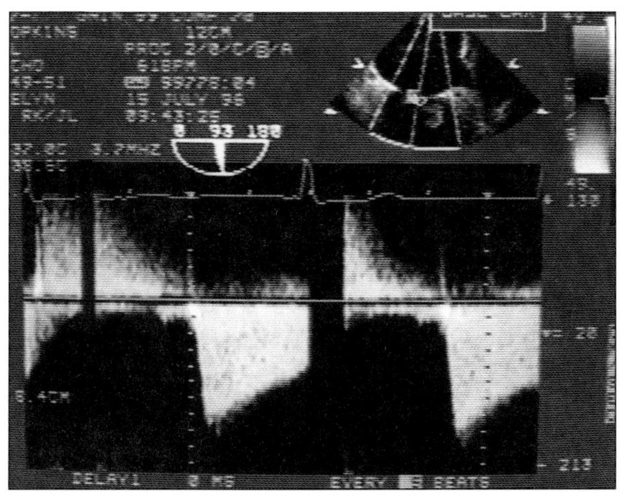

a

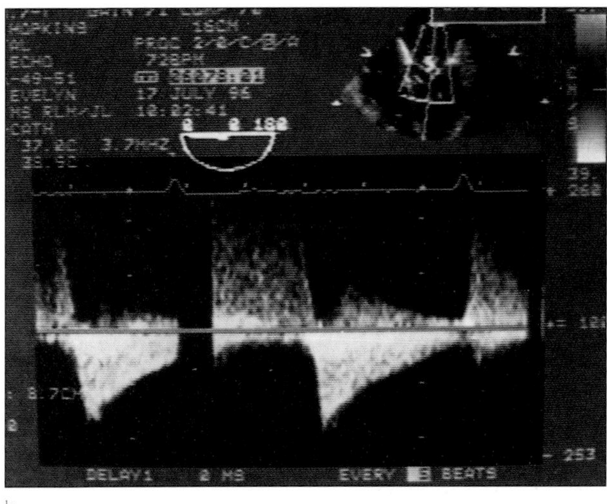

b

Figure 7.4
(a) Doppler echocardiographic mitral inflow pattern. Peak diastolic flow early in diastole is elevated, but this feature does not distinguish mitral stenosis from conditions of high inflow volume through a normal mitral valve such as mitral regurgitation and atrial septal defect. The mean diastolic gradient, measured as the average of gradients obtained at different time points throughout the diastolic period is a more reliable index of mitral stenosis. Similarly, the rate of reduction in transmitral flow velocity during the diastolic period is a better discriminator between stenotic and non-stenotic valve orifices than the peak diastolic flow gradient.
(b) The rate of descent of mitral inflow velocity during diastole can be quantified as the slope of the mitral valve inflow envelope (pressure half time), and compared with the slope generated by a hypothetical mitral valve with a 1.0 cm^2 area (see text for formula).

mentioned above, but its rate of fall in early diastole is decreased. One may estimate mitral valve area in patients with mitral stenosis by quantifying the rate of diastolic decay by the pressure half-time method.[21] In brief, the pressure half-time ($P_{1/2t}$) is the time interval required for the peak flow velocity to fall to one-half its initial level (Fig. 7.4). This is calculated by using the slope of the diastolic spectral envelope from the mitral valve continuous wave Doppler tracing, and averaging 5–10 beats at paper speeds of 50–100 mm/s. This value correlates well with the mitral valve area (MVA) for a wide range of mitral inflows and thus may be related to the half-time interval obtained empirically from a 1 cm^2 mitral valve using the formula:

$$MVA = 220/P_{1/2t}$$

Normally, the mitral valve area is 4–6 cm^2. In mild mitral stenosis, valve area is typically within 1.6 to 2 cm^2, and in moderate stenosis between 1.1 and 1.5 cm^2. Severe mitral stenosis is characterized by a mitral valve area equal to or below 1.0 cm^2. Mitral area assessed by this method correlates well with that found at cardiac catheterization[22] and is now routinely used to assess results from valvuloplasty by catheter-based[23] and surgical interventions.

Color flow Doppler echocardiography demonstrates mitral stenosis as a brilliant mosaic pattern of mitral valve inflow, the area of which increases with the pressure gradient (Fig. 7.5). Moreover, in some patients with severe subvalvular apparatus disease, the inflow jet may be quite eccentric in direction, and require color flow Doppler for proper alignment of continuous wave flow measurements. Finally, this modality is also particularly useful in patients with mitral valve rheumatic disease, to assess the degree of combined mitral regurgitation as the relative area of the left atrium subtended by the jet in two orthogonal planes.

Role of transesophageal echocardiography

TEE is a technique that has recently gained increased usage among cardiologists. As experience grows with this

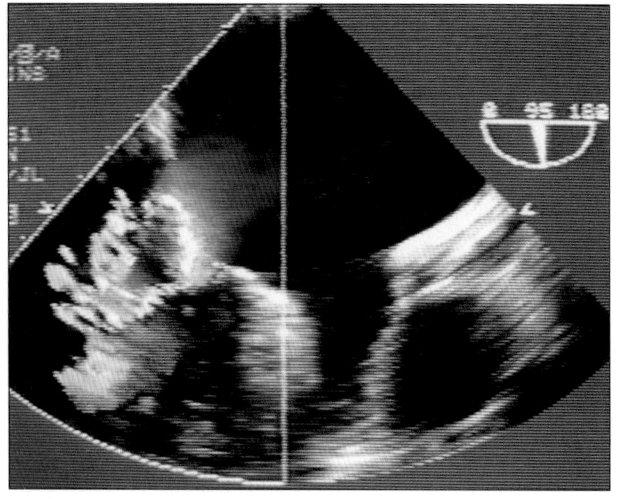

a

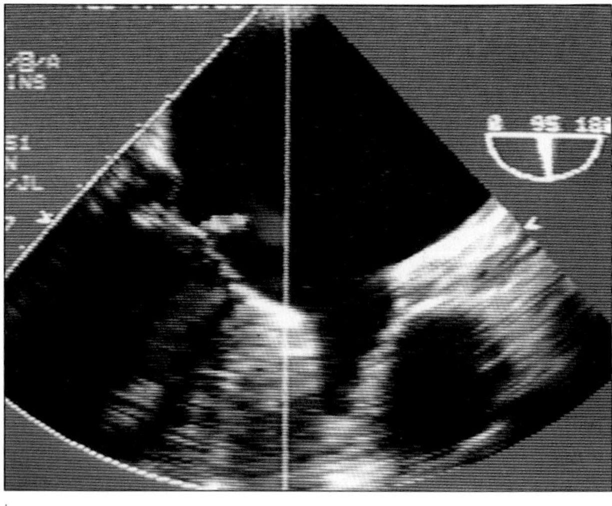

b

Figure 7.5
Four-chamber view with color flow Doppler showing accelerated inflow pattern across the mitral valve in diastole, typical of mitral valve inflow obstruction by rheumatic or any other type of mitral stenotic disease.

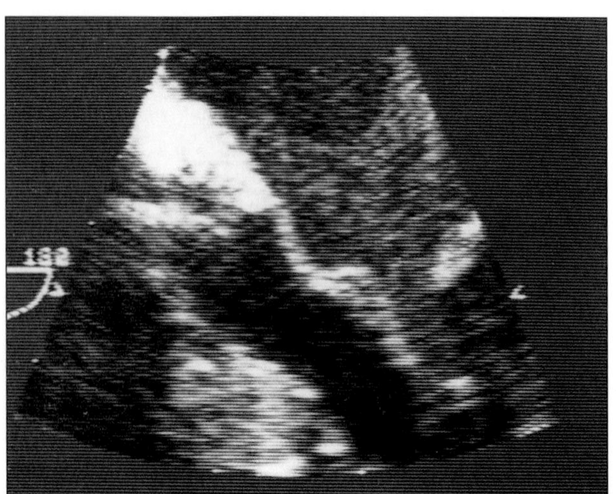

a

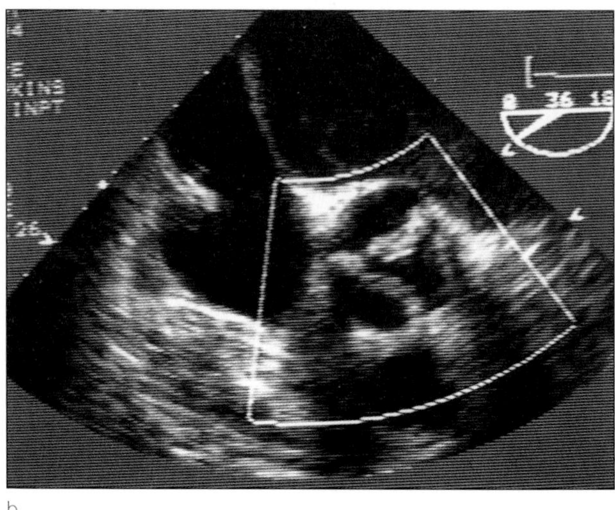

b

Figure 7.6
Transesophageal echocardiogram depicting thickened mitral valve and subvalvular chordae tendineae. Typically, in patients with rheumatic mitral stenosis the proximal portions of valve leaflets and chordae are thickened and more affected by the fibrotic process as in this patient. The transesophageal approach allows a direct view into the left atrium and the mitral valve, since the transducer is located in the esophagus, in close proximity with the left atrium.

technique and technology progresses toward esophageal probes of lesser and lesser diameter, its clinical applications will likewise continue to expand. The high resolution views of valvular anatomy, the left atrial appendage, and the aorta make this tool superior to the transthoracic approach for a number of specific situations in the case of patients with mitral stenosis (Fig. 7.6). As the use of percutaneous valvuloplasty grows, it is clear that TEE may evolve to play a greater role in the assessment of patients prior to, during and after that procedure.

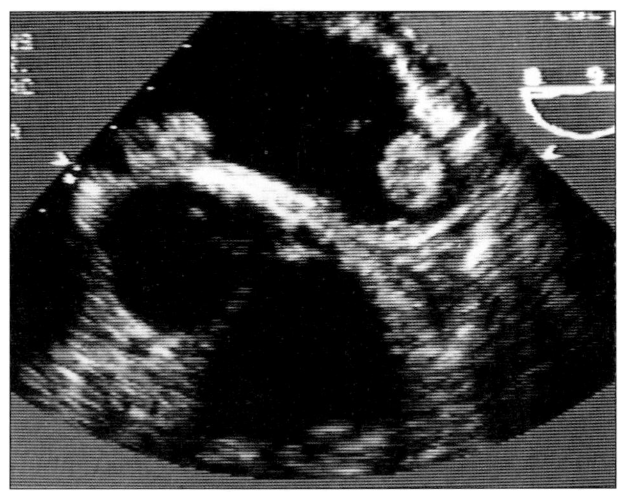
a

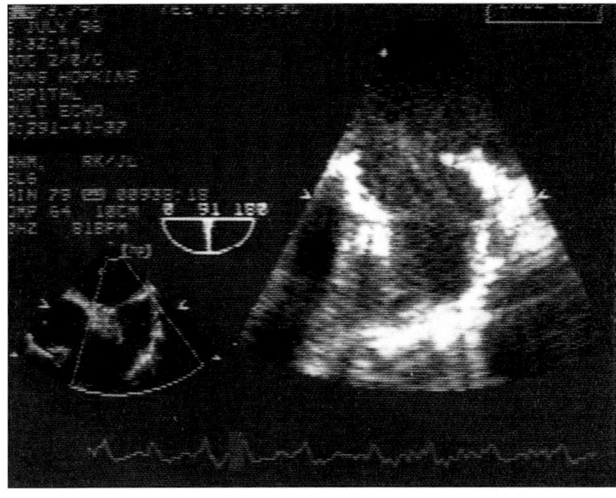
b

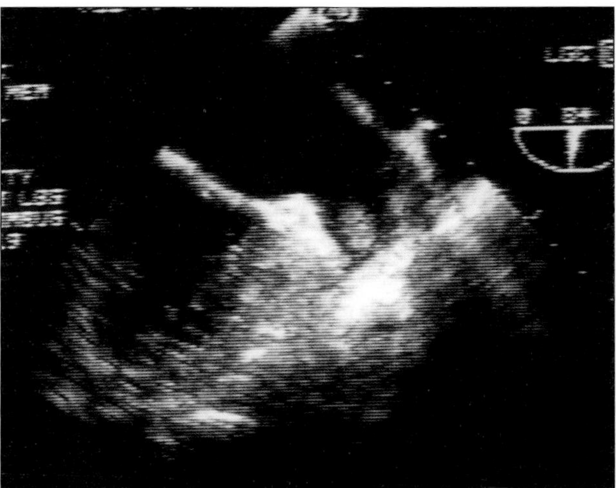
c

Figure 7.7
Transesophageal echocardiogram showing left atrial thrombus within the left atrial appendage. Intra-atrial thrombus formation is particularly common in patients with mitral stenosis with enlarged left atria and diminished transmitral flow causing intra-atrial blood stasis characterized as spontaneous echocardiographic contrast. Patients with such finding are at particularly high risk of suffering cerebral embolic ischemic events.

The TEE approach probably does not add important new information or a more detailed assessment of mitral valve morphology when compared to the conventional transthoracic non-invasive approach in patients with mitral stenosis (TTE). Both Marwick et al[24] and Cormier et al[25] have found the modalities to be of equal value in assessing leaflet mobility. The former study suggested that TEE may actually underestimate subvalvular disease and calcification because of shielding by the echo-dense valve leaflets. Similarly, the degree of commissural fusion is probably best assessed by TTE in the parasternal short-axis view. The valve orifice and degree of commissural fusion may be poorly visualized with the biplane TEE probe. Subvalvular structures may be distant, as the ultrasound beam traverses the enlarged left atrium and then becomes attenuated by the echodense valve leaflets and annulus. Yet, the transgastric view of the left ventricle allows a particularly nice view of the chordae and papillary muscles with the biplane or omniplane TEE probes. For these reasons, TEE is not superior to TTE in patients with mitral stenosis, but complementary to assessment with TTE in specific disease settings, as discussed later.[26]

Perhaps the most important role for TEE in patients with mitral stenosis is the detection of left atrial thrombus formation, a potential source for cerebral and systemic embolization (Fig. 7.7). TEE allows superior visualization of the left atrium, atrial septum, and left atrial appendage, all common sites for thrombus formation that are traditionally poorly visualized by the standard transthoracic approach. The presence of spontaneous echocardiographic

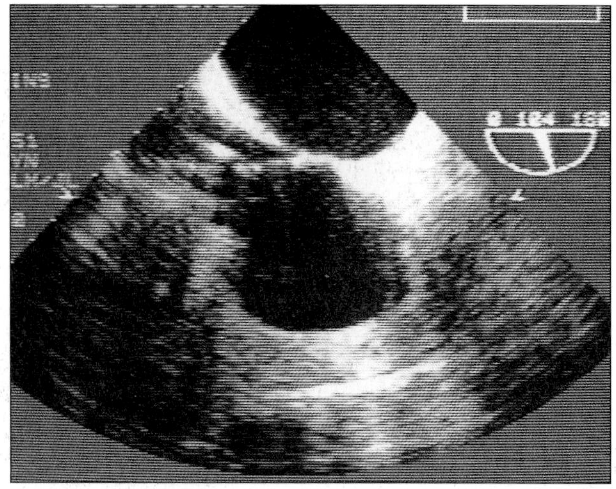

a

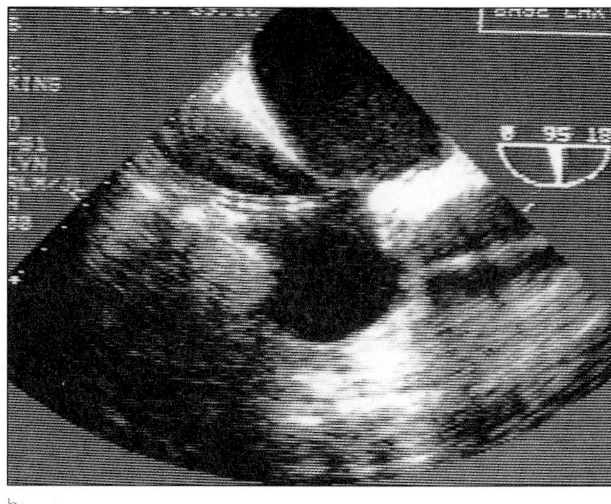

b

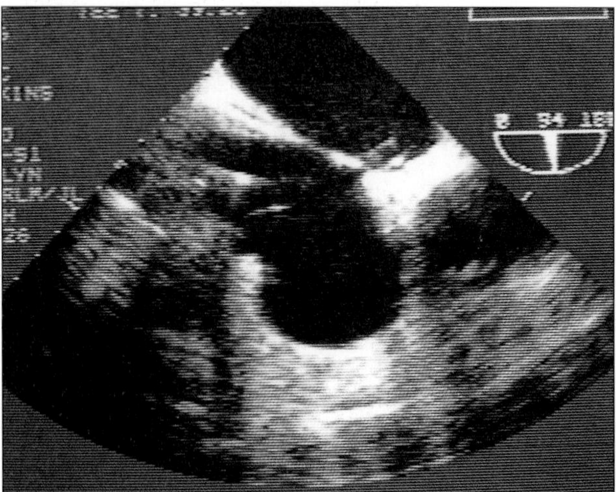

c

Figure 7.8
Transseptal puncture prior to mitral valvuloplasty, guided by transesophageal echocardiography. (a) The catheter/needle positioned against the foramen ovale. (b) The tip of the catheter within the left atrium having successfully crossed the septum at the level of the foramen ovale.

contrast, which represents a marker of reduced blood flow within the left atrium, can be clearly demonstrated by TEE, and indicates risk of cerebral embolization, particularly in patients who are not receiving anticoagulants. Because TEE is clearly superior to TTE for detecting left atrial thrombi, and given the risks of embolization during balloon valvuloplasty due to intra-atrial catheter manipulation, it is recommended that all patients considered for this procedure should undergo TEE.[27,28] Similarly, the quantification of mitral regurgitation can be performed in a superior fashion by TEE, which can be particularly useful in patients with poor precordial images by TTE, or in those with regurgitant jets which are masked by heavy valvular or annular calcification. Continuous wave Doppler can also be performed during the TEE examination, and mitral valve area and valve gradients can be assessed precisely by this approach. When obtained by TEE, mitral valve gradients and area correlate well with those obtained by conventional transthoracic Doppler echocardiography.[29]

One of the most useful potential applications of TEE in patients undergoing balloon valvuloplasty is for guidance of transseptal puncture.[26] TEE is technically feasible during valvuloplasty, but not always well tolerated because of the natural difficulty for patients with mitral stenosis to lie supine during concomitant transesophageal and catheterization procedures. However, in patients who have enlarged right and left atria or aortic root dilatation, the placement of the Brokenbrough needle may be difficult and lead to inadvertent puncture of either atrial wall, the coronary sinus, the right ventricle, or the aorta despite fluoroscopic

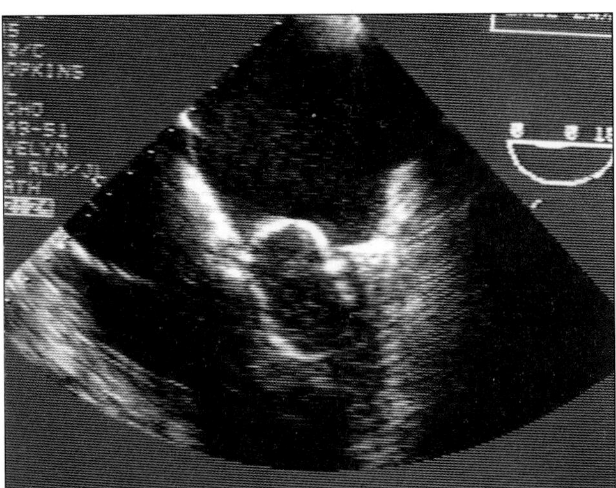

Figure 7.9
Transesophageal echocardiogram with color flow Doppler from the same patient shown in Figure 7.8 depicting the residual atrial septal defect created by the transseptal crossing of the valvuloplasty catheter. While such defects are of no hemodynamic consequence, they can sometimes predispose patients to peripheral embolic events caused by venous thrombi reaching the left heart through the atrial septal defect.

guidance.[30] Biplane and omniplane probes can be very helpful as the tip of the needle can be well visualized in the longitudinal plane (Fig. 7.8). Goldstein and Campbell[26] report that TEE guidance can also help to avoid transseptal punctures that are too high or too low, and allow appreciation of 'tenting' of the midportion of the septum, which may be difficult to appreciate by feel and fluoroscopy alone. Moreover, the assessment of iatrogenic left-to-right shunts caused by transseptal puncture is best performed by TEE with color flow Doppler and contrast echocardiography (Fig. 7.9). Finally, another useful application of TEE in patients undergoing balloon valvuloplasty is in crossing the mitral valve. In patients in whom the mitral valve funnel is oblique rather than perpendicular to the mitral valve annulus, the angle for catheter advancement is quite different, and TEE guidance is quite helpful.[26] Theoretically, TEE could reduce the incidence of chordal rupture leading to severe mitral regurgitation during valvuloplasty by the Inoue balloon.[31]

While it is unlikely that the transesophageal approach will supplant the conventional transthoracic approach in the routine evaluation of patients with mitral stenosis, the above indications make TEE a useful adjunct to TTE, particularly in patients with evidence or suspicion of cerebral or peripheral embolism. In patients who are candidates for balloon valvuloplasty, TEE may be useful to exclude left atrial thrombi prior to the procedure, in the immediate assessment of the efficacy of valvuloplasty, and for the detection of complications secondary to this procedure.

Selection of patients for mitral valvuloplasty

Immediate outcome

The best-defined role for echocardiography in balloon valvuloplasty is in the evaluation of mitral valve morphology in patients with mitral stenosis. Abascal and colleagues[9] described an echocardiographic grading score that allows assessment of four features: leaflet mobility, leaflet thickening, subvalvular thickening, and calcification (Table 7.1). Each feature is graded on a scale of 1–4 based on the appearance of the valve on two-dimensional echocardiography, with higher scores indicative of more severe involvement. Scores for each factor are added, for a possible total score of 4–16.[12] Block and colleagues[14] found that the immediate outcome of percutaneous balloon valvuloplasty was best predicted by the echocardiographic score prior to the procedure. Patients with an echo score of 8 or less have a >90% chance of a good result with this procedure. Additionally, patients with scores of 11 or greater have a lower chance of success. Patients with scores between 8 and 11 fall into a 'gray zone', wherein results frequently are influenced by the amount of calcification and subvalvular fibrosis affecting the valve. Of the four components of the total echocardiographic score, valvular thickening consistently correlates best with the change in mitral valve area by univariate and multiple regression analysis techniques. However, the dichotomy of clinical outcomes has not been as predictable by echocardiographic scores in other studies.[32,33]

Long-term outcome

Long-term outcome of percutaneous balloon valvuloplasty, likewise, seems to be influenced by the echocardiographic score. Abascal et al[9] reported that the occurrence of restenosis of the mitral valve, defined as a decrease of 25% of the mitral valve area 6–11 months after valvuloplasty, was more likely to occur in patients with higher echo scores (11 or greater). Other factors that may influence outcomes and restenosis include age, balloon size, and the presence of atrial fibrillation, mitral regurgitation, or heavy fluoroscopic calcification.[2] All of these factors, except for

Table 7.1 Echocardiographic grading of mitral valve characteristics in MS.

Mobility
- Grade 1: Highly mobile valve with leaflet only tips restricted
- Grade 2: Leaflet mid and base portions have reduced mobility
- Grade 3: Valve continues to move forward in diastole, mainly from the base
- Grade 4: No or minimal diastolic forward movement of the leaflets

Thickening
- Grade 1: Leaflets near normal in thickness (4–5 mm)
- Grade 2: Midleaflets normal, marked thickening of margins (5–8 mm)
- Grade 3: Thickening extending through the entire leaflet (5–8 mm)
- Grade 4: Marked thickening of all leaflet tissue (>8–10 mm)

Subvalvular thickening
- Grade 1: Minimal thickening just below the mitral leaflets
- Grade 2: Thickening of chordal structures extending up to one-third of the chordal length
- Grade 3: Thickening extending to the distal third of the chords
- Grade 4: Extensive thickening and shortening of all chordal structures extending down to the papillary muscles

Calcification
- Grade 1: A single area of increased echo brightness
- Grade 2: Scattered areas of brightness confined to single leaflet margins
- Grade 3: Brightness extending into the midportion of the leaflets
- Grade 4: Extensive brightness throughout much of the leaflets

balloon size, are also associated with higher echocardiographic scores.

Reid et al[32] reported a similar association between mitral valve morphology and clinical outcome immediately after and 6 months after valvuloplasty in 555 patients enrolled in the NHLBI Balloon Valvuloplasty Registry. However, multiple regression analysis did not find the total morphology score to be an independent predictor in that series. They correctly suggested that leaflet mobility is influenced by numerous pathologic processes affecting the valve apparatus, which together reflect the severity and duration of disease in acquired mitral stenosis. In essence, the echocardiographic score's predictive power is a manifestation of the severity of the disease.

Experience with the Inoue single-balloon catheter valvuloplasty has revealed that commissural splitting is the primary mechanism by which the mitral valve area is increased. In a series of 30 patients, Faitkin et al[33] reported that a good outcome of >25% increase in mitral valve area was achieved in 96% of those who underwent valvuloplasty with the Inoue single-balloon catheter and had documented splitting of one or both commissures. Good outcomes were not achieved in any of the six patients who did not develop commissural splitting. Absence of splitting could be accurately predicted when marked fibrosis or calcification was present in both commissures, reflecting the utility of assessing valve morphology prior to the procedure.

In comparison to the double-balloon experience, Herrmann et al[34] found a weaker correlation between total echocardiographic score and immediate outcome in the North American Multicenter Registry of 200 patients who underwent percutaneous valvuloplasty with the Inoue balloon catheter. However, only 7% of the selected patients had scores >11, reflecting the utilization of echocardiographic data to identify prospective candidates for the procedure. In addition, there was potential for greater variability in the subjective echocardiographic scoring, given the multicenter nature of the registry. Cohen et al[8] treated mitral stenosis with single-balloon valvuloplasty in 102 patients and with the double-balloon technique in 36 patients obtaining good long-term results. Event-free survival rate was directly related to the echocardiographic score, left ventricular end-diastolic pressure, and New York Heart Association functional class.

In summary, in patients with mitral stenosis, echocardiography also provides important information which can help predict patients likely to have better immediate and long-term outcomes from percutaneous balloon valvuloplasty. A standardized echocardiographic score can be used to assess mitral valve morphology prior to the procedure. Those with lower scores tend to be younger patients who have less atrial fibrillation, leaflet calcification and mitral regurgitation. It is likely, therefore, that the echocardiographic score is a semi-quantitative reflection of the duration and severity of acquired rheumatic mitral valve disease.

Concomitant and subsequent mitral regurgitation

Another determinant of outcome in percutaneous valvuloplasty is the severity of mitral regurgitation, both before and after the procedure (Fig. 7.10). The presence of

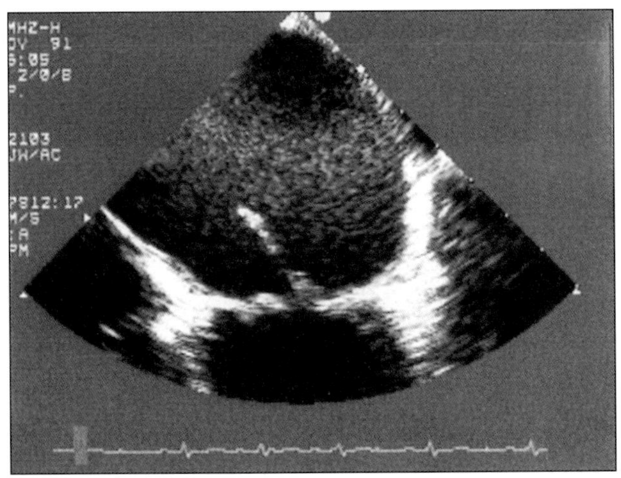
a

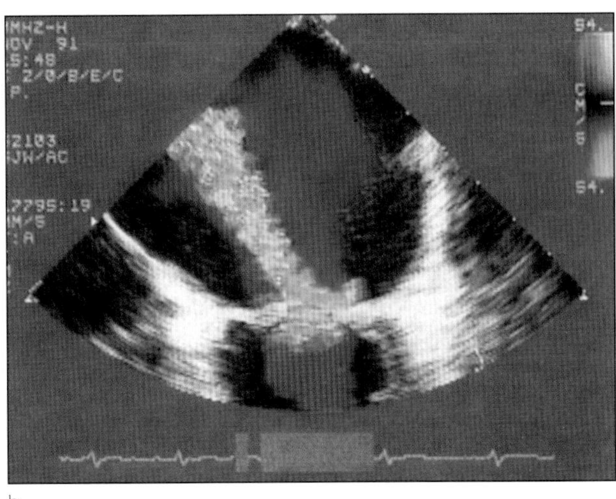
b

Figure 7.10
Sequence of frames from a transesophageal echocardiogram obtained immediately before mitral valve replacement in a patient with severe mitral regurgitation after Inoue balloon valvuloplasty. (a) Prolapse of the posterior leaflet with an attached chord into the left atrium during systole. (b) A central and septally directed Doppler color flow jet of severe mitral regurgitation.

moderate or severe mitral regurgitation (>2+/4) is a widely accepted contraindication to balloon valvuloplasty, because the development of worsened mitral regurgitation occurs in up to 50% of patients who undergo the procedure to treat mitral stenosis. Equally important is the fact that significant mitral regurgitation clearly will not be ameliorated by balloon valvuloplasty; therefore, clinical improvement is unlikely even if the stenotic valve area is increased. In patients with trivial or mild mitral regurgitation at baseline, the increase in magnitude is usually small and does not significantly alter the clinical improvement achieved by widening the valve orifice. Severe mitral regurgitation may occur in up to 15% of procedures and usually requires medical therapy followed by elective valve replacement. Studies have suggested that a high echocardiographic score may be associated with the development of worsened mitral regurgitation by left ventriculography or pulsed Doppler echocardiography[35–37] when patients are treated with double-balloon valvuloplasty. The mechanism of regurgitation with that technique is very often widening at the site of commissural splitting secondary to poor coaptation of the opened but immobile leaflets.[35] Posterior leaflet rupture and anterior leaflet tears have also been described as a result of double-balloon procedures.[36]

New mitral regurgitation associated with the Inoue single-balloon catheter is a slightly different entity, particularly when related to echocardiographic scores. Feldman and colleagues[38] found that patients who developed the greatest increases in mitral regurgitation when treated with the Inoue catheter did not differ significantly with respect to echocardiographic score. The reason for this is probably related to the mechanism of the worsened mitral regurgitation with the Inoue balloon technique. Herrmann et al[31] described the mechanisms of severe mitral regurgitation in patients undergoing percutaneous valvuloplasty with the Inoue catheter. Chordal rupture was the most common cause, and most often involved the anterior leaflet. The chordae of this leaflet may become entangled when the catheter is steered across the valve, causing leaflet disruption during balloon inflation. Posterior leaflet tears are also frequent causes of severe mitral regurgitation with the Inoue balloon, and appear to be related to heavy calcification of the posterior leaflet. In addition, changes in the direction of the regurgitant jet associated with worsened mitral regurgitation frequently provided insight into the mechanism of leaflet damage during valvuloplasty by the Inoue balloon technique (Fig. 7.10). Anterior leaflet rupture frequently results in regurgitant jets oriented laterally and posteriorly, whereas posterior leaflet fracture due to advanced disease with leaflet calcification commonly generates jets oriented medially, along the posterior wall of the ascending aorta.[31]

In summary, in addition to providing information on the likelihood of valvular restenosis, echocardiography is a useful modality for excluding patients with moderate or severe mitral regurgitation and for predicting which patients may be at greatest risk for developing severe mitral regurgitation as a result of the valvuloplastic procedure. Those patients who develop severe regurgitation may ultimately require valve replacement and should be followed with serial echocardiograms. In patients undergoing valvuloplasty by the Inoue balloon technique, careful placement of the catheter may play an important role in avoiding the development of severe mitral regurgitation.

Other echocardiography and ultrasound applications

As hemodynamic parameters may not necessarily correlate with the symptomatic status of the patient after mitral valvuloplasty, mitral valve reserve capacity as assessed by the response to dobutamine echocardiography may be a more useful indicator of restenosis. Dobutamine stress echocardiography has been used to assess mitral valve orifice variability in patients with mitral stenosis who have undergone balloon valvuloplasty. Okay et al[39] demonstrated that significant variability in the mitral valve orifice exists in patients with symptomatic improvement after balloon valvotomy, but not in those with symptomatic recurrence. If this can be demonstrated to be consistently true, dobutamine stress echocardiography may become a useful adjunct in evaluating restenosis in mitral stenosis patients treated with percutaneous valvuloplasty.

Another exciting potential future application of ultrasound techniques in mitral stenosis patients undergoing valvuloplasty may be the use of intravascular ultrasound catheters during the procedure. These small caliber catheters could be placed in the right atrium or right ventricle and be used for guidance of transseptal puncture, and may allow accurate balloon sizing and placement. They may also prove to be useful in eventually assessing flow across the valve, providing information regarding the immediate outcome of the procedure without the need for additional echocardiographic studies.[40] As experience with these devices grows, other interesting applications are likely to evolve, facilitating the accurate assessment of valvular structure and function in patients with mitral stenosis.

Summary

Mitral stenosis can be evaluated thoroughly with the many echocardiographic modalities now available, including M-mode, two-dimensional echocardiography, continuous wave Doppler, and transesophageal echocardiography. The rheumatic process starts at the distal portions of the mitral valve involving the leaflet edges and causing commissural fusion and chordal thickening. Echocardiography can detect the process at its early stages and demonstrate its progression to involve both the proximal portions of the valve leaflets and the subvalvular apparatus. Leaflet and chordal inflammation lead to fibrosis and calcification, ultimately causing mitral stenosis combined or not with mitral regurgitation. Advanced rheumatic disease involves the mitral valve ring with fibrosis and calcification to the point of muffling the first heart sound and mitral opening snap. Surgical or catheter-based mitral valvuloplasty is indicated to relieve mitral inflow obstruction in patients with rheumatic mitral stenosis, but advanced leaflet calcification and/or severe subvalvular involvement are best treated by mitral valve replacement in symptomatic patients. Because cerebral embolization is frequently a catastrophic consequence of mitral stenosis, aggressive investigation to detect the presence of left atrial thrombus, and/or anticoagulation to prevent its formation, should be considered in every patient with more than mild mitral stenosis.

The use of cardiac imaging techniques enhances patient selection for percutaneous balloon mitral valvuloplasty or mitral valve surgical replacement, as important questions about the morphology of the diseased valve can be answered noninvasively. Standardized echocardiographic scores have been devised and validated and have been useful in predicting immediate and long-term outcomes. However, it is important to understand that the utility of these scoring systems stems from the fact that they reflect the severity of acquired rheumatic mitral valve disease.

Percutaneous transvenous balloon mitral valvuloplasty with the Inoue single-balloon catheter is now an established alternative to surgical commissurotomy for many patients with mitral stenosis. Transesophageal echocardiography can assess the presence of thrombus hidden within the left atrial appendage or elsewhere in the left atrium before mitral valvuloplasty, or at any time during the time course of the disease. It may also be of assistance during the procedure by providing better anatomical landmarks than fluoroscopy, thus facilitating transseptal puncture and positioning of the dilating balloon catheter across heavily diseased and atypical valves. Finally, transesophageal echocardiography may better delineate the magnitude and mechanism of mitral regurgitation following mitral valvuloplasty and assess the need for mitral valve replacement.

References

1 Palacios IF, Block PC, Brandi S et al: Percutaneous balloon mitral valvotomy for patients with severe mitral stenosis. *Circulation* 1987; **75**: 778.

2 Palacios IF, Block PC, Wilkins GT et al: Follow-up of patients undergoing percutaneous mitral balloon

valvotomy: analysis of actors determining restenosis. *Circulation* 1989; **79**: 573.

3 Patel JJ, Sharma JJ, Mithu AS et al: Balloon valvuloplasty versus closed commissurotomy for pliable mitral stenosis: a prospective hemodynamic study. *J Am Coll Cardiol* 1991; **18**: 1318.

4 Turi ZG, Reyes VP, Raju BS et al: Percutaneous balloon versus surgical closed commissurotomy for mitral stenosis: a randomized trial. *Circulation* 1991; **83**: 1179.

5 Vahanian A, Michel PL, Cormier B et al: Results of percutaneous mitral commissurotomy in 200 patients. *Am J Cardiol* 1989; **64**: 847.

6 Herrmann HC, Kleaveland JP, Hill JA et al: The M-heart percutaneous balloon mitral valvuloplasty registry: initial results and early follow-up. *J Am Coll Cardiol* 1990; **15**: 1221.

7 Wilkins GT, Weyman AE, Abascal VM et al: Percutaneous balloon dilation of the mitral valve: an analysis of echocardiographic variables related to outcome and the mechanism of dilatation. *Br Heart J* 1988; **60**: 299.

8 Cohen DJ, Kuntz RE, Gordon SPF et al: Predictors of long-term outcome after percutaneous mitral valvuloplasty. *N Engl J Med* 1991; **327**: 1329.

9 Abascal VM, Wilkins GT, Choong CY et al: Echocardiographic evaluation of mitral valve structure and function in patients followed for at least 6 months after percutaneous balloon mitral valvuloplasty. *J Am Coll Cardiol* 1988; **12**: 606.

10 Abascal VM, Wilkins GT, O'Shea JP et al: Prediction of successful outcome in 130 patients undergoing percutaneous balloon mitral valvotomy. *Circulation* 1990; **82**: 448.

11 Herrmann HC, Wilkins GT, Abascal VM et al: Percutaneous balloon mitral valvotomy for patients with mitral stenosis: analysis of factors influencing early results. *J Thorac Cardiovasc Surg* 1988; **96**: 33.

12 Abascal VM, Wilkins GT, Choong CY et al: Mitral regurgitation after percutaneous balloon mitral valvuloplasty in adults; evaluation by pulsed doppler echocardiography. *J Am Coll Cardiol* 1988; **11**: 257.

13 Rusted IE, Scheifley CH, Edwards JE: Studies of the mitral valve: certain anatomic features of the mitral valve and associated structures in mitral stenosis. *Circulation* 1956; **14**: 398.

14 Block PC: Who is suitable for percutaneous balloon mitral valvotomy? *Int J Cardiol* 1988; **20**: 9 (editorial).

15 Nanda NC, Gramiak R, Shah PM et al: Mitral commissurotomy versus replacement: preoperative evaluation by echocardiography. *Circulation* 1975; **51**: 263.

16 Edler I: Ultrasound cardiogram in mitral valve disease. *Acta Chir Scand* 1956; **111**: 230.

17 Feigenbaum H: Echocardiography. In: Braunwald E, ed. *Heart Disease: A Textbook of Cardiovascular Medicine,* 4th edn (WB Saunders: Philadelphia, 1992); 81–2.

18 Holen J, Aaslic R, Landmark K, Simonsen S: Determination of pressure gradients in mitral stenosis with a non-invasive ultrasound doppler technique. *Acta Med Scand* 1979; **199**: 455.

19 Holen J, Simonsen S: Determination of pressure gradient in mitral stenosis with Doppler echocardiography. *Br Heart J* 1979; **41**: 529.

20 Hatle L, Brubakk A, Tromsdal A, Angelsen B: Non-invasive assessment of pressure drop in mitral stenosis by Doppler ultrasound. *Br Heart J* 1978; **40**: 131.

21 Hatle L, Angelsen B, Tromsdal A: Noninvasive assessment of atrioventricular pressure half-time by Doppler ultrasound. *Circulation* 1979; **60**: 1096.

22 Motro M, Schneeweiss A, Lehrer E et al: Correlation between cardiac catheterization and echocardiography in assessing the severity of mitral stenosis. *Int J Cardiol* 1981; **1**: 25.

23 Chen C et al: Reliability of the Doppler pressure half-time method for assessing effects of percutaneous mitral balloon valvuloplasty. *J Am Coll Cardiol* 1989; **13**: 1309.

24 Marwick TH, Torelli J, Obarski T et al: Assessment of the mitral valve splitability score by transthoracic and transesophageal echocardiography. *Am J Cardiol* 1991; **68**: 1106.

25 Cormier B, Vahanian A, Michel PL et al: Transesophageal echocardiography in the assessment of percutaneous mitral commissurotomy. *Eur Heart J* 1991; **12** (suppl B): 61.

26 Goldstein SA, Campbell AN: Mitral stenosis: evaluation and guidance of valvuloplasty by transesophageal echocardiography. *Cardiol Clin* 1993; **11**: 409.

27 Casale PN, Whitlow P, Currie PJ et al: Transesophageal echocardiography in percutaneous balloon valvuloplasty for mitral stenosis. *Cleve Clin J Med* 1989; **56**: 597.

28 Chan KL, Marquis JF, Ascah C et al: Rise of transesophageal echocardiography in percutaneous balloon mitral valvuloplasty. *Echocardiography* 1990; **7**: 115.

29 Chan K, Sochowski R: Comparison of transesophageal continuous wave Doppler with transthoracic Doppler in the assessment of mitral stenosis. *J Am Coll Cardiol* 1992; **19**: 201A (abstract).

30 Baim DS, Grossman W: Percutaneous approach and transseptal catheterization. In: Grossman W, ed. *Cardiac Catheterization and Angiography,* 3rd edn (Lea & Febiger: Philadelphia, 1974); 59–75.

31 Herrmann HC, Lima JAC, Feldman T et al: Mechanisms and outcome of severe mitral regurgitation after Inoue balloon valvuloplasty. *J Am Coll Cardiol* 1993; **22**: 783.

32 Reid CL, Otto CM, Davis KB et al: Influence of mitral valve morphology on mitral balloon commissurotomy: immediate and 6 month results from the NHLBI balloon valvuloplasty registry. *Am Heart J* 1992; **124**: 657.

33 Faitkin D, Roy P, Morgan JJ et al: Percutaneous balloon mitral valvotomy with the Inoue single balloon catheter: Commissural morphology as a determinant of outcome. *J Am Coll Cardiol* 1993; **21**: 390.

34 Herrmann HC, Ramaswamy K, Isner JM et al: Factors influencing immediate results, complications, and short-term follow-up status after Inoue balloon mitral valvotomy: a North American multicenter study. *Am Heart J* 1992; **124**: 160.

35 Essop MR, Wisenbaugh T, Skoularigis J et al: Mitral regurgitation following mitral balloon valvotomy. *Circulation* 1991; **84**: 1669.

36 O'Shea JP, Abascal VM, Wilkins GT et al: Unusual sequelae after percutaneous mitral valvuloplasty: a doppler echocardiographic study. *J Am Coll Cardiol* 1992; **19**: 186.

37 Roth RB, Block PC, Palacios IF: Predictors of increased mitral regurgitation after percutaneous mitral balloon valvotomy. *Cathet Cardiovasc Diagn* 1990; **20**: 17.

38 Feldman T, Carroll JD, Isner JM et al: Effect of valve deformity on results and mitral regurgitation after Inoue balloon commissurotomy. *Circulation* 1992; **85**: 180.

39 Okay T, Deligonul U, Sancaktar O et al: Contribution of mitral valve reserve capacity to sustained symptomatic improvement after balloon valvulotomy in mitral stenosis: implications for restenosis. *J Am Coll Cardiol* 1993; **22**: 1691.

40 Follman DF, Levin TN, Lang RM et al: Low-frequency intra-cardiac ultrasonographic imaging before and after balloon pulmonary valvuloplasty. *Am Heart J* 1993; **125**: 259.

8

Echocardiography of the aortic valve

Susan E Wiegers, Ted Plappert and Martin St John Sutton

The structure and function of the aortic valve can be completely characterized by echocardiography. The anterior position of the valve affords excellent visualization of the anatomy and motion of the valve. Doppler echocardiographic techniques allow hemodynamic assessment that is comparable to invasive techniques.

Two-dimensional views

The aortic valve is visualized in the parasternal long-axis view (Fig. 8.1). The right coronary cusp is imaged anteriorly as a thin line, while the posterior echo is the non-coronary cusp. Depending on the angulation of the transducer, the left coronary cusp may also be seen posteriorly. The coaptation point of the leaflets is directly in the center of the aortic root and parallel to its walls. In systole, the leaflets may be difficult to separate from the aortic walls. From the parasternal view, the continuity between the anterior mitral valve leaflet and the aortic valve can be appreciated. The anterior mitral annulus and the posterior aortic annulus are also seen as continuous structures. The normal aortic root is wider at the level of the sinuses than is the proximal ascending aorta. When the transducer is rotated 90° the aortic valve is imaged in cross-section (Fig. 8.2). The right coronary cusp is anterior and the non-coronary cusp posterior and to the left. The coronary ostia arise from the corresponding sinus, and a short portion of their proximal course may be followed. Enlargement of the sinuses of Valsalva is best appreciated from this view.

The aortic valve structures are more difficult to visualize from the apical views. The apical long-axis view is along the same axis as the parasternal long-axis view. However, the aortic valve is imaged at a greater distance and is less well seen. The advantage of the apical view lies in the fact that the direction of aortic outflow is parallel to the long axis, making this an appropriate view for Doppler interrogation. Similarly, the apical five-chamber view is useful for hemodynamic assessment. In this view in particular, the motion of the aortic valve leaflets may appear artifactually

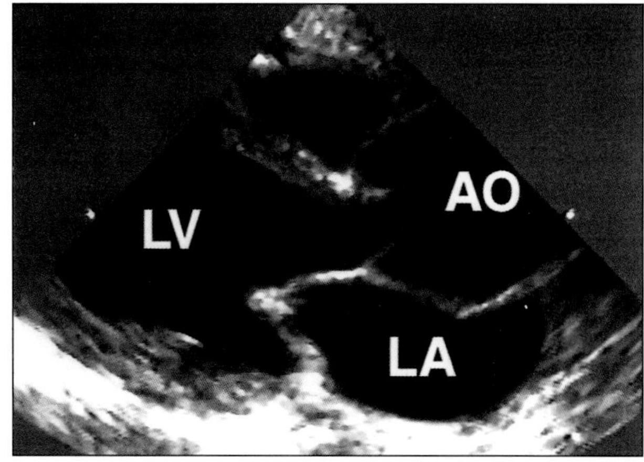

Figure 8.1
Two-dimensional echocardiogram of the parasternal long-axis view. The aorta (AO) is markedly dilated and the left atrium (LA) appears compressed. The aortic leaflets are seen in early systole and are partially opened. The leaflets themselves are essentially normal but the patient had severe aortic insufficiency (not seen here) due to the aortic root dilatation. The left ventricle (LV) is dilated.

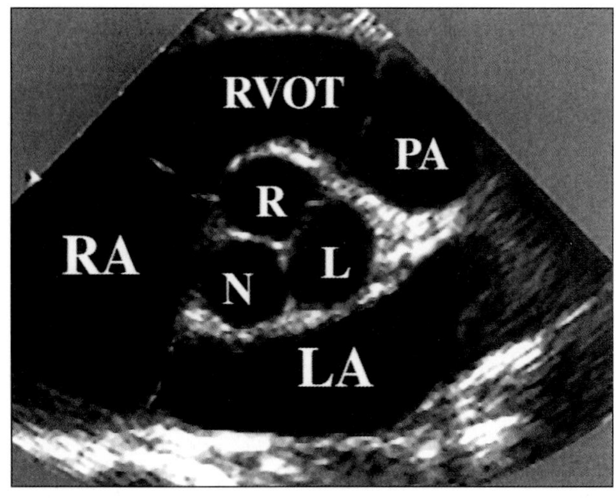

a

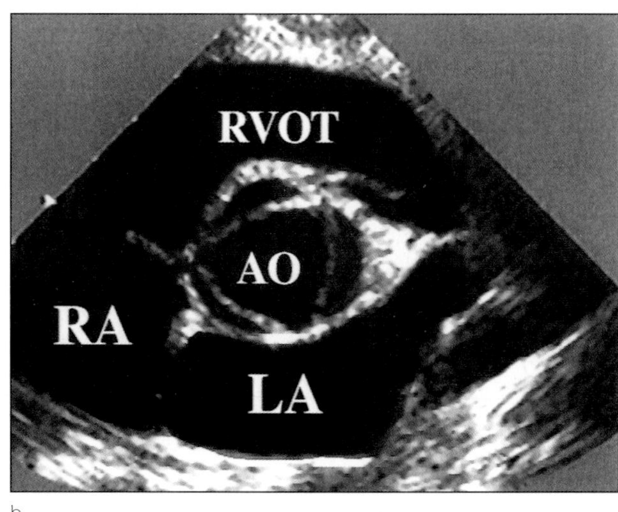

b

Figure 8.2
(a) Two-dimensional echocardiogram of the parasternal short axis at the level of the aortic valve in diastole. The commissures between the right coronary (R), non-coronary (N), and left coronary (L) cusps are clearly visualized. The pulmonic valve is not labeled, but is seen between the right ventricular outflow tract (RVOT) and the pulmonary artery (PA). RA, right atrium; LA, left atrium. (b) The same view in systole. Note the triangular shape of the aortic valve orifice (AO). One of the pulmonary valve cusps is seen in the right ventricular outflow tract. It is at the level of the right and left coronary cusps' commissures.

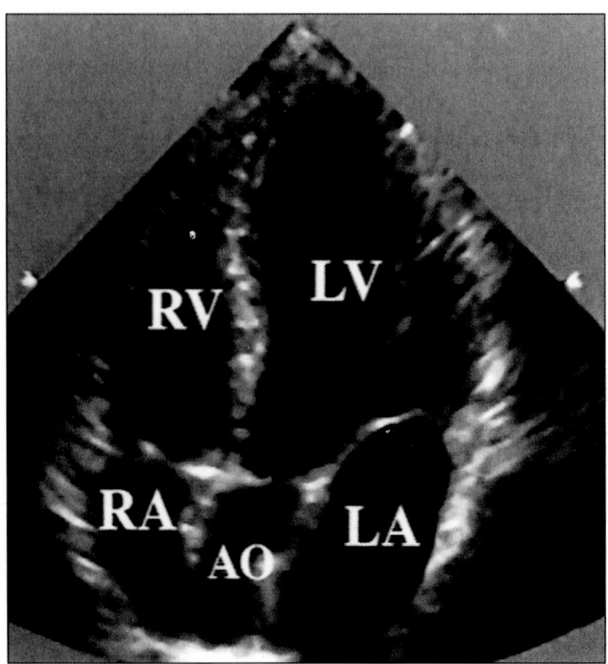

Figure 8.3
Two-dimensional echocardiogram of the apical five-chamber view. The aortic valve is seen in the left ventricular outflow tract. A small portion of the ascending aorta (AO) is also visualized. LV, left ventricle; LA, left atrium; RA, right atrium; RV, right ventricle.

reduced (Fig. 8.3). Short axis views of the aortic valve may also be obtained from the subcostal short axis.

Biplane transesophageal echocardiograms image the aortic valve in transverse and longitudinal planes. The multiplane transducers allow for easier imaging of short- and long-axis views, although these can usually be obtained with manipulation of the biplane probe (Fig. 8.4). Transesophageal imaging is invaluable in the patient with poor transthoracic windows. Occasionally, a mitral valve prosthesis or mitral annular ring may obscure imaging of the aortic valve with this approach.

M-mode images are important for timing of cardiac events and optimize accurate measurements. The aortic valve motion is recorded from the parasternal long-axis view (Fig. 8.5). The leaflets are again seen to coapt in the center of the root. Their motion describes a box-like pattern due to vigorous opening of the leaflets in systole. Their closing should be as abrupt.

Doppler examination

Color flow Doppler examination of the valve should be performed in every view. Abnormal flows will usually be identified as high velocity, turbulent jets. Although spectral Doppler is assessed only from the apical views, color flow

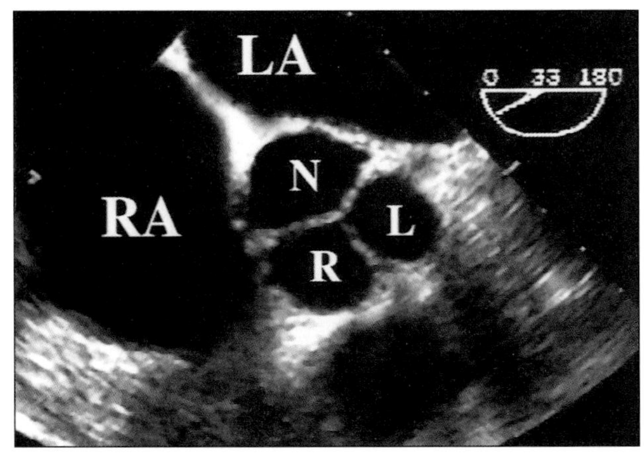

a

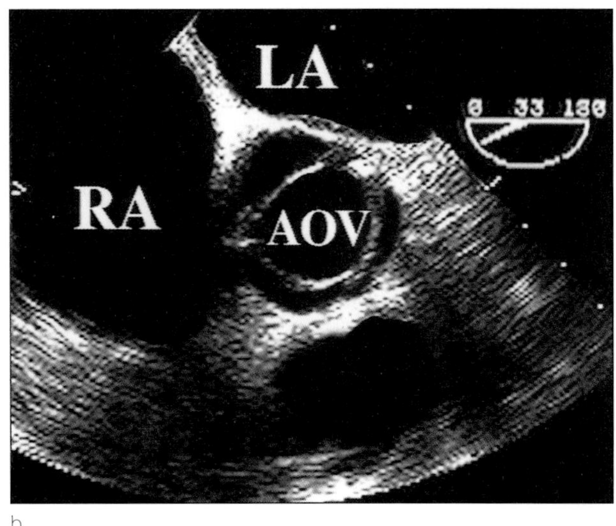

b

Figure 8.4
(a) Transesophageal two-dimensional echocardiogram of the aortic valve in diastole. The left atrium (LA) is the most superior structure. Angulation of the multiplane probe to approximately 30° allows for short-axis visualization of the coronary cusps. The non-coronary (N), right coronary (R), and left coronary (L) cusps are marked. RA, right atrium. (b) The same view in systole. The aortic valve area (AOV) may be planimetered from this view.

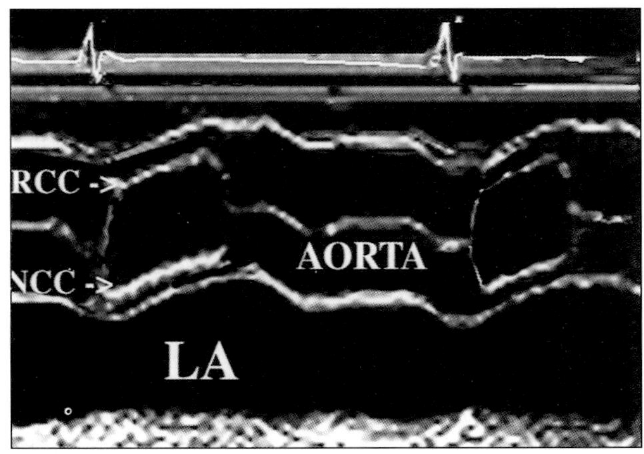

Figure 8.5
M-mode echocardiogram from the parasternal long axis at the level of the aortic valve. The right coronary cusp (RCC) is seen anteriorly and the non-coronary cusp (NCC) is posterior. The systolic opening is abrupt as is the valve closure at the end of systole. The coaptation of the two leaflets in this normal valve is seen to be midline and parallel to the walls of the aortic root.

Doppler in the parasternal views may image eccentric regurgitant jets that would otherwise be missed.

The velocity spectra of the left ventricular outflow can be recorded across the aortic valve from either the apical long-axis or the five-chamber views. Normally, the maximum velocity of the outflow is 1.5 m/s. Pulsed wave Doppler is used to sample the velocity spectra along the septum. The peak velocity increases as the sample volume approaches the aortic valve. The maximum systolic velocity obtained with continuous wave Doppler represents the velocity across the aortic valve (Fig. 8.6a). Velocity spectra across the aortic valve may also be recorded from other views. In both the right parasternal and the suprasternal regions, the jet flow direction is towards the transducer, and the velocity spectra will be a positive deflection above the baseline (Fig. 8.6b). The flow across the aortic valve may be eccentric when the aorta is ectatic or when the aortic valve is calcified. Non-standard transducer positioning may be required to measure the highest velocity. Color flow Doppler imaging can be helpful in identifying the direction of the jet. An imaging Doppler transducer can then be used to align the Doppler ultrasound beam.

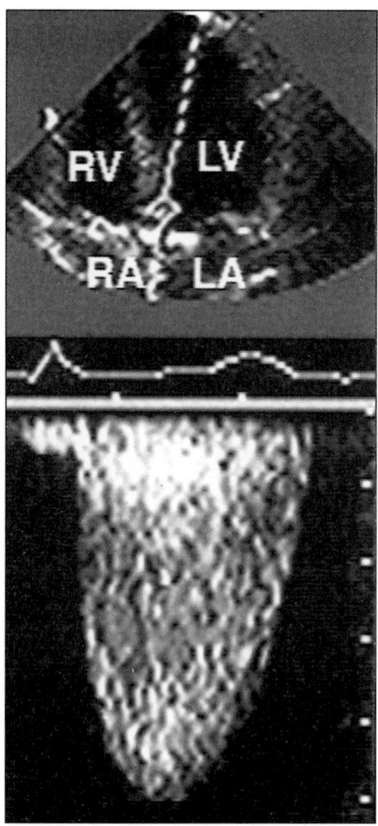

a

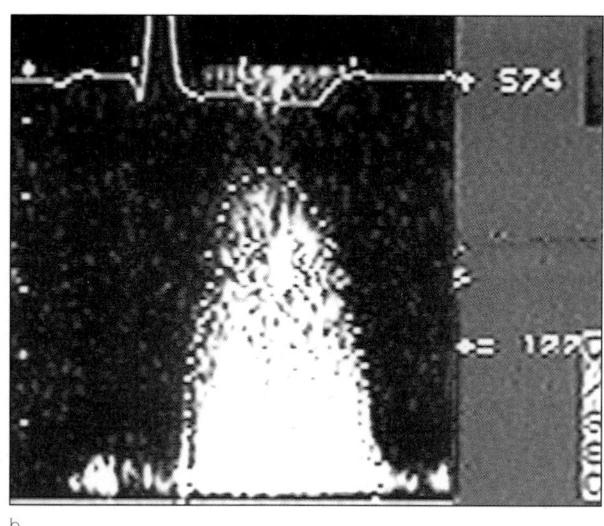

b

Figure 8.6
(a) Continuous wave Doppler tracing from the apical position. The imaging transducer demonstrates correct positioning of the ultrasound beam across the aortic valve from the apical five-chamber view. The peak velocity of almost 5 m/s predicts a transaortic gradient of approximately 100 mmHg. The patient had severe aortic stenosis. Scale: each dot represents 1 m/s or 100 cm/s. (b) Continuous wave Doppler tracing using a non-imaging (Pedoff) transducer in the suprasternal position. The spectral pattern is above the baseline because the flow is towards the transducer. This patient had approximately a 64 mmHg gradient across the valve. Scale as (a).

Bicuspid aortic valve

Bicuspid aortic valve is the most common congenital anomaly in the adult population.[1] An eccentric coaptation point may be demonstrated by M-mode echocardiography. Two-dimensional echocardiogram views from the parasternal short-axis position demonstrate the size and orientation of the leaflets (Fig. 8.7). The leaflets are usually of the same size with the single commissure running obliquely from left to right. An off-axis view may image only two leaflets of a normal trileaflet valve. However, the presence of three leaflets may be inferred by the location of the visible commissures which will be configured as two points of a triangle. The bicuspid valve by contrast has a systolic orifice that is elliptical in shape, resembling a football. Bicuspid valves may be categorized by the relation of the commissures to the coronary ostia. If both coronary arteries arise from the same anterior sinus, the commissure is said to be horizontal. If the commissure is vertical, the coronary arteries arise from opposite sinuses and the leaflets have a right–left orientation. The horizontal commissure is more common, and may have a greater tendency to calcify and become stenotic.[2] This is presumably due to the orientation of normal ejection jets from the ventricle. Either of the leaflets may contain raphe or ridges of tissue at the site of the missing commissure representing partial development. In diastole, the raphe may be mistaken for a commissure. The systolic shape of the orifice and the abnormal motion of the leaflet will distinguish the bileaflet valve with a raphe from an anatomically normal one.

In younger patients, the bicuspid valve is more likely to be regurgitant than stenotic.[3] However, bicuspid valves tend to calcify prematurely and present as aortic stenosis in the fourth or fifth decade. Coarction of the aorta is the congenital anomaly most frequently associated with bicuspid aortic valves. It is essential that the transverse and descending thoracic aorta be carefully imaged from the suprasternal position. Careful Doppler interrogation should be performed from the suprasternal position in the descending aorta to rule out a step up in gradient. The abdominal aorta may also be interrogated from the subcostal view. Coarctation of the descending thoracic aorta is associated with persistent forward diastolic flow.

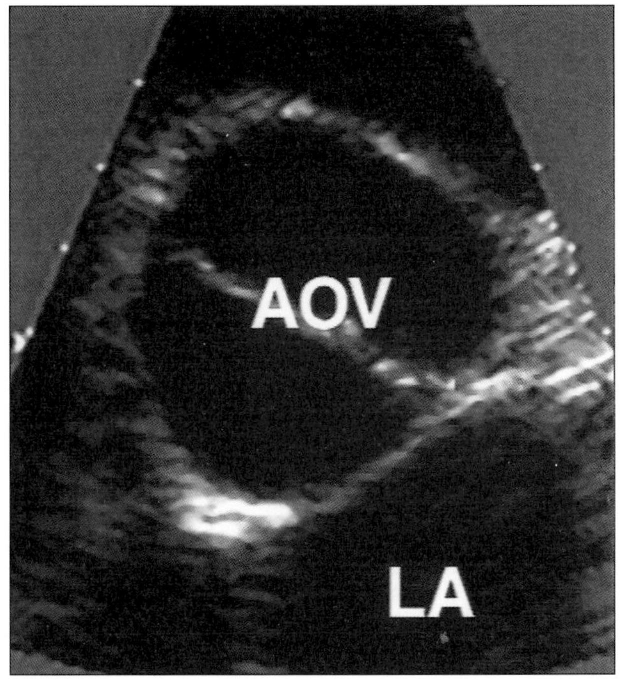

a

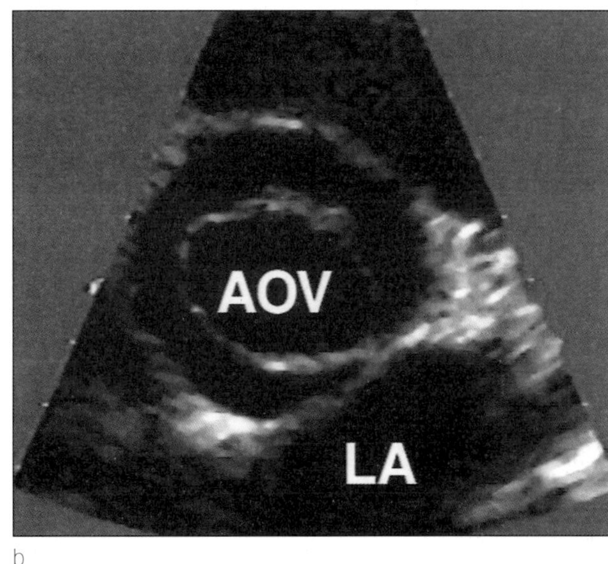

b

Figure 8.7
(a) Two-dimensional echocardiogram of a bicuspid aortic valve (AOV) in diastole taken from the parasternal short axis. The single commissure runs obliquely. The anterior leaflet is slightly larger than the posterior leaflet. Both coronary arteries (not imaged in this reproduction) arose from the anterior sinus. The valve would thus be characterized as having a horizontal commissure. (b) The elliptical shape of the orifice of the bicuspid valve is appreciated in this echocardiogram. LA, left atrium.

Aortic stenosis

Two-dimensional echocardiography

The etiology of aortic stenosis can usually be ascertained from the transthoracic study. The parasternal short-axis view is often the most helpful in this regard. Congenital aortic stenosis usually presents in infancy. Congenitally stenotic valves may be unicuspid or bicuspid and rarely tricuspid or quadracuspid. Systolic doming of the leaflets is best seen in the parasternal long-axis view. Bicuspid valves calcify with time and can present in the fourth or fifth decade with severe aortic stenosis. Senile calcific aortic stenosis begins with calcium deposits at the base of the cusps with slowly progressive involvement of the leaflets. The calcium deposits become large enough to restrict motion of the valves and may extend from the annulus to the tips of the leaflets (Fig. 8.8). Degenerative calcific aortic stenosis is often associated with calcification of the mitral annulus and presents in the sixth or seventh decades of life. Rheumatic disease results in fusion and calcification of the commissures beginning at the annulus. The cusps also

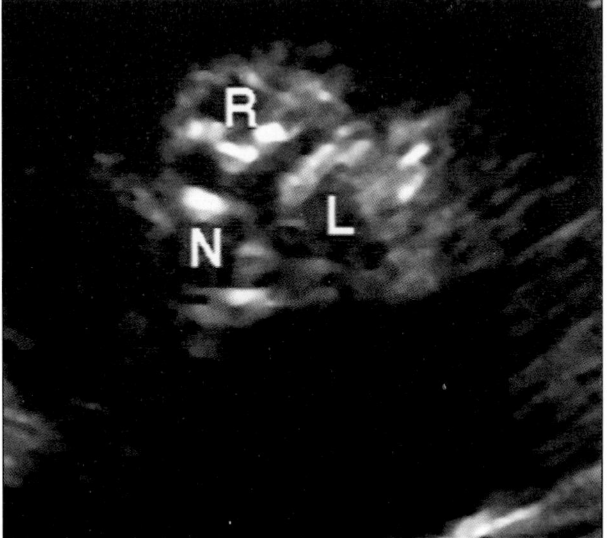

Figure 8.8
Two-dimensional echocardiogram of an aortic valve in the parasternal short-axis view. The cusps are labeled. R, right coronary cusp; N, non-coronary cusp; L, left coronary cusp. Dense calcific deposits are seen at the base of the leaflets, particularly the left coronary cusp. These deposits restricted leaflet motion and caused severe calcific aortic stenosis.

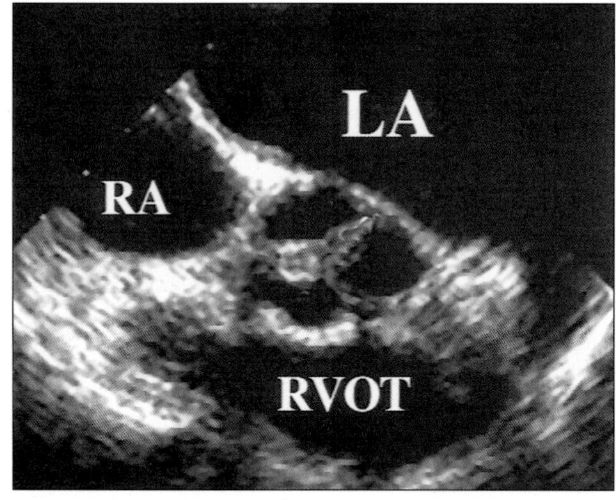

a

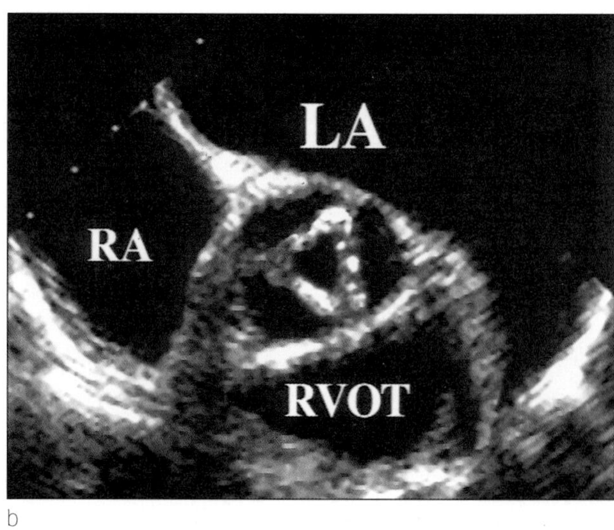

b

Figure 8.9
(a) Transesophageal two-dimensional echocardiogram of the aortic valve in diastole. The patient had rheumatic fever several times as a young adult. The commissures are markedly thickened. In contrast to calcific aortic stenosis, the root and the leaflets are relatively unaffected. LA, left atrium; RA, right atrium; RVOT, right ventricular outflow tract. (b) The same view in systole. The opening of the valve is shown to be restricted due to partial fusion of the commissures.

thicken and scar. The process is always associated with involvement of the mitral valve (Fig. 8.9).

It is not always possible to determine reliably the severity of the stenosis from the two-dimensional images. Pre-Doppler studies attempted to correlate the separation of the aortic valve leaflets on M-mode and two-dimensional echocardiographic images with the severity of stenosis measured at catheterization.[4,5] The correlations have been poor, although an opening of <8 mm is conventionally thought to be associated with significant stenosis. Planimetry of the valve orifice from the short-axis view is often difficult because of ultrasound artifacts arising from the calcification and thickening of the valve. Color flow Doppler imaging sometimes allows better definition of the orifice.[6] Clearly visualized movement of two of three cusps to the aortic wall in systole rules out significant aortic stenosis. Conversely, in critical aortic stenosis the valve leaflets usually do not appear to move throughout the cardiac cycle. Occasionally, the short-axis image of the valve is obtained at the level of pliable but congenitally stenotic cusps making the orifice appear much larger than is actually the case. As previously mentioned, the apical five-chamber view should not be used to assess aortic valve motion. Transesophageal echocardiography usually allows more precise imaging of the size of the aortic valve orifice, and the planimetered area correlates well with invasive measurements of aortic valve area (Fig. 8.10).[7,8] The imaging plane must be oriented to image the cross-section of the valve. If not, a portion of the left ventricular outflow tract may appear to be part of the valve orifice adjacent to the left coronary cusp. Multiplane imaging provides a better assessment of the aortic valve area than monoplane transesophageal imaging because multiplane transesophageal transducers allow optimal positioning.[9] A cross-section of the aortic valve can usually be obtained with the transducer rotated to approximately 30° from the transverse plane. An aortic valve area of <0.5 cm^2 can be inferred

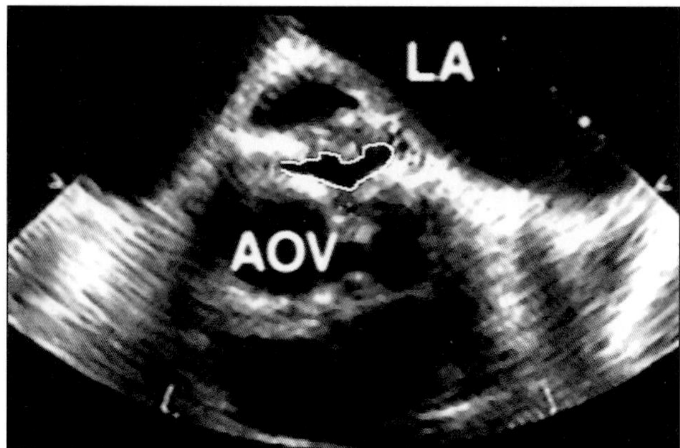

Figure 8.10
Transesophageal two-dimensional echocardiogram of a stenotic aortic valve in systole. The valve is imaged in short axis. The aortic valve area has been planimetered off line and the area computed. This can be done on line with most current equipment. AOV, aortic valve; LA, left atrium.

if there is no motion of the valve and no identifiable orifice on the transesophageal images.[10]

Chronic outflow obstruction results in progressive left ventricular hypertrophy and reduction in cavity size so that end-systolic wall stress is normalized. Severe aortic stenosis can be excluded in a ventricle with normal contracile function and no significant hypertrophy. The progression of aortic stenosis is a gradual process. The development of left ventricular dilatation and worsening mitral regurgitation also indicates progression of the stenosis and failure of the compensatory mechanisms.[11] Gender differences in the ventricular response to aortic stenosis have been described. Women are more likely to have hyperdynamic function, more severe hypertrophy and more abnormal indices of diastolic dysfunction.[12,13] Severe hypertrophy and hyperdynamic ventricular function predict a high morbidity and mortality after aortic valve replacement. Hyperdynamic function may cause intraventricular cavity obstruction characterized by cavity obliteration and abnormal dagger-shaped spectral Doppler velocity signal in the mid-cavity. When postoperative hypotension caused by intracavitary obstruction is treated with ionotropes, profound hypotension and death may result.

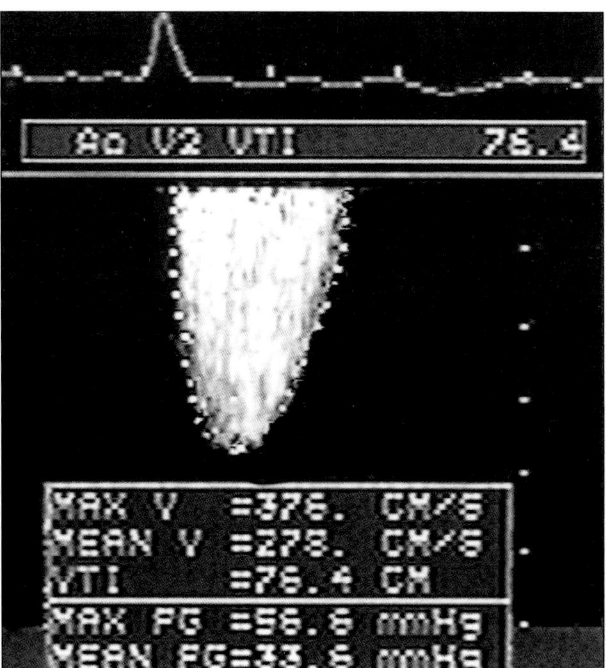

Figure 8.11
Continuous wave Doppler spectral flow velocity tracing across a stenotic aortic valve. The transducer is positioned in the apical five-chamber position. The spectral signal has been traced on line. The peak gradient is calculated from the maximum velocity. The mean gradient is calculated by integrating the velocity flow tracing over the systolic time interval. In this example, the maximum velocity (MAX V) = 376 cm/s, mean velocity (MEAN V) = 278 cm/s and the velocity time integral (VTI) = 76.4 cm. The maximum gradient (MAX PG) = 56.6 mmHg and the mean gradient (MEAN PG) = 33.6 mmHg.

Doppler measurements

Aortic valve gradient

Development of continuous wave Doppler allows assessment of the severity of aortic stenosis with a degree of accuracy comparable to cardiac catheterization. The modified Bernoulli equation relates the velocity of blood across the valve to the pressure gradient between the left ventricle and the aorta.[14]

$$P_1 - P_2 = 4(v_1^2 - v_2^2) \qquad \text{(Equation 1)}$$

where $P_1 - P_2$ represents the gradient across the valve, v_1 represents the peak velocity across the aortic valve measured by continuous wave Doppler, and v_2 is the velocity in the left ventricular outflow tract measured by pulsed Doppler. In a further simplification, the velocity of blood in the outflow tract may be ignored since it is usually less than 1 m/s. In that case, the equation becomes:

$$P_1 - P_2 = 4v^2 \qquad \text{(Equation 2)}$$

When the spectral velocity tracing is integrated over the systolic interval, the mean pressure gradient can be calculated (Fig. 8.11). Both peak and mean pressure gradients obtained by Doppler have correlated well with gradients obtained at catheterization.[14,15] The correlations are best when the measurements are performed simultaneously (or nearly so) since hemodynamic conditions affecting the gradients, particularly cardiac output, may vary from day to day.[16,17] Furthermore, the peak gradient obtained by Doppler echocardiography is an instantaneous gradient, while the peak-to-peak gradient is conventionally used in the catheterization laboratory (Fig. 8.12).

The accuracy of the Doppler-derived gradients depends on various technical and theoretical factors. Most importantly, the ultrasound beam should be parallel to the direction of blood flow. If not, the measured velocity will vary from the true velocity by the cosine of the incidence angle, and the estimated gradient will be less than the true gradient. The blood flow may be eccentric in stenotic valves or ectactic aortas so that the direction of flow may not be parallel to the walls of the aortic root. Continuous wave Doppler velocity should be measured in the apical five-chamber, the apical long-axis, the right parasternal and the suprasternal positions, and the highest velocity used. It is not acceptable to average the velocities obtained, rather the highest recorded velocity after a

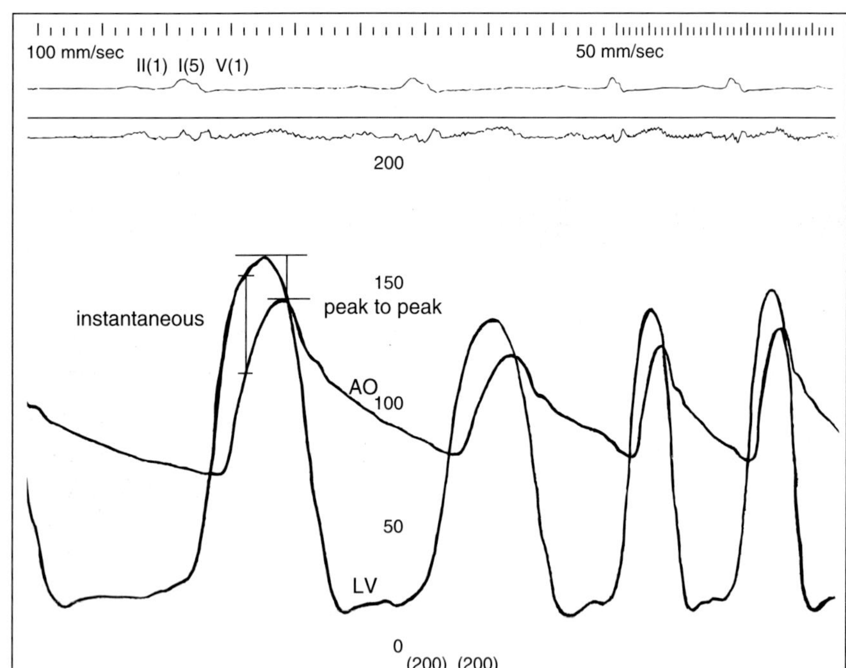

Figure 8.12
Simultaneous pressure tracings of the left ventricle (LV) and aorta (AO) in a patient with moderate aortic stenosis. The peak-to-peak gradient reported by the catheterization laboratory is seen to be different than the instantaneous gradient obtained by echocardiography.

normal beat should be used. It is not possible to overestimate the aortic valve gradient by malalignment of the interrogating Doppler ultrasound beam. However, if a mitral regurgitation jet (or any other high velocity jet) is mistaken for the aortic velocity, the aortic valve gradient may be overestimated. Imaging continuous wave transducers make this error easier to avoid, as does knowledge of the magnitude, duration, and acceleration times of the spectral contours of valvular jets.

The gradient across a valve depends not only on the orifice size but also on the flow across the valve. Conditions which increase the cardiac output will produce higher gradients for the same orifice size. Similarly, aortic regurgitation will increase the flow across the valve and may increase the aortic systolic gradient for a given orifice size. In this case, the velocity of blood in the left ventricular outflow tract may be considerably higher than 1 m/s and may not be a negligible factor in the modified Bernoulli equation (see Equation 1). Better correlation with invasively measured gradients has been obtained by taking this factor into account.[18,19] The left ventricular outflow velocity is measured in the apical long-axis or the apical five-chamber views by placing the sample volume several centimeters proximal to the valve and sampling towards the valve. The highest velocity obtained with clearly laminar flow should be used.

Aortic valve area

The continuity equation has been established as the echocardiographic 'gold standard' for assessment of aortic stenosis. The theoretic basis of the equation is the conservation of mass. The volume of blood flow across the aortic valve orifice must equal the volume of blood flow across the left ventricular outflow tract. The velocity time integral of a Doppler velocity signal is equal to the flow past a given point in one cardiac cycle. The product of the velocity time integral and the cross-sectional area both measured at a given point is equal to the total flow past that level during the cardiac cycle. Thus the continuity equation is:

$$CSA_{AV} \times VTI_{AV} = CSA_{LVOT} \times VTI_{LVOT} \quad \text{(Equation 3)}$$

where CSA_{AV} is the cross-sectional area of the aortic valve, VTI_{AV} is the velocity time integral of the peak velocity spectral envelope measured by continuous wave, CSA_{LVOT} is the cross-sectional area of the left ventricular outflow tract, and VTI_{LVOT} is the velocity time integral of the velocity spectral envelope measured in the left ventricular outflow tract by pulsed Doppler.

The area of the left ventricular outflow tract can be calculated by measuring the left ventricular outflow diameter (*D*) and applying the formula for the area of a circle. Solving for the aortic valve area gives the continuity equation:

$$CSA_{AV} = \pi(D_{LVOT}/2)^2 \times VTI_{LVOT}/VTI_{AV} \quad \text{(Equation 4)}$$

(Fig. 8.13). Aortic valve areas calculated by the continuity equation show excellent correlation with invasively obtained areas calculated with the Gorlin equation.[20,21]

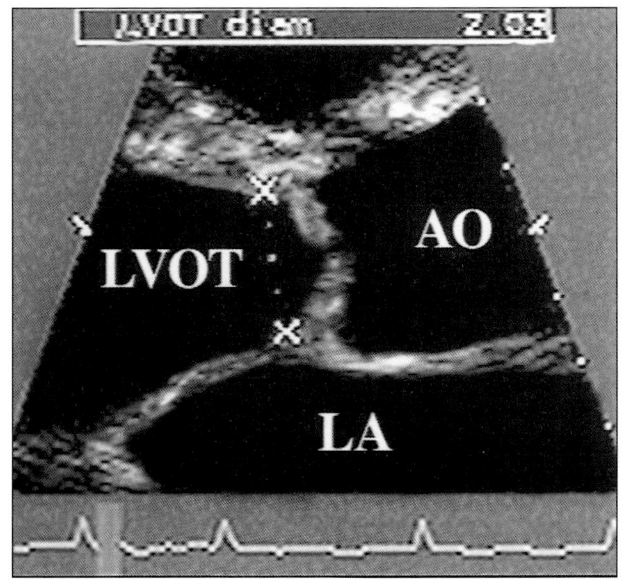

a

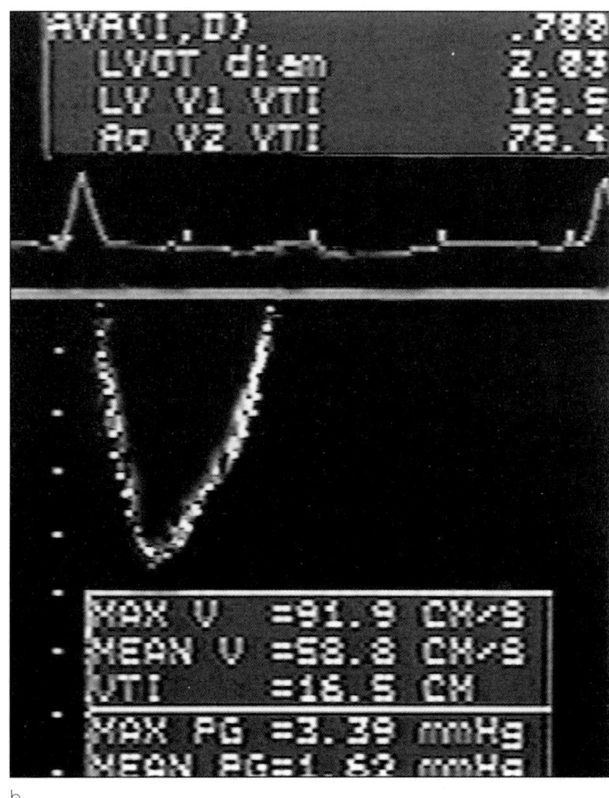

b

Figure 8.13
An example of the continuity calculation in a patient with rheumatic aortic stenosis. (a) The diameter of the left ventricular outflow tract is measured in the parasternal long-axis view and is seen to be 2.03 cm, which is rounded to the nearest tenth (2.0 cm). (b) The velocity time integral in the left ventricular outflow tract is measured from the apical five-chamber view by pulsed Doppler. The velocity spectral envelope was planimetered on line and has a velocity time integral (VTI) = 16.5 cm. The continuous wave Doppler interrogation of the aortic valve in this patient is shown in Figure 8.11. The velocity time integral is 76.4 cm. Substituting these numbers into the continuity equation (Equation 4) yields: AVA = 3.14 × 1 × 16.5/76.4 = 0.678 cm^2, which is rounded to the nearest tenth (0.7 cm^2).

Peak velocities can be substituted for the flow velocity time integrals in the continuity equation.[22]

The accuracy of the aortic valve area calculation by the continuity equation is dependent on a number of factors. As noted in the discussion on aortic valve gradients, the ultrasound beam must be aligned as close to parallel to the direction of blood flow as possible to measure the maximum flow velocities. The diameter of the left ventricular outflow tract should only be measured in the parasternal long-axis view in systole immediately below the level of the aortic annulus. In the average adult patient, the diameter is approximately 2 cm.[23] Because the diameter measurement is squared in the calculation of the cross-sectional area (area = $\pi(\text{diameter}/2)^2$), an error in the left ventricular outflow tract diameter measurement is propagated as a larger quadratic error in the continuity equation. In cases in which the diameter cannot be measured accurately, it may be useful to use the arbitrary value of 2 cm while noting the inherent inaccuracy. The left ventricular outflow velocity may be difficult to resolve in the setting of very high velocities associated with subvalvular obstruction. In this setting, the outflow tract diameter cannot be easily measured and the continuity equation cannot be applied. The peak gradient obtained represents the pressure drop across both the subvalvular and the valvar obstruction. Planimetry of the orifice area from the transesophageal approach may provide an assessment of the contribution of the valvar stenosis to the overall gradient.

The aortic valve area calculated by continuity equation should be independent of cardiac output. Recently, the aortic valve area measured by the Gorlin equation has been shown to be dependent on transvalvular flow rates.[24–26] The continuity equation has not been dependent on the flow rate in some studies,[24,26] but not all.[25] The continuity equation has proven to be a reliable tool in multiple clinical settings and can be used with confidence if the echocardiographic variables have been correctly measured. There is evidence that the preoperative use of catheterization is declining after diagnosis by echocardiography.[27] However, catheterization is necessary for the assessment of coronary anatomy in patients who are at increased risk for clinically significant coronary artery disease. Initial studies indicate that aortic valve areas obtained by planimetry of the aortic valve via the transesophageal approach are not dependent on transvalvular flow rates.[28]

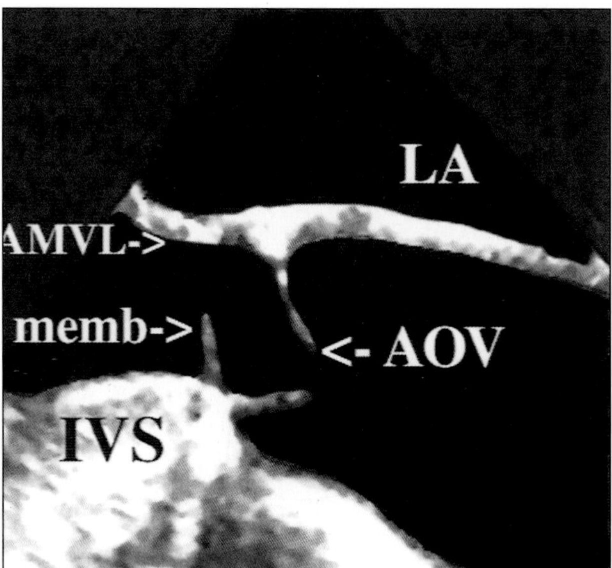

Figure 8.14
Transesophageal two-dimensional echocardiogram in the longitudinal plane. A subaortic membrane (memb) arises from the interventricular septum (IVS). Its attachment to the anterior mitral valve leaflet (AMVL) is not seen in this view. The membrane is seen to be closely associated with the right coronary cusp of the aortic valve (AOV).

Surgical options

The decision to replace a stenotic aortic valve is largely a clinical one. However, echocardiography may be useful in identifying high-risk patients. Left ventricular failure is a poor prognostic sign as is a severely hypertrophied, hyperdynamic left ventricle with a high intracavitary gradient and a small cavity.[29] Women appear to have a greater tendency to develop severe hypertrophy with the same degree of stenosis.[12,13]

The Ross procedure involves the placement of a pulmonary autograft in the aortic site and a bioprosthesis in the pulmonary position. The aortic and pulmonic annulus can both be sized during intraoperative transesophageal echocardiographic study to determine if the autograft will be an appropriate size.[30,31] Follow-up echocardiographic studies of autografts as well as of prosthetic valve replacements are essential for optimal postoperative patient care.

Subvalvular aortic stenosis

Fixed subaortic stenosis is usually due to a discrete subaortic membrane or shelf which partially obstructs the left ventricular outflow tract. The membrane may encircle the entire left ventricular outflow tract with an ostium of varying size. Alternatively, a crescent-shaped thick shelf arises from the interventricular septum. The obstructing structure may be a thin membrane, but is often a thick ridge of tissue arising as a bulge from the interventricular septum (Fig. 8.14). Subaortic stenosis most frequently presents in infancy or childhood. If the subvalvular obstruction is present for any length of time, damage to the aortic valve from the high velocity jet may result in aortic insufficiency. The membrane may also interfere with leaflet function if it is contiguous with the valve leaflets. Associated lesions include aortic obstructions (coarctation of the descending thoracic aorta, interrupted aortic arch, and supravalvular aortic stenosis) as well as primum atrial septal defects. Accessory mitral tissue may cause subaortic stenosis.[32] Turbulent flow in the left ventricular outflow tract is thought to predispose to the development of the abnormal subvalvular tissue.[33,34]

The subaortic membrane may be very difficult to visualize but is generally best seen in the parasternal long-axis view or the apical five-chamber view. The membrane appears as a bright echodensity in the left ventricular outflow tract 1–8 mm below the valve. The attachment to the ventricular surface of the anterior mitral valve leaflet may cause concomitant mitral regurgitation.[35] Sometimes the turbulent flow caused by the left ventricular outflow tract obstruction can be appreciated by color flow Doppler imaging even when the membrane is not visualized. Transesophageal echocardiography provides better visualization of the attachments of the valve and can be used to direct surgical therapy.[36–38] Transesophageal studies can be safely undertaken in children by trained clinicians, with appropriate transducers. Continuous wave Doppler can measure the outflow tract pressure gradient.[39–41] The surgical approach in discrete subaortic stenosis can be simple resection of the membrane, although aortic valve replacement may be required for significant aortic regurgitation or concurrent aortic stenosis. However, regrowth of the membrane has been described in a significant minority of patients, occasionally many years after the original surgery.[42] Balloon angioplasty of discrete membranes is most successful with membranes <3 mm thick. Results of the procedure can be assessed and followed serially by transthoracic studies.[43] Complex diffuse subaortic stenosis requires a more complicated surgical approach which often involves aortic root reconstruction and aortic valve replacement, usually with a homograft. Recently, the use of the pulmonary autograft and left ventricular outflow tract enlargement with allograft aortic or Dacron patches has been described.[44,45]

Supravalvular aortic stenosis

Supravalvular aortic stenosis can be recognized as an hourglass narrowing of the ascending aorta usually immediately above the aortic root. It is best visualized in the parasternal long axis with a high window so that the proximal ascending aorta is imaged (Fig. 8.15). Williams' syndrome is the most common cause of obstruction at this level and is characterized by abnormal and typical facies, mental retardation, hypercalcemia and supravalvular aortic and pulmonic stenosis.[46] Patients with familial homozygous hypercholesterolemia may develop supravalvular stenosis with the deposition of atherosclerotic plaques along the root and ascending aorta. The gradients are usually low and can be followed by Doppler echocardiography.[47,48] When concomitant aortic valve stenosis is suspected, imaging of the valve may exclude significant obstruction. The aorta proximal to the level of obstruction can be interrogated with pulsed Doppler echocardiography to rule out the presence of a high velocity jet. As in the case of subvalvular obstruction, if both levels of obstruction are present, only the total transtenotic gradient can be obtained. It may be impossible to determine the contribution of each level of the obstruction to the total gradient. Transesophageal imaging of the aortic valve and planimetry of the valve area may be helpful in this case.

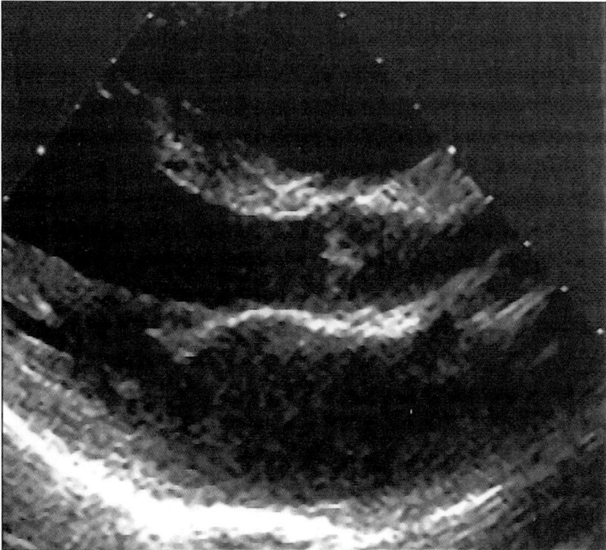

Figure 8.15
Two-dimensional echocardiogram from the parasternal long axis in a patient with supravalvular stenosis. The ascending aorta is narrowed to <1 cm in diameter (distance markings are at 1-cm intervals). Doppler echocardiogram demonstrated a mild step-up in velocity across this narrowing (not shown).

Aortic regurgitation

Chronic aortic regurgitation

Two-dimensional echocardiography

All the processes which result in aortic stenosis may also produce aortic regurgitation. Calcific degeneration is unlikely to cause severe insufficiency, but as the valvular architecture is disrupted, the initial lesion may be regurgitation. Regurgitation may lessen as the disease process continues and the orifice becomes smaller and more stenotic. Almost all congenitally abnormal valves are at least mildly regurgitant. Both calcific degeneration and rheumatic disease can produce a fixed orifice that is both stenotic and regurgitant.

Aortic valve prolapse has been identified as an infrequent but increasingly recognized cause of aortic regurgitation.[49-51] It is most easily visualized in the parasternal long-axis view (Fig. 8.16). The body of at least one cusp will be seen to prolapse past the aortic annulus into the left ventricular outflow tract in diastole. Prolapse may also be appreciated in transesophageal views particularly in the longitudinal axis which parallels the parasternal long axis. Aortic valve prolapse may be associated with bicuspid valves, myxomatous changes of the aortic leaflets, and mitral valve prolapse. Damage to the leaflets or the supporting structures may occur with endocarditis or traumatic disruption. High velocity jets associated with subvalvar obstruction may be directed onto a cusp and cause progressive damage. The high velocity jet associated with a perimembranous ventricular septal defect will pass immediately below the right coronary cusp. A Venturi force may cause the cusp to prolapse into the left ventricular outflow tract or even through the septal defect. The danger of developing severe aortic insufficiency is the basis

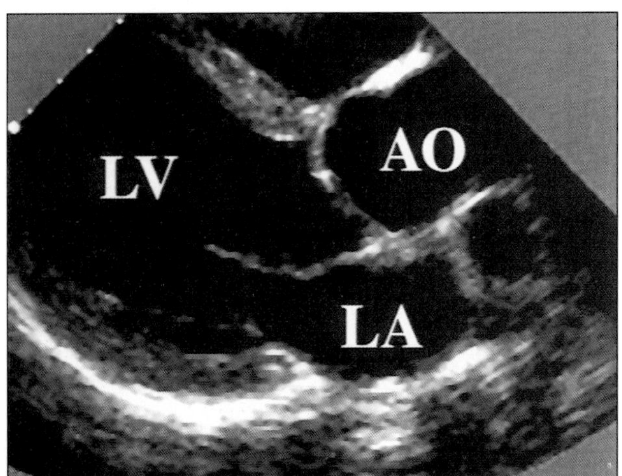

Figure 8.16
Two-dimensional echocardiogram of the parasternal long axis in diastole demonstrating prolapse of both the right and non-coronary cusps of the aortic valve below the level of the aortic annulus.

for the recommendation that all perimembranous defects be closed. The familiar maxim that 'aortic regurgitation begets aortic regurgitation' emphasizes the role of aortic root dilatation in the development of valvular insufficiency. Many processes primarily involving the aorta may result in aortic regurgitation. Transesophageal echocardiography has a special role in the diagnosis of aortic dissection and aneurysm (see later).

Chronic severe aortic regurgitation always leads to left ventricular dilatation associated with concentric hypertrophy. The globular shape peculiar to this etiology of ventricular remodeling is most easily recognized from the apical four-chamber view. Hypertrophy of the walls initially normalizes the wall stress but eventually the hypertrophy cannot keep up with the increased volume. Wall stress rises and contractile function falls. The decrease in systolic function may be permanent, accounting for increased surgical mortality in patients who undergo valve replacement after the development of systolic dysfunction. Echocardiography has demonstrated its usefulness in predicting the optimal timing of valve replacement. There is no consensus that a stenotic valve should ever be replaced in an asymptomatic patient. However, it is quite clear that irreversible but asymptomatic left ventricular function may occur in the course of chronic severe aortic insufficiency.[52] Patients with decreased systolic function have a higher morbidity and mortality associated with aortic valve replacement.[53] An end-systolic dimension >55 mm or a fractional shortening of <25% have been suggested as indications for valve replacement in patients with chronic regurgitation.[54,55] These measurements were made with M-mode echocardiography in the early literature, but similar dimensions may be measured from the two-dimensional parasternal long-axis view. However, repetitive measurements of the end-systolic dimension of the volume-loaded and globular left ventricle can be variable.[56,57] The left ventricular end-systolic dimension is also extremely sensitive to afterload which may vary depending on hemodynamic conditions.[58] Attempts have been made to develop load-independent indices of left ventricular function which can predict incipient contractile failure. End-systolic stress, calculated from two-dimensional imaging and peripheral systolic blood pressure, can be plotted against ventricular systolic diameter at rest and with changing afterloads. The slope of the line is independent of left ventricular loading conditions and is theoretically related to myocardial contractility.[59,60] Although useful in the research setting, these methods are labor-intensive and therefore have not been widely used in clinical practice.

M-mode demonstration of early mitral valve closure is a sign of acute severe decompensated aortic insufficiency (Fig. 8.17).[61] Other M-mode signs of aortic insufficiency such as diastolic fluttering of the anterior mitral valve leaflet and the septum are unnecessary for the diagnosis of aortic insufficiency, do not relate to its severity, and thus are of largely historical interest.

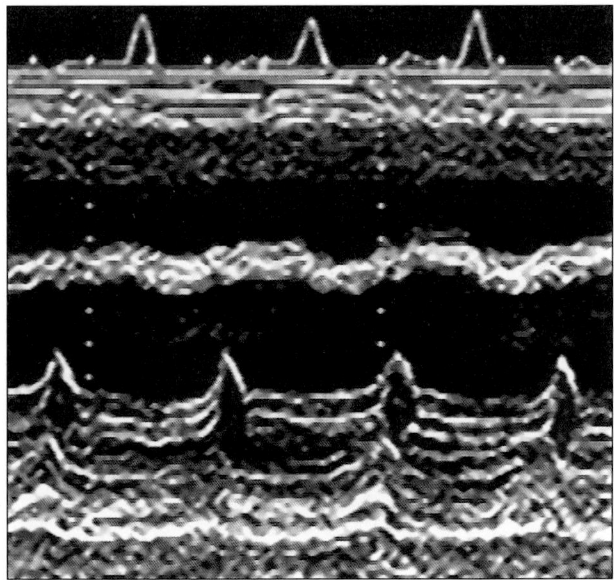

Figure 8.17
M-mode echocardiogram from the parasternal long-axis position demonstrating early closure of the mitral valve. The mitral valve is opened for only a small portion of diastole and closes well before the onset of the QRS complex on the simultaneous EKG tracing.

Doppler assessment of aortic regurgitation

Color flow Doppler

A few quantitative methods have been developed, but the evaluation of the severity of aortic insufficiency remains largely qualitative, both echocardiographically and angiographically. Aortic insufficiency appears as a turbulent, high velocity diastolic jet which originates in the left ventricular outflow tract at the level of the valve itself (Fig. 8.18). The size of the color flow Doppler jet would appear intuitively to be linked to the degree of aortic insufficiency. Both jet length and area correlate with the degree of insufficiency estimated by aortic root injection. The most commonly used criteria rate the degree of aortic insufficiency depending on the length of aortic insufficiency jet. These criteria grade 1+ (mild) regurgitation as a jet identified only in the proximal left ventricular outflow tract. Grade 2+ extends to the tips of the mitral leaflets; grade 3+ to the papillary muscles and grade 4+ to the ventricular apex. This grading system was originally established for pulsed Doppler flow mapping but has been applied to color flow Doppler echocardiography. Similarly, the jet area may be digitized to grade the degree of insufficiency. However, the jet area as well as apparent jet length may vary depending on the view, the gain setting, initial jet velocity, the compliance of the ventricle, the pulse repetition frequency and the transmission frequency.[62–64] These inherent technical inaccuracies have led to the search for other methods of quantifying aortic insufficiency.

The width of the regurgitant jet at its origin has a closer correlation with invasively measured values. A simple technique relates the height of the color jet immediately subjacent to the valve to the height of the ventricular outflow tract in the parasternal long-axis view[65,66] (Fig. 8.19). A ratio of 25% or less correlates with mild aortic insufficiency and a ratio >40% with severe insufficiency. However, it is easy to understand that this ratio will be affected by the shape of the regurgitant orifice and also the orientation of the regurgitant defect to the long axis of the left ventricular outflow tract.[67] To avoid this dependency, the parasternal short-axis view may be used to digitize the cross-sectional area of the regurgitant jet and compare it to the area of the high left ventricular outflow tract. In this case, a ratio of <25% correlates with angiographic 1+ or 2+ insufficiency. However, there is less agreement on the criteria for severe insufficiency, but a ratio of >50% indicates severe aortic insufficiency. An inexperienced sonographer may have difficulty obtaining the short axis of the left ventricular outflow tract.[66] Substituting the area of the root for that of the outflow tract will result in an erroneously small ratio. Jet widths may also be assessed in the transesophageal approach, although the orientation of the beam is less optimal.[68]

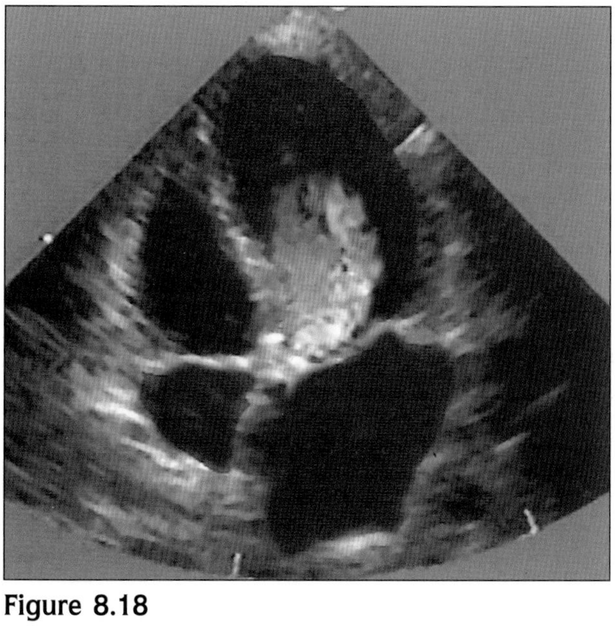

Figure 8.18
Two-dimensional echocardiogram with color Doppler flow imaging in the apical four-chamber view. The left ventricle and left atrium are enlarged. The high velocity turbulent jet of aortic insufficiency is seen in diastole to reach to the papillary muscle level of the left ventricular cavity.

Spectral Doppler

The spectral pattern of the aortic regurgitant jet may be measured by continuous wave Doppler. The peak velocity should be at least 4 m/s representing an initial diastolic gradient of approximately 60 mmHg between the aorta and the left ventricle since pressure difference and velocity are related by a quadratic function in the modified Bernoulli equation. If the aortic insufficiency is mild, the contribution of the regurgitation to ventricular filling will be negligible and the gradient between the aorta and the left ventricle will remain high and relatively constant throughout diastole. This will be represented by a spectral pattern with a flat deceleration slope. On the other hand, severe aortic insufficiency will cause the left ventricular diastolic pressure to rise quickly. The gradient between the aorta and the left ventricle may begin at a normal level but will quickly fall off. This will be represented by a rapid deceleration slope as the velocity of the regurgitant jet falls towards zero (Fig. 8.20). A deceleration slope <200 cm/s^2 is indicative of mild aortic insufficiency. A slope of >400 cm/s^2 correlates with severe insufficiency.[69–72] A direct comparison of deceleration slope to color flow Doppler methods favored the ratio of jet height in the parasternal long-axis view to the height of the outflow tract as the more reliable method in one study.[65] Pressure half

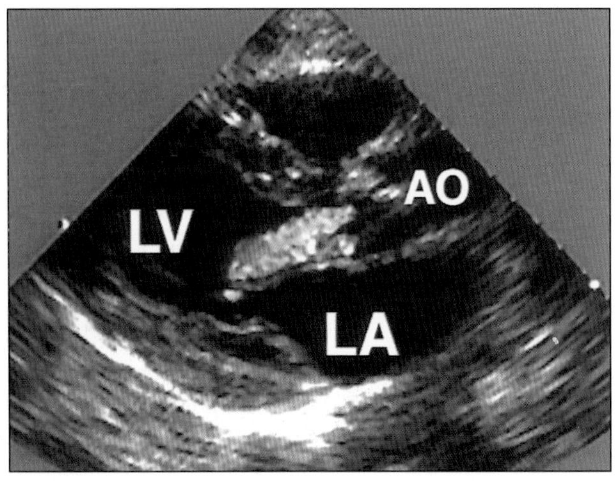

a

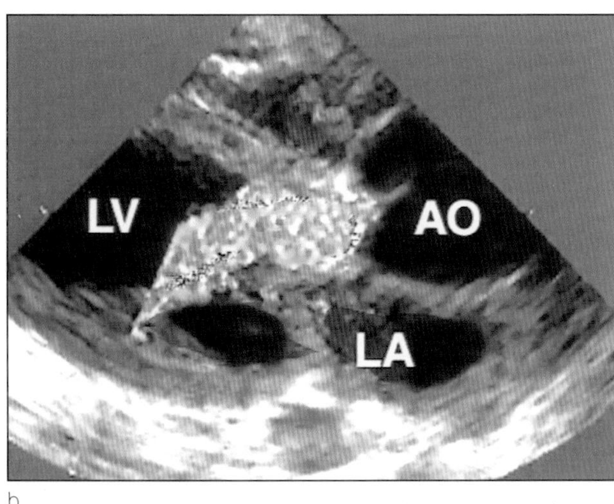

b

Figure 8.19
(a) and (b) Two-dimensional echocardiogram with color Doppler flow imaging from the parasternal long-axis position in two different patients with aortic insufficiency. (a) The aortic valve is thickened and calcified. Two narrow jets of aortic insufficiency are seen immediately below the level of the valve and widen in the outflow tract. The patient had mild aortic insufficiency. (b) The aortic root and ascending aorta are markedly dilated. The jet of aortic insufficiency fills the area below the valve and the entire outflow tract. This patient had severe aortic insufficiency.

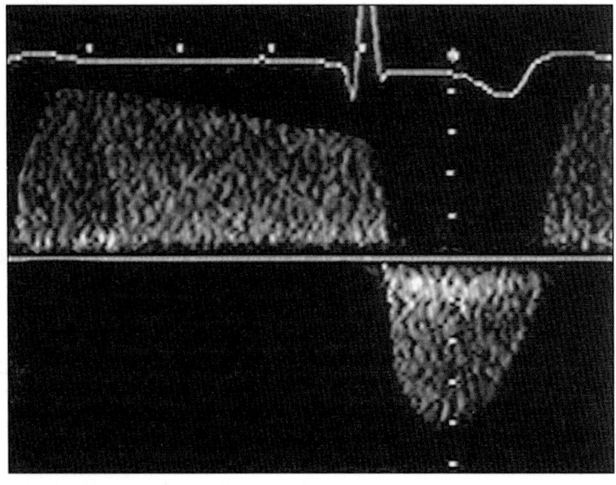

a

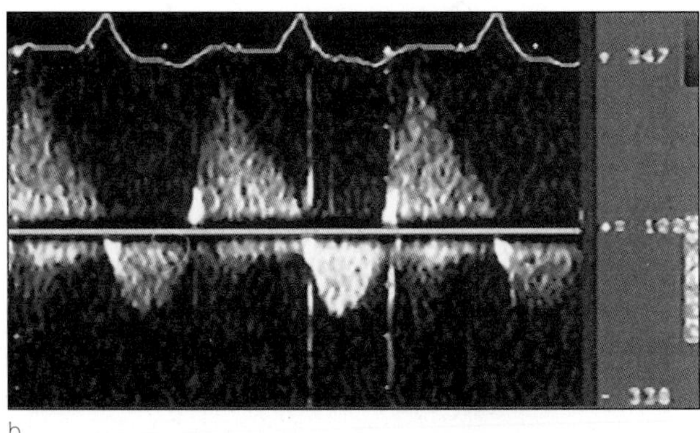

b

Figure 8.20
(a) Continuous wave Doppler spectral tracing in a patient with mild aortic insufficiency. The velocity of the aortic regurgitant jet is initially 3.9 m/s and falls to only 2.8 m/s at the end of diastole. The deceleration slope which can be measured on line (not shown here) is approximately 150 cm/s^2, which is predictive of mild aortic insufficiency. (b) Continuous wave Doppler spectral tracing in a patient with severe and decompensated aortic insufficiency. The velocity of the aortic regurgitant jet is initially only 3.2 m/s and falls to nearly zero by systole. The deceleration slope in this patient is greater than 800 cm/s^2. The left ventricular end-diastolic pressure is extremely high in this patient who was in cardiogenic shock.

time can also be calculated from the continuous wave spectra, but deceleration slope has proved to be a better discriminator of severe insufficiency.[65,70] A direct comparison of deceleration slope to color flow Doppler methods favored the ratio of jet height in the parasternal long-axis view to the height of the outflow tract as the more reliable method in one study.[65] Concomitant mitral stenosis may occasionally limit the assessment of aortic insufficiency by color flow Doppler by imposing a second turbulent diastolic jet in the region of the left ventricular outflow tract. Deceleration slope of the continuous wave spectral Doppler may be more reliable in this situation.[71]

The aorta can be interrogated from the suprasternal notch with the patient's head extended by placing a small roll under the neck. The ascending aorta, transverse arch and descending thoracic aorta can be seen in this view. In the normal patient, there is a brief signal of flow reversal in the proximal ascending aorta as the aortic valve closes. As the degree of aortic insufficiency worsens, the diastolic flow reversal is seen in the transverse aorta and in the descending thoracic aorta. The area under the curve of the diastolic pulsed wave spectral display should be at least one-third the area under the systolic curve to be considered significant (Fig. 8.21). Only the descending thoracic aorta should be assessed by pulsed wave Doppler to detect flow reversal. If the sample volume is too high in the transverse aorta, the ultrasound beam may be more perpendicular than parallel to blood flow and fail to detect flow reversal. Use of continuous wave Doppler will eliminate the range gating and make analysis of the signal unreliable. Flow reversal in the descending thoracic aorta may also be assessed by transesophageal echocardiography.[73] Artifactual diastolic flow reversal may be seen if the sample volume is placed too close to the origin of the left subclavian or the left carotid arteries. Normal diastolic runoff towards the transducer in the suprasternal notch may be misinterpreted as evidence of aortic regurgitation. An arteriovenous fistula in the left arm may also cause reversal of diastolic flow in the descending thoracic aorta in the absence of aortic insufficiency. Evidence of reversal of flow in the abdominal aorta is suggestive of severe aortic insufficiency.[74,75]

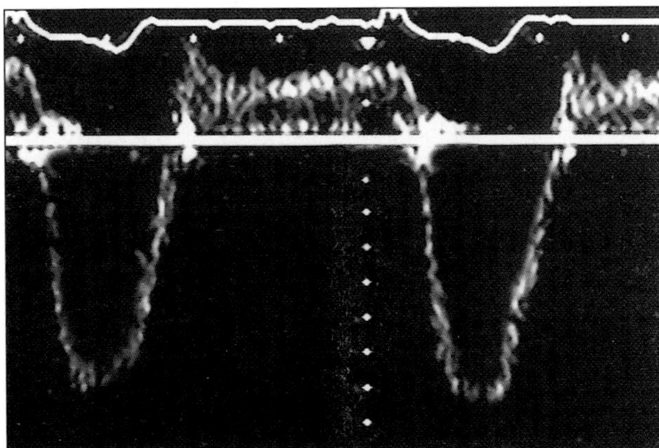

Figure 8.21
Pulsed wave Doppler spectral flow tracing from the descending thoracic aorta. The transducer is in the suprasternal notch. There is continuous retrograde flow towards the transducer indicative of severe aortic insufficiency.

Several other methods have been described which attempt to quantify aortic regurgitation. Regurgitant fractions may be calculated by determining the difference between the right-sided and left-sided stroke volume using spectral Doppler flow patterns.[76] The velocity time integrals of the pulmonary artery and the left ventricular outflow tracts are measured in a method similar to the calculation of shunt ratios or Qp/Qs. However, the regurgitant fraction is given by the formula:

$$\text{Regurgitant fraction} = Qp - Qs$$

As in the calculation of shunt ratios, the method is dependent on the measurement of the pulmonary artery diameter which may be problematic. In an attempt to find a flow-independent measure of the degree of valvular insufficiency, the 'regurgitant orifice' has recently been described.[77–80] One of the major difficulties with these newer methods is the lack of an invasive standard to judge their correctness.

In our laboratory, we assess the degree of aortic insufficiency by routinely evaluating the area and height of color Doppler jets in all relevant views to calculate the ratio of jet height to left ventricular outflow tract height, measuring the deceleration slope of the continuous wave Doppler spectral pattern and assessing flow velocity reversal in the descending thoracic aorta. A synthesis of all of these Doppler and two-dimensional parameters usually provides an accurate evaluation of the extent of aortic insufficiency.

Acute severe aortic insufficiency

The methods used to assess chronic aortic insufficiency may not be relevant to the evaluation of acute aortic insufficiency leading to hemodynamic compromise. The most severe insufficiency will lead to rapid equilibration of aortic and left ventricular diastolic pressures in a normal size ventricle. Thus the color Doppler jet may be very small or not visible. The spectral pattern of the continuous wave Doppler will have a low peak velocity and an extremely rapid deceleration slope (Fig. 8.20b). These phenomena are related to the inaudibility of the murmur of acute severe aortic insufficiency. In the most severe case, complete disruption or avulsion of the valve, the aorta and left ventricle are a continuous chamber and there is little diastolic flow into the ventricle. As previously noted, early closure of the mitral valve as seen on two-dimensional or M-mode echocardiography is an ominous sign, as is diastolic mitral regurgitation in the absence of first degree aortic valve block.[61] Furthermore, the left ventricular function will be reduced rather than hyperdynamic due to the severe acute volume overload. Two-dimensional echocardiography may demonstrate one or more flail aortic cusps, with or without vegetations involving the valve. Transesophageal echocardiography may be necessary to demonstrate disruption of valvular or annular architecture from endocarditis, aortic dissection or trauma. Since acute severe aortic insufficiency is rapidly fatal, there should be little delay in transport to the operating room where the valvular abnormality can be addressed.

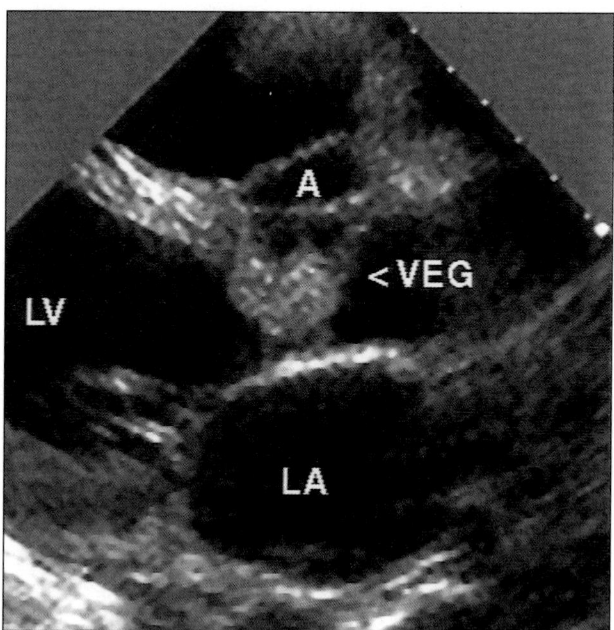

Figure 8.22
Two-dimensional echocardiogram in the parasternal long-axis view of a patient with aortic valve endocarditis. The large vegetation (VEG) involves all of the aortic valve leaflets and partially fills the aortic root. A large annular abscess (A) is seen in the anterior aortic root. The left atrium (LA) is mildly dilated. The left ventricle (LV) is of normal size.

Endocarditis of the aortic valve

Echocardiography should be performed in any patient suspected of having endocarditis. It is no longer acceptable to view endocarditis as a purely clinical and laboratory diagnosis that does not require an imaging study. In addition, potentially lethal complications such as abscess formation may be apparent only on echocardiographic examination, necessitating early and definitive surgical treatment. However, it would be inappropriate to perform echocardiography on every patient with a single positive blood culture or bacteremia from another identifiable source which is rarely associated with endocarditis (e.g. pneumococcal pneumonia). Transthoracic echocardiography should be the initial study except in patients with mitral valve prosthesis, in which case it may be more efficient to proceed directly to transesophageal study. The resolution of the transthoracic study is approximately 2 mm. Smaller vegetations may not be visualized transthoracically. Studies have reported detection of vegetations in 50–80% of patients with proven bacterial endocarditis.[81] Vegetations appear as polypoid masses with independent or chaotic motion. They usually involve the ventricular surface of aortic valve cusps and are associated with some degree of aortic insufficiency (Fig. 8.22). Nonspecific abnormalities of the valve may be present. It is well known that the failure to visualize definite vegetations on transthoracic echocardiography does not rule out the diagnosis of endocarditis. Thickening of the aortic root is a sign of possible abscess formation and requires immediate follow-up with transesophageal echocardiography. The presence of a pericardial effusion is suggestive of valve ring abscess or concurrent purulent pericarditis and requires immediate further evaluation.

Transesophageal echocardiography has revolutionized the evaluation of endocarditis. Numerous studies have documented the improved sensitivity and specificity of this approach for the detection of vegetations and the complications of endocarditis (Fig. 8.23).[81–84] Similarly, biplane and multiplane imaging have been shown to be superior to monoplane imaging, particularly in the evaluation of aortic valve involvement.[85] Serial studies are indicated for the detection of progression of the infection with the development of worsening valvular disease or the appearance of abscess despite apparent clinical response. The presence of a valve ring abscess warrants immediate surgical intervention. Pseudoaneurysms of the mitral–aortic intervalvular fibrosa also occur with valvular endocarditis and are distinguished from abscess by the lack of cavity echodensities and systolic expansion.[86]

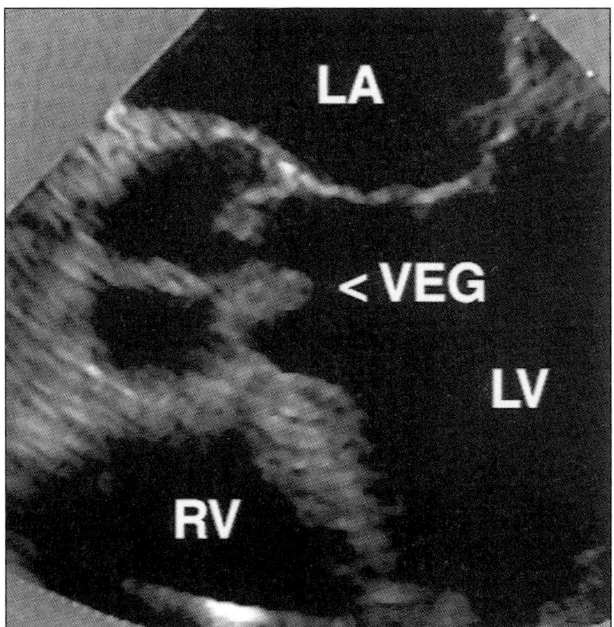

Figure 8.23
Transesophageal two-dimensional echocardiogram in the transverse plane. A vegetation (VEG) is attached to the right coronary cusp of the aortic valve and prolapses into the left ventricular outflow tract in diastole. LA, left atrium; LV, left ventricle; RV, right ventricle.

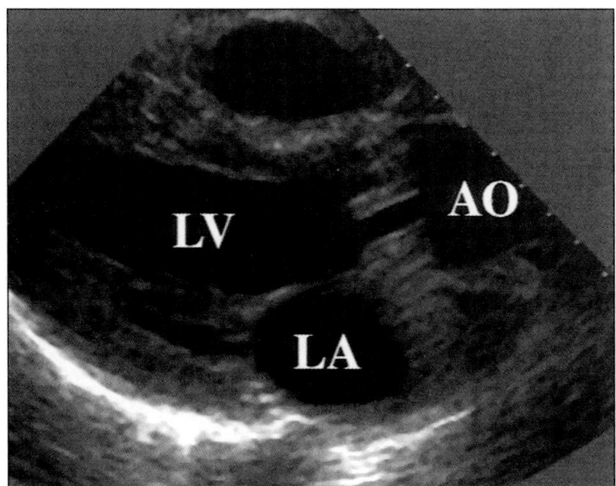

Figure 8.24
Two-dimensional echocardiogram in the parasternal long-axis view of a patient with a St Jude's prosthetic valve in the aortic position. The disks of the St Jude's valve are open in systole. The echodense leaflets can be seen parallel to the aortic (AO) walls. LA, left atrium; LV, left ventricle.

Prosthetic aortic valves

There are several prosthetic valves available today and it is difficult to be familiar with the echocardiographic characterizations of each of these. However, there are several broad principles which apply to evaluation of the aortic prosthetic valves.

The valves with the highest profiles are mechanical valves with a central occluder (Beall–Surgitool) or ball and cage variety (Starr–Edwards). The supporting structures and sewing ring may completely obscure the motion of the ball in the case of the Starr–Edwards valve. Tilting disk valves have either a single disk (Björk–Shiley) or are bileaflet valves (St Jude's or Carbomedics). The most commonly used bioprosthesis in the aortic position is the pericardial or Carpentier–Edwards valve. While bioprostheses have a lower profile than the mechanical valves, the stents may cause confusion. It may be difficult or impossible to image the leaflets of a bioprosthesis on a transthoracic echocardiogram unless the leaflets are thickened or calcified.

The prosthetic aortic valve is imaged in the same planes as a native valve. The valve should be stable at the sewing ring. As opposed to prosthetic mitral valves which may be sewn to a small portion of the posterior mitral valve leaflet, there should be no motion of the aortic sewing ring. Instability of the valve should be immediately investigated with transesophageal echocardiography and may require surgical intervention. The parasternal long-axis view is often best for visualization of the movement of tilting disk valves (Fig. 8.24), and M-mode of the valve may be helpful in verifying the timing of opening and closing of the valve. Irregular intervals of opening from the onset of the QRS complex in normal sinus rhythm suggest obstruction of the valve. Movement of the ball in the Starr–Edwards valve may be difficult to appreciate from the parasternal view and is best seen in the apical five-chamber plane. In this view, both the anterior and posterior surfaces of the ball will reflect ultrasound waves and the two resultant echodense lines will have parallel motion. In the transthoracic study, the posterior aortic root is generally obscured by the valve itself. The posterior root can be imaged via the transesophageal approach. Conversely, the anterior aortic root is generally best visualized in the transthoracic study and may not be clearly seen on the transesophageal study. Transesophageal echocardiography is essential if endocarditis or abscess is suspected (Fig. 8.25). The transesophageal study may not be as valuable in detecting obstruction of the valve since both visualization of leaflet movement and measurement of gradients are not optimal.

Aortic valve homografts have recently become available as an alternative to prosthetic valve replacement. Transthoracic and transesophageal echocardiography can be used to measure the aortic annulus size so that an appropriately sized homograft may be placed.[87] Similarly, pulmonary

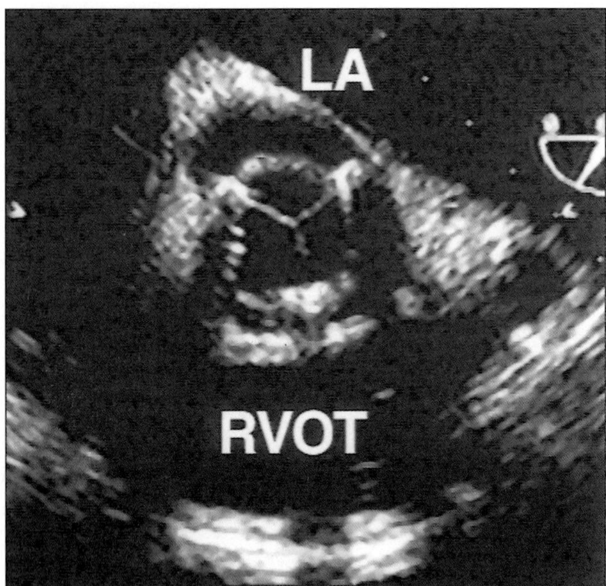

Figure 8.25
Transesophageal two-dimensional echocardiogram in a patient with a bioprosthetic aortic valve replacement. The imaging plane is oriented at approximately 25° from the transverse plane. The leaflets of the valve are clearly seen in this diastolic frame. The stents of the valve are imaged at the three commissures. The sinuses of Valsalva are markedly dilated due to severe preoperative aortic insufficiency. This dilatation results in the echo lucent area between the valve sewing ring and the aortic root. The valve was competent and there was no aortic insufficiency. LA, left atrium; RVOT, right ventricular outflow tract.

autografts should be sized prior to the procedure to ensure compatible dimensions.[30,88]

Measurement of transvalvular gradients are accomplished in a similar manner as in the native valve. Immediate or early postoperative baseline Doppler recordings are important for evaluation of any subsequent change in valvular function.[89] Acceptable peak and mean gradients across prosthetic valves depend on the size of the prosthesis as well as the type of valve.[90,91] Occasionally, unexpectedly large peak gradients can be recorded across prosthetic valves with small annular sizes. The phenomenon of 'pressure recovery' has been suggested as an explanation of the high gradients across these apparently normally functioning valves.[92–94] Gradients which take into account the left ventricular outflow tract velocity may also be more reliable in this situation.[93] Calculation of the 'effective' aortic valve area is theoretically better for serial comparison because of the dependence of the gradient on transvalvular flow. However, the left ventricular outflow tract diameter may be impossible to measure because of the artifacts arising from the valve. Substitution of the prosthesis size is not an acceptable alternative.[95]

References

1 Roberts W: The congenitally bicuspid aortic valve: a study of 85 autopsy cases. *Am J Cardiol* 1970; **26**: 72–83.

2 Beppu S et al: Rapidity of progression of aortic stenosis in patients with congenital bicuspid aortic valves. *Am J Cardiol* 1993; **71**: 322–7.

3 Pachulski R, Chan K: Progression of aortic valve dysfunction in 51 adult patients with congenital bicuspid aortic valve: assessment and follow up by Doppler echocardiography. *Br Heart J* 1993; **69**: 237–40.

4 Williams D, Sahn D, Friedman W: Cross-sectional echocardiographic localization of sites of left ventricular outflow tract obstruction. *Am J Cardiol* 1976; **37**: 250–5.

5 Lesbre J, Scheuble C, Kalisa A: Echocardiography in the diagnosis of severe aortic valve stenosis in adults. *Arch Mal Mil Coeur* 1983; **76**: 1–12.

6 Veyrat C et al: Assessment of number of cusps in aortic lesions by Doppler imaging: surgical correlations. *J Thorac Cardiovasc Surg* 1994; **107**: 319–21.

7 Stoddard M et al: Two-dimensional transesophageal echocardiographic determination of aortic valve area in adults with aortic stenosis. *Am Heart J* 1991; **122**: 1415–22.

8 Hofmann T et al: Determination of aortic valve orifice area in aortic valve stenosis by two-dimensional transesophageal echocardiography. *Am J Cardiol* 1987; **59**: 330–5.

9 Tribouilloy C et al: Quantitation of aortic valve area in aortic stenosis with multiplane transesophageal echocardiography: comparison with monoplane transesophageal approach. *Am Heart J* 1994; **128**: 526–32.

10 Hoffman R, Flachskampf F, Hanrath P: Planimetry of orifice area in aortic stenosis using multiplane transesophageal echocardiography. *J Am Coll Cardiol* 1993; **22**: 529–34.

11 Brener S et al: Progression of aortic stenosis in 394 patients: relation to changes in myocardial and mitral valve dysfunction. *J Am Coll Cardiol* 1995; **25**: 305–10.

12 Legget M et al: Gender differences in left ventricular function at rest and with exercise in asymptomatic aortic stenosis. *Am Heart J* 1996; **131**: 94–100.

13 Carroll J et al: Sex-associated differences in left ventricular function in aortic stenosis of the elderly. *Circulation* 1992; **86**: 1099–107.

14 Hatle L, Angelson B, Tromsdal A: Non-invasive assessment of aortic stenosis by Doppler ultrasound. *Br Heart J* 1980; **43**: 284–92.

15 Berger M, Berdoff RL, Gallerstein PE et al: Evaluation of aortic stenosis by continuous wave Doppler ultrasound. *J Am Coll Cardiol* 1984; **3**: 150–6.

16 Currie PJ, Seward JB, Reeder GS et al: Continuous wave Doppler echocardiographic assessment of severity of calcific aortic stenosis: a simultaneous Doppler–catheter correlative study in 100 adult patients. *Circulation* 1985; **71**: 1162–9.

17 Kosturakis D, Allen H, Goldberg, S: Noninvasive quantification of stenotic semilunar valve areas by Doppler echocardiography. *J Am Coll Cardiol* 1984; **33**: 1256–62.

18 Panidis I, Mintz G, Ross J: Value and limitations of Doppler ultrasound in the evaluation of aortic stenosis: a statistical analysis of 70 consecutive patients. *Am Heart J* 1986; **112**: 150–8.

19 Krafchek J, Robertson JH, Radford M et al: A reconsideration of Doppler assessed gradients in suspected aortic stenosis. *Am Heart J* 1985; **110**: 765–73.

20 Otto CM, Pearlman AS, Commess KA et al: Determination of the stenotic aortic valve area in adults using Doppler echocardiography. *J Am Coll Cardiol* 1986; **7**: 509–17.

21 Skjaerpe T, Hegrenaes L, Hatle L: Noninvasive estimation of valve area in patients with aortic stenosis by Doppler ultrasound and two-dimensional echocardiography. *Circulation* 1985; **72**: 810–18.

22 Zoghbi W, Galan A, Quinones M: Accurate noninvasive quantification of stenotic aortic valve area by Doppler echocardiography. *Circulation* 1986; **73**: 452–9.

23 Dittmann H, Voelker W, Karsch KR et al: Influence of sampling site and flow area on cardiac output measurements by Doppler echocardiography. *J Am Coll Cardiol* 1987; **10**: 818–23.

24 Blackshear J et al: Beat-by-beat aortic valve area measurements indicate constant orifice area in aortic stenosis: analysis of Doppler data with varying RR intervals. *J Am Soc Echocardiogr* 1992; **5**: 414–20.

25 Burwash IG, Thomas DD, Sadahiro M et al: Dependence of Gorlin formula and continuity equation valve areas on transvalvular volume flow rate in valvular aortic stenosis. *J Am Coll Cardiol* 1994; **89**: 827–35.

26 Casale PN, Palacios IF, Abascol VM et al: Effects of dobutamine on Gorlin and continuity equation valve areas and valve resistance in valvular aortic stenosis. *Am J Cardiol* 1992; **70**: 1175–9.

27 Roger VL, Tajik AL, Reeder GS et al: Effect of Doppler echocardiography on utilization of hemodynamic cardiac catheterization in the preoperative evaluation of aortic stenosis. *Mayo Clinic Proc* 1996; **71**: 141–9.

28 Tardif JC, Miller DS, Pandean NG et al: Effects of variations in flow on aortic valve area in aortic stenosis based on in vivo planimetry of aortic valve area by multiplane transesophageal echocardiography. *Am J Cardiol* 1995; **76**: 193–8.

29 Aurigemma G, Battista S, Orsinelli D et al: Abnormal left ventricular intracavitary flow acceleration in patients undergoing aortic valve replacement for aortic stenosis. *Circulation* 1992; **86**: 926–36.

30 Gerosa G et al: Aortic valve replacement with pulmonary homografts. *J Thorac Cardiovasc Surg* 1994; **107**: 424–37.

31 Koughoukos N et al: Replacement of the aortic root with a pulmonary autograft in children and young adults with aortic-valve disease. *N Engl J Med* 1994; **330**: 1–6.

32 Ow EP, DeLeon SY, Freeman JE et al: Recognition and management of accessory mitral tissue causing severe subaortic stenosis. *Ann Thorac Surg* 1994; **57**: 952–5.

33 Gewillig M, Daenon W, Dumoulen M et al: Rheologic genesis of discrete subvalvular aortic stenosis: a Doppler echocardiographic study. *J Am Coll Cardiol* 1992; **19**: 818–24.

34 Borow K, Glagov S: Discrete subvalvular aortic stenosis: is the presence of upstream complex blood flow disturbances an important pathogenic factor? *J Am Coll Cardiol* 1992; **19**: 825–7.

35 Frommelt MA, Snider AR, Bove EL et al: Echocardiographic assessment of subvalvular aortic stenosis before and after operation. *J Am Coll Cardiol* 1992; **19**: 1018–23.

36 Essop M, Skudicky D, Sareli P: Diagnostic value of transesophageal versus transthoracic echocardiography in discrete subaortic stenosis. *Am J Cardiol* 1992; **70**: 962–3.

37 Decoodt P, Kacenilenbogen R, Viart P et al: Evaluation of membranous subaortic stenosis using biplane transesophageal echocardiography. Report of two cases. *Acta Cardiol* 1991; **46**: 479–84.

38 Gnanapragasam JP, Houston AB, Doig WB et al: Transoesophageal echocardiographic assessment of fixed subaortic obstruction in children. *Br Heart J* 1991; **66**: 281–4.

39 Kinney EL, Machado H, Cortada X et al: Diagnoses of discrete subaortic stenosis by pulsed and continuous wave Doppler. *Am Heart J* 1985; **110**: 1069–71.

40 Hatle L: Noninvasive assessment and differentiation of left ventricular outflow obstruction with Doppler ultrasound. *Circulation* 1981; **64**: 381–7.

41 Valdes-Cruz LM, Jones M, Scagnelli et al: Prediction of gradients in fibrous subaortic stenosis by continuous wave two-dimensional Doppler echocardiography: animal studies. *J Am Coll Cardiol* 1985; **5**: 1363–7.

42 Maron BJ, Graham KJ, Poliac LC et al: Recurrence of a discrete subaortic membrane 27 years after operative resection. *Am J Cardiol* 1995; **76**: 104–5.

43 Shrivastava S, Den V, Bahl VK et al: Echocardiographic determinants of outcome after percutaneous transluminal balloon dilatation of discrete subaortic stenosis. *Am Heart J* 1991; **122**: 1323–6.

44 Daenen W, Vanhove M, Gewillig M: Extended aortic root replacement with pulmonary autografts: experience in 14 cases. *Ann Thorac Surg* 1995; **60** (suppl): S180–4.

45 Reddy V, Rajasinghe HA, Teitel DF et al: Aortoventriculoplasty with the pulmonary autograft; the 'Ross-Konno' procedure. *J Thorac Cardiovasc Surg* 1996; **111**: 158–65.

46 Wren C, Oslizlok P, Bull C: Natural history of supravalvular aortic stenosis and pulmonary artery stenosis. *J Am Coll Cardiol* 1990; **15**: 1625–30.

47 Braunstein PW Jr, Sade RM, Crawford FA Jr et al: Repair of supravalvular aortic stenosis: cardiovascular morphometric and hemodynamic results. *Ann Thorac Surg* 1990; **50**: 700–7.

48 French J: Aortic and pulmonary artery stenosis: improvement without intervention? *J Am Coll Cardiol* 1990; **15**: 1631–2.

49 Shapiro LM, Thivoites B, Westgate C et al: Prevalence and clinical significance of aortic valve prolapse. *Br Heart J* 1985; **54**: 179–83.

50 Shiu M, Coltart D, Braimbridge M: Echocardiographic findings in prolapsed aortic cusps with vegetations. *Br Heart J* 1979; **41**: 118–20.

51 Kai H, Koyanagi S, Takeshita A: Aortic valve prolapse with aortic regurgitation assessed by Doppler color-flow echocardiography. *Am Heart J* 1992; **124**: 1297–304.

52 Bonow RO, Lakatus E, Maron BJ et al: Serial long-term assessment of the natural history of asymptomatic patients with chronic aortic regurgitation and normal left ventricular systolic function. *Circulation* 1991; **84**: 1625–35.

53 Tornos M et al: Clinical evaluation of a prospective protocol for the timing of surgery in chronic aortic regurgitation. *Am Heart J* 1990; **120**: 649–57.

54 Tornos M et al: Clinical outcome of severe asymptomatic chronic aortic regurgitation: a long-term prospective follow-up study. *Am Heart J* 1995; **130**: 333.

55 Henry WL, Bonow RO, Rosing DR et al: Observations on the optimum time for operative intervention for aortic regurgitation: II. Serial echocardiographic evaluation of asymptomatic patients. *Circulation* 1980; **61**: 484–92.

56 Abdulla AM, Frank MJ, Canedo MI et al: Limitations of echocardiography in the assessment of left ventricular size and function in aortic regurgitation. *Circulation* 1980; **61**: 148–55.

57 Crawford M, Grant D, O'Rourke, R: Accuracy and reproducibility of new M-mode recommendations for measuring left ventricular dimensions. *Circulation* 1980; **66**: 137–43.

58 St John Sutton MG, Plappert TA, Hirschfield JW et al: Assessment of left ventricular mechanics in patients with asymptomatic aortic regurgitation. *Circulation* 1984; **69**: 259–68.

59 Borow K, Green L, Mann T: End-systolic volume as a predictor of postoperative left ventricular function in volume overload from valvular regurgitation. *Am J Med* 1980; **68**: 655.

60 Carabello G, Spann J: The uses and limitations of end-systolic indices of left ventricular function. *Circulation* 1984; **69**: 1058.

61 Eusebio J, Louie EK, Edwards LC III et al: Alterations in transmitral flow dynamics in patients with early mitral valve closure and aortic regurgitation. *Am Heart J* 1994; **128**: 941–47.

62 Wong M, Matsumura M, Suzuki K et al: Technical and biologic sources of variability in the mapping of aortic, mitral and tricuspid color flow jets. *Am J Cardiol* 1987; **69**: 847–51.

63 Spain M, Smith M: Effect of isometric exercise on mitral and aortic regurgitation as assessed by color Doppler flow imaging. *Am J Cardiol* 1990; **65**: 78–83.

64 Smith MD, Kuan OL, Spain MG et al: Temporal variability of color Doppler jet areas in patients with mitral and aortic regurgitation. *Am Heart J* 1992; **123**: 953–60.

65 Dolan MS, Castello R, St Vrain JA et al: Quantitation of aortic regurgitation by Doppler echocardiography: a practical approach. *Am Heart J* 1995; **129**: 1014–20.

66 Perry G, Helmoke F, Nanda NC et al: Evaluation of aortic insufficiency by Doppler color flow mapping. *J Am Coll Cardiol* 1987; **9**: 952–9.

67 Taylor AL, Eichhorn EJ, Brickner ME et al: Aortic valve morphology: an important in vitro determinant of proximal regurgitant jet width by Doppler color flow mapping. *J Am Coll Cardiol* 1990; **16**: 405–12.

68 Castello R, Fagan L Jr, Lenzen P et al: Comparison of transthoracic and transesophageal echocardiography for assessment of left-sided valvular regurgitation. *Am J Cardiol* 1991; **68**: 1677–80.

69 Vanoverschelde JL, Taymans-Robert AA, Raphael DA et al: Influence of transmitral filling dynamics on continuous-wave Doppler assessment of aortic regurgitation by half-time methods. *Am J Cardiol* 1989; **64**: 614–9.

70 Beyer RW, Ramirez M, Josephson MA et al: Correlation of continuous-wave Doppler assessment of chronic aortic regurgitation with hemodynamics and angiography. *Am J Cardiol* 1987; **60**: 852–6.

71 Masuyama T, Kitabatke A, Kodama K et al: Semiquantitative evaluation of aortic regurgitation by Doppler echocardiography: effects of associated mitral stenosis. *Am Heart J* 1989; **117**: 133–9.

72 Labovitz AJ, Ferran RP, Kern MJ et al: Quantitative evaluation of aortic insufficiency by continuous wave Doppler echocardiography. *J Am Coll Cardiol* 1986; **8**: 1341–7.

73 Sutton D, Kluger R, Ahmed SU et al: Flow reversal in the descending aorta: a guide to intraoperative assessment of aortic regurgitation with transesophageal echocardiography. *J Thorac Cardiovasc Surg* 1994; **108**: 576–82.

74 Nishimura RA, Vonk GD, Rumberger JA et al: Semiquantitation of aortic regurgitation by different Doppler echocardiographic techniques and comparison with ultrafast computed tomography. *Am Heart J* 1992; **124**: 995–1001.

75 Tribouilloy C, Avinec P, Shen WF et al: End diastolic flow velocity just beneath the aortic isthmus assessed by pulsed Doppler echocardiography: a new predictor of the aortic regurgitant fraction. *Br Heart J* 1991; **65**: 37–40.

76 Kitabatake A, Ito H, Inoue M: A new approach to noninvasive evaluation of aortic regurgitant fraction by two-dimensional Doppler echocardiography. *Circulation* 1985; **72**: 523–29.

77 Yeung A, Plappert T, Sutton MSJ: Calculation of aortic regurgitation orifice area by Doppler echocardiography: an application of the continuity equation. *Br Heart J* 1992; **68**: 236–40.

78 Reimold SC, Ganz P, Bittl JA et al: Effective aortic regurgitant orifice area: description of a method based on the conservation of mass. *J Am Coll Cardiol* 1991; **18**: 761–8.

79 Reimold SC, Maier SE, Fleischmann KE et al: Dynamic nature of the aortic regurgitant orifice area during diastole in patients with chronic aortic regurgitation. *Circulation* 1994; **89**: 2085–92.

80 Enriquez-Sarano M, Miller FA Jr, Hayes SN et al: Effective regurgitant orifice area: a noninvasive Doppler development of an old hemodynamic concept. *J Am Coll Cardiol* 1994; **23**: 443–51.

81 Mugge A, Daniel WG, Frank G et al: Echocardiography in infective endocarditis: reassessment of prognostic implications of vegetation size determined by the transthoracic and the transesophageal approach. *J Am Coll Cardiol* 1989; **14**: 631–8.

82 Daniel W, Mugge A, Martin RP et al: Improvement in the diagnosis of abscesses associated with endocarditis by transesophageal echocardiography. *N Engl J Med* 1991; **324**: 795–800.

83 Taams MA, Gussenhoven EJ, Bos E et al: Enhanced morphological diagnosis in infective endocarditis by transoesophageal echocardiography. *Br Heart J* 1990; **63**: 109–13.

84 Karalis D, Bansal RC, Hauck AJ et al: Transesophageal echocardiographic recognition of subaortic complications in aortic valve endocarditis: clinical and surgical implications. *Circulation* 1992; **86**: 353–62.

85 Job FP, Frank S, Lethen H et al: Incremental value of biplane and multiplane transesophageal echocardiography for the assessment of active infective endocarditis. *Am J Cardiol* 1995; **75**: 1033–37.

86 Alfridi I, Apostioliclou MA, Saad RM et al: Pseudoaneurysms of the mitral-aortic fibrosa: dynamic characterization using transesophageal echocardiographic and Doppler techniques. *J Am Coll Cardiol* 1995; **25**: 137–45.

87 Moscucci M, Weinert L, Karp RB et al: Prediction of aortic annulus diameter by two-dimensional echocardiography. Application in the preoperative selection and preparation of homograft aortic valves. *Circulation* 1991; **84** (suppl): III76–80.

88 Rubay JE, Raphael D, Sluysmans T et al: Aortic valve replacement with allograft/autograft: subcoronary versus intraluminal cylinder or root. *Ann Thorac Surg* 1995; **60** (suppl): S78–82.

89 Wiseth R, Hegrenaes L, Rossvoll O et al: Validity of an early postoperative baseline Doppler recording after aortic valve replacement. *Am J Cardiol* 1991; **67**: 869–72.

90 Reisner S, Meltzer R: Normal values of prosthetic valve Doppler echocardiographic parameters: a review. *J Am Soc Echocardiogr* 1988; **1**: 201–10.

91 Iwasaka T, Naggar CZ, Sugiura T et al: Doppler echocardiographic assessment of prosthetic aortic valve function. Findings in normal valves. *Chest* 1991; **99**: 399–403.

92 Baumgartner H, Khan S, DeRobertis M et al: Discrepancies between Doppler and catheter gradients in aortic prosthetic valves in vitro: a manifestation of localized gradients and pressure recovery. *Circulation* 1990; **82**: 1467–75.

93 Laske A, Jenni R, Maloigne M et al: Pressure gradients across bileaflet aortic valves by direct measurement and echocardiography. *Ann Thorac Surg* 1996; **61**: 48–57.

94 Laskey W, Kussmaul W: Pressure recovery in aortic valve stenosis. *Circulation* 1994; **89**: 116–21.

95 Pibarot P, Honos GN, Durand LG et al: Substitution of left ventricular outflow tract diameter with prosthesis size is inadequate for calculation of the aortic prosthetic valve area by the continuity equation. *J Am Soc Echocardiogr* 1995; **8**: 511–17.

9

Imaging in infective endocarditis

Simon Ray and Chris Ward

Typical cases of infective endocarditis can be confidently diagnosed on the basis of pyrexia, a heart murmur, emboli and bacteremia or fungemia plus immunological phenomena. However, changes in the pattern and presentation of infective endocarditis, first documented in 1966, have resulted in many cases presenting atypically, making the diagnosis more difficult.[1] The main changes have been:

1. An increase in the average age of the affected population, many of whom have multiple pathologies. Such patients often have nosocomial infection, fewer symptoms than younger patients, a diminished febrile response and a high mortality.[2]
2. An increased number of cases caused by staphylococci.
3. Prosthetic valve endocarditis. These latter two factors are interrelated in that 40–50% of cases of prosthetic valve endocarditis are caused by staphylococci, notably coagulase negative organisms.[3]

Diagnostic delays and difficulties also occur in culture negative endocarditis and in patients whose presentation is dominated by one of the major complications such as an embolism or cardiac failure.

As a result of these changes, the mortality of infective endocarditis has remained at 25–30% despite the introduction of open heart surgery and new antibiotics: nowadays approximately 75% of deaths are caused by cardiac failure and most of the remainder result from cerebral emboli or hemorrhage. The mortality of infective endocarditis will only fall if these complications can be pre-empted or diagnosed early and treated promptly.[4]

Until recently, attempts to identify high risk patients, and to establish diagnostic criteria, have lacked sensitivity and specificity. However, in 1994, Durack et al devised new criteria (the Duke criteria) which have been shown to have a high specificity for the clinical diagnosis of infective endocarditis.[5] These recommendations, based on a combination of major and minor criteria, give a pivotal role to echocardiography. The echocardiographic detection of vegetations, an abscess or new partial dehiscence of a prosthetic valve is one of their major criteria, and in the presence of positive blood cultures merits a diagnosis of endocarditis. In a series of 106 patients from five studies with pathological confirmation of the diagnosis, 82% would have been classified as definite infective endocarditis with the Duke criteria and none would have been excluded.[6] In other studies, the criteria had a specificity of 99% and a negative predictive accuracy for rejected cases of 98%.[7]

Cardiac involvement in infective endocarditis includes the primary endocardial lesion and its local complications: valve cusp destruction or rupture, cordal rupture, valve ring abscess, mycotic aneurysm of the aorta or sinus of Valsalva, purulent pericarditis, and coronary emboli. The mitral and aortic valves are most commonly involved. The tricuspid valve is less frequently affected; the pulmonary valve rarely. The commonest susceptible congenital lesions are bicuspid aortic valve, ventricular septal defect and patent ductus arteriosus.

Echocardiography in the diagnosis of endocarditis

Whichever diagnostic criteria are employed, evidence of endocardial involvement is essential for the diagnosis of infective endocarditis. Before the introduction of echocardiography this was assumed from the presence of new or changing regurgitant murmurs or demonstrated directly at surgery or autopsy. Echocardiography is uniquely able to identify endocardial lesions noninvasively and should be performed in all suspected cases. However the diagnostic yield depends on the pre-test likelihood of endocarditis, and speculative imaging of all patients with fever is inappropriate. Questions that can be addressed by echocardiography include:

- the presence, size, extent and mobility of vegetations;
- the severity of valve destruction and consequent regurgitation;
- the occurrence of extravalvular extension of infection; i.e. valve ring abscesses, mycotic aneurysms and fistulae;
- the assessment of ventricular function.

Imaging of suspected native valve endocarditis: mitral and aortic valves

A vegetation is defined in the Duke criteria as: 'An oscillating intracardiac mass, on a valve or supporting structure, or in the path of a regurgitant jet, or on implanted material, in the absence of an alternative anatomic explanation'.[5] The physical appearance of vegetations varies from highly mobile pedunculated masses to smaller almost sessile structures. On native valves, vegetations are usually attached on the regurgitant side of the valve, i.e. on the atrial aspect of the mitral valve and on the ventricular aspect of the aortic valve (Figs 9.1 and 9.2). The overall sensitivity of transthoracic echocardiography (TTE) for the detection of vegetations is approximately 60–70%.[8,9] TTE has several limitations. Images may be technically inadequate in obese patients or in those with obstructive airways disease and, depending on the operating frequency of the transducer (typically 2.5 MHz in adults), structures smaller than 2–5 mm may not be visualized. Transesophageal echocardiography (TEE) overcomes the problems of poor ultrasound windows and allows the use of higher frequency transducers (typically 5 MHz) which have improved resolution to structures of 1–2 mm (Figs 9.3, 9.4 and 9.5). Numerous papers confirm the improved diagnostic sensitivity of TEE.[8–10] The vast majority of these studies used monoplane TEE which has now largely been superseded by biplane and multiplane imaging.

A practical echocardiographic approach to endocarditis is summarized in Table 9.1. A transthoracic echo should be performed first and must include an assessment of valvular integrity and ventricular function. If vegetations are clearly present or clearly absent and ventricular function and valve integrity can be adequately assessed, there is no need for TEE.[11,12] TEE is indicated in patients with a technically inadequate transthoracic study, in those with equivocal findings suggestive but not diagnostic of vegetations, and in patients with a negative transthoracic study but a strong clinical suspicion of endocarditis. It is also indicated where there is a discrepancy between TTE

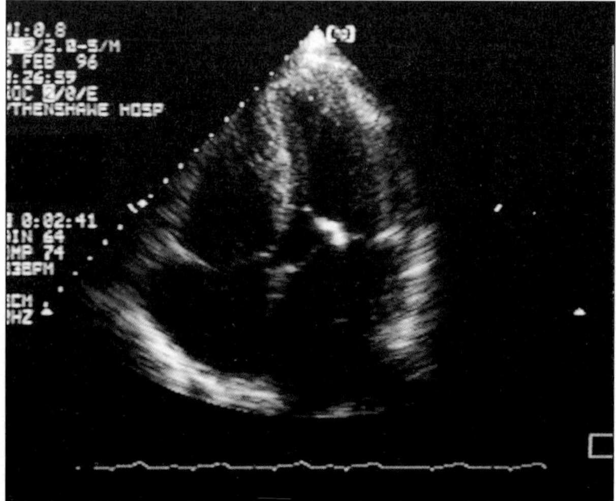

Figure 9.1
TTE, apical four-chamber view. There is a bright mass of vegetations attached to the anterior mitral leaflet.

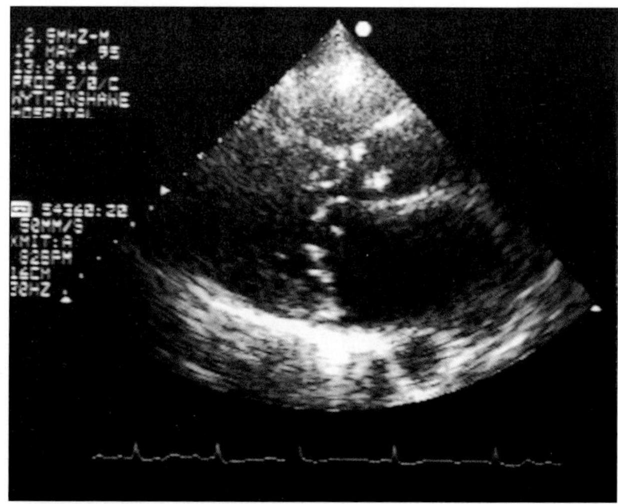

Figure 9.2
TTE, long-axis parasternal view. Vegetations are present on both the mitral and aortic valves.

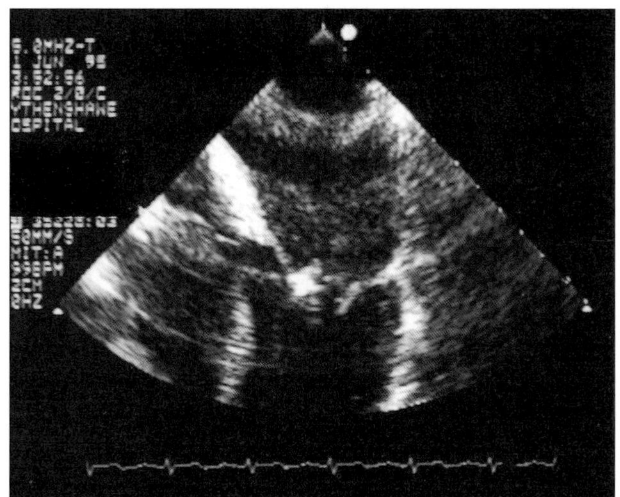

Figure 9.3
TEE, four-chamber view. There is a large mass of vegetations attached to the atrial aspect of the mitral valve.

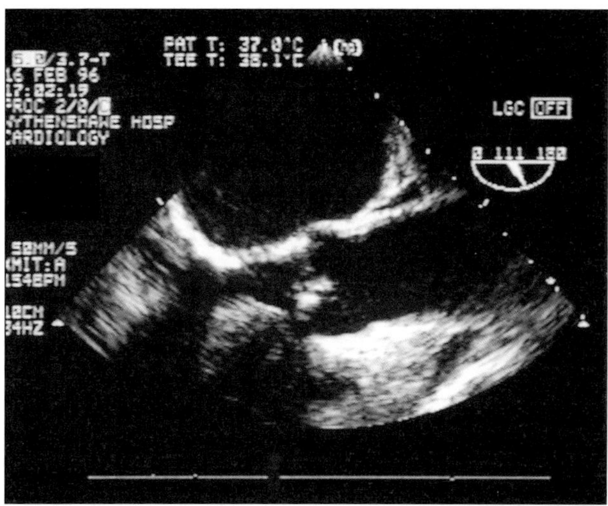

Figure 9.4
TEE, long-axis view of the aorta. There are vegetations attached to the aortic valve.

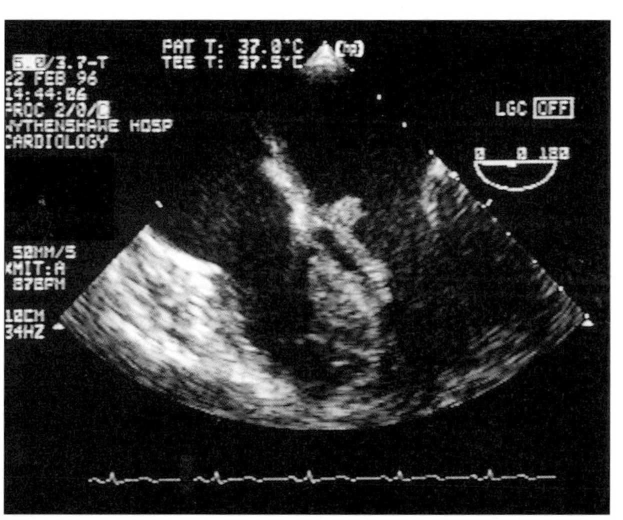

a

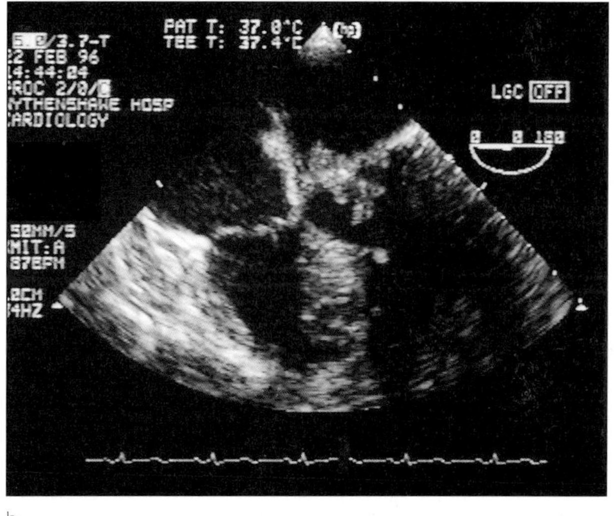

b

Figure 9.5
(a) TEE, four-chamber view in diastole. This patient with hypertrophic cardiomyopathy was successfully treated for streptococcal endocarditis but later developed increasing breathlessness with clinical signs of mitral regurgitation. TEE demonstrated a very abnormal mitral valve with a large mass of vegetations on the anterior mitral leaflet. (b) In the same view in systole a probable vegetation attached to the interventricular septum is also apparent.

Table 9.1

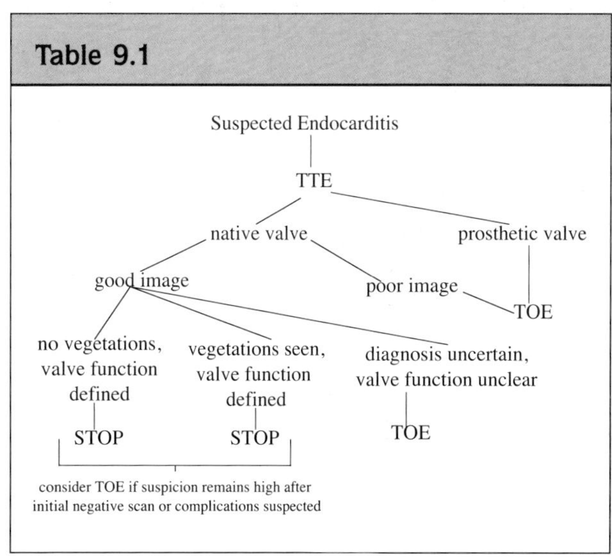

and clinical findings. The sensitivity of multiplane TEE is sufficiently high that a negative study virtually excludes vegetative endocarditis of a native valve. However, since vegetations may take 2 weeks to appear after symptom onset a repeat study should be performed in patients where the clinical suspicion remains high after an initially negative study.[13] A small minority of patients with endocarditis never develop visible vegetations.

Echocardiography is particularly useful in confirming the diagnosis in suspected culture negative endocarditis.[4]

Right sided endocarditis

Tricuspid endocarditis is a particular concern in intravenous drug abusers.[14] It often presents with a combination of arthralgia, myalgia, cough, hemoptysis and rigors. Clinical examination often suggests pulmonary embolism or pneumonia, but evidence of tricuspid valve involvement is frequently lacking. In general, tricuspid vegetations are larger than those on the mitral and aortic valves (Fig. 9.6). Monoplane TEE is equivalent to TTE for the detection of tricuspid vegetations, but multiplane imaging is probably superior, allowing visualization of the valve in both transverse plane four-chamber views and a variety of longitudinal short-axis views.[10]

Multiplane TEE is the best imaging technique for the detection of vegetations associated with pacing leads or indwelling cannulae in the right heart. Multiple imaging planes are necessary to track the path of these structures from the superior vena cava into the right heart chambers.

Pulmonary valve endocarditis is rare. Visualization of the pulmonary valve by TTE is difficult in many adults and transesophageal longitudinal short-axis scanning of the right ventricular outflow tract is the best imaging technique.

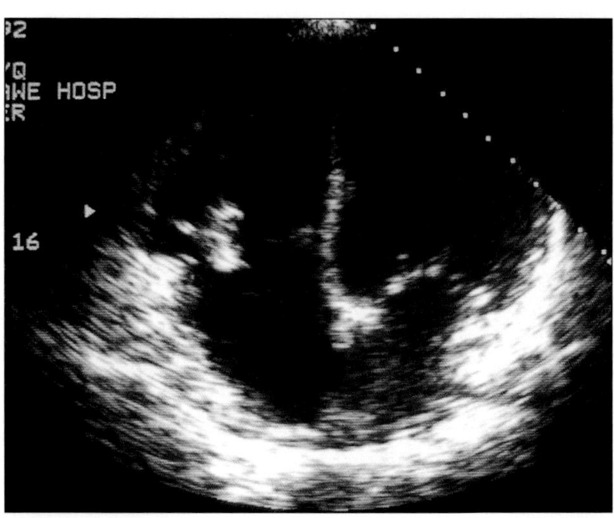

Figure 9.6
TTE, apical four-chamber view. Bulky vegetations on the posterior leaflet of the tricuspid valve. This patient was an intravenous drug abuser.

Prosthetic valve endocarditis

Prosthetic valve material is highly reflective and the resulting acoustic shadowing limits TTE visualization of the valve and perivalvular structures, particularly in the mitral position. The sensitivity of TTE for the detection of vegetations on prosthetic valves is unacceptably low.[8] The sensitivity of monoplane TEE for the detection of prosthetic valve vegetations is around 80% and biplane and particularly multiplane TEE are better still.[15,16] Consequently TEE should be performed in all patients with suspected prosthetic valve endocarditis (Fig. 9.7).

Vegetations may occur on any part of the prosthetic apparatus but are most commonly attached to the sewing ring of mechanical valves and to the leaflets of degenerating bioprostheses. Because the echocardiographic appearance of vegetations varies considerably, all aspects of the prosthetic valve should be inspected from all possible views.

The atrial aspect of mitral prostheses is usually well visualized from standard midesophageal transverse and longitudinal planes, but imaging of the ventricular aspect of mechanical prostheses is limited by acoustic shadowing. Acoustic interference is minimized by short- and long-axis imaging from the transgastric window.

Aortic prostheses are usually well visualized by a combination of transverse plane long-axis imaging of the aortic outflow tract and longitudinal long-axis and short-axis views. Acoustic shadowing from a mechanical prosthesis in the mitral position limits visualization of the aortic valve. This can be difficult to overcome, but transgastric long-axis imaging often allows good visualization of the left ventricular outflow tract.

Endocarditis in congenital heart disease

Congenital lesions with high velocity jets are susceptible to endocarditis. Totally corrective surgery such as complete closure of a VSD or division and ligation of an arterial duct virtually abolishes the risk of endocarditis, but patients with either a residual defect or a prosthetic valve or conduit remain susceptible.[17] TEE is necessary for the complete evaluation of suspected endocarditis in adolescents or

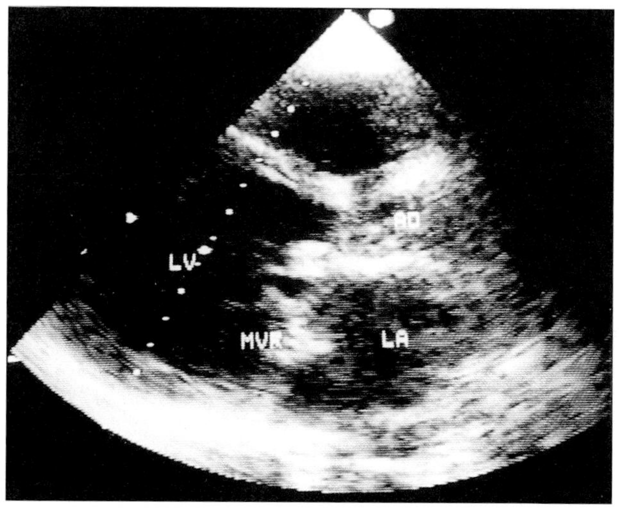

a

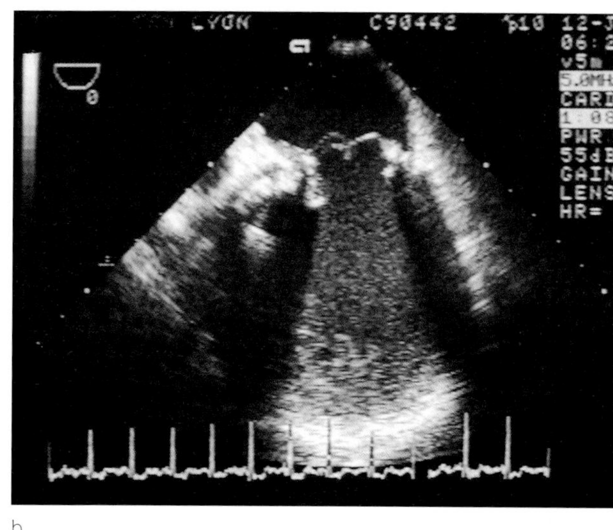

b

Figure 9.7
(a) TTE, parasternal long-axis view. Suspected endocarditis of a Carpentier–Edwards bioprosthesis. The structure of the valve is not clearly seen on TTE and endocarditis cannot be ruled out. (b) TEE, transverse long-axis view. With TEE the structure of bioprostheses can be visualized in detail. In this case there was mild leaflet prolapse but no evidence of endocarditis.

adults with complex congenital heart disease. Even in skilled hands it is sometimes difficult to obtain optimal images of aortic coarctation or a patent arterial duct, and in these instances magnetic resonance imaging is indicated.

Need for repeat echocardiography

We do not feel that routine repeat scanning to assess progression of vegetations during treatment is necessary or useful. In patients who are responding clinically to antibiotics and who remain hemodynamically stable, we do not repeat echocardiography routinely until the end of the course of antibiotics when a repeat scan is performed to allow future comparisons. A repeat scan is indicated during treatment if a patient remains pyrexial, biochemical markers of infection fail to improve, or a new murmur or hemodynamic instability develop.

Potential pitfalls of echocardiographic diagnosis of endocarditis

The increased resolution of TEE has removed much of the uncertainty from the diagnosis of vegetations in thickened or distorted native valves, but several potential pitfalls remain. Normal cardiac structures may be mistaken for features of endocarditis. The Eustachian valve may appear as a highly mobile structure in the right atrium mimicking a vegetation (Fig. 9.8). The transverse sinus is a fold of

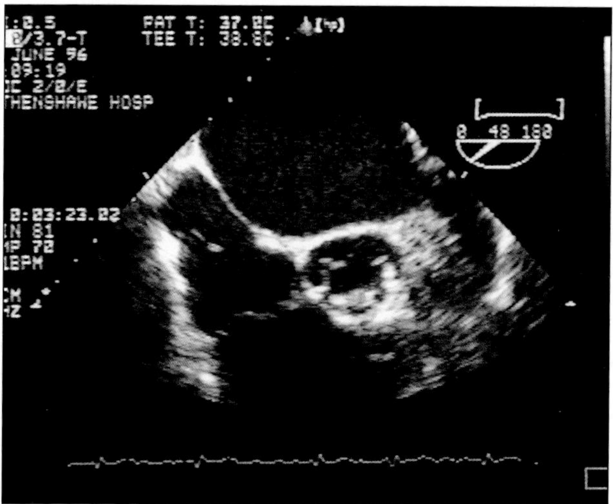

Figure 9.8
TEE, longitudinal short-axis scan at 48°. The Eustachean valve is visible as a membranous structure in the right atrium. In real time the Eustachean valve undulates and can be mistaken for a vegetation.

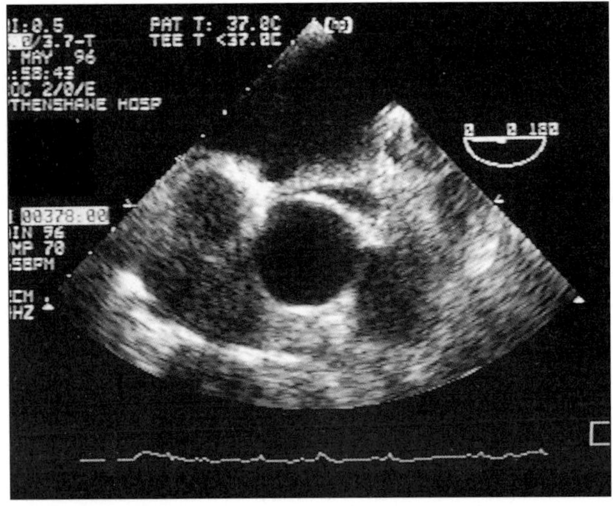

a

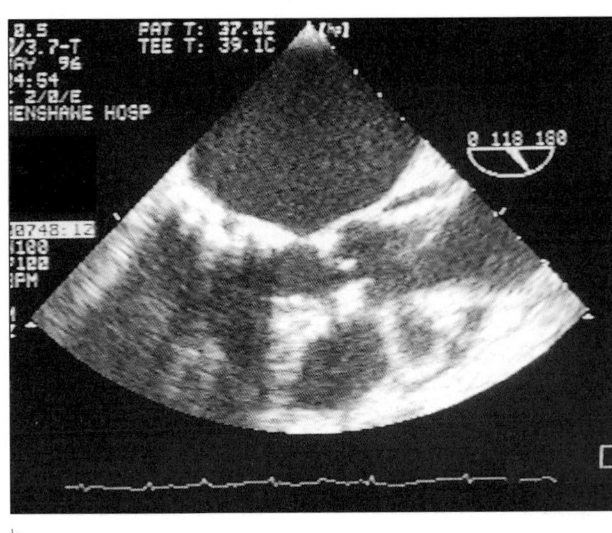

b

Figure 9.9

(a) TEE, transverse plane, basal short-axis view. The transverse sinus is visible as an echo-free space immediately anterior to the left atrium and posterior to the aortic root. (b) TEE, longitudinal long-axis scan of the aortic root. In this view the transverse sinus is visible as a slit-like echo-free space anterior to the left atrium and posterior to the ascending aorta.

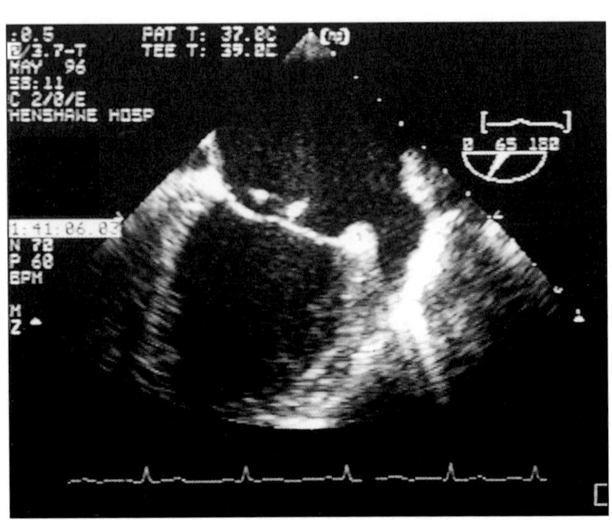

a

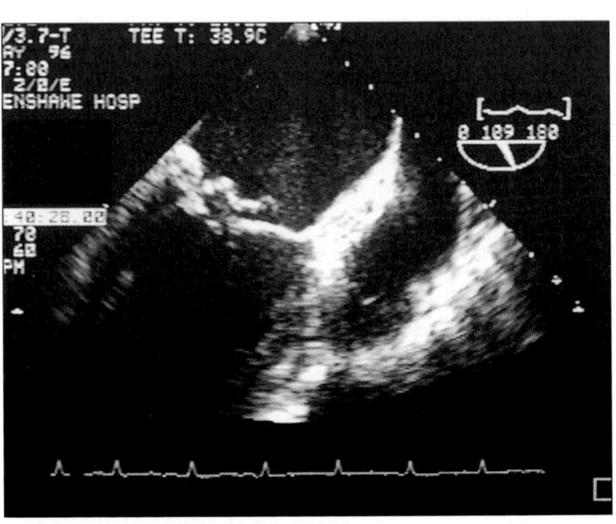

b

Figure 9.10

(a) TEE, long-axis view at 65°. Two mobile structures, possibly vegetations, are present on the atrial aspect of the mitral valve in a patient with severe mitral regurgitation and a fever. (b) TEE, long-axis view at 109°. With adjustment of the scan plane it is apparent that the mobile structures are part of a flail posterior leaflet. This patient had bronchopneumonia, not endocarditis.

pericardium which appears as an echo-free space between the aorta and the left atrium and may be mistaken for an abscess cavity (Fig. 9.9). Lambl's excrescences are fine filamentous strands which form on the surface of heart valves, particularly the ventricular surface of the aortic valve. They are about 1 mm in diameter and 1 cm long. They are more delicate than vegetations and may be a normal finding, although there is a suggestion that they may be associated with thromboembolic events.[18]

Myxomatous mitral valves appear thickened and irregular and are often associated with ruptured chordae tendineae. Chronically ruptured chordae tend to contract and may closely mimic mobile vegetations attached to a flail segment of the valve (Fig. 9.10). Papillary fibroelastomas

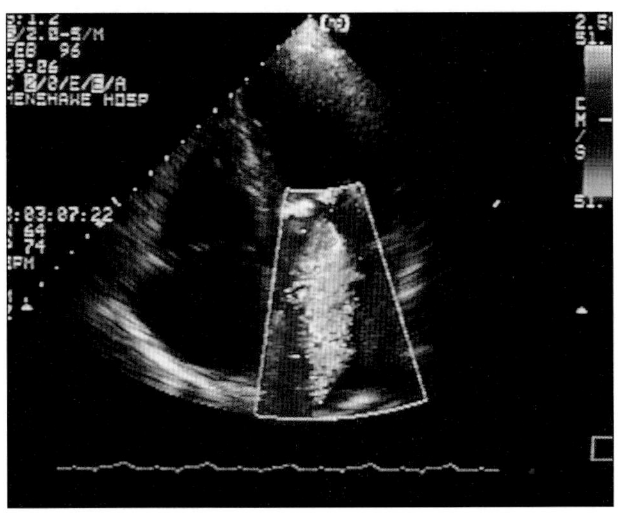

a

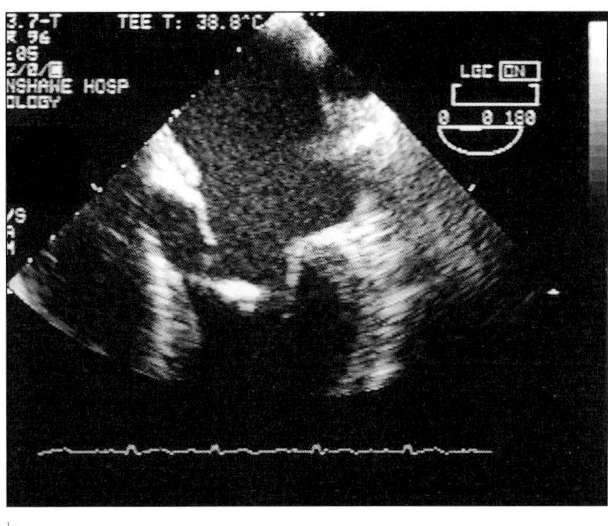

b

Figure 9.11
(a) TTE, apical four-chamber view. This is taken from the same patient as in Figure 9.1. There is severe mitral regurgitation which cannot be completely explained by the TTE appearances. TEE is indicated in this situation. (b) TEE, transverse long-axis view. TEE demonstrated a large perforation in the anterior mitral leaflet adjacent to a large vegetation. The severity of the regurgitation was explained allowing surgical repair to be planned.

are benign nodular tumors usually attached to valves or their support structures and may sometimes be mistaken for sessile vegetations. A number of conditions including uremia, systemic lupus erythematosus, and malignancy are associated with sterile thrombotic vegetations. These may be indistinguishable echocardiographically from infected vegetations.

Strands of torn sewing ring or suture material are sometimes seen in association with prosthetic valves and may be very difficult to distinguish from vegetations. The degenerating leaflets of bioprostheses may contain highly mobile torn segments that oscillate in a similar way to vegetations.

Old vegetations may be extremely hard to distinguish from current infection. Comparison with previous echoes is essential in patients with suspected recurrent endocarditis.

Echocardiographic assessment of complications of endocarditis

Valvular destruction

Valvular destruction is common in patients with endocarditis, particularly when the infecting organism is *Staphylococcus aureus*.[4] The endocarditic process typically begins along the closure line of the valve and may progress rapidly, distorting normal valve coaptation with consequent regurgitation. Cusp perforation, most commonly of the mitral valve, occurs in 8–20% of cases, sometimes within days of the onset of symptoms in virulent infections.[19] TEE is superior to TTE in detecting mitral perforations (Fig. 9.11).[20] A regurgitant jet through an infected aortic valve may impinge on the anterior mitral leaflet, leading to metastatic infection and mitral perforation (Fig. 9.12). Severe mitral regurgitation may also occur secondary to rupture of chordae tendineae. Very uncommonly, massive vegetations may obstruct a native valve.

Infection of the sewing ring of prosthetic valves may spread to the surrounding tissues, leading to valve dehiscence and a paravalvular leak (Fig. 9.13). Echocardiographically, dehiscence is recognized as a rocking motion of the valve, analogous to that seen on fluoroscopy. Destruction or perforation of the leaflets of bioprostheses can occur, leading to valvular regurgitation. Occasionally mechanical valves may be impeded by large masses of vegetations, leading to either obstruction or to failure of closure, both resulting in severe hemodynamic deterioration.

The sudden onset of valvular regurgitation leads to acute severe cardiac failure, but the physical signs characteristic of chronic regurgitation may be absent. This is because acute valve incompetence causes a dramatic rise

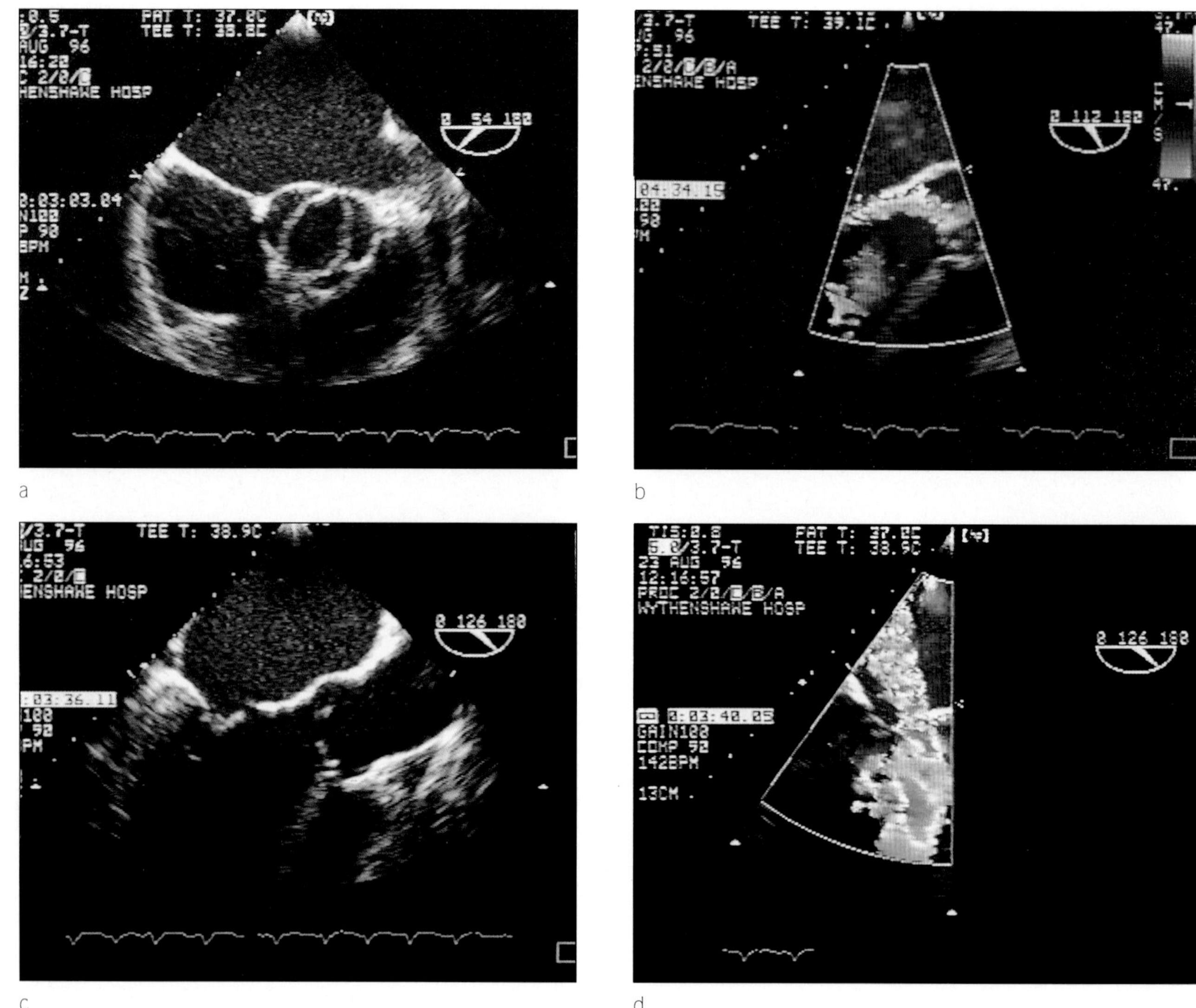

Figure 9.12
(a) TEE, short-axis view at 54°. Short-axis view of a bicuspid aortic valve during systole. The patient had previously been treated for aortic endocarditis and now presented with pulmonary edema. (b) TEE, long-axis view at 112°. An eccentric jet of aortic regurgitation impinges on the anterior mitral leaflet. (c) TEE, long-axis view at 126°. There is a perforation in the anterior mitral leaflet at the site of impingement of the aortic regurgitant jet. (d) TEE, long-axis view at 126°. There is severe regurgitation through the perforation in the anterior mitral leaflet. This defect was closed with a pericardial patch.

in pressure behind the regurgitant valve causing the regurgitant murmur to be abbreviated. Tachycardia makes auscultation difficult, and in acute aortic regurgitation the pulse, instead of being collapsing, is of low volume.

The onset of cardiac failure in a patient with endocarditis is an indication for urgent echocardiography. The same general principles apply. A TEE should be performed if a TTE does not provide all the information necessary to guide management, particularly decisions on surgery, and is mandatory in suspected prosthetic valve dysfunction. Paraprosthetic jets and regurgitation through perforations may be very eccentric and great care should be taken to inspect the valve thoroughly from all possible windows. TTE is usually adequate for monitoring ventricular size and function.

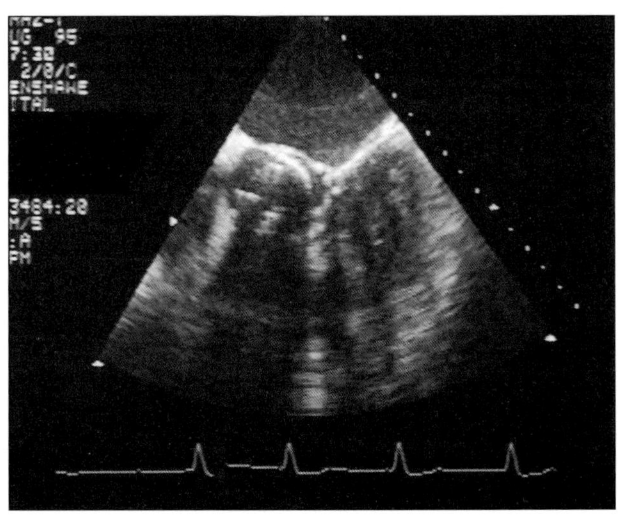

a

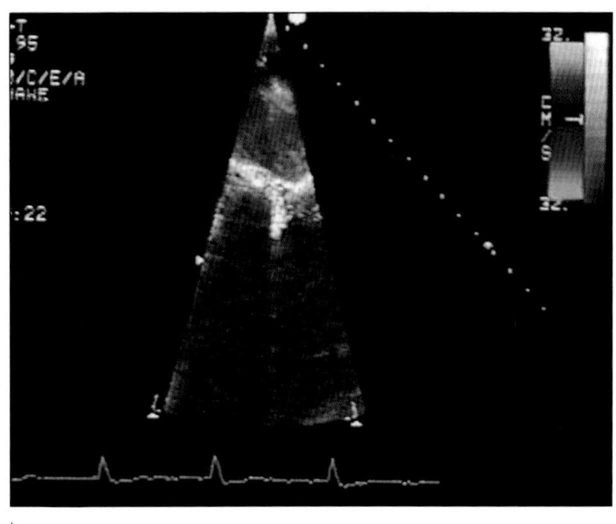

b

Figure 9.13
(a) TEE, transverse, basal short-axis view. This patient had had a mechanical aortic valve replacement 3 years previously and presented with a pyrexia and non-specific malaise. Transthoracic echo was technically inadequate. On TEE the aortic prosthetic valve appears to have partially dehisced posteriorly. (b) Color flow mapping demonstrates a paraprosthetic flow jet from the aortic root to the left ventricular outflow tract. Abscess formation and partial dehiscence of the valve was confirmed at surgery.

Detection of extravalvular spread of infection

Periannular abscesses are detected in up to 30% of patients undergoing surgery or at autopsy in native valve endocarditis and are more common with aortic valve infection.[20,21] Abscess formation is almost universal in endocarditis of mechanical prostheses as the infection invariably involves the sewing ring and adjacent tissues (Fig. 9.14). It is associated with persistent pyrexia and a poor clinical response to antibiotics. A purulent pericardial effusion is strongly suggestive of abscess formation. Abscess formation is associated with a poor outcome and any patient who fails to respond as expected to appropriate antibiotics should have a TEE performed to exclude the presence of an abscess.[4,21,22]

Abscesses have been defined echocardiographically as abnormal echolucent areas within the valvular annulus or perivalvular tissue in the setting of an infected valve.[22] Abscesses which communicate with the left ventricular outflow tract are expansile and intracavity blood flow may be demonstrated on color flow Doppler. Since abscesses can be difficult to visualize and are sometimes multifocal, the entire perivalvular region should be scanned carefully. Patients with abscesses complicating endocarditis are at high risk and have a poor prognosis if treated medically. The detection of a perivalvular abscess is an indication for early valve surgery.

Endocarditis of the aortic valve may spread to involve subvalvular structures. Metastatic infection and perforation of the anterior mitral leaflet has already been mentioned. Rarely a mycotic aneurysm of the anterior leaflet is seen. Infection may spread into the mitral–aortic intervalvular fibrosa producing an abscess or mycotic aneurysm which may then rupture into the left atrium producing a fistula.[23] The resulting eccentric jet into the left atrium should raise the possibility of a leaflet perforation or fistula, and suspicion of either should prompt a TEE to define the anatomy prior to surgery.

Spread of infection from the aortic valve into an adjacent sinus of Valsalva may lead to a mycotic aneurysm (Fig. 9.15) which may rupture into the right atrium, right ventricle or left ventricle producing a continuous murmur and worsening cardiac failure. Aneurysms of the sinuses of Valsalva can be visualized on TTE, but multiplane TEE is indicated to define the anatomy prior to surgical repair.

Vegetation size and embolization

Embolization to the brain, skin, kidney and viscera is a frequent complication of endocarditis with the average reported incidence about 30%.[4] Vegetation size >10 mm, mobility and mitral valve involvement have all been associated with an increased risk of embolism in some but not all reports.[8,24,25] Spontaneous echo contrast on TEE has

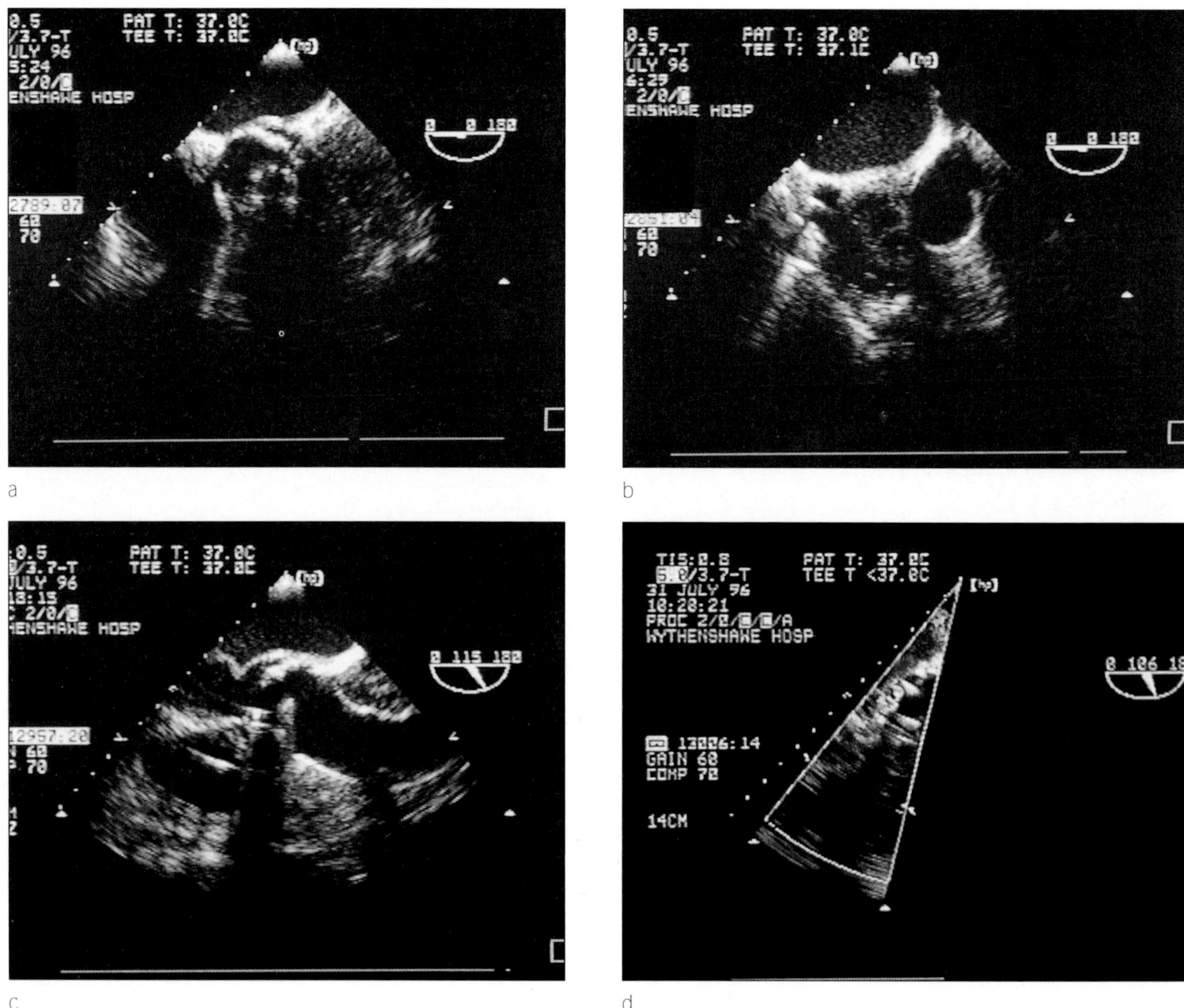

Figure 9.14
(a) TEE, transverse, basal short-axis view. This patient had previously had a replacement of his aortic valve and root. He represented with overwhelming sepsis and hemodynamic collapse. TTE suggested a paraprosthetic leak. TEE confirmed partial dehiscence of the aortic valve posteriorly. (b) Withdrawing the TEE probe slightly brought into view a large abscess cavity situated to the right of the aorta. (c) TEE, long-axis view at 115°. In this view the abscess cavity is well seen lying between the aortic root and the left atrium and is displacing the aorta anteriorly. (d) Color flow mapping demonstrates a paraprosthetic leak at the posterior aspect of the aortic prosthesis.

been reported to be a risk factor for embolization in patients with endocarditis.[26] The incidence of embolization decreases markedly after the initiation of antibiotic therapy.[27]

Vegetations on right-sided valves or indwelling lines may embolize to the lungs. The chest X-ray is abnormal in 75% of cases of tricuspid endocarditis showing areas of atelectasis or, characteristically, multiple pulmonary abscesses (Fig. 9.16). A sterile pleural effusion is often present. A V/Q scan will confirm the presence of pulmonary embolization.

It is controversial whether surgery is indicated in patients with large mobile vegetations to decrease the risk of embolism. We do not believe that routine surveillance of vegetation size contributes to the management of endocarditis in patients who are responding clinically to antibiotics, and do not refer such patients for surgery solely on the basis of vegetation size or mobility. However, enlargement of vegetations in a patient with a poor clinical response is indicative of a poor prognosis and is a factor favoring prompt surgery.

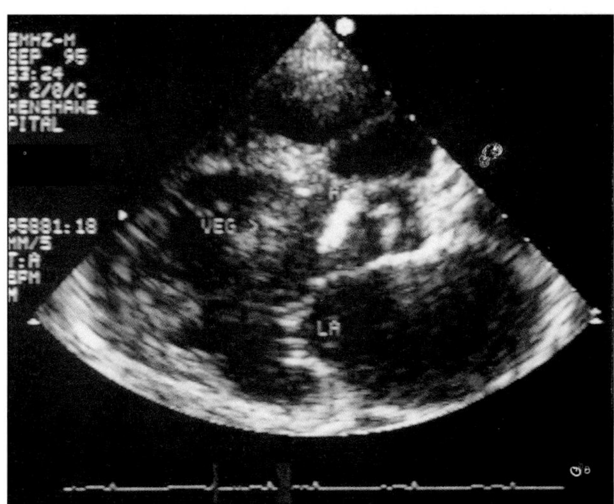

Figure 9.15
TTE, long-axis parasternal view of the aortic valve in an intravenous drug abuser with aortic valve endocarditis. There is a mass of vegetations attached to the ventricular surface of the aortic valve which is very abnormal. There is an echo-free space anterior to the aortic valve which was confirmed at operation as a mycotic aneurysm of the right sinus of Valsalva.

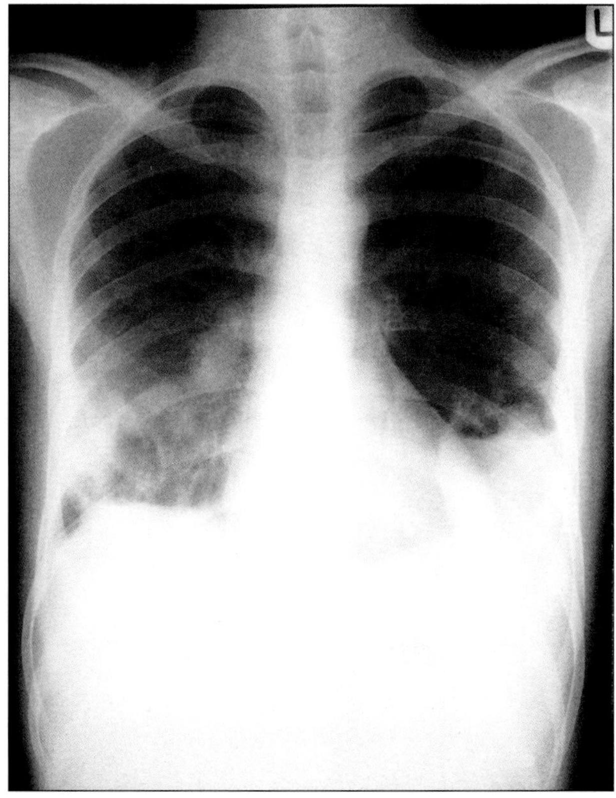

Figure 9.16
Chest X-ray showing lung abscesses and pleural effusions in a patient with tricuspid endocarditis.

Role of cardiac catheterization

Cardiac catheterization has a less important diagnostic role since the introduction of two-dimensional, color flow and TEE. While angiography accurately demonstrates valvular regurgitation, vegetations are usually not visualized. Although it may help to define and locate aortic root abscesses, almost half of annular lesions will be undetected.[28] Coronary angiography may be required prior to open heart surgery. Claims that cardiac catheterization should not be performed because of the risk of dislodging emboli are largely apocryphal; certainly a number of series report no such incidents.[29] However, in patients with severe acute valvular regurgitation, the risk that a large volume of contrast medium may worsen cardiac failure should be considered.

Non-cardiac involvement

Neurological symptoms, usually the result of embolism or hemorrhage, occur in an average of 30% of cases of endocarditis, and in one report were the presenting symptom in 20%.[30] They may occur after the commencement of antibiotics although rarely after 2 weeks of treatment. However, rupture of a mycotic aneurysm may occur after many years. Central nervous system (CNS) involvement results from mitral or aortic valve endocarditis with equal frequency. Focal neurological events have been reported in 11–44% of cases of prosthetic valve endocarditis. Major neurological features in both native and prosthetic valve endocarditis are associated with an increased mortality.[4,30,31]

Cerebral emboli are the commonest cause of CNS involvement and often occur in conjunction with peripheral embolism.[31] The embolus most often lodges in a middle cerebral artery and the presentation is usually that of an acute ischemic or hemorrhagic infarction, either of which may cause seizures. A hemorrhagic infarction is likely if the patient is anticoagulated. Emboli may occasionally (approximately 5% of cases) cause a cerebral abscess or mycotic aneurysm. When there are multiple small emboli, confusion, psychoses or coma can occur. Patients with focal neurological findings or seizures should have computed tomography (CT) scanning or magnetic resonance imaging performed. These will distinguish hemorrhagic from non-hemorrhagic lesions and from cerebral abscess and may indicate the possibility of a mycotic aneurysm (Fig. 9.17). Cerebral angiography is the only reliable investigation for mycotic aneurysm, and because these lesions are often multiple, angiography of all four cerebral vessels is required. Mycotic aneurysms are usually asymptomatic until rupture occurs but if the lesion is expanding or leaking, it can cause

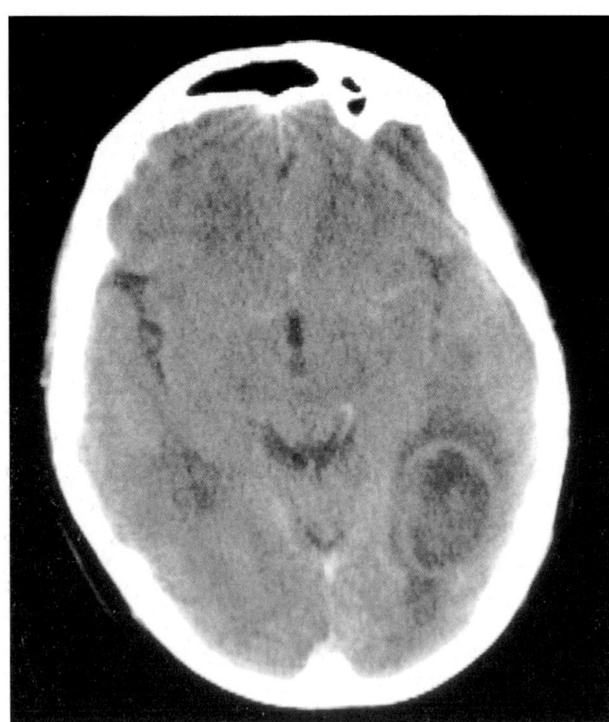

Figure 9.17
CT scan of the brain in a patient with a left cerebellar abscess secondary to aortic valve endocarditis.

headache (although this is a feature in up to 45% of all cases of infective endocarditis) and neck stiffness. If this situation is confirmed by angiography, prompt surgery will be needed.[30,31]

Peripheral emboli have been reported in 22–49% of cases and may be more common with large vegetations such as are produced by fungi, *Haemophilus influenzae* and variant streptococci. Splenic emboli are found in 50% of cases at post-mortem but most are asymptomatic. Rupture may occur. Three different CT patterns have been described:[32]

- a low density peripheral wedge shaped lesion;
- multiple heterogeneous lesions;
- massive low density lesions.

Contrast enhancement may be required to demonstrate a splenic embolism and even then, it may not be possible to distinguish mycotic aneurysm from an abscess without angiography.

Renal emboli are common but usually silent, producing hematuria or red cell casts. If multiple and recurrent, 'flea bitten' kidneys result. If large with associated significant infarction, there is loin pain. CT scanning with contrast enhancement will demonstrate renal infarcts.

Summary

Echocardiography has had an enormous impact on the diagnosis and treatment of endocarditis. It has not replaced clinical and microbiological assessment but is a complementary technique. In many cases a TTE will provide all the information required, but in those where the diagnosis remains uncertain, those with prosthetic valves in situ, and those where complications are suspected, then TEE should be performed. The absence of vegetations on a multiplane TEE effectively rules out vegetative endocarditis at that instant, but vegetations take time to develop and may be present on a repeat examination.

References

1 Hughes P, Gauld WRC: Bacterial endocarditis: a changing disease. *Q J Med* 1966; **35**: 511–20.

2 Terpenning MS, Buggy BP, Kauffman CA: Infective endocarditis: clinical features in young and elderly patients. *Am J Med* 1987; **83**: 626–34.

3 Douglas JL, Cobbs CG: Prosthetic valve endocarditis. In: *Infective Endocarditis* (Raven Press: New York, 1992); 375–96.

4 Erbel R, Liu F, Ge J et al: Identification of high risk subgroups in infective endocarditis and the role of echocardiography. *Eur Heart J* 1995; **16**: 588–602.

5 Durack DT, Lukes AS, Bright DK: New criteria for diagnosis of infective endocarditis: utilisation of specific echocardiographic findings. *Am J Med* 1994; **96**: 200–9.

6 Bayer AS: Revised diagnostic criteria for infective endocarditis. *Cardiol Clin* 1996; **14**: 345–50.

7 Dodds GA, Sexton DJ, Durack DT et al: Negative predictive value of the Duke criteria for infective endocarditis. *Am J Cardiol* 1996; **77**: 403–7.

8 Mugge A, Daniel WG, Frank G, Lichtlen PR: Echocardiography in infective endocarditis: reassessment of prognostic implications of vegetation size determined by the transthoracic and the transoesophageal approach. *J Am Coll Cardiol* 1989; **14**: 631–8.

9 Erbel R, Rohman S, Drexler M et al: Improved diagnostic value of echocardiography in patients with infective endocarditis by transoesophageal approach. A prospective study. *Eur Heart J* 1988; **9**: 43–53.

10 Shively BK, Gurule FT, Rolden CA et al: Diagnostic value of transoesophageal compared with transthoracic echocardiography in infective endocarditis. *J Am Coll Cardiol* 1991; **18**: 391–7.

11 Lindner JR, Case A, Dent JM et al: Diagnostic value of echocardiography in suspected endocarditis. *Circulation* 1996; **93**: 730–6.

12 Irani WN, Grayburn PA, Afridi I: A negative transthoracic echocardiogram obviates the need for transoesophageal echocardiography in patients with suspected native valve active endocarditis. *Am J Cardiol* 1996; **78**: 101–3.

13 Sochowski RA, Chan K-L: Implication of negative results on a monoplane transoesophageal echocardiographic study in patients with suspected infective endocarditis. *Am J Cardiol* 1993; **21**: 216–21.

14 Hecht SR, Berger M: Right sided endocarditis in intravenous drug abusers. *Ann Intern Med* 1992; **117**: 562–6.

15 Daniel WG, Mugge A, Grote J et al: Comparison of transthoracic and transoesophageal echocardiography for detection of abnormalities of prosthetic and bioprosthetic valves in the mitral and aortic positions. *Am J Cardiol* 1993; **71**: 210–15.

16 Job FP, Franke S, Lethen H et al: Incremental value of biplane and multiplane transoesophageal echocardiography for the assessment of active infective endocarditis. *Am J Cardiol* 1995; **75**: 1033–7.

17 Child JS, Perloff JK: Infective endocarditis. In: Perloff JK, Child JS, eds, *Congenital Heart Disease in Adults* (WB Saunders: Philadelphia, 1991); 111–123.

18 Morris D, Kenny A: Lambl's excrescences: a transoesophageal study. *Eur Heart J* 1996; **17** (suppl): 148 (abstract).

19 Buchbinder NA, Roberts WC: Left sided valvular active infective endocarditis. A study of 45 necropsy patients. *Am J Med* 1972; **53**: 20–35.

20 Cziner DG, Rosenwig BP, Katz ES et al: Transoesophageal versus transthoracic echocardiography for diagnosing mitral valve perforation. *Am J Cardiol* 1992; **69**: 1495–7.

21 Arnett EN, Roberts WC: Valve ring abscess in active infective endocarditis: frequency, location, and clues to clinical diagnosis from the study of 95 necropsy patients. *Circulation* 1976; **54**: 140–5.

22 Daniel WG, Mugge A, Martin R et al: Improvement in the diagnosis of abscesses associated with endocarditis by transoesophageal echocardiography. *N Engl J Med* 1991; **324**: 795–800.

23 Karalis DG, Bansal RC, Hauck AJ et al: Transoesophageal echocardiographic recognition of subaortic complications in aortic valve endocarditis. *Circulation* 1992; **86**: 353–62.

24 Jaffe WM, Morgan DE, Pearlman AS, Otto CM: Infective endocarditis, 1983–1988: echocardiographic findings and factors influencing morbidity and mortality. *J Am Coll Cardiol* 1990; **15**: 1227–33.

25 Sanfilippo AJ, Picard MH, Newell JB et al: Echocardiographic assessment of patients with infective endocarditis: prediction of risk for complications. *J Am Coll Cardiol* 1991; **18**: 1191–9.

26 Rohmann S, Erbel R, Darius H et al: Spontaneous echo contrast imaging in infective endocarditis: a predictor of complications? *Int J Card Imaging* 1992; **8**: 197–207.

27 Steckelberg JM, Murphy JG, Ballard D et al: Emboli in infective endocarditis: the prognostic value of echocardiography. *Ann Intern Med* 1991; **114**: 635–40.

28 Mills J, Abbott J, Utley JR, Ryan C: Role of cardiac catheterisation in infective endocarditis. *Chest* 1977; **72**: 576–82.

29 Hosenpud JD, Greenberg BH: The preoperative evaluation in patients with endocarditis. Is cardiac catheterisation necessary? *Chest* 1983; **84**: 690–4.

30 Tunkel AR, Kaye D: Neurologic complication in infective endocarditis. *Neurol Clin* 1993; **11**: 419–40.

31 Jones HR, Siekert RG: Neurological manifestations of infective endocarditis. *Brain* 1989; **112**: 1295–315.

32 Balcar I, Seltzer SE, Davis S, Geller S: CT patterns of splenic infarction: a clinical and experimental study. *Radiology* 1984; **151**: 723–9.

10

Cardiomyopathy and cardiac transplantation

Mark D Kelemen and Edward K Kasper

Overview

In 1980, the World Health Organization (WHO) and the International Society and Federation of Cardiology (ISFC) defined cardiomyopathy as a 'heart muscle disease of unknown cause' grouped into dilated, hypertrophic, and restrictive subtypes.[1] They also defined specific heart muscle disease, formerly known as 'secondary cardiomyopathies', as being 'of known cause or associated with disorders of other systems'. In addition, the WHO/ISFC excluded from specific heart muscle disease 'disorders of the myocardium caused by systemic or pulmonary hypertension, coronary artery disease, valvular heart disease, or congenital cardiac anomalies'. While there have been objections to this classification,[2] it continues to be a useful framework in which to consider clinical cardiomyopathy.

The prevalence of cardiomyopathy has increased as treatment, including cardiac transplantation, has improved, and better cardiac imaging can diagnose early or subclinical cases. The list of causes is long and is reviewed elsewhere.[2,3] In this chapter, we focus on the most common cardiomyopathies and an approach for initial evaluation and follow-up using clinical signs and noninvasive imaging techniques. Two-dimensional echocardiography is generally the imaging modality of choice to confirm the diagnosis of cardiomyopathy, although there are specific examples of cases in which nuclear cardiac imaging is preferable, and these will be highlighted. Further, magnetic resonance imaging (MRI) may soon be able to combine structural and physiological data in a single noninvasive test. In this chapter, emphasis will be placed on how the findings by echocardiography or Doppler ultrasound reflect the underlying pathophysiology of the disease.

Hypertrophic cardiomyopathy

Hypertrophic cardiomyopathy (HCM) is a primary myocardial disorder characterized by gross morphologic hypertrophy of the left ventricle, enhanced left ventricular function, diminished left ventricular cavity size and systolic outflow gradients. Although the classic descriptions are of asymmetric septal hypertrophy, the current definition includes all forms of left ventricular hypertrophy without an obvious cause. In fact, the wall thickness is often heterogeneous and discontinuous, although 55% of cases will have septal hypertrophy.[4] About 50% of familial cases of the disorder are associated with missense mutations of the β myosin heavy chain gene.[5] Clinical and genetic variability in this disorder is great, and echocardiography has become the imaging procedure of choice. Echocardiography also helps to guide and assess therapy. Symptoms can be vague and do not always reflect the degree of hypertrophy. These can include exertional dyspnea or angina, fatigue, lightheadedness or presyncope. Because it is an autosomal dominant disorder with high penetrance, all first degree relatives of patients with HCM should be screened with a clinical examination and echocardiography.

Asymmetric hypertrophy of the ventricular septum was long considered the hallmark of hypertrophic cardiomyopathy. Figure 10.1 shows a patient with marked septal hypertrophy but a normal posterior wall. The degree and the location of the septal hypertrophy can vary greatly. In general, there are septal, mid-ventricular, and apical forms of hypertrophy. The apical form is generally seen only in people of Asian descent and is one of the most prevalent forms of HCM in Japan.[6] It should be remembered that hypertrophy, even asymmetric hypertrophy, is not specific for HCM. Hypertension and aortic stenosis can cause

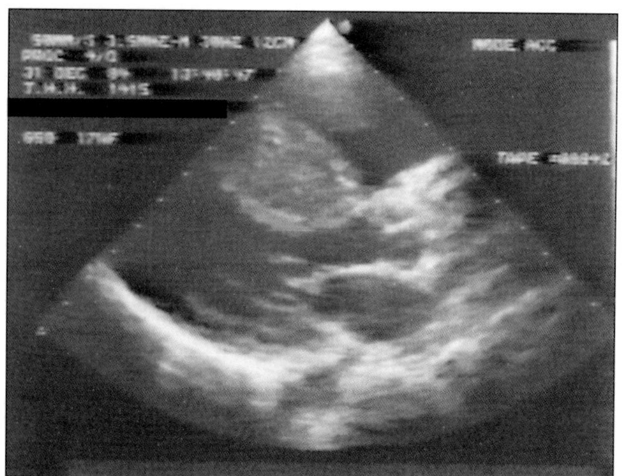

Figure 10.1
Parasternal long-axis (PL) view at end-diastole of a patient with hypertrophic cardiomyopathy and profound septal hypertrophy. Septal thickness is 2.8 cm while the posterior wall thickness is normal.

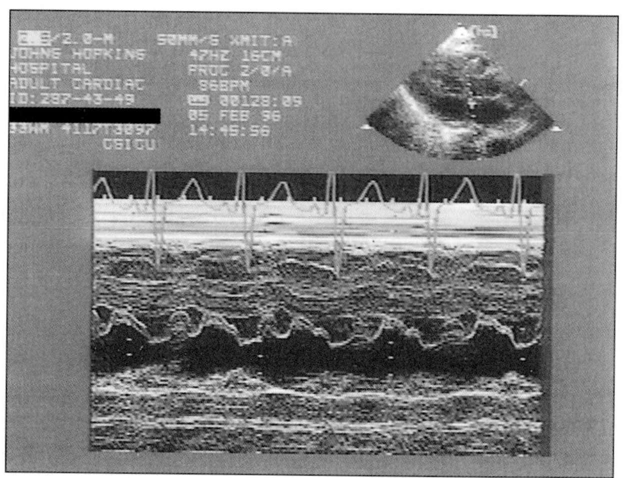

Figure 10.2
M-mode echocardiogram of systolic anterior motion (SAM) of the mitral valve. The anterior leaflet moves toward the septum in early systole and returns to normal position just before diastole.

profound left ventricular hypertrophy and diastolic dysfunction; well-conditioned athletes can also have markedly enlarged ventricles.[7] Further, elderly patients will often have proximal septal hypertrophy on echocardiogram, the so-called 'sigmoid septum', which is often mistaken for HCM, but is not associated with outflow gradients or lethal ventricular arrhythmias.[8]

It is important to differentiate between obstructive and nonobstructive varieties of HCM. Obstruction to left ventricular outflow is a common finding in this disorder. The obstruction is usually caused by systolic anterior motion of the mitral valve with mitral valve leaflet–septal contact (Figure 10.2), best visualized by M-mode echocardiography.[9] Notice how the leaflet moves toward the septum just after the onset of systole and returns to normal position before diastole. A pressure gradient between the left ventricle and the proximal aorta is often produced which may be latent but provocable, variable, or persistent. Doppler echocardiography is the noninvasive procedure of choice to determine the presence and severity of left ventricular outflow tract obstruction. Figure 10.3 shows the continuous wave Doppler findings in a patient with HCM and concentric hypertrophy and a resting systolic gradient of 136 mmHg. There is a relatively slow increase in the velocity in early systole with peaking in late systole, the characteristic 'ski slope' appearance of a dynamic gradient. The continuous wave Doppler velocities accurately reflect the hemodynamic obstruction and may be used to follow interventions. Drugs or maneuvers that decrease preload or afterload, or increase contractility may provoke or increase the pressure gradient. Gradients measured by catheterization are often falsely elevated because of cavity obliteration with direct pressure on the tip of the catheter. Apical cavity obliteration and midventricular hypertrophy may also cause dynamic outflow gradients.

Mitral regurgitation commonly accompanies obstructive HCM. With systolic anterior motion (SAM) of the mitral valve, there can be failure of mitral valve coaptation with a resultant regurgitant jet directed posteriorly into the left atrium. The degree of regurgitation is often related to the degree of outflow tract obstruction. Transesophageal echocardiography (TEE) has been shown to be superior to two-dimensional echocardiography in defining the coaptation point of the mitral valve and is being used intraoperatively to make decisions on the extent and success of ventricular resection.[10] In these studies, SAM has been shown to resolve and mitral regurgitation disappear despite persistent abnormalities of mitral closure.

HCM is associated with diastolic dysfunction and the mitral inflow pattern of early hypertrophic disease is characterized by E to A reversal. Normally, the E wave is taller than the A wave, reflecting the dominance of passive,

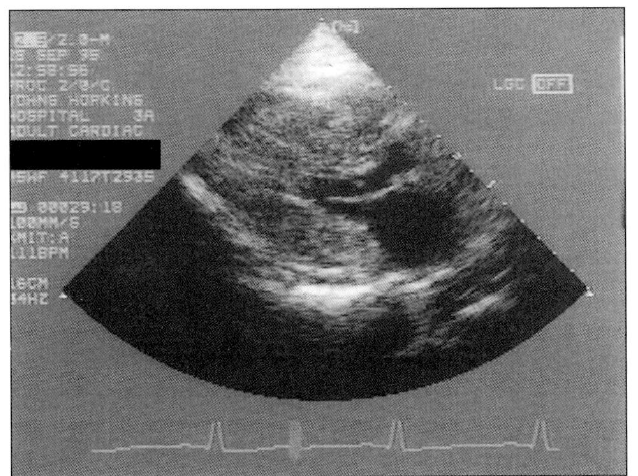

a

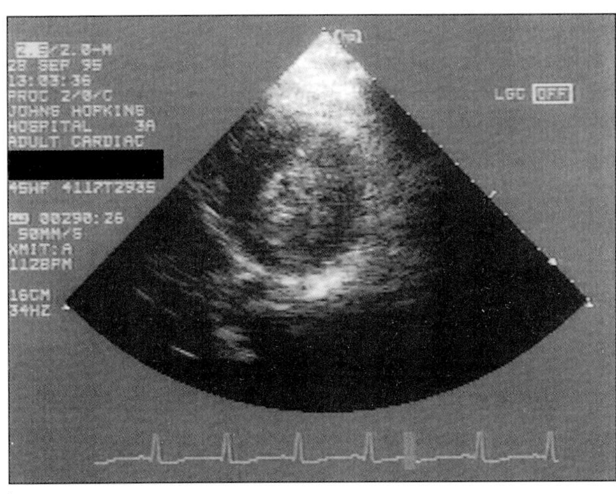

b

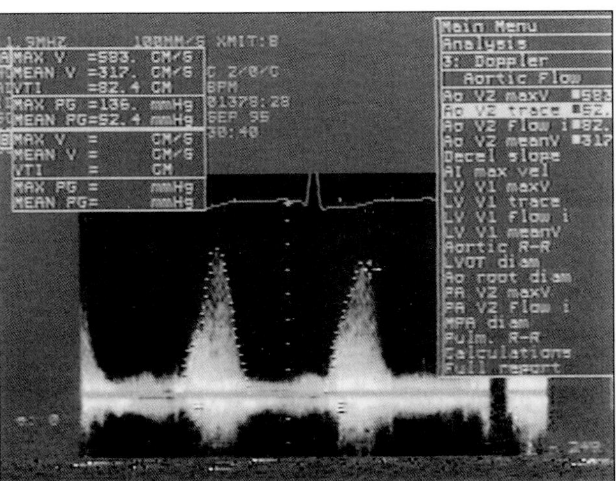

c

Figure 10.3
Parasternal long-axis (a), short-axis (b) and continuous wave Doppler at the aortic outflow tract (c) in a patient with hypertrophic cardiomyopathy and a resting outflow gradient of 136 mmHg (5.8 m/s). In this case, the hypertrophy was concentric.

early diastolic filling over the contribution of atrial systole. When diastolic function is abnormal, the E wave may be reduced and atrial systole becomes proportionally more important (Fig. 10.4). In patients with HCM, left ventricular relaxation is impaired and left ventricular diastolic pressures are elevated. In nonobstructive HCM, there is no systolic gradient at rest or with provocation. Diastolic dysfunction predominates, with systolic function impaired only in the late stages of disease.

The treatment of HCM depends upon the pathophysiology. If obstruction predominates, medical therapy consists of administering negative inotropic agents such as β blockers, calcium channel blockers, or disopyramide. Drugs which increase the obstruction (such as digoxin, diuretics, and afterload reducing agents) should be avoided. Left ventricular septal myectomy[11] and mitral valve replacement are surgical means to decrease the gradient and accompanying symptoms. Dual-chamber pacing to interrupt the activation pattern of the septum has been effective in reducing symptoms and increasing exercise duration in patients refractory to medical therapy.[12] Treatment can be monitored with echocardiography as in a patient who underwent ventricular myectomy for symptomatic HCM with intraoperative TEE (Fig. 10.5), revealing a marked improvement in resting systolic gradient. Once left ventricular systolic function becomes impaired, negative inotropic drugs must be discontinued. Treatment then becomes similar to patients with dilated cardiomyopathy with resultant congestive heart failure. Cardiac transplantation is an alternative at this stage.

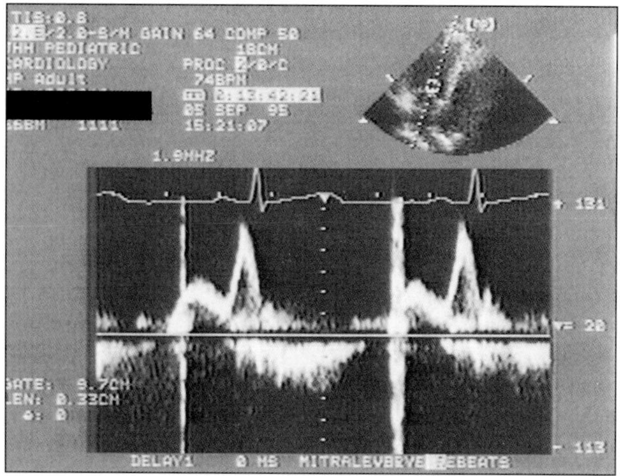

Figure 10.4
Pulse wave Doppler echocardiogram of mitral inflow in a patient with hypertrophic cardiomyopathy. Notice the dominant A wave reflecting the added importance of atrial contraction in left ventricular filling. This is termed 'E to A reversal'. In the small insert, the two-dimensional echo confirms the location of the Doppler signal at the opening of the mitral valve within the left ventricle.

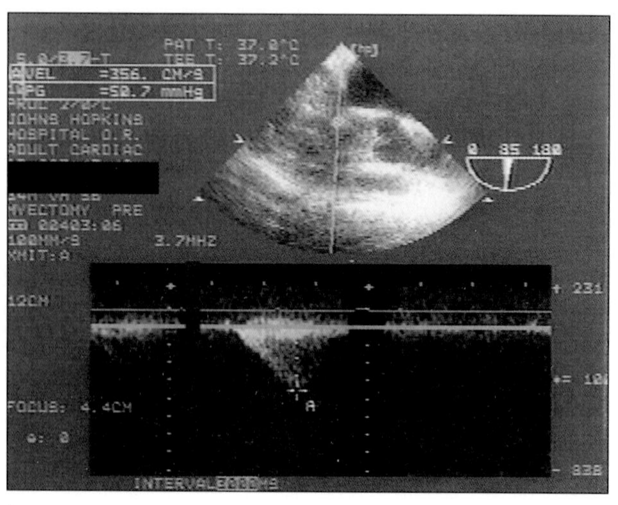

a

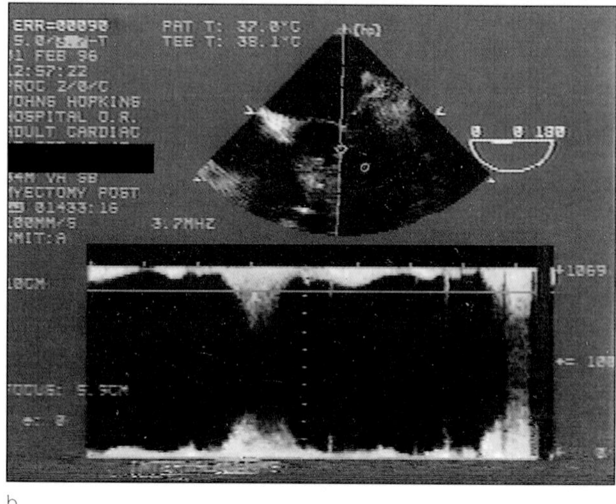

b

Figure 10.5
Continuous wave Doppler echocardiograms before (a) and after (b) ventricular myectomy for hypertrophic cardiomyopathy (HCM). The study was obtained during intraoperative TEE monitoring of the same patient as Figure 10.2 and reveals a significant decrease in the resting left ventricular outflow gradient.

Dilated cardiomyopathy

The WHO/ISFC define dilated cardiomyopathy (DCM) as a condition recognized by ventricular dilatation and systolic dysfunction of unknown cause.[1] The dilatation is usually accompanied by eccentric hypertrophy and symptoms of congestive heart failure. Arrhythmias are common, and death may occur at any stage. In a series of 673 endomyocardial biopsies at this institution, about 50% of them were of idiopathic origin.[3] Although this is clearly a selected population, epidemiological studies report an incidence of five to eight new cases per 100 000 per year and a prevalence of 36/100 000.[13] Patients often present with subacute symptoms of congestive heart failure and warrant an evaluation of possible causes, including ischemia, drugs/toxins, infectious causes and rheumatologic diseases. Dyspnea,

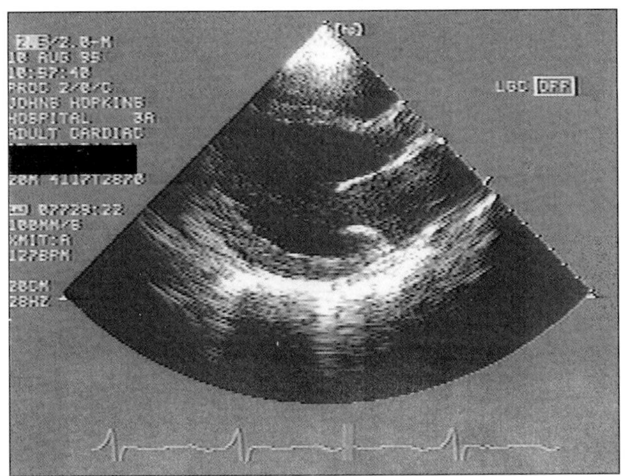

a

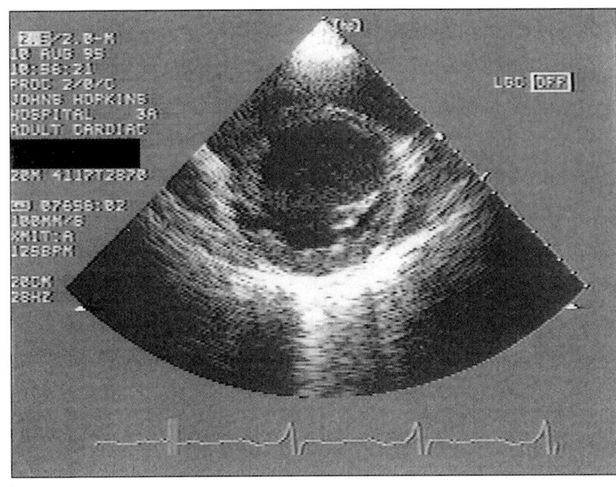

b

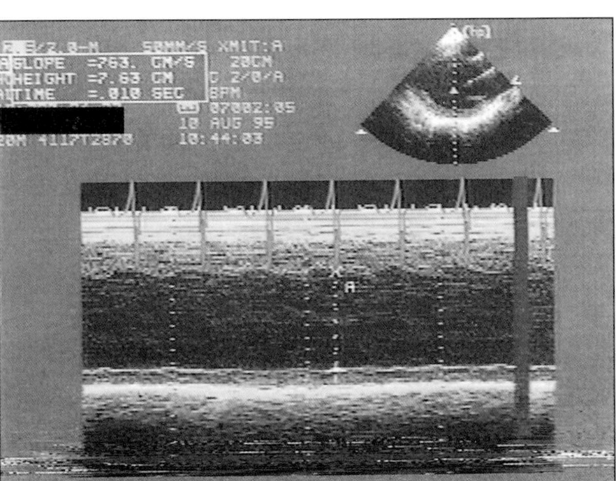

c

Figure 10.6
Parasternal long-axis (a), short-axis (b) and M-mode (c) echocardiograms of a 22-year-old patient with an idiopathic dilated cardiomyopathy and an ejection fraction of 10%. Wall thickness is normal although the left ventricular cavity is markedly dilated at 7.6 cm.

orthopnea, peripheral edema, paroxysmal nocturnal dyspnea, palpitations, syncope, fatigue, poor exercise tolerance or chest pain can be presenting complaints of patients with any form of cardiomyopathy. The physical examination can similarly be rather nonspecific with elevated jugular venous pressure, rales, a diffuse apical impulse, third or fourth heart sounds, and regurgitant murmurs. Therefore, patients with signs or symptoms of congestive heart failure should undergo either echocardiography or radionuclide ventriculography (MUGA) to define the presence and type of cardiomyopathy.

Impaired systolic function is reflected by several indices, including ejection fraction, fractional shortening, or the end-systolic pressure–volume relationship (ESPVR). ESPVR is the best measure of overall cardiac performance, but requires catheterization with high-fidelity catheters. MUGA is superior to echocardiography in precise calculation of ejection fraction, but both techniques require geometric assumptions of left ventricular shape that are violated in markedly dilated ventricles. For this reason, we generally use MUGA for following patients receiving adriamycin-based chemotherapy where subtle changes in ejection fraction can predict more severe cardiotoxicity. However, echocardiography (two-dimensional and Doppler) remains the test of choice for most patients with dilated cardiomyopathy in which estimates of systolic dysfunction are adequate for making therapeutic decisions. The additional information that echocardiography brings, including valvular abnormalities and estimates of right-sided intracardiac pressure, make it a better single test than MUGA. Figure 10.6 is the echo of a 22-year-old patient with dilated cardiomyopathy revealing several typical features. Ventricular dilatation is noted

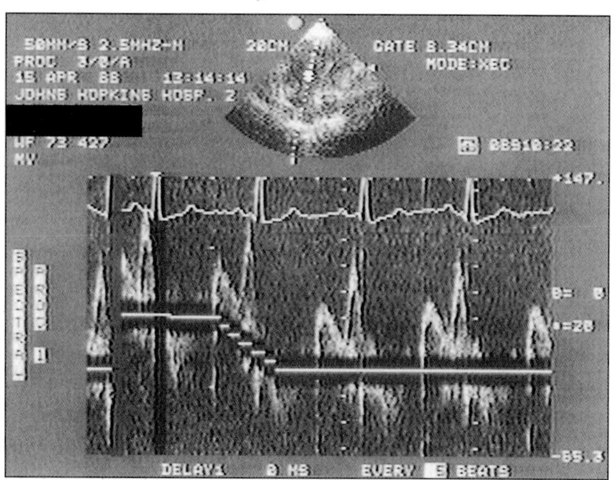

Figure 10.7
Pulse wave Doppler echocardiogram of mitral inflow in a 73-year-old women with an ischemic dilated cardiomyopathy showing E to A reversal, similar to the early changes in hypertrophic cardiomyopathy. In the late stages of dilated cardiomyopathy, when diastolic pressures are markedly elevated, the E to A wave ratio often normalizes. This is called 'pseudonormalization' of mitral inflow.

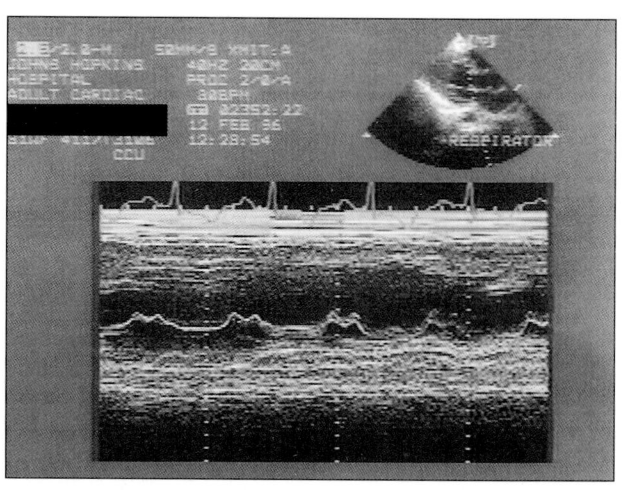

Figure 10.8
M-mode echocardiogram of an 81-year-old woman who suffered an anterior wall myocardial infarction complicated by pulmonary edema. Mitral valve motion is limited, reflecting a low output state and a B-notch is present, indicating elevated end-diastolic pressure.

and can be easily quantified with M-mode echocardiography. The dilatation occurs primarily in the short axis rather than in length and thus the ventricle becomes globular in shape. The ventricular walls are usually normal in thickness. There is little difference in systolic and diastolic left ventricle (LV) cavity dimension reflecting severe left ventricular dysfunction.

Left ventricular systolic dysfunction is almost always accompanied by both abnormal ventricular diastolic function and elevated left ventricular end-diastolic pressure (LVEDP). In the early stages of dilated and hypertrophic cardiomyopathy, this may be reflected as E to A reversal of mitral inflow (Fig. 10.7). If the left atrial pressure is markedly elevated, and ventricular compliance markedly reduced, ventricular filling may occur early with atrial contraction contributing relatively little to the final ventricular volume. In such cases, the E wave may predominate. This phenomenon is termed 'pseudonormalization' of mitral inflow velocity and is a poor prognostic sign. Elevated left ventricular end-diastolic pressure is sometimes reflected in a B notch on the M-mode tracing of mitral valve motion (Fig. 10.8). Right ventricular overload due to pulmonary hypertension can also be seen on echocardiography. The shape of the left ventricle in the short axis is normally circular with the right ventricle having a surrounding arc shape. With pressure elevation in the right ventricle, the septum may assume a flat shape or even curve into the left ventricle (Fig. 10.9). Right ventricular systolic pressure (RVSP) can be calculated from the velocity of regurgitant flow across the tricuspid valve which is found in most people by using the modified Bernoulli equation[14] and peak systolic velocity to determine the pressure drop across the valve. Pulmonary artery pressure is estimated by adding 10 mmHg to reflect the additional contribution of right atrial pressure. Right ventricular function may play an important role in the development of symptoms and in prognosis of DCM.[15] Therapy in this instance is directed at the proximate cause of the pulmonary hypertension, namely left ventricular systolic dysfunction.

With increased ventricular filling pressures, tricuspid or mitral regurgitation are commonly seen. This is most typically due to annular dilatation, and is usually associated with atrial dilatation (Fig. 10.10). Mitral regurgitation can also be a cause of dilated cardiomyopathy. In this instance, the regurgitation must occur prior to the development of the cardiomyopathy. Improvement in the degree of mitral regurgitation in response to therapy may imply better prognosis.[16] In cases of severe left ventricular dysfunction, color Doppler often overestimates the severity of mitral regurgitation.

Thrombotic complications of dilated cardiomyopathy may be detected using echocardiography.[17] Thrombi are common in DCM and can be seen in the atrium or in the ventricular apex (Fig. 10.11). Unusual locations for ventricular clot include the left ventricular outflow tract (Fig. 10.12). Owing to abnormal blood flow patterns seen in a

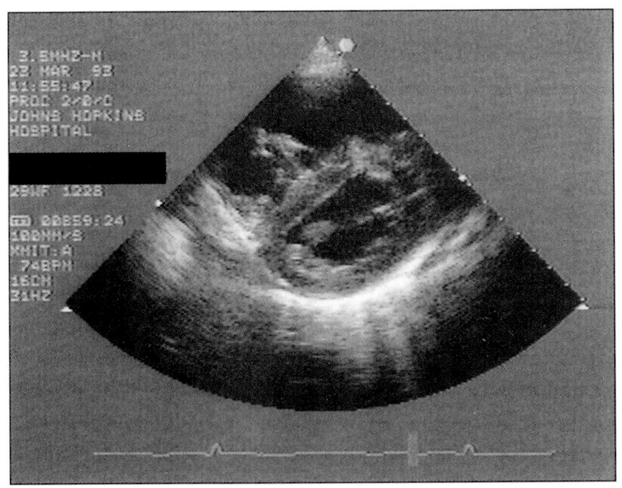

Figure 10.9
Short-axis echocardiogram of a patient with severe pulmonary hypertension. Although the left ventricular walls are moderately thickened, the right ventricle is markedly dilated and the septum is flattened, almost bowing into the left ventricle (LV).

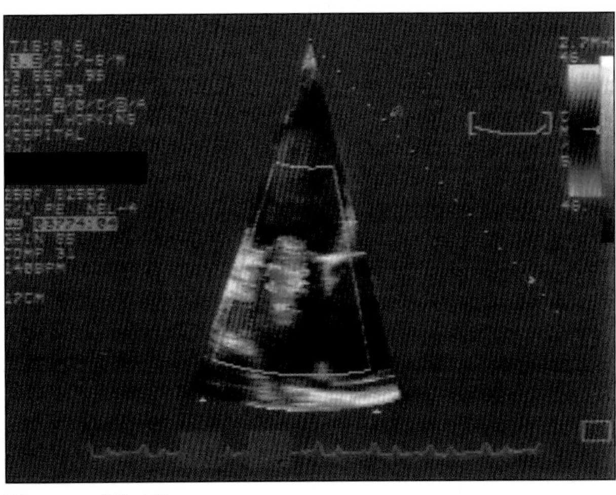

Figure 10.10
Color Doppler echocardiogram in the apical four-chamber view of a 25-year-old woman with dilated cardiomyopathy and secondary mitral regurgitation. Both atria are dilated and annular dilatation is thought to be the mechanism for valvular regurgitation. In patients with severe left ventricular dysfunction and diminished cardiac output, color Doppler often overestimates the degree of valvular regurgitation.

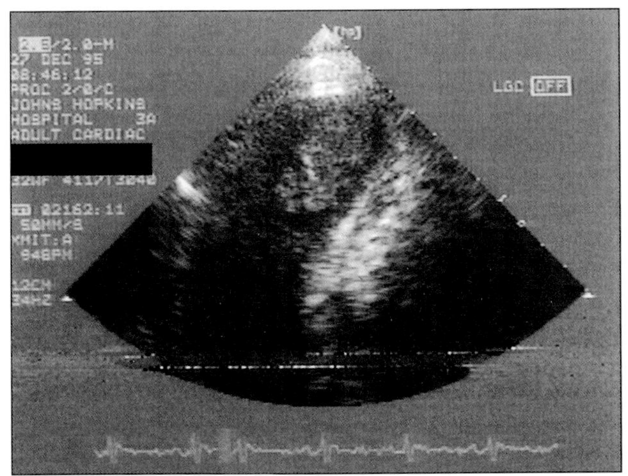

a

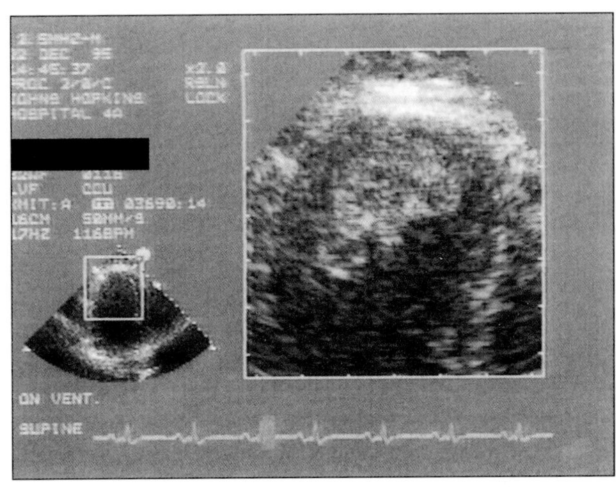

b

Figure 10.11
Two-chamber echocardiogram (a) and close-up of the ventricular apex (b) of a 32-year-old woman with a dilated cardiomyopathy (DCM) and a huge apical thrombus. Patients with DCM and without contraindications should be anticoagulated.

poorly contracting and dilated ventricle, spontaneous contrast can sometimes be seen by echo, although it is fairly commonly seen by TEE. Patients with DCM are at higher risk for stroke and peripheral embolization and should be anticoagulated with warfarin if they have no contraindications. TEE is now commonly performed in patients who present with stroke; however, in the setting of DCM, the etiology is likely to be embolic from the heart. We do not recommend routine TEE in patients with cardiomyopathy who have embolic events.

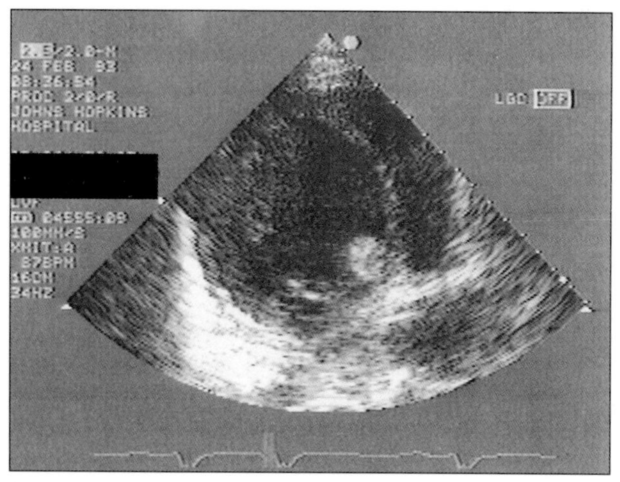

a

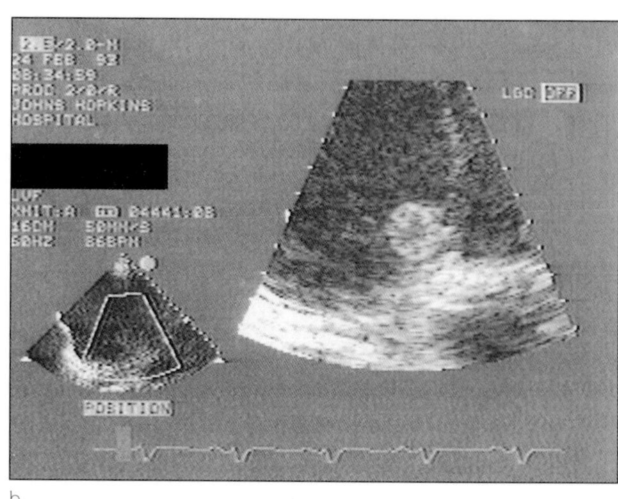

b

Figure 10.12
Short-axis echocardiogram (a) and close-up of the left ventricular outflow tract (b) of a 33-year-old man with dilated cardiomyopathy (DCM) awaiting cardiac transplantation. The echogenic mass in the outflow tract is an organized thrombus.

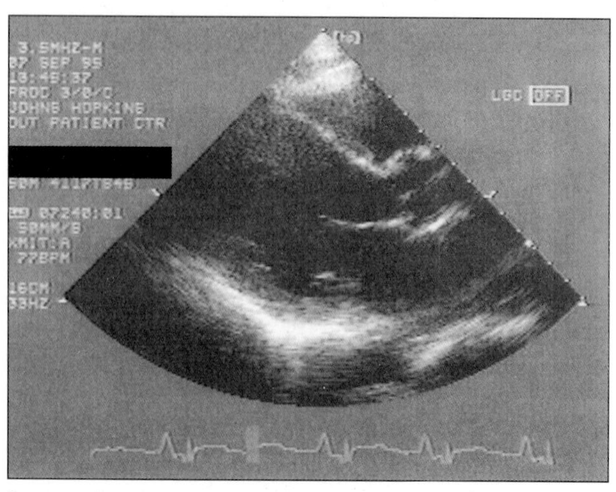

a

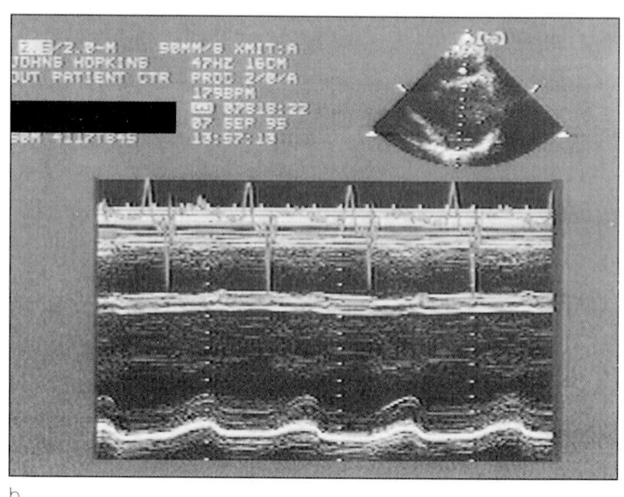

b

Figure 10.13
Parasternal long-axis (a) and M-mode echocardiogram (b) of a 50-year-old man who suffered an anterior wall myocardial infarction and presented later with an ischemic cardiomyopathy. The septum is thinned and displaced anteriorly, representing ventricular remodeling. The posterior wall has normal thickness and contractility as seen in the M-mode tracing.

In the differential diagnosis of heart failure with a dilated left ventricle, the most important distinction to be made is between ischemic and idiopathic cardiomyopathy, since coronary revascularization may improve cardiac function (Fig. 10.13). Unfortunately, efforts to distinguish the two using echocardiographic wall motion indices have been disappointing. In one study of 50 patients with DCM and normal coronary arteries, 64% had segmental wall motion abnormalities.[18] Thallium imaging, with or without exercise, often reveals perfusion abnormalities in patients with no coronary artery disease (CAD). Patients have to undergo coronary angiography to exclude significant CAD in many cases.

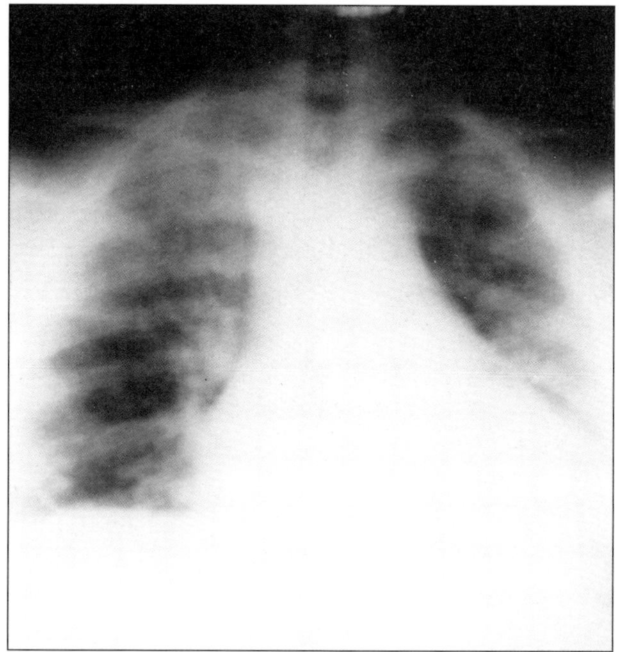

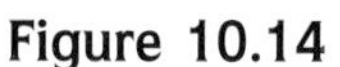

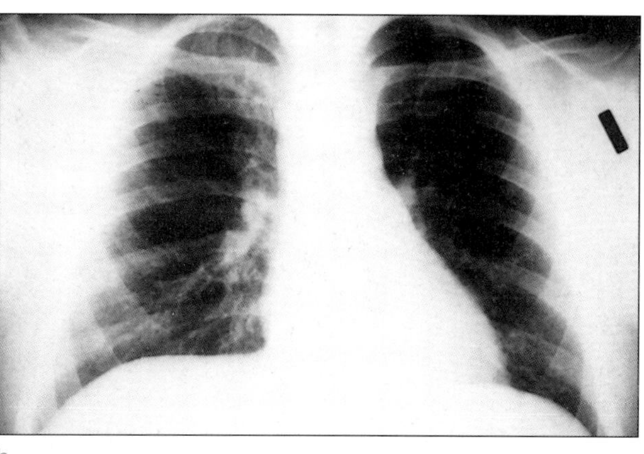

b

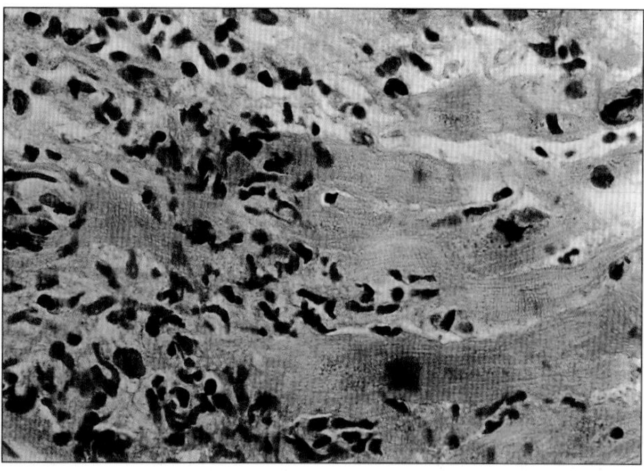

c

Figure 10.14
(a) and (b) Chest X-rays in the AP projection in a patient with fulminant myocarditis who presented with heart failure and resolved completely after a course of corticosteroids.
(c) Endomyocardial biopsy of another patient with myocarditis revealing destruction of myocytes by an intense inflammatory reaction.

Recent studies suggest that dobutamine stress echocardiography (DSE) can localize ischemic tissue as well as viable, hibernating myocardium,[19] allowing us the ability to predict who will benefit the most from revascularization. In the future, cardiac MRI with perfusion techniques or TEE with attention to aortic atherosclerosis may reduce the number of angiograms performed in the evaluation of DCM.[20]

DCM may rarely improve either spontaneously or with therapy. Standard therapy consists of loop diuretics, digoxin, and afterload reducing agents (preferably angiotensin converting enzyme inhibitors). The abnormalities described may resolve completely or partially. Figure 10.14 shows spontaneous resolution of left ventricular dysfunction in a patient with fulminant myocarditis. Routine use of echocardiography in the follow-up of patients with dilated cardiomyopathy is not warranted. Repeat testing is only indicated if there is a sudden change in the patient's symptoms or physical examination.

Restrictive cardiomyopathy

The WHO/ISFC defined restrictive cardiomyopathy (RCM) as a scarring affecting either or both ventricles which restricts filling.[1] It is a rare disorder characterized by diastolic dysfunction with rapid left ventricular inflow and abrupt cessation of flow early in diastole. The left ventricle has normal or near normal systolic function, but never supernormal function. The left ventricle may be hypertrophied, but never dilated. Figure 10.15 shows an example of mitral valve inflow velocities in a patient with an RCM caused by cardiac amyloidosis. The tall early diastolic velocities, E wave, and short late diastolic velocities, A wave, are characteristic but not specific.

The natural history of idiopathic RCM in adults is often a prolonged, progressive decline. Severe symptoms of congestive heart failure and low cardiac output predominate. Cardiac cirrhosis and systemic embolization are relatively

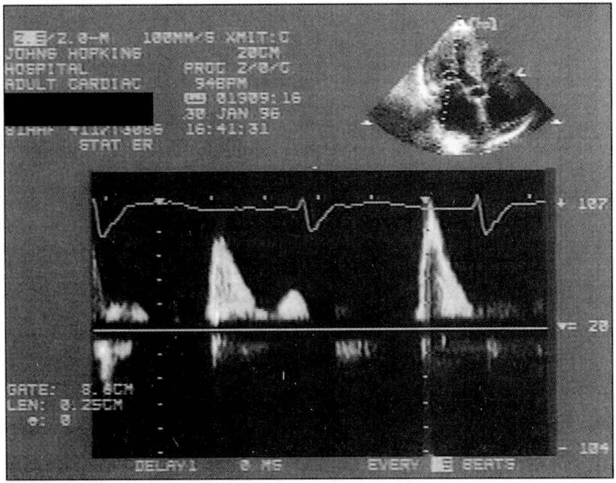

Figure 10.15
Continuous wave Doppler echocardiogram of a patient with a 'restrictive filling pattern'. The mitral inflow Doppler reveals a dominant E wave with little or no A wave. Almost all left ventricular filling is occurring in early diastole.

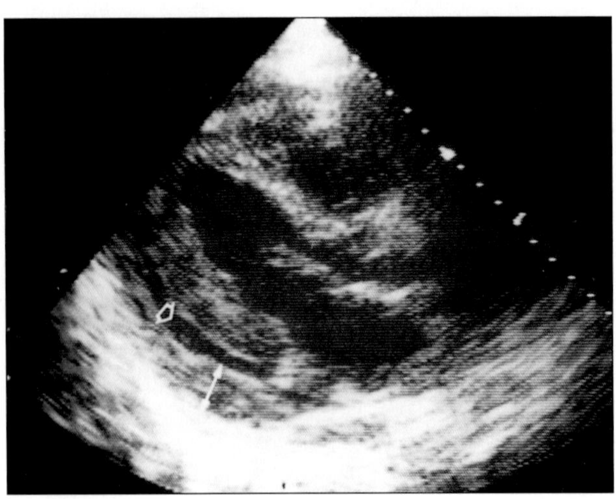

a

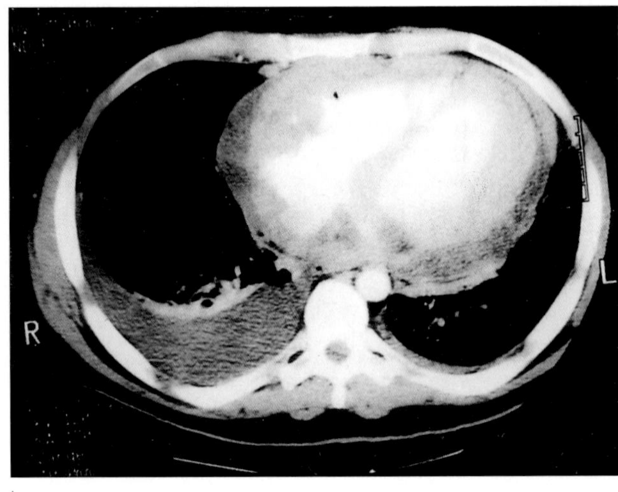

b

Figure 10.16
Parasternal long-axis echocardiogram (a) and CT of the chest (b) of a 34-year-old patient who presented with right sided heart failure and was found to have constrictive pericarditis caused by pericardial lymphoma. The thickened pericardium noted here should prompt an aggressive diagnostic approach and an attempt at pericardial stripping which relieved the symptoms in this case. Small arrow = thickened pericardium; large arrowhead = pericardial effusion.

common complications. Therapy is similar to patients with dilated cardiomyopathy. Digoxin, however, should be used with caution. Cardiac transplantation is a viable alternative.

RCM may be difficult to differentiate from constrictive pericarditis. The diagnosis of constrictive pericarditis should not be missed as this disorder is surgically correctable. There is no specific therapy for RCM. Constrictive pericarditis is established if pericardial thickening or calcification is present. Echocardiography, CT, or MRI may be used to diagnose pericardial thickening. Figure 10.16 shows the thickened pericardium of a patient with constrictive pericarditis due to pericardial lymphoma, a rare malignancy. This patient had severe symptoms of right heart failure, which were relieved by pericardial stripping. In the catheterization laboratory, LVEDP more than 12 mmHg higher than right ventricular end-diastolic pressure (RVEDP)[21] suggests the diagnosis of RCM. Noninvasive measures of left ventricular filling rate as determined by the E to A ratio on the mitral inflow velocity (Doppler echocardiography) or first-pass filling rates as determined

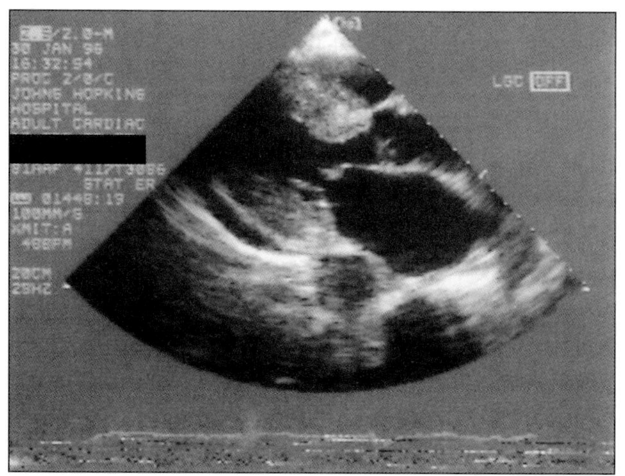

a

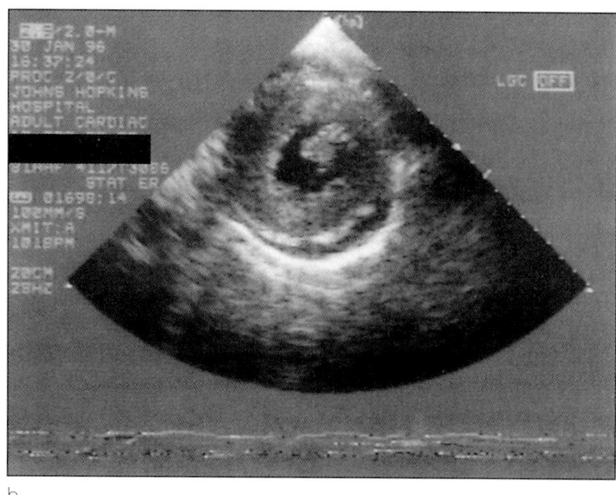

b

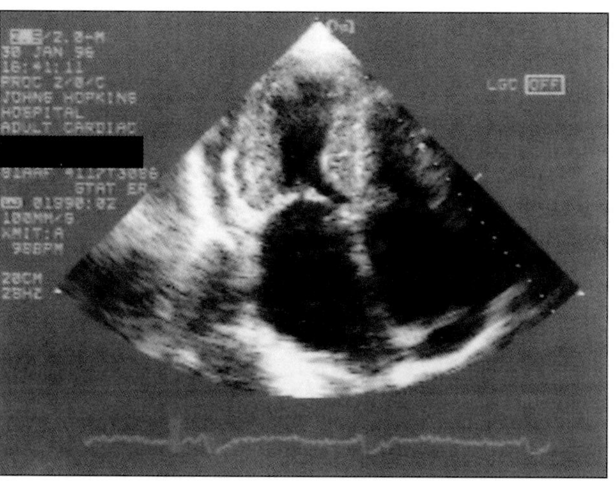

c

Figure 10.17
Parasternal long-axis (a), short-axis (b) and apical four-chamber echocardiograms (c) of a patient with cardiac amyloidosis revealing left ventricular hypertrophy with diffuse myocardial speckling and thickening of the mitral valve apparatus. There is a moderate pericardial effusion and severe systolic dysfunction which is a poor prognostic sign.

by gated blood pool analysis are variably helpful in making the distinction. A constrictive pattern is suggested by: (a) rapid early diastolic filling; (b) an inspiratory decrease in left ventricular filling; and (c) limitation of right ventricular filling with expiration.[22] Respiratory variation in pulmonary venous flow can be measured by TEE and can aid in distinguishing constrictive pericarditis from RCM.[23]

Specific heart muscle diseases

Amyloidosis

The most common type of RCM is due to amyloid heart disease. Differentiation from idiopathic RCM can be made on clinical grounds. Patients with idiopathic RCM are more likely to have a family history of heart failure, complete heart block or a concurrent skeletal myopathy.[21] Ultimately, however, the diagnosis is confirmed with endomyocardial biopsy. Figure 10.17 shows several echocardiographic features of cardiac amyloidosis. Thickening of the myocardium and valves is noted. Amyloid infiltrates all parts of the heart. The myocardium itself may have a fairly characteristic speckled pattern. The interatrial septum can be thickened as well, although this is not a universal feature. Left atrial enlargement is common and due to left ventricular diastolic dysfunction. A small pericardial effusion can be seen with infiltrative cardiomyopathies. The systolic function is usually normal, but when systolic function is impaired or the patient has heart failure symptoms, the prognosis is poor.[24] Doppler echo reflects abnormal left ventricular relaxation in the early stages; pseudonormalization of the mitral inflow pattern is a late finding and a poor prognostic sign.[25]

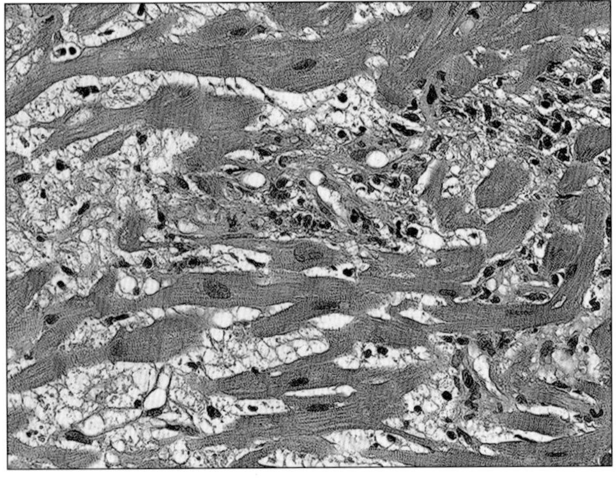

a

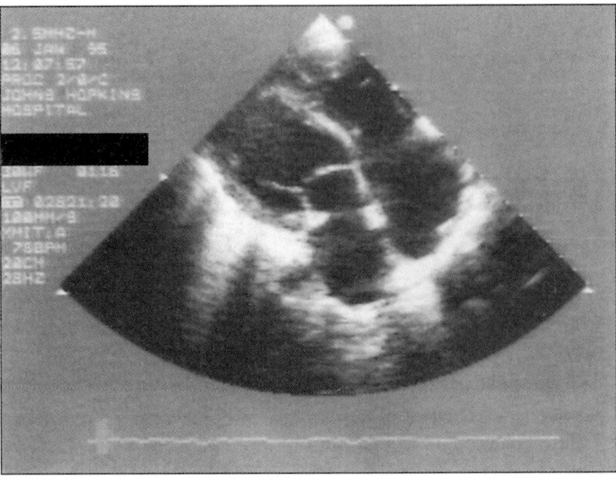

b

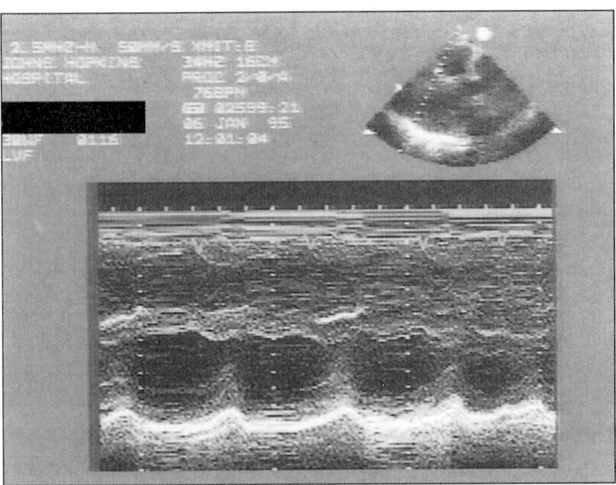

c

Figure 10.18
(a) Endomyocardial biopsy specimen of a patient with acute rejection. Note the intense lymphocytic infiltrate. (b) Apical four-chamber echocardiogram of a patient after cardiac transplantation. Notice the prominent atrial suture lines that resemble the thrombus seen in previous examples. (c) M-mode echo in the parasternal long-axis of the same patient revealing normal left ventricular function.

Sarcoidosis

Sarcoid heart disease can have features of both a dilated or restrictive cardiomyopathy. It is characterized by localized thinning and dilatation of the myocardium, usually toward the base of the heart.[26] A pseudoinfarction or focal aneurysm formation is common. Doppler echo findings reflect abnormal left ventricular filling. Myocardial involvement can cause heart block and ventricular arrhythmias; right heart failure accompanies severe lung involvement with pulmonary hypertension. Left ventricular dysfunction is a poor prognostic sign, although some patients will have improvement with corticosteroid therapy.

Cardiac transplantation

Since the first heart transplant was performed in 1967, cardiac transplantation has become a viable alternative to conventional therapy for a variety of end-stage cardiac conditions. Current 1-year survival is about 90%, and the 5-year survival is 70%. Infection and cardiac rejection remain major problems following cardiac transplantation. Endomyocardial biopsy is the gold standard for the diagnosis of cardiac rejection. Rejection is often manifested as alterations in ventricular filling. The typical echocardiographic finding is a restricted filling pattern. Systolic dysfunction is a late finding in cardiac rejection, and represents a

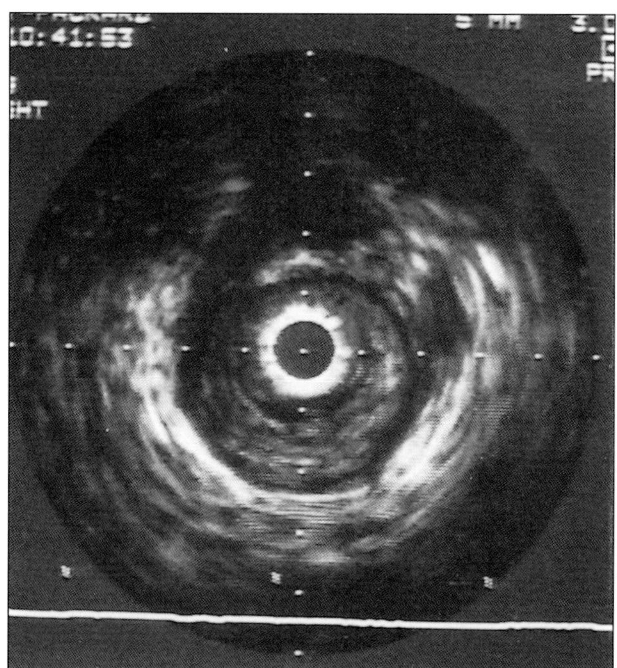

Figure 10.19
Intracoronary ultrasonography (ICUS) image of a transplant coronary artery with accelerated arthrosclerosis. The central dark zone is the catheter with a bright halo artifact. The lesion is circumferential and involves most of the lumen of the aorta.

true emergency. Figure 10.18 shows an endomyocardial biopsy of cardiac allograft rejection, although left ventricular cavity size and systolic function remain normal. A characteristic echocardiographic finding in cardiac transplant recipients is a prominent atrial suture line (Figure 10.18b). The suture lines can be fairly large and can be mistaken for a cardiac mass. Pericardial effusions are occasionally seen in the early postoperative period.

With the improved early survival of cardiac transplant recipients, accelerated graft arteriosclerosis has emerged as a major cause of morbidity and mortality. As many as 50% of heart transplant recipients develop angiographically detectable accelerated graft arteriosclerosis 3–5 years following the transplant. Almost all recipients will have histologic evidence of this disorder within the first year. Accelerated graft arteriosclerosis is characterized by diffuse, concentric narrowing of the coronary arteries. Histologically, the internal and external elastic laminae are usually intact. The intima is thickened by an accumulation of smooth muscle cells, lipid-laden macrophages, and lymphocytes. These microscopic changes are different from the changes seen in patients with natural atherosclerosis. Unfortunately, the central mechanisms responsible for the development of accelerated graft arteriosclerosis are unknown.

Because the allograft is denervated, this disorder may strike without the development of angina. Therefore, many programs perform routine, annual cardiac angiography. Intracoronary ultrasonography has become the gold standard for the diagnosis of early coronary lesions, and may be predictive of future mortality (Fig. 10.19).

References

1 Brandenburg RO, Chazov E, Cherian G et al: Report of the WHO/ISFC task force on the definition and classification of cardiomyopathies. *Br Heart J* 1980; **44**: 672–3.

2 Abelmann WH: Classification and natural history of primary myocardial disease. *Prog Cardiovasc Dis* 1984; **27**: 73–94.

3 Kasper EK, Agema WRP, Hutchins GM et al: The causes of dilated cardiomyopathy: a clinicopathologic review of 673 consecutive patients. *J Am Coll Cardiol* 1994; **23**: 586–90.

4 Codd MB, Sugrue DD, Gersh BJ, Melton LJ: Epidemiology of idiopathic dilated and hypertrophic cardiomyopathy. *Circulation* 1989; **80**: 564–72.

5 Watkins H, Rosenzweig A, Hwang D et al: Characteristics and prognostic implications of myosin missense mutations in familial hypertrophic cardiomyopathy. *N Engl J Med* 1992; **326**: 1108–14.

6 Maron BJ, Gottdiener JS, Epstein SE: Patterns and significance of distribution of left ventricular hypertrophy in hypertrophic cardiomyopathy: a wide angle, two-dimensional echocardiographic study of 125 patients. *Am J Cardiol* 1981; **48**: 418–28.

7 Shapiro LM, McKenna WJ: Distribution of left ventricular hypertrophy in hypertrophic cardiomyopathy: A two dimensional echocardiographic study. *J Am Coll Cardiol* 1983; **2**: 437–44.

8 Topol EJ, Traill TA, Fortuin NJ: Hypertensive-hypertrophic cardiomyopathy of the elderly. *N Engl J Med* 1985; **312**: 277–83.

9 Ballester M, Rickards A, Rees S, McDonald L: Systolic anterior motion of the mitral valve in hypertrophic cardiomyopathy. A cross-sectional echocardiographic study. *Eur Heart J* 1983; **4**: 846–53.

10 Grigg LE, Wigle ED, Williams WG et al: Transesophageal Doppler echocardiography in obstructive hypertrophic cardiomyopathy: clarification of pathophysiology and importance in intraoperative decision making. *J Am Coll Cardiol* 1992; **20**: 42–52.

11 Morrow AG, Reitz BA, Epstein SE et al: Operative treatment in hypertrophic subaortic stenosis: techniques and

the results of pre- and postoperative assessment in 83 patients. *Circulation* 1975; **52**: 88–102.

12 Fananapazir L, Cannon RO, Tripodi D, Panza JA: Impact of dual-chamber permanent pacing in patients with obstructive hypertrophic cardiomyopathy with symptoms refractory to verapamil and β-adrenergic blocker therapy. *Circulation* 1992; **85**: 2149–61.

13 Dec GW, Fuster V: Idiopathic dilated cardiomyopathy. *N Engl J Med* 1994; **331**: 1564–75.

14 Stevenson JG: Comparison of several non-invasive methods for estimation of pulmonary artery pressure. *J Am Soc Echocardiogr* 1989; **2**: 157–71.

15 DiSalvo TG, Mathier M, Semigran MJ, Dec GW: Preserved right ventricular ejection fraction predicts exercise capacity and survival in advanced heart failure. *J Am Coll Cardiol* 1995; **25**: 1143–53.

16 Hamilton MA, Stevenson LW, Child JS et al: Sustained reduction in valvular regurgitation and atrial volumes with tailored vasodilator therapy in advanced congestive heart failure secondary to dilated (ischemic or idiopathic) cardiomyopathy. *Am J Cardiol* 1991; **67**: 259–63.

17 Siostrzonek P, Kuppensteiner R, Gossinger H et al: Hemodynamic and hemorheologic determinants of left atrial spontaneous echo contrast and thrombus formation in patients with idiopathic dilated cardiomyopathy. *Am Heart J* 1993; **125**: 430–34.

18 Wallis DE, O'Connell JB, Henkin RE et al: Segmental wall motion abnormalities in dilated cardiomyopathy: a common finding and good prognostic sign. *J Am Coll Cardiol* 1984; **4**: 674–79.

19 Williams MJ, Odabashian J, Lauer MS et al: Prognostic value of dobutamine echocardiography in patients with left ventricular dysfunction. *J Am Coll Cardiol* 1996; **27**: 132–39.

20 Fazio GP, Redberg RF, Winslow T, Schiller NB: Transesophageal echocardiographically detected atherosclerotic aortic plaque is a marker for coronary artery disease. *J Am Coll Cardiol* 1993; **21**: 144–50.

21 Katritsis D, Wilmshurst PT, Wendon JA et al: Primary restrictive cardiomyopathy: clinical and pathologic characteristics. *J Am Coll Cardiol* 1991; **18**: 1230–35.

22 Oh JK, Hatle LK, Seward JB et al: Diagnostic role of Doppler echocardiography in constrictive pericarditis. *J Am Coll Cardiol* 1994; **23**: 154–62.

23 Klein AL, Cohen GI, Pietrolungo JF et al: Differentiation of constrictive pericarditis from restrictive cardiomyopathy by Doppler transesophageal echocardiographic measurements of respiratory variations in pulmonary venous flow. *J Am Coll Cardiol* 1993; **22**: 1935–43.

24 Siqueira-Filho AG, Cunha CL, Tajik AJ et al: M-Mode and two dimensional echocardiographic features in cardiac amyloidosis. *Circulation* 1981; **63**: 188–96.

25 Klein AL, Hatle LK, Taliercio CP et al: Prognostic significance of Doppler measures of diastolic function in cardiac amyloidosis. *Circulation* 1991; **83**: 808–16.

26 Lorell B, Alderman EL, Mason JW: Cardiac sarcoidosis. *Am J Cardiol* 1978; **42**: 143–46.

11

Hypertrophic heart disease

Wendy S Post and Edward P Shapiro

Left ventricular hypertrophy (LVH) is a heterogeneous disorder that is characterized by an increase in the mass of the ventricular myocardium. LVH may occur primarily owing to systemic or environment stimuli, such as hypertension, or may be the result of a genetic mutation, leading to hypertrophic cardiomyopathy. Since nonembryonic cardiac myocytes are incapable of cell division, increased myocardial mass is due to an increase in cell size (hypertrophy) rather than due to an increase in cell number (hyperplasia). LVH can occur through either an increase in wall thickness with a small or normal ventricular chamber (concentric hypertrophy), an increase in the volume of the left ventricular chamber (eccentric hypertrophy), or an increase in both wall thickness and chamber size.

Factors associated with left ventricular hypertrophy

Left ventricular mass (LVM) follows a normal bell shaped distribution in the general population. The strongest predictors of LVH include valvular heart disease, obesity, hypertension, advanced age, and coronary heart disease. In addition, alcohol intake,[1] plasma viscosity,[2] physical activity,[3] genetics,[4,5] insulin resistance,[6] and arterial stiffness[7] have been shown to impact on LVM. In the elderly, hypertrophy often develops predominantly in the proximal septum, referred to as a 'sigmoid septum'. A dramatic increase in LVM with age, especially in hypertensive women, has been termed 'hypertensive hypertrophic cardiomyopathy of the elderly'.[8] Long-term, vigorous physical activity may lead to an 'athlete's heart'. It may sometimes be difficult to distinguish this from genetic hypertrophic cardiomyopathy, which is the most common cause of sudden death in young competitive athletes. This physiologic hypertrophy is not associated with the abnormalities of diastolic filling typically associated with pathologic hypertrophy.

Left ventricular hypertrophy is an adverse prognostic sign

It has been clearly demonstrated that LVM is an important predictor of adverse events in the general population. In the Framingham Heart Study, the association between LVM and the development of cardiovascular disease and mortality was studied in 3220 men and women who were free of clinically apparent cardiovascular disease.[9] After adjusting for blood pressure and other risk factors, the relative risk for all-cause mortality during 4 years of follow-up in men was 1.49 for each 50 g increment of LVM (indexed to height), and 2.01 in women. Increased LVM was also significantly associated with an increased incidence of cardiovascular events and cardiovascular mortality (Fig. 11.1). The risk associated with increased LVM persisted during 10 years of follow-up of 253 hypertensive men and women studied by Koren et al.[10] Possible mechanisms for the increased risk associated with LVH include an increased risk of cardiac arrhythmias (including sudden death),[11] endothelial dysfunction leading to an impairment in coronary flow reserve[12] with an increase in demand due to increased myocardial mass and diastolic dysfunction leading to congestive heart failure.

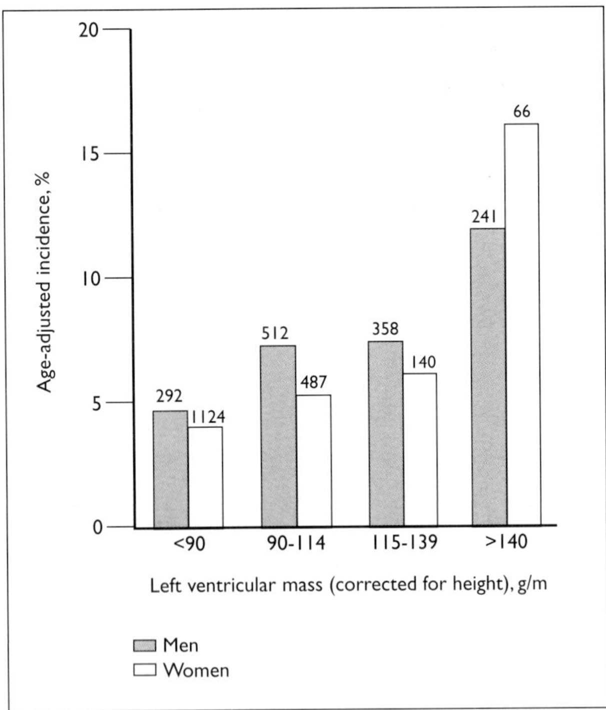

Figure 11.1
Four-year age adjusted incidence of cardiovascular disease, according to quartiles of left ventricular mass (corrected for height), from the Framingham Heart Study. Rates for men – grey bars – and women – white bars. The numbers at the top of the bars indicate the numbers of subjects at risk in each quartile. Reprinted with permission from Levy et al.[9]

Measuring left ventricular mass

M-mode echocardiographic methods

There are a variety of electrocardiographic criteria that have been established to diagnose LVH. These methods are insensitive compared with echocardiography and therefore often lead to false negative diagnoses. Therefore, LVM is often measured with M-mode echocardiography.

Using diastolic measurements of left ventricular wall thickness and chamber size obtained using the Penn convention, LVM can be estimated with the following formula:

$$\text{LVM(g)} = 1.04\,[(\text{VST} + \text{LVID} + \text{PWT})^3 - \text{LVID}^3] - 13.6$$

where VST is ventricular septal thickness, LVID is left ventricular internal dimension, and PWT is posterior wall thickness. Devereux et al[13] have shown with autopsy studies that this modified cubed formula is a valid estimate of LVM in subjects with symmetrically contracting ventricles. The Penn convention excludes the endocardial echoes from the measurement of wall thickness, and includes the endocardial echoes in the internal dimension measurement. If M-mode measurements are made with the American Society of Echocardiography criteria (leading edge to leading edge) then the following equation can be used:

$$\text{LVM(g)} = 0.8 \times 1.04\,[(\text{VST} + \text{LVID} + \text{PWT})^3 - \text{LVID}^3] + 0.6$$

It is important when obtaining M-mode images that the beam is directed perpendicular to the ventricular septum. If the beam is placed at an angle, the values obtained for VST, PWT and LVID will be artifactually increased.

LVM can be indexed to body surface area or height to account for differences in body size. Since LVM increases with obesity, indexation of LVM to body surface area can result in underestimation of LVM in obese individuals. Levy et al[14] have suggested indexation to height to prevent this 'forgiveness' of obesity.

Criteria for LVH have been developed, based on two standard deviations above the mean, in a healthy reference population at the Framingham Heart Study.[9] Using the Penn convention, when LVM is indexed to body surface area or to height, the cut-points for LVH are 131 g/m^2 and 143 g/m, respectively, in men, and 100 g/m^2 and 102 g/m, respectively, in women. These criteria are similar to those derived from a working population in New York, 134 g/m^2 in men, and 110 g/m^2 in women.[15]

Two-dimensional echocardiographic methods

M-mode measurement of LVM is relatively accurate and simple to acquire, and therefore is used extensively in population based studies. However, since M-mode measurements require assumptions regarding left ventricular shape, these measurements may not be accurate in individuals in whom the left ventricle is asymmetric or is distorted due to cardiac disease. Two-dimensional methods of measuring LVM require fewer assumptions about left ventricular geometry and therefore may be more accurate.

Many standard echocardiogram software packages are now equipped with the capability to measure two-dimensional LVM using the 5/6 area–length method.[16] The cross-sectional area of the myocardium is determined from tracing the epicardial (A_1) and endocardial (A_2) borders at the papillary muscle tip-level from a short-axis image. The long-axis dimension (L) is measured from an apical view (two- or four-chamber) starting from the mitral annulus to the apex. LVM is then calculated using the machine's software with the following formula:

$$\text{LVM(g)} = 1.05\,[5/6(A_1(L + t)) - 5/6(A_2L)]$$

in which t is the mean wall thickness.

Three-dimensional methods

In addition, LVM can be measured with three-dimensional techniques such as magnetic resonance imaging (MRI), in which the volume of the left ventricular myocardium is measured by tracing sequential parallel short-axis images. These analyses are more time-consuming than two-dimensional or M-mode measurements; however, they do not require any assumptions about the geometry of the ventricle. Several validation studies in experimental animals have addressed the accuracy and reproducibility of mass measurements by MRI. In comparing the LVM measured in animals by MRI and at autopsy, the correlation has uniformly been excellent[17–19] with 'r' values ranging from 0.95 to 0.98 and standard errors of the estimate (SEE) ranging from 6.1 g to 13.1 g. Intraobserver and interobserver correlations were also excellent. Shapiro et al[20] used intracoronary injection of a viscous polymer to occlude collateral flow and create dense transmural infarcts, which expanded into large aneurysms. These ventricles are distorted in shape. In this situation, formulas used with echocardiography, which assume cylindrical or ellipsoid geometry, cannot be relied on. Correlation between MRI mass and post-mortem weight was again excellent, with r = 0.95 and SEE = 6.5 g.

Ostrzega et al[21] imaged 20 normal male humans, and found the expected correlation of mass with body surface area (r = 0.83), body weight (r = 0.82), and body height (r = 0.75). The relationship between body weight and LV mass in that study corresponded closely to values published from autopsy data. The average mass was 146 ± 23.1 g. Katz et al[22] tested the reproducibility of MRI LV mass in humans, and found excellent intraobserver (r = 0.96, SEE = 11.1 g) and interobserver (r = 0.91, SEE = 17.8) variability.

MRI measurement of LVM has been used for testing of physiological hypotheses. Milliken et al[23] tested the effect of dynamic exercise on human male LV mass by imaging nonathletic control (189 ± 6 g), skiers (239 ± 9 g) and cyclists (258 ± 11 g) and found a highly significant difference, even after adjustment for body weight, surface area, and lean body mass. Eichstadt et al[24] documented regression of pathological hypertrophy after treatment with ramipril, an angiotensin converting enzyme inhibitor.

Cine-CT is another high resolution tomographic method that can be used to measure LVM with high accuracy,[25] but is less feasible than MRI because of the need for contrast material and irradiation, and because rapid CT units are less readily available for use than are MRI systems.

Three-dimensional echocardiography is an evolving technology in which multiple two-dimensional views are reconstructed into a three-dimensional data set from which multiple short-axis images may be derived and digitized, for determination of LVM. Preliminary data from our laboratory suggest that this method is accurate, but with currently available equipment, offers little advantage over two-dimensional echocardiography.[26]

Hypertrophic cardiomyopathy

Hypertrophic cardiomyopathy (HCM) is a genetic disorder, characterized by pathologic, often severe, myocardial hypertrophy. The disease prevalence is thought to be about 2 per 1000 young adults.[27] It typically follows an autosomal dominant pattern of inheritance; however, the penetrance (the likelihood that an individual with the genetic mutation will develop disease) is variable. Angiotensin-I converting enzyme genotypes may influence the phenotypic expression of hypertrophy in HCM.[28] The disease may also occur due to spontaneous mutation. A variety of mutations have been identified in the β-myosin heavy chain gene (chromosome 14q1) in individuals with HCM. Preliminary studies suggest that the type of mutation within the β-myosin heavy chain gene can predict the risk of sudden death. Additional genes for which mutations have been associated with hypertrophic cardiomyopathy include the cardiac troponin-T gene (chromosome 1q3), alpha-tropomyosin gene (chromosome 15q2), and the myosin binding protein C gene (chromosome 11q11).

HCM has been identified by a variety of names including idiopathic hypertrophic subaortic stenosis (IHSS), obstructive hypertrophic cardiomyopathy (OHCM), and asymmetric septal hypertrophy (ASH), owing to the common presence of a dynamic outflow tract gradient, and predominant hypertrophy in the septal region (Fig. 11.2). However, some patients with HCM do not have asymmetric septal hypertrophy, and may have either concentric hypertrophy, or hypertrophy involving the apex of the left ventricle. In addition, not all patients with HCM have evidence of a dynamic outflow tract gradient. In contrast to the microscopic appearance of left ventricular hypertrophy due to hypertension, the myofibrils in familial HCM are characterized by myofibrillary disarray (Fig. 11.3).

Individuals with HCM may be asymptomatic and manifest the disease only through abnormalities on the electrocardiogram and/or echocardiogram, or only through genetic testing due to a family history of the disease. Others may be severely symptomatic. The most common symptoms include dyspnea, fatigue, syncope and

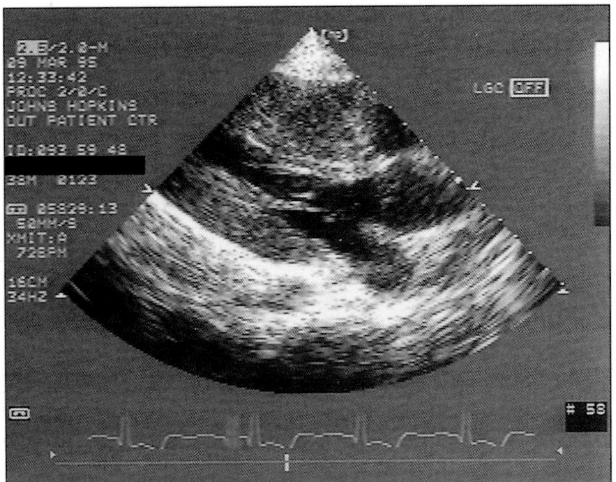

Figure 11.2
Asymmetric septal hypertrophy in a patient with hypertrophic cardiomyopathy. Note the marked increase in septal wall thickness relative to the posterior wall.

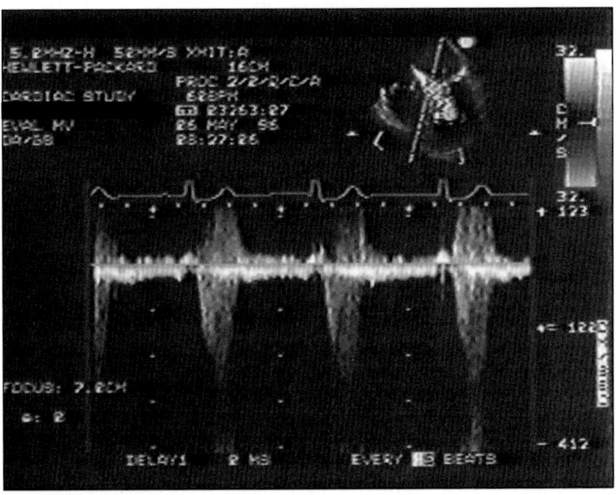

Figure 11.4
Continuous wave Doppler recording from the aortic outflow tract in a patient with severe hypertrophic cardiomyopathy. Note the increased velocity (2.5 m/s) which peaks in mid–late systole.

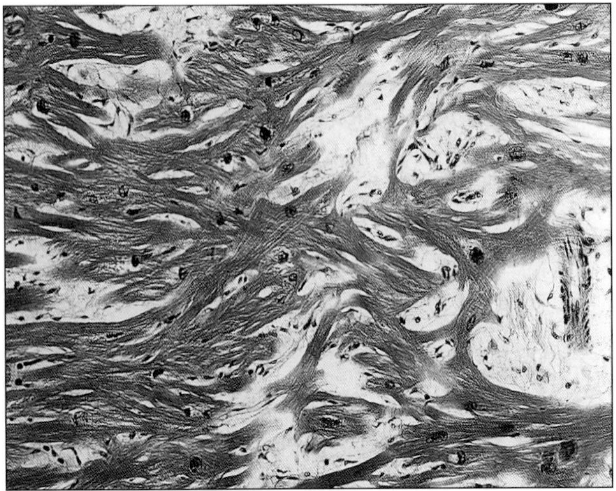

Figure 11.3
Characteristic myocyte disarray and enlargement of interstitial spaces in the myocardium of a heart with idiopathic hypertrophic subaortic stenosis. Note, in the center of the field, that there is disarray of contractile elements as well as of myocytes. Hematoxylin and eosin, ×160.

chest pain. Dyspnea often is due to diastolic dysfunction which may lead to congestive heart failure. Diastolic dysfunction is a result of impaired relaxation, and decreased compliance (chamber stiffness), which leads to increased diastolic pressures. Ventricular arrhythmias may lead to lightheadedness, or syncope, and place these patients at an increased risk for sudden death. Left atrial enlargement, due to diastolic dysfunction and mitral regurgitation, may lead to atrial fibrillation. Since these patients are dependent on the atrial 'kick' for left ventricular filling, atrial fibrillation is often poorly tolerated. Chest pain may be caused by subendocardial ischemia resulting from an increased demand due to extreme myocardial mass (sometimes in the setting of abnormal coronary arteries due to intimal-medial hypertrophy) leading to decreased blood supply.

Importance of the dynamic outflow tract gradient

Patients with HCM often have an intracavitary pressure gradient which peaks in mid-to-late systole (Fig. 11.4). In some patients this pressure gradient may be present intermittently or only with provocation, such as adrenergic stimulation, exercise, or decreased blood volume. Classically, after a premature ventricular contraction, which is followed by postextrasystolic potentiation, the intracavitary gradient develops or increases and the aortic pressure fails to rise. This is known as the Brockenbrough phenomenon. Most authors have suggested that the intraventricular pressure gradient reflects obstruction of LV outflow and that this is the major contributor to the pathophysiology of the syndrome. In obstructive HCM, systolic anterior

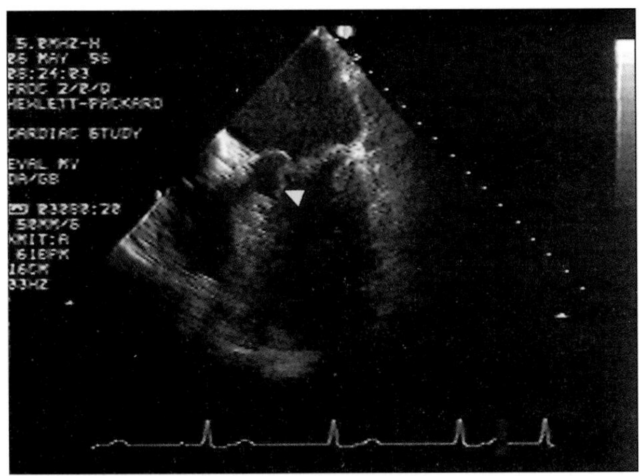

a

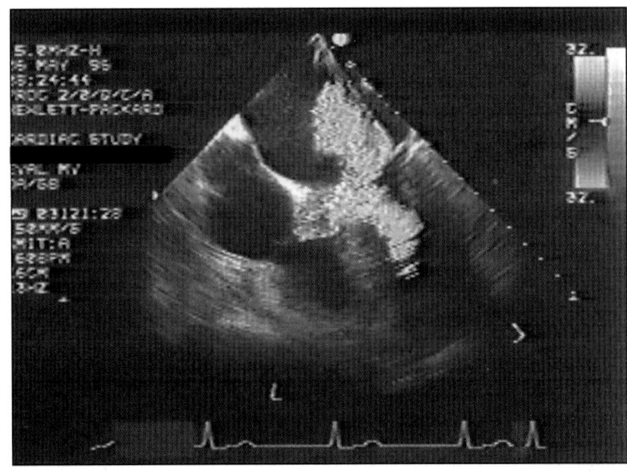

b

Figure 11.5
Transesophageal echocardiographic images during systole from a patient with hypertrophic cardiomyopathy. (a) Note the systolic anterior motion (SAM) of the anterior leaflet of the mitral valve (arrow). (b) Color flow Doppler during systole in the same patient. Note the mitral regurgitant jet which is probably secondary to the SAM of the mitral valve.

motion (SAM) of the mitral valve leads to mitral valve leaflet–ventricular septal contact (Fig. 11.5) as the anterior mitral valve leaflet is pulled forward, leading to both obstruction to flow and to mitral regurgitation.

Other authors have argued that the high ejection fractions and the very rapid rate of ejection characteristic of hypertrophic cardiomyopathy are inconsistent with important obstruction to outflow.[29,30] The intracavitary gradient in 'obstructive' HCM might represent an artifact of cavity obliteration. If the ventricular space is obliterated and the myocardium continues to contract isometrically, a catheter in the empty space will record high pressures. In this case, although there appears to be a pressure gradient within the ventricular cavity, there is no obstruction to flow per se, since the cavity has already emptied by the time the gradient has developed. These authors suggest that cavity obliteration and diastolic dysfunction, rather than obstruction, are the main contributors to the pathophysiology of the syndrome.

Assessment by echocardiography

Echocardiography remains the mainstay for the diagnosis and characterization of hypertrophic cardiomyopathy. The classic M-mode findings of asymmetric septal hypertrophy, SAM of the mitral valve, and aortic valve 'pre-closure' have withstood the test of time, but two-dimensional, Doppler, and transesophageal imaging have demonstrated that a wide variety of patterns of hypertrophy exist, and have shed light on the pathophysiology of mitral valve motion and ejection flow in the syndrome.

Wall thickness and motion

Early studies[31,32] suggested that a septal to free wall thickness ratio of ≥1.3 was characteristic of HCM. However, it is now understood that while focal hypertrophy of the proximal and mid septum is the most common site of involvement, the syndrome often results in asymmetric hypertrophy involving other regions. In a study of 600 patients with HCM, Klues et al[33] found multiple patterns of hypertrophy involving various combinations of the anterior and posterior septum, the lateral free wall, and the posterior free wall. Hypertrophy localized to the apex is a common pattern in Japan[34] (Fig. 11.6) but is infrequently seen in North America.[33] A space-like configuration of the left ventricular cavity at end-diastole is typically seen in the right anterior oblique ventriculogram.[35] This form of the disease is often associated with giant T wave inversion in the left precordial leads (Fig. 11.7). At times the hypertrophy can involve so many regions that it becomes concentric, and the syndrome can be distinguished from severe secondary forms of hypertrophy only by the presence of SAM or Doppler evidence of an intracavitary gradient. Likewise, asymmetric septal hypertrophy is not truly specific for HCM, and is occasionally seen in other situations, the most common being concentric LVH with occurrence of infarction and thinning of the posterior wall, which returns posterior wall thickness toward normal. A sigmoid shape

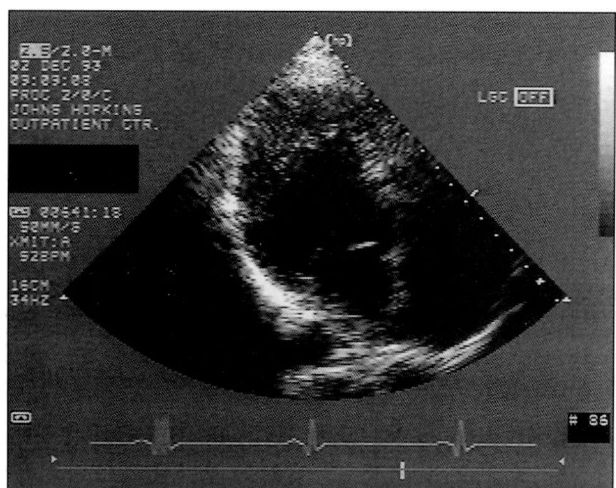

Figure 11.6
Apical four-chamber view from a patient with apical hypertrophy. Note the marked increase in myocardial thickness in the apical region relative to the rest of the myocardium.

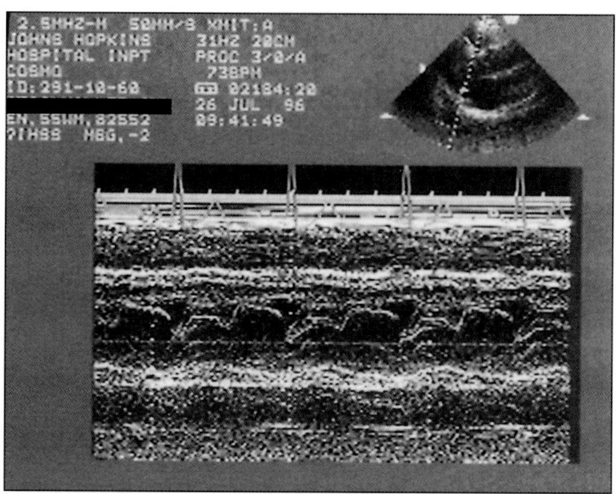

Figure 11.8
M-mode echocardiographic images from a parasternal long-axis view. Note the systolic anterior motion (SAM) of the mitral valve.

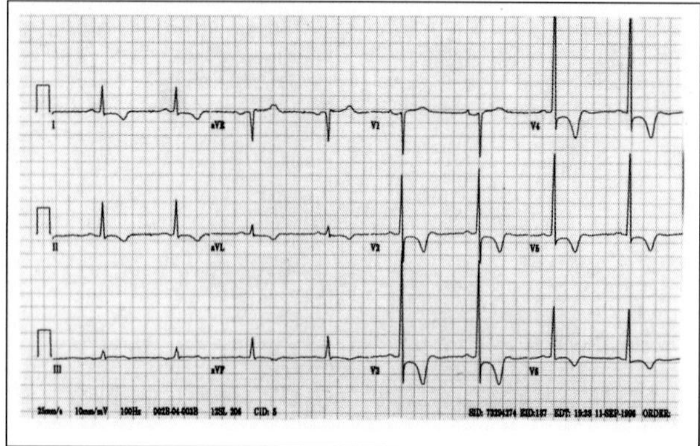

Figure 11.7
Electrocardiogram from the same patient as Figure 11.6 with apical hypertrophy. Note the 'giant' inverted T waves in the precordial leads.

of the septum without other features of HCM is sometimes present in the elderly, and appears to be of little physiological significance.[36] Right ventricular hypertrophy, amyloidosis, and septal tumors can cause asymmetric septal hypertrophy and resemble HCM.

In HCM, LV cavity size is normal or small at end-diastole and nearly always abnormally small at end-systole. Endocardial motion is hyperdynamic with the appearance of cavity obliteration or near cavity obliteration, particularly of the apical portion of the LV.

Echocardiography often reveals bright stippled regions in the septum or other regions involved with the pathologic hypertrophy. Tissue characterization by integrated backscatter consistently shows increased backscatter in hearts with hypertrophy compared to normals,[37] and may even allow a distinction to be made between HCM patients and patients with hypertensive LVH.[38]

Mitral valve

The mitral valve characteristically displays SAM, moving toward the septum and often striking it, providing the substrate for dynamic LV outflow tract obstruction. This pattern is easily seen using M-mode (Fig. 11.8). Using two-dimensional echo, the motion is evident to the trained eye, but may be missed by an inexperienced observer since the SAM may involve only a small segment of the mitral leaflets. SAM is typically seen in the parasternal views, but if those views are suboptimal, the apical four-chamber view is usually quite helpful, and reveals an unapposed portion of the anterior leaflet moving toward the septum. SAM may also involve chordae near the MV leaflet tip. The presence of SAM correlates with the presence of a murmur and of an outflow gradient detectable by Doppler or catheterization. The duration of mitral–septal apposition predicts the magnitude of the gradient.[39] SAM may be absent at rest but inducible by the administration of amyl nitrite.

Two mechanisms for SAM have been proposed. Early theories suggested that hyperdynamic LV ejection, in combination with a narrowed outflow tract due to the hypertrophied septum, and anterior displacement of the mitral valve, resulted in very rapid flow in the outflow tract, with a Venturi effect sucking the mitral leaflet into the septum.[40] More recently, anatomic variations in the mitral apparatus have been noted, including increased area and length of the leaflets[41] with large unapposed sections of leaflet,[42] and anterior and medial displacement of the papillary muscles.[43] SAM may be due to these structural abnormalities allowing portions of the mitral apparatus to protrude into areas of flow where they can be caught up and dragged toward the septum.[44] Much anatomic evidence now supports this concept.

In situations when the LV is hyperdynamic in response to catecholamines, tachycardia, or volume overload, the entire heart may move anteriorly with systole. SAM should therefore only be considered pathological if the motion is exaggerated with respect to the motion of the posterior wall. Even true SAM is not specific for HCM and has been reported in other situations characterized by cavity obliteration including hemorrhagic shock and catecholamine stimulation.[45]

Mitral regurgitation is usually present in HCM, especially if SAM is present, and is probably due to disruption of normal leaflet coaptation.

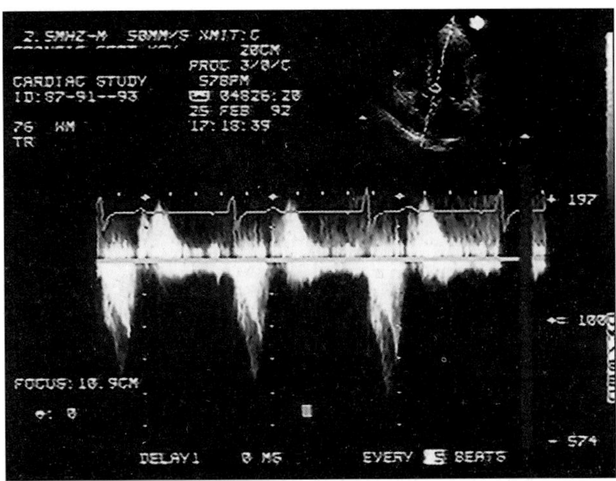

Figure 11.9
Fluctuation in the gradient in a patient with hypertrophic cardiomyopathy during counting from 1 to 5.

Gradient

A gradient across the LV outflow tract can usually be measured in patients with HCM and SAM. This is best recorded from an apical four-chamber or two-chamber view, using continuous wave Doppler. The outflow tract should then be interrogated using color flow mapping and/or pulsed Doppler, to detect regions of aliasing, to demonstrate the subaortic localization of the obstruction.[46] The continuous wave Doppler tracing is characteristically asymmetric in shape, with a slow rise in early systole followed by further acceleration of flow and an abrupt peak in mid systole[47,48] (Fig. 11.4). This differs from the pattern in aortic stenosis, where the peak (instantaneous) gradient is earlier. Sherrid et al[44] have presented evidence that the increasing acceleration of flow is due to an unapposed portion of a mitral leaflet being driven further toward the septum as systole progresses, further constricting the orifice and increasing the gradient.

The magnitude of the gradient is calculated by using the simplified Bernoulli equation, in which the pressure drop equals four times the square of the velocity. Estimates of gradient by Doppler and catheterization correlate extremely well at rest, and moderately well during increased gradients provoked by maneuvers such as isoproterenol administration and induced PVCs.[48] Care must be taken to distinguish the Doppler envelope of the outflow gradient from that of a mitral regurgitant jet (which is wider and more rounded). Caution is advised in interpreting jets of more than about 5.5 m/s (estimated gradient >120 mmHg) as representative of an outflow tract signal because a velocity of such magnitude is most consistent with mitral regurgitation.

The dynamic nature of the gradient can be demonstrated by the Valsalva maneuver, or by the administration of amyl nitrite. Surprisingly wide fluctuations in the gradient occur simply during talking. We often have the patient count to 20 during recording (Fig. 11.9).

Doppler assessment of diastolic function

Left ventricular filling in HCM may show the characteristic changes of hypertrophy: reduced velocity of early diastolic filling (E wave) due to a reduced rate of relaxation, with a compensatory increase in the velocity of late diastolic filling during atrial systole (A wave) (Fig. 11.10). This usually results in a marked reduction in E/A ratio below that which would be expected for the patient's age.[49] However, it must be realized that many hemodynamic factors, to which patients with HCM are susceptible, can affect left ventricular filling patterns. The left atrial pressure has a major influence on the E/A ratio and if congestive heart failure with a concomitant elevation of LA pressure develops, the E/A ratio may become 'pseudonormalized'.[50] The presence of mitral regurgitation may have a similar effect. Finally, if left atrial enlargement results in intermittent or episodic atrial fibrillation, the atrial component of filling may be very small, even during sinus rhythm.[51] Because of these factors,

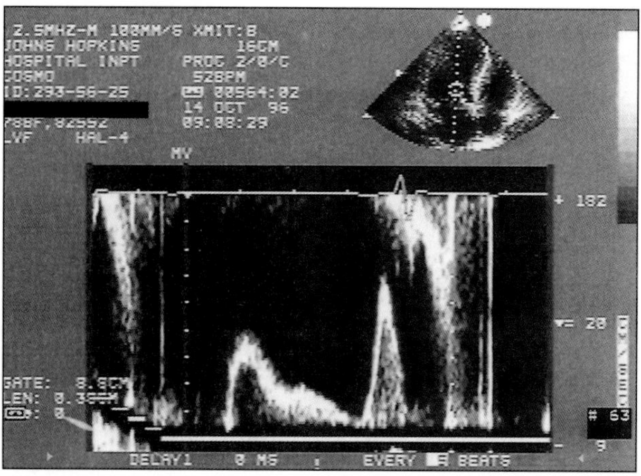

Figure 11.10
Pulsed wave Doppler of the mitral valve inflow from a patient with hypertrophic cardiomyopathy. Note the increased velocity of the A wave (atrial contraction) relative to the E wave (early diastolic filling), suggesting impaired early diastolic filling.

Doppler filling patterns have not been reliable predictors of symptoms or prognosis in patients with HCM.[52,53] The isovolumic relaxation time, an indirect measure of left ventricular relaxation that is also influenced by aortic and left atrial pressure, is often prolonged in HCM.

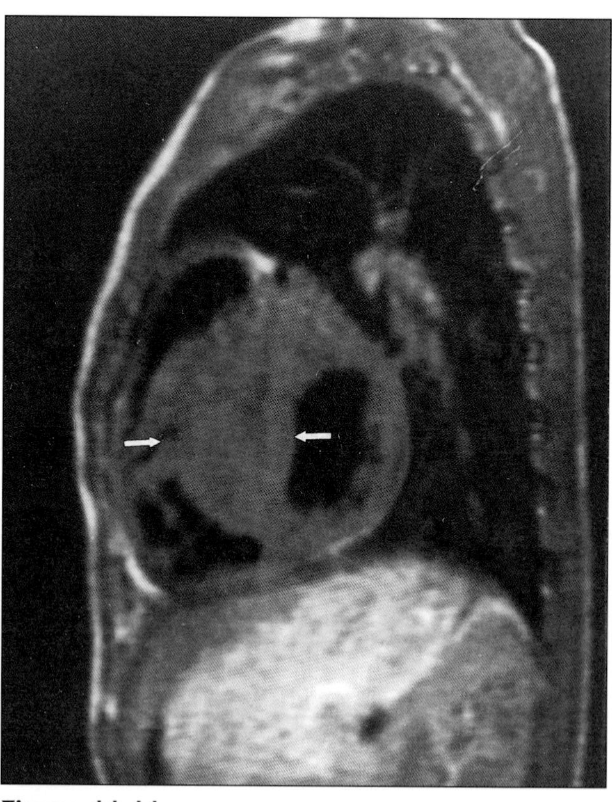

Figure 11.11
Short-axis magnetic resonance image of a patient with hypertrophic cardiomyopathy and massive septal hypertrophy.

Use of transesophageal echo

Transesophageal echo (TEE) is indicated in patients with suspected HCM if poor acoustic windows prevent adequate transthoracic assessment of the extent of hypertrophy and gradient. TEE has been a useful tool for visualizing the improvement in septal thickness, SAM, and outflow gradients that occur after myotomy–myectomy. Patients in whom myotomy–myectomy is planned should have a preoperative and intraoperative TEE so that the extent of the resection can be planned and the immediate results assessed.[54,55]

Assessment by MRI

Cardiac MRI is becoming an increasingly popular method for clinical evaluation of patients with structural heart disease, since it allows the visualization of the entire heart in a series of tomographic sections (Fig. 11.11) and is not limited to specific views by acoustic windows. Small areas of localized hypertrophy can be detected, probably with greater sensitivity than by echocardiography. A more extensive distribution of hypertrophy is sometimes seen by MRI in patients thought to have hypertrophy localized to the septum by echo.

MRI investigation of patients with HCM has resulted in better understanding of morphologic variants of the syndrome. For example, Suzuki et al[56] described a variant of the apical form of HCM in which the typical spade-like pattern of the left ventricular cavity did not appear on the right anterior oblique (RAO) ventriculogram, because the hypertrophy involved a very localized area of the apical septum or lateral wall, that could not be seen in the RAO projection. These very thick but very focal regions were best seen on short-axis apical views, which are very difficult to obtain by echo. Typical giant negative T waves were present in these patients.

MRI with tissue tagging[57] is a unique method that allows noninvasive markers to be placed onto the myocardium, and then tracked throughout the cardiac cycle. These markers are created by presaturation of myocardial tissue by RF pulses at end-diastole, and appear as signal voids that move along with the myocardium onto which they are

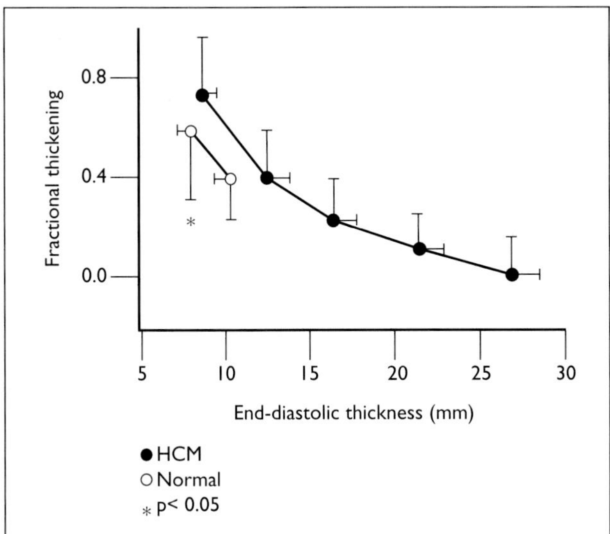

Figure 11.12
Correlation of end-diastolic thickness (x-axis) and thickening (y-axis) in 17 patients with hypertrophic cardiomyopathy (solid points). Note that thickening is markedly reduced at higher wall thicknesses. Open points represent six normal controls. Reprinted with permission from Dong et al.[58] 1994.

placed, allowing details of myocardial deformation to be defined in three dimensions.[58,59] Dong et al[60] made a crucial observation that explains much about the pathophysiology of hypertrophy, using MRI tagging. While the hypertrophied ventricle in HCM demonstrates exaggerated systolic emptying, and appears to manifest *hyper*dynamic systolic function, hypertrophied segments are actually *hypo*contractile. Regional endocardial and epicardial shortening in HCM were measured using tagging, and an inverse relationship between end-diastolic wall thickness and regional shortening, and between end-diastolic thickness and regional thickening (Fig. 11.12). This was a clear demonstration that the abnormally thick regions of the LV shorten and thicken poorly. Endocardial motion is preserved, however, since the large bulk of myocardium that is present needs only to thicken slightly to cause a normal amount of endocardial motion. This concept also applies to myocardial function in hypertensive LVH. Palmon et al,[61] also using MRI tagging techniques, demonstrated reduced intramural shortening in patients with hypertensive LVH despite preserved pump function. Again, this observation was consistent with geometric considerations, since these patients have increased myocardial mass, so less shortening is necessary for the same absolute increase in wall thickness and endocardial cavity shrinkage. That is, the fibers are larger, and can achieve the same systolic effect by shortening less.

Measurements of principal strain by MRI tagging,[62] and strain rates by velocity encoding of myocardial motion by MRI,[63] have confirmed that systolic contractile activity is affected by hypertrophy, and have emphasized the marked regional heterogeneity of systolic function in this syndrome. Nakatani et al[64] demonstrated that regional function is further reduced because local hypertrophy distorts the endocardial wall curvature, making it more convex toward the left ventricular cavity. This increases regional wall stress, as predicted by the Laplace equation, and reduces endocardial intramyocardial shortening.

Treatment

Management of patients with HCM depends on the degree of hypertrophy and symptoms. Negative inotropic and chronotropic drugs, such as calcium channel blockers and beta blockers, may be beneficial by decreasing the force of ejection in systole and prolonging the diastolic filling time. However, caution must be used in patients with obstructive HCM, since it has been reported that calcium channel blockers with vasodilatory properties can increase the degree of obstruction, and cause cardiogenic shock and pulmonary edema. Disopyramide, a type IA antiarrhythmic with negative inotropic properties has also been used successfully in patients with HCM.

In patients with severe symptomatic HCM, unresponsive to medical therapy, myotomy–myectomy is often performed to decrease the mass of the ventricular septum in the ventricular outflow tract. This surgery can relieve the obstruction and is associated with an improvement in symptoms.[65] An implantable cardiac defibrillator may be placed in patients who have survived sudden death or have been observed to have life threatening ventricular arrhythmias.

Preliminary results have been favorable with dual chamber pacemaker implantation.[66,67] Preexcitation of the interventricular septum leads to discoordinate septal motion, and a less effective ventricular contraction. Pacing has been shown to decrease the left ventricular outflow tract gradient (Fig. 11.13), decrease heart failure symptoms, and decrease left ventricular mass in the anterior septum, and distal anterior wall. However, pacing results in reduced diastolic function,[68] and its use in patients on a non-experimental basis is still controversial.[69] Studies comparing the outcome of pacemaker therapy with that of myectomy have not yet been performed.

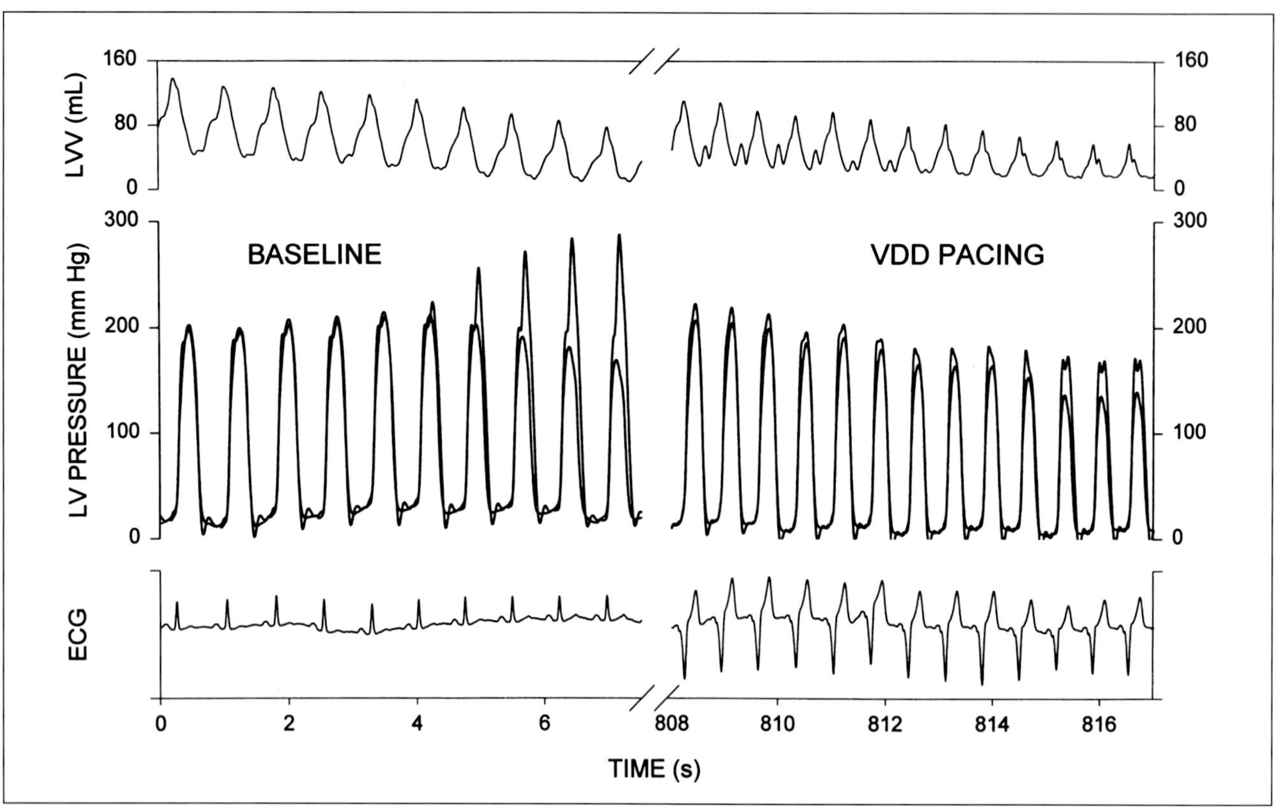

Figure 11.13
Effect of VDD pacing on the intraventricular pressure gradient in hypertrophic cardiomyopathy. In a patient with no resting intraventricular gradient, simultaneous pressures were measured at the apex and the base of the left ventricle before and during VDD pacing. Left ventricular volume (LVV) was measured continuously using a multi-electrode conductance catheter. Intraventricular pressure gradient was provoked by gradual decrease in the LV preload volume by obstructing inferior vena caval inflow through the use of a balloon catheter (top panel). A 130 mmHg pressure gradient was produced by this maneuver at baseline (middle panel, left). However, VDD pacing reduced the provokable pressure gradient to 40 mmHg (middle panel, right) at a comparable preload volume.

A few patients may progress to endstage HCM, in which the left ventricle becomes dilated with systolic dysfunction. When hypertrophic cardiomyopathy leads to intractable heart failure or cardiac arrhythmias, cardiac transplantation may become the only therapeutic option available.

Acknowledgements

We thank Peter Pak MD and Grover Hutchins MD for their gracious assistance with the preparation of figures.

References

1 Manolio TA, Levy D, Garrison RJ et al: Relation of alcohol intake to left ventricular mass. *J Am Coll Cardiol* 1991; **17**: 717–21.

2 Devereux RB, Drayer JIM, Chien S et al: Whole blood viscosity as a determinant of cardiac hypertrophy in systemic hypertension. *Am J Cardiol* 1984; **54**: 592–5.

3 Savage DD, Levy D, Dannenberg AL et al: Association of echocardiographic left ventricular mass with body size, blood pressure and physical activity (The Framingham Study). *Am J Cardiol* 1990; **65**: 371–6.

4 Harshfield GA, Grim CE, Hwang C et al: Generic and environmental influences on echocardiographically determined left ventricular mass in black twins. *Am J Hypertens* 1990; **3**: 538–43.

5 Adams TD, Yanowitz FG, Fisher AG et al: Heritability of cardiac size: an echocardiographic and electrocardiographic study of monozygotic and dizygotic twins. *Circulation* 1985; **71**: 39–44.

6 Sasson Z, Rasooly Y, Bhesani T et al: Insulin resistance is an important determinant of left ventricular mass in the obese. *Circulation* 1993; **88**: 1431–6.

7 Saba PS, Roman NJ, Pini K et al: Relation of arterial pressure waveform to left ventricular and carotid anatomy in normotensive subjects. *J Am Coll Cardiol* 1993; **22**: 1873–80.

8 Topol EJ, Traill TA, Fortuin NJ: Hypertensive hypertrophic cardiomyopathy of the elderly. *N Engl J Med* 1985; **312** (5): 277–83.

9 Levy D, Garrison RJ, Savage DD et al: Prognostic implications of echocardiographically determined left ventricular mass in the Framingham Heart Study. *N Engl J Med* 1990; **322**: 1561–6.

10 Koren MJ, Devereux RB, Casale PN et al: Relation of left ventricular mass and geometry to morbidity and mortality in the uncomplicated essential hypertension. *Ann Intern Med* 1991; **114**: 345–52.

11 Levy D, Anderson KM, Savage DD et al: Risk of ventricular arrhythmias in left ventricular hypertrophy. *Am J Cardiol* 1987; **60**: 560–5.

12 Treasure CB, Klein JL, Vita JA et al: Hypertension and left ventricular hypertrophy are associated with impaired endothelium mediated relaxation in human coronary resistance vessels. *Circulation* 1993; **87**: 86–93.

13 Devereux RB, Alopnso DR, Lutas EM et al: Echocardiographic assessment of left ventricular hypertrophy: comparison to necropsy findings. *Am J Cardiol* 1986; **57**: 450–8.

14 Levy D, Savage DD, Garrison RJ et al: Echocardiographic criteria for left ventricular hypertrophy. *Am J Cardiol* 1987; **59**: 956–60.

15 Hammond IW, Devereux RB, Alderman MH et al: The prevalence and correlates of echocardiographic left ventricular hypertrophy among employed patients with uncomplicated hypertension. *J Am Coll Cardiol* 1986; **7**: 639–50.

16 Reichek N, Helak J, Plappert T et al: Anatomic validation of left ventricular mass estimates from clinical two dimensional echocardiography: initial results. *Circulation* 1983; **67**: 348–52.

17 Maddahi J, Crues J, Berman DS et al: Noninvasive quantification of left ventricular mass by gated proton nuclear magnetic resonance imaging. *J Am Coll Cardiol* 1987; **10**: 682–92.

18 Florentine MS, Grosskreutz CL, Chang W et al: Measurement of left ventricular mass in vivo using gated nuclear magnetic resonance imaging. *J Am Coll Cardiol* 1986; **8**: 107–12.

19 Keller AM, Peshock RM, Malloy CR et al: In vivo measurement of myocardial mass using nuclear magnetic resonance imaging. *J Am Coll Cardiol* 1986; **8**: 113–17.

20 Shapiro EP, Rogers WJ, Beyar R et al: MRI determination of left ventricular mass in hearts deformed by acute infarction. *Circulation* 1989; **79**: 706–11.

21 Ostrzega E, Maddahi J, Honma H et al: Quantification of left ventricular myocardial mass in humans by nuclear magnetic resonance imaging. *Am Heart J* 1989; **117**: 444–52.

22 Katz J, Milliken MC, Stray-Gundersen J et al: Estimation of human myocardial mass with MR imaging. *Radiology* 1988; **169**: 495–8.

23 Milliken MC, Stray-Gundersen J, Peshock RM et al: Left ventricular mass as determined by magnetic resonance imaging in male endurance athletes. *Am J Cardiol* 1988; **62**: 301–5.

24 Eichstadt HW, Felix R, Langer M et al: Use of nuclear magnetic resonance imaging to show regression of hypertrophy with ramipril treatment. *Am J Cardiol* 1987; **59**: 98D–103D.

25 Feiring AJ, Rumberger JA, Reiter SJ et al: Determination of left ventricular mass in dogs with rapid-acquisition cardiac computed tomographic scanning. *Circulation* 1985; **72**: 1355–64.

26 Post WS, Lugo-Olivieri CH, Lima JA et al: Is 3D echocardiography necessary for measurement of left ventricular mass? *Circulation* 1996; **94**: I–688.

27 Maron BJ, Gardin JM, Flack JM et al: Prevalence of hypertrophic cardiomyopathy in a general population of young adults. Echocardiographic analysis of 4111 subjects in the CARDIA Study. Coronary Artery Risk Development in (Young) Adults. *Circulation* 1995; **92**: 785–9.

28 Lechin M, Quinones MA, Omran A et al: Angiotensin-I converting enzyme genotypes and left ventricular hypertrophy in patients with hypertrophic cardiomyopathy. *Circulation* 1995; **92**: 1808–12.

29 Criley JM, Lewis KB, White RI: Pressure gradients without obstruction: a new concept of 'hypertrophic subaortic stenosis'. *Circulation* 1965; **32**: 881–7.

30 Criley JM, Siegel RJ: Has 'obstruction' hindered our understanding of hypertrophic cardiomyopathy? *Circulation* 1985; **72**: 1148–54.

31 Clark CE, Henry WL, Epstein CE: Familial prevalence and genetic transmission of idiopathic hypertrophic subaortic stenosis. *N Eng J Med* 1973; **289**: 709–14.

32 Henry WL, Clark CE, Epstein SE: Assymetric septal hypertrophy. Echocardiographic identification of the pathognomonic anatomic abnormality of IHSS, *Circulation* 1973; **47**: 225–33.

33 Klues HG, Schiffers A, Maron BJ: Phenotypic spectrum and patterns of left ventricular hypertrophy in hypertrophic cardiomyopathy: morphologic observations and significance as assessed by two-dimensional echocardiography in 600 patients. *JACC* 1995; **26**: 1699–708.

34 Koga Y, Itaya KI, Toshima H: Prognosis in hypertrophic cardiomyopathy. *Am Heart J* 1984; **108**: 351–9.

35 Yamaguchi H, Ishimura T, Nishiyama S et al: Hypertrophic nonobstructive cardiomyopathy with giant negative T waves (apical hypertrophy): ventriculographic and echocardiographic features in 30 patients. *Am J Cardiol* 1979; **44**: 401–12.

36 Swinne C, Shapiro EP, Jamart J, Fleg J: Age-associated anatomic and functional changes in left ventricular outflow geometry in normal subjects. *Am J Cardiol* 1996; **78**: 1070–3.

37 Lattanzi F, De Bello V, Picano E et al: Normal ultrasonic myocardial reflectivity in athletes with increased left ventricular mass. A tissue characterization study. *Circulation* 1992; **85**: 1828–34.

38 Naito J, Masuyama T, Tanouchi J et al: Analysis of transmural trend of myocardial integrated ultrasound backscatter for differentiation of hypertrophic cardiomyopathy and ventricular hypertrophy due to hypertension. *J Am Coll Cardiol* 1994; **24**: 517–24.

39 Pollick C, Rakowski H, Wigle ED: Muscular subaortic stenosis: quantitative relationship between systolic anterior motion and the pressure gradient. *Circulation* 1984; **69**: 43–9.

40 Wigle ED: Hypertrophic cardiomyopathy: a 1987 viewpoint. *Circulation* 1987; **75**: 311–22.

41 Klues HG, Roberts WC, Maron BJ: Morphological determinants of echocardiographic patterns of mitral valve systolic anterior motion in obstructive hypertrophic cardiomyopathy. *Circulation* 1993; **87**: 1570–9.

42 Shah PM, Taylor RD, Wong M: Abnormal mitral valve coaptation hypertrophic obstructive cardiomyopathy: proposed role in systolic anterior motion of mitral valve. *Am J Cardiol* 1981; **48**: 258–62.

43 Jiang L, Levine RA, King ME et al: An integrated mechanism for systolic anterior motion of the mitral valve in hypertrophic cardiomyopathy based on echocardiographic observations. *Am Heart J* 1987; **113**: 633–44.

44 Sherrid MV, Chu CK, Delia E: An echocardiographic study of the fluid mechanics of obstruction in hypertrophic cardiomyopathy. *JACC* 1993; **22**: 816–25.

45 Bulkley BH: Idiopathic hypertrophic subaortic stenosis afflicted: idols of the cave and the marketplace. *Am J Cardiol* 1977: **40**: 476–9.

46 Schwammenthal E, Block M, Schwartzkopff B et al: Prediction of the site and severity of obstruction in hypertrophic cardiomyopathy by color flow mapping and continuous wave Doppler echocardiography. *J Am Coll Cardiol* 1992; **20**: 964–72.

47 Yock PG, Hatle L, Popp RL: Patterns and timing of Doppler-detected intracavitary and aortic flow in hypertrophic cardiomyopathy. *J Am Coll Cardiol* 1986; **8**: 1047–58.

48 Panza JA, Petrone RK, Fananapazir L: Utility of continuous wave Doppler echocardiography in the noninvasive assessment of left ventricular outflow tract pressure gradient in patients with hypertrophic cardiomyopathy. *J Am Coll Cardiol* 1992; **19**: 91–9.

49 Downes TR, Abdel-Mohsen N, Smith KM et al: Mechanism of altered pattern of left ventricular filling with aging in subject without cardiac disease. *Am J Cardiol* 1989; **64**: 523–7.

50 Marino P, Destro G, Barbieri E et al: Early left ventricular filling: an approach to its multifactorial nature using a combined hemodynamic-Doppler technique. *Am Heart J* 1991; **122**: 132–41.

51 Shapiro EP, Effron MB, Lima S et al: Transient atrial dysfunction after conversion of chronic atrial fibrillation to normal sinus rhythm. *Am J Cardiol* 1988; **62**: 1202–7.

52 Maron BJ, Spirito P, Green KJ et al: Noninvasive assessment of left ventricular diastolic function by pulsed Doppler echocardiography in patients with hypertrophic cardiomyopathy. *J Am Coll Cardiol* 1987; **10**: 733–42.

53 McCully RB, Nishimura RA, Bailey KR: Hypertrophic obstructive cardiomyopathy: preoperative echocardiographic predictors of outcome after septal myectomy. *J Am Coll Cardiol* 1996; **27**: 1491–6.

54 Grigg LE, Wigle ED, Williams WG et al: Transesophageal Doppler echocardiography in obstructive hypertrophic cardiomyopathy: clarification of pathophysiology and importance in intraoperative decision making [see comments]. *J Am Coll Cardiol* 1992; **20**: 42–52.

55 Marwick TH, Stewart WJ, Lever HM et al: Benefits of intraoperative echocardiography in the surgical management of

hypertrophic cardiomyopathy. *J Am Coll Cardiol* 1992; **20**: 1066–72.

56 Suzuki J, Watanabe F, Takenaka K et al: New subtype of apical hypertrophic cardiomyopathy identified with nuclear magnetic resonance imaging as an underlying cause of markedly inverted T waves. *J Am Coll Cardiol* 1993; **22**: 1175—81.

57 Zerhouni EA, Parish DM, Rogers WJ et al: Human heart: tagging with MR images – a method for noninvasive assessment of myocardial motion. *Radiology* 1988; **169**: 59–63.

58 Azhari H, Weiss JL, Rogers WJ et al: Non-invasive quantification of principal strains in normal canine hearts using tagged MRI in 3D. *Am J Physiol* 1993; **264**: H205–16.

59 Rademakers FE, Rogers WJ, Guier WH et al: Relationship of regional cross-fiber shortening to wall thickening in the intact heart. *Circulation* 1994; **89**: 1174–82.

60 Dong SJ, MacGregor JH, Crawley AP et al: Left ventricular wall thickness and regional systolic function in patients with hypertrophic cardiomyopathy. A three-dimensional tagged magnetic resonance imaging study. *Circulation* 1994; **90**: 1200–9.

61 Palmon LC, Reichek N, Clark NR et al: Intramural myocardial shortening in hypertensive left ventricular hypertrophy with normal pump function. *Circulation* 1994; **89**: 122–31.

62 Young AA, Kramer CM, Ferrari VA et al: Three-dimensional left ventricular deformation in hypertrophic cardiomyopathy. *Circulation* 1994; **90**: 854–67.

63 Beache FM, Wedeen VJ, Weisskoff RM et al: Intramural mechanics in hypertrophic cardiomyopathy: functional mapping with strain-rate MR imaging. *Radiology* 1995; **197**: 117–24.

64 Nakatani S, White RD, Powell KA et al: Dynamic magnetic resonance imaging assessment of the effect of ventricular wall curvature on regional function in hypertrophic cardiomyopathy. *Am J Cardiol* 1996; **77**: 618–22.

65 ten Berg JM, Suttorp MJ, Knaepen PJ et al: Hypertrophic obstructive cardiomyopathy. Initial results and long-term follow-up after Morrow septal myectomy [see comments]. *Circulation* 1994; **90**: 1781–5.

66 Fananapazir L, Cannon RO, Tripodi D et al: Impact of dual-chamber permanent pacing in patients with obstructive hypertrophic cardiomyopathy with symptoms refractory to verapamil and β-adrenergic blocker therapy. *Circulation* 1992; **85**: 2149–61.

67 Fananapazir L, Epstein ND, Curiel RV et al: Long-term results of dual-chamber (DDD) pacing in obstructive hypertrophic cardiomyopathy. *Circulation* 1994; **90**: 2731–42.

68 Nishimura RA, Hayes DL, Ilstrup DM et al: Effect of dual-chamber pacing on systolic and diastolic function in patients with hypertrophic cardiomyopathy. *JACC* 1996; **27**: 421–30.

69 Maron BJ: Appraisal of dual-chamber pacing therapy in hypertrophic cardiomyopathy: too soon for a rush to judgement? *JACC* 1996; **27**: 431–2.

12

Restrictive cardiomyopathy: a non-invasive diagnostic approach and the differentiation from constrictive pericarditis

Edmundo J Nassri Câmara

Introduction

Restrictive cardiomyopathy is a form of myocardial disease in which the main problem is related to a diastolic restriction of ventricular filling. It is much less common than the other forms of myocardial disease (dilated and hypertrophic cardiomyopathy),[1,2] but it must always be remembered in the differential diagnosis of a patient with heart failure of unknown cause, especially when the diagnosis of constrictive pericarditis is considered. The usual clinical picture is one of severe, refractory congestive heart failure, with both pulmonary and systemic venous congestion. The systolic ventricular function is usually preserved, the ventricles are of normal size and the atria enlarged.

In the past few years, with the new methods of Doppler Echocardiography, Computed Tomography (CT) and Magnetic Resonance Imaging (MRI), it is possible to diagnose restrictive cardiomyopathy and to differentiate it from constrictive pericarditis and from other causes of heart failure, noninvasively in the majority of cases.

Table 12.1 Etiology

Restrictive cardiomyopathy (%)		*Constrictive pericarditis (%)*	
Idiopathic	35.1	Cardiac surgery	39.0
Amyloid	32.4	Idiopathic	14.6
Endomyocardial	29.7	Infection	11.0
Fibrosis		Post-MI	2.4
		Tumor	1.2
		Radiation	1.2
		Lupus	1.2
		Trauma	1.2
		Unstated	28.0

Source: Vaitkus PT, Kussmaul WG. Constrictive pericarditis versus restrictive cardiomyopathy: a reappraisal and update of diagnostic criteria. *Am Heart J* 1991; **122**: 1431–41.

Etiology

The pathologic basis for most cases of restrictive cardiomyopathy includes infiltrative disease such as amyloidosis, sarcoidosis, hemochromatosis, endomyocardial fibrosis, Löffler endocarditis, endocardial fibroelastosis, glycogen storage disease, mucopolysaccharidoses and scleroderma. However, in many cases, the clinical syndrome and the restrictive hemodynamic profile may occur in the absence of specific infiltrative disorders or other associated conditions, and it is described as an idiopathic restrictive cardiomyopathy. Most of the cases reported in the literature are idiopathic or caused by amyloidosis or endomyocardial fibrosis (Table 12.1).[3]

In the classification of myocardial diseases proposed by WHO/ISFC task force in 1980, in which cardiomyopathy was defined as a heart muscle disease of unknown origin, restrictive cardiomyopathy included only endomyocardial fibrosis and fibroblastic parietal endocarditis (Löffler).[4] Obviously, that classification needs to be reviewed. In the new classification reported by WHO/ISFC, it is no longer necessary to be of 'unknown' cause, and restrictive

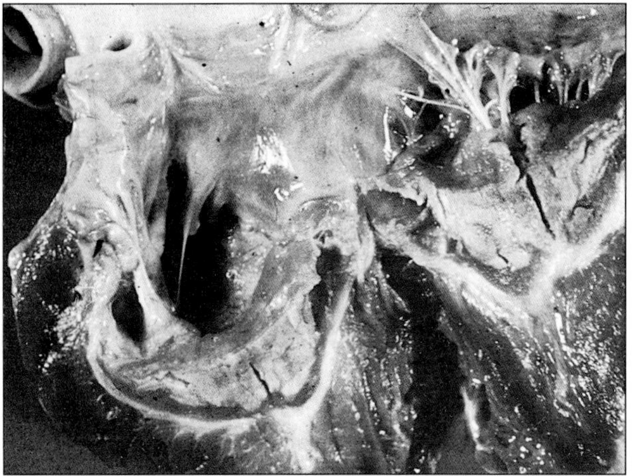

a

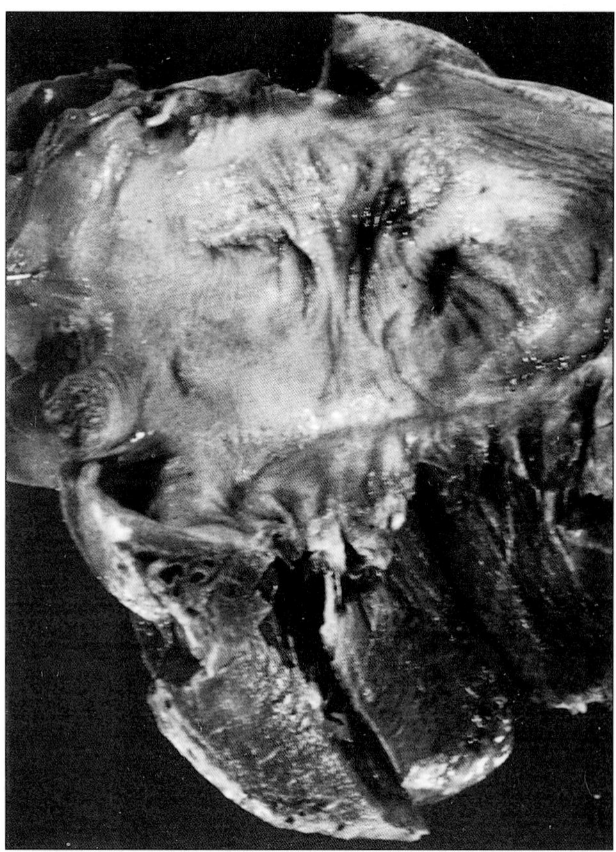

b

Figure 12.1
Macroscopic findings of endomyocardial fibrosis (a), showing the characteristic layer of fibrosis covering the internal surface of the ventricles and involving the mitral and tricuspid valves, and amyloidosis (b) with very thick left and right ventricular walls, small ventricles and large atria.

cardiomyopathy may be idiopathic or associated with other disease (e.g. amyloidosis; endomyocardial fibrosis with or without hypereosinophilia).[5]

In many tropical countries, such as Brazil,[6–9] Uganda,[10] Nigeria,[11] India,[12,13] and others,[14,15] endomyocardial fibrosis is a common cause of restrictive cardiomyopathy, but a good number of operated cases have been reported from temperate climate countries (Switzerland, U.S.A., France, Great Britain).[16–18]

Other conditions which may manifest a restrictive hemodynamic pattern are: post heart transplantation,[19] diabetes cardiomyopathy,[20] carcinoid, radiation anthracycline toxicity and metastatic malignancies.[21]

Pathology

Characteristically the atria are enlarged without ventricular dilatation.[22,23] The ventricular walls may be thickened, as in amyloidosis.

In endomyocardial fibrosis, there is a typical obliteration of the ventricular cavity, usually the apex, by a mass of fibrous tissue and thrombus (Fig. 12.1a).[6] One or both ventricles may be involved. Calcifications of the ventricular endocardium and cardiac fibrous skeleton have been described.[24] Thrombi have been found in 58% of autopsy cases, usually at the atrial cavities. Microscopically, the involved endocardium demonstrates a thick layer of collagen tissue, and septa of fibrous and granulation tissue are seen extending for variable distances into the myocardium.[6] In amyloidosis, deposits of amyloid are present between the myocardial fibers, in the atrial and ventricular endocardium, and and can be demonstrated by an endomyocardial biopsy of the right ventricle. The ventricular walls and septum are thickened, as well as the interatrial septum while the ventricular cavities are usually small (Fig. 12.1b).[25,26]

In the idiopathic form of restrictive cardiomyopathy, no infiltrative disorder is present, and microscopic studies demonstrate only interstitial fibrosis of the myocardium without inflammatory cells.[22]

Pathophysiology

Initially, the systolic function is preserved in most cases, but may become severely impaired[21] later in the course of disease.[22] Diastolic dysfunction, due to a marked decrease in ventricular chamber compliance, is the hallmark of restrictive cardiomyopathy. The increased myocardial stiffness limits cardiac filling, from the beginning of diastole, whereas, in constrictive pericarditis, ventricular chamber compliance is likely to be normal in the first third of the diastole.[23,27,28] The abnormal impedance to ventricular filling throughout diastole leads to a reduction in the proportion of filling due to atrial contraction and, ultimately, atrial enlargement and failure.[29]

In restrictive cardiomyopathy, as well as in constrictive pericarditis, an increased filling in the first third of the diastole is observed, along with a sudden decrease in the mid and late diastole. This filling pattern is reflected in pressure recordings as an early diastolic dip in pressure, immediately followed by a quick rise and a plateau (dip and plateau pattern). In normal individuals, the right atrial pressure and caval veins flow display X (systolic) and Y (diastolic) descent, the X descent usually being more prominent.[30] In patients with restriction, in opposition, the Y descent becomes more prominent and is the predominant wave.[30,31]

In restrictive cardiomyopathy, contrary to constrictive pericarditis, the intrathoracic pressure is transmitted to the atria and ventricles and there is no interventricular dependence. This explains the lesser respiratory variation in vena cava, pulmonary veins, mitral and tricuspid flows in restrictive than in constrictive pathophysiology.[32]

Clinical features

Patients with restrictive cardiomyopathy usually present with severe biventricular failure, i.e., dyspnea, jugular venous distention, hepatomegaly, ascites and pedal edema, which have been present for months or years.[17,22] Fatigue, palpitations and right upper quadrant pain may also be reported.[7] The symptoms and signs of right-sided heart failure often predominate, characteristically with refractory ascites. However, in some cases, for example, in endomyocardial fibrosis and amyloidosis, heart failure may be either left-sided only or left-sided failure preceding right-sided failure. Endomyocardial fibrosis may involve mainly the right ventricle.[6] The clinical picture is very similar to the patients with biventricular disease but with predominant right ventricular failure. The finding of a mitral regurgitation murmur may help to indicate the left ventricular involvement. The chronic hepatic congestion may lead to icterus, high AST, ALT, protrombin time and low serum albumin, and the differential diagnosis with hepatic cirrhosis is often important in clinical practice.

Chest pain typical of angina pectoris with normal coronary arteries, arrhythmias and sudden death can occur in amyloidosis and can precede the onset of heart failure.[23] Amyloidosis may also mimic hypertrophic cardiomyopathy and can cause asymmetrical septal hypertrophy and even systolic anterior movement of the mitral valve.[33,34]

The cardiovascular examination shows prominent jugular venous distention with a marked early diastolic Y descent. Kussmaul's sign may occasionally be present. The apical impulse is not prominent, and is usually unpalpable. A prominent fourth heart sound is usual in restrictive cardiomyopathy, and a third sound (protodiastolic) is less frequent. Mitral and tricuspid insufficiency murmurs are very common in restrictive cardiomyopathy and may be helpful in distinguishing from constrictive pericarditis, because in this latter condition murmurs are uncommon.

Diagnostic methods

M-mode and two-dimensional echocardiography

The clues to the diagnosis of restrictive cardiomyopathy are normal left and right ventricular end-diastolic dimension, with enlarged (sometimes huge) atria, normal or near normal systolic function and abnormal ventricular diastolic filling. Left ventricular posterior wall and interventricular septal thickness are usually normal, but concentric hypertrophy may be present, as in amyloidosis and infiltrative myocardial disease.

The abnormal left ventricular posterior wall endocardial flatness in diastole, characteristically described in constrictive pericarditis, has not been found in restrictive cardiomyopathy.[35,36] It has been reported that patients with restrictive amyloid cardiomyopathy have no plateau in the diastolic left ventricular filling volume curve, studied with computer analysis of digitized left ventriculograms, and that left ventricular filling rate is slower than normal during the first half of diastole.[37] This has also been described from digitised M-mode echocardiograms.[36] The same authors found that patients with restrictive cardiomyopathy had a slower left ventricular filling rate than controls and that patients with constrictive pericarditis had a faster ventricular filling rate than controls and than patients with restrictive cardiomyopathy. However, this is not uniformly reported. In endomyocardial fibrosis, for example, a rapid early diastolic posterior motion and flatness of the left ventricular posterior wall is commonly seen.[17,38]

The two-dimensional (2D) study shows indirect findings such as normal sized ventricles, enlarged atria and dilatation with diminished or absent inspiratory collapse of the inferior vena cava (Fig. 12.2). These findings indicate restrictive physiology.

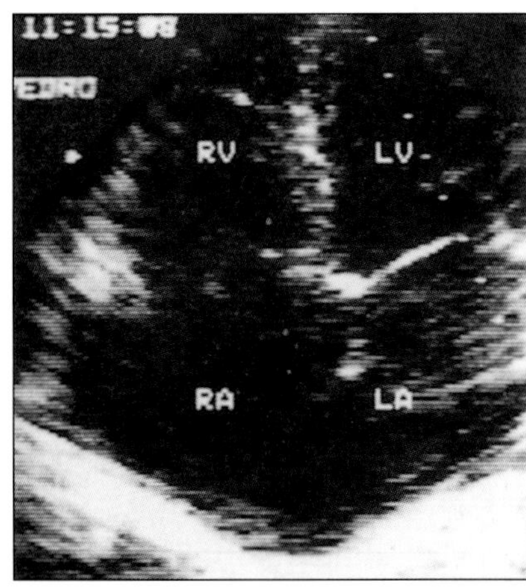

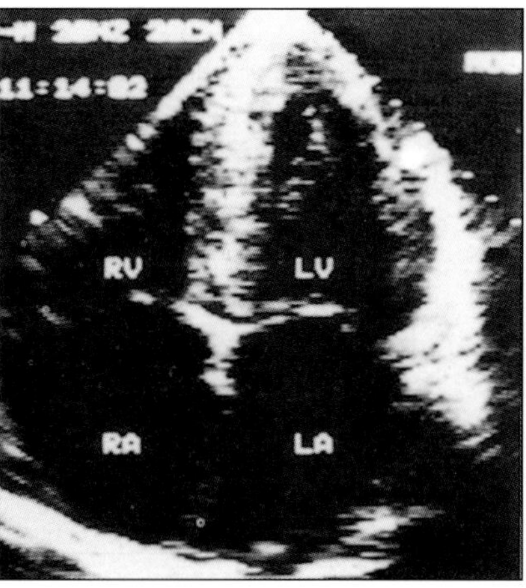

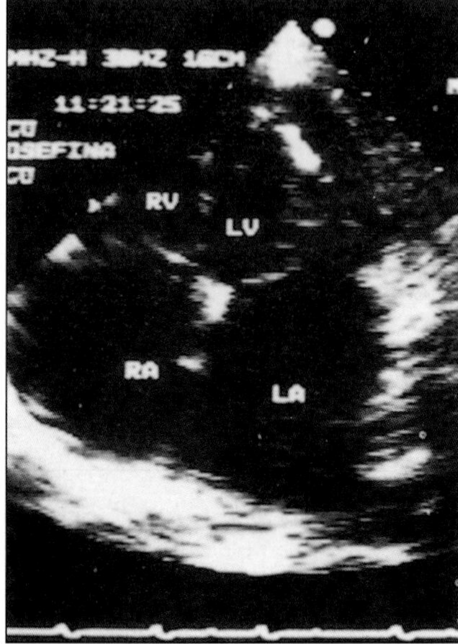

Figure 12.2
Four-chamber two-dimensional echocardiographic apical view of three patients that shows findings suggestive of restriction. These features are normal to small ventricular size and normal to mildly reduced systolic function, with dilated atria.

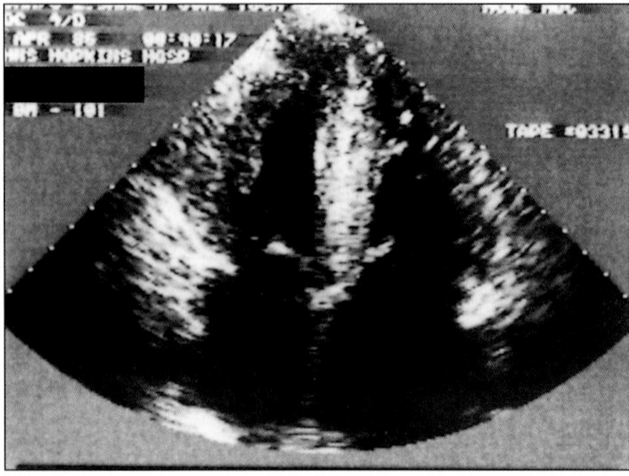

Figure 12.3
Bidimensional echocardiogram (4-chamber view) in a case of amyloidosis, showing a severely thickened septum, left and right ventricular walls, with the characteristic granula sparkling, and thickened mitral and tricuspid valves.

In addition, 2D echo may suggest the etiology. In amyloidosis, the increased myocardial echogenicity with a 'granular sparkling' appearance seen throughout all walls of the left ventricle (Fig. 12.3), that persist with a low gain, is fairly characteristic if not diagnostic.[26] It has been described in 45% of patients.[39] All cardiac structures may be thickened: left and right ventricular walls, papillary muscles, valves and the interatrial septum, the last one being typical of this pathology.[25,26,40–42] Cardiac amyloidosis can also sometimes mimic hypertrophic obstructive cardiomyopathy, even with systolic anterior motion of mitral valve and early systolic aortic valve closure.[33,34,43,44] The association of a thickened left ventricle on echocardiogram with low voltage on ECG is very suggestive of amyloidosis.[39,45] The systolic function usually remains intact until late in the course of this disease. While the left ventricular cavity decreases in amyloidosis, the right ventricular cavity tends to increase with the severity of the disease, and a LV/RV area <2 predicts a markedly shortened survival.[46] Pericardial effusion, usually small, is also common.

In endomyocardial fibrosis, the apex of one or both ventricles is obliterated by a homogeneous, fixed, fibrotic mass, which is very characteristic of this condition (Fig. 12.4).[47,48] Furthermore, when one compares the severity of the left and right ventricular obliteration by echocardiography against contrast angiography, there is excellent concordance.[48] Papillary muscles and atrioventricular valves may be involved by the fibrotic process. In one of our patients with severe right ventricular disease (inflow tract completely obliterated by fibrotic mass), it was not possible to identify the tricuspid valve. Paradoxical septal motion was found in 50% of our patients, always in association with tricuspid regurgitation. We have also described a 'sinusoid' type of septal motion, where the septum had an S form at end-diastole, because only the proximal portion is subjected to the volumetric overload caused by tricuspid regurgitation.[48] The peculiar motion of the interventricular septum has also captured the attention of other authors. Acquatella described it as a 'sail type' motion of the upper two-thirds, while the lower septal third was 'anchored' into the apical

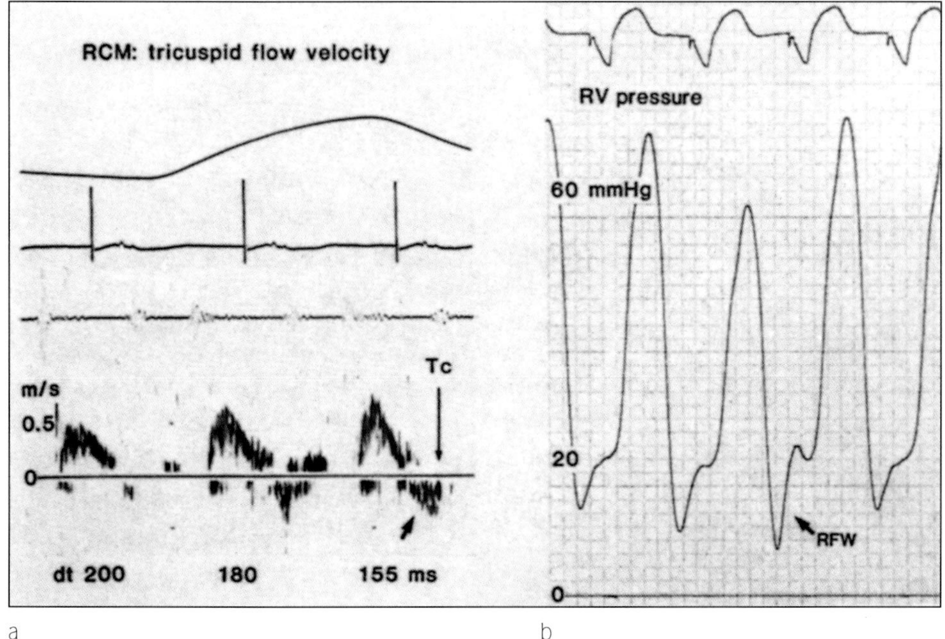

Figure 12.4
Mitral and tricusoid flow velocity recordings from patients with restrictive cardiomyopathy. (a) mitral flow velocity and left ventricular (LV) and pulmonary capillary (PCW) tracings. Note the shortened mitral deceleration time (dt), minimal flow with atrial contraction and increased left ventricular rapid filling wave (RFW) and end diastolic pressure. (b) tricuspid flow velocity and right ventricular (RV) pressure recordings in a patient with atrial-paced rhythm. With inspiration, peak tricuspid flow velocity increases, but there is abnormal shortening of the tricuspid deceleration tome (dt) with a reversal flow in late diastole (arrow). Right ventricular diastolic pressure (nonsimultaneous) shows a corresponding more abrupt and larger increase in the rapid filling wave (RFW, arrow) with inspiration. Tc = tricuspid closure.

obliterative process.[47] Calcifications can be seen at the endocardial surface or within the obliterative fibrotic mass. Pericardial effusion was seen in 42% of our patients (5 of 12), being large in only one, without signs of tamponade.

In sarcoidosis, localized thinning of the left ventricular wall with dilatation of the left ventricle may be found by echocardiography, resembling myocardial infarction with aneurysm formation.

Doppler and color flow findings

The restrictive hemodynamic pattern of cardiac filling can be recognized noninvasively by Doppler echocardiography.[30] This is usually done by the transthoracic approach, the analysis of mitral, tricuspid, superior vena cava and hepatic vein flow velocities. More recently, typical pulmonary venous flow velocity patterns recorded by transesophageal echocardiography have been described in restrictive cardiomyopathy and constrictive pericarditis. These Doppler patterns may help in the differentiation between the two conditions, and are described below:

Mitral and tricuspid flows

In restrictive cardiomyopathy, pulsed Doppler interrogation at the tip of the mitral or tricuspid valves shows normal or increased peak E wave velocity, diminished or absent A wave and increased E/A ratio (≥1.5). In addition, there is generally marked shortened deceleration time of E wave (usually less than 160 ms) (Fig. 12.4a), with further shortening of the tricuspid deceleration time (and sometimes of the mitral as well) with inspiration (Fig. 12.4b).[29,30] However, these findings may be subtle. For example, the early stages of amyloidosis may produce abnormal left ventricular relaxation with a mitral flow pattern characterized by a short E wave and tall A wave. Furthermore, in restrictive cardiomyopathy, respiratory variation of Doppler inflow velocities is not significant, with less than 15% difference between respiratory values of the early diastolic mitral filling wave.[29] The Doppler findings described

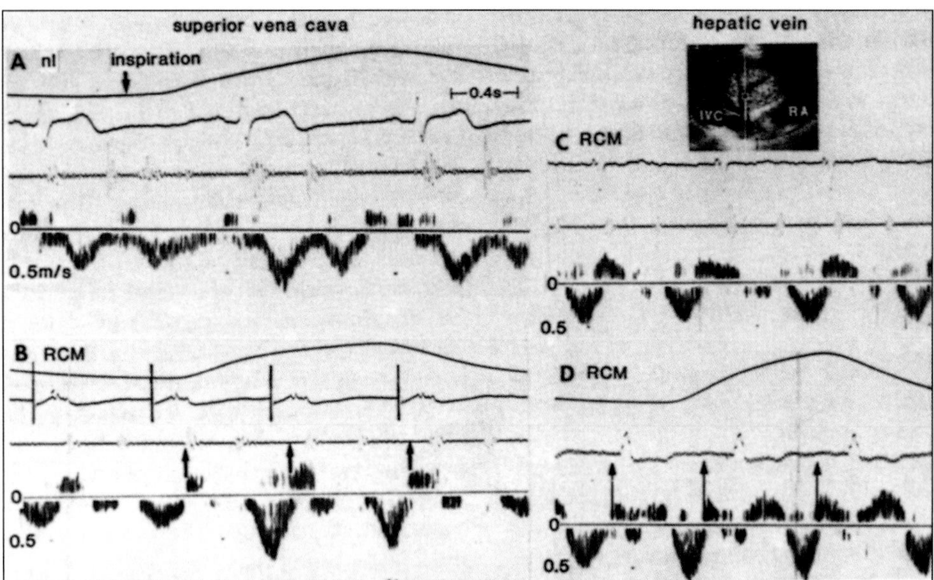

Figure 12.5
Superior vena cava (*left*) and hepatic veing (*right*) flow velocity recordings from a normal (nl) subject (panel A) and three patients with restrictive cardiomyopathy (RCM) (panels B through D). Panel A shows systolic forward flow greater than diastolic forward flow (below zero baseline), and small flow reversals at atrial contraction during apnea withut any increase on inspiration (above zero baseline). Panel B is a superior vena cava recording from a patient with restrictive cardiomyopathy with atrial-paced rhythm, showing diastolic forward flow followed by presystolic flow reversals that become larger and begin earlier with inspiration (arrows). Panel C is a hepatic veing tracing from a patient with atrial fibrillation, showing only diastolic forward flow, followed by diastolic reversal of flow. Panel D is a hepatic veing tracing from a patient in sinus rhythm with moderately severe tricuspid regurgitation. There is forward flow only during diastole, followed by presystolic flow reversals that increase and occur earlier in diastole with inspiration, as shown by the arrows. IVC = inferior vena cava; RA = atrium.

above, however, are not specific for restrictive cardiomyopathy, since patients with left ventricular dysfunction due to dilated cardiomyopathy, hypertrophic cardiomyopathy, ischemic or hypertensive heart disease, may present with similar mitral flow patterns. Indeed, in patients with dilated cardiomyopathy, the finding of restrictive physiology (with shortened deceleration time of mitral E wave) has been established as an independent marker of poor survival.[49] Furthermore, serial Doppler assessment has shown that patients with heart failure and persistent restrictive left ventricular filling pattern despite therapy for CHF have a high mortality, while disappearance of this pattern is associated with a better prognosis.[50,51]

Mitral and tricuspid diastolic regurgitation may be seen in restrictive cardiomyopathy.

It is important to notice that, for the correct recording of velocities and deceleration times, it is necessary to use pulsed instead of continuous wave Doppler, since the latter may prolong the deceleration time. Moreover, the sample volume must be located between the tips of the mitral or tricuspid valve leaflets.

Color Doppler flow mapping is useful to demonstrate and assess the severity of mitral and tricuspid regurgitation (usually moderate to severe), both very common in restrictive cardiomyopathy.

Superior vena cava and hepatic vein flow velocities

There has been much interest in characterizing the systemic venous flow in restriction, and to distinguish restrictive cardiomyopathy from constrictive pericarditis using its respiratory variation. The usually interrogated flows are from hepatic vein and superior vena cava, because of their parallel direction to the Doppler cursor and easiness to obtain. In normal individuals, there are bimodal systolic (X) and diastolic (Y) forward flow waves, with a predominant systolic wave (X>Y). Inspiratory or expiratory diastolic reversals are less than 20% of forward flow velocities (Fig.12.5).[30,52] In restrictive cardiomyopathy the predominant forward flow is during diastole (Y>X), with a small or absent X wave (Fig. 12.6). Moreover, there is an increase in diastolic reversal with inspiration compared with the expiratory phase, which differentiate it from constrictive pericarditis.[30,53] This is caused by a sudden reduction in right ventricular filling at end diastole owing to decreased ventricular compliance. Using these criteria Oh et al reported a sensitivity of 88% and specificity of 96% for the diagnosis of restrictive cardiomyopathy.[53]

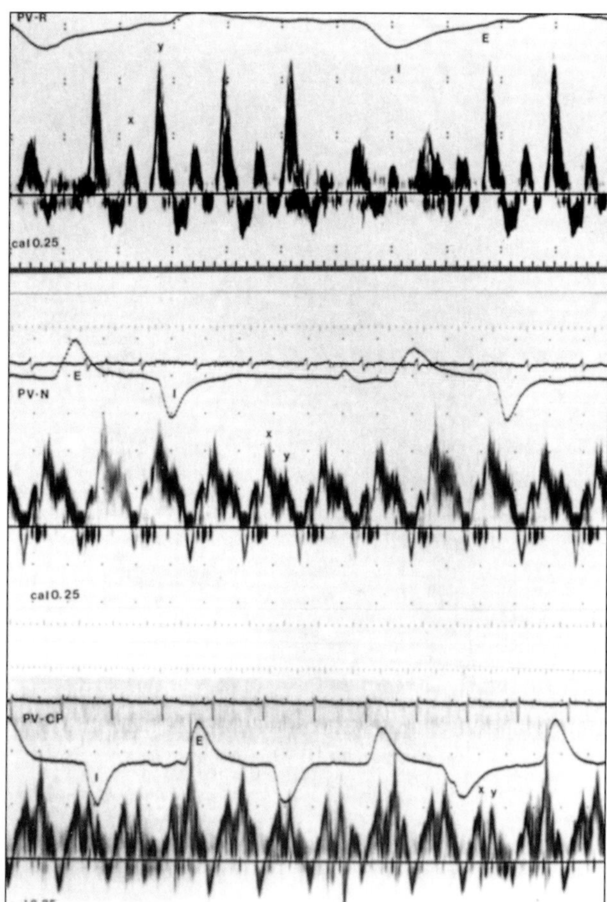

Figure 12.6

Pulmonary venous flow

Measurements of pulmonary venous flow velocities may add to the evaluation of left ventricular diastolic filling. It cannot be reliably obtained in many patients with transthoracic Doppler echocardiography, thus it is necessary to use transesophageal echocardiography in most cases. In normals, the pulmonary venous flow is also bimodal, as in hepatic vein, with greater systolic (X) than diastolic (Y) flow waves (Fig. 12.6). In restriction, there is an inversion of systolic/diastolic flow, with a significantly greater Y and X wave (Fig. 12.6), as reported by Schiavone[54] and Klein,[32] causing a small X/Y flow ratio (0.4 ± 0.2).[32] It is important to analyse respiratory variations in pulmonary venous flow to distinguish restriction from constriction. In restrictive cardiomyopathy a mild increase in both X (10 ± 12%) and Y (16 ± 14%) waves from inspiration to expiration has been found, and diastolic flow velocities (Y) persisted greater than systolic (X) in all respiratory phases. This differed from constrictive pericarditis,[32] as will be discussed later.

Radionuclide ventriculography

Diastolic filling may be evaluated by radionuclide ventriculography. Gerson et al measured peak filling rate, time to peak filling rate, corrected first third filling fraction, corrected first half filling fraction and Fourier ratio of peak left ventricular filling rate-to-peak emptying rate in patients with restrictive cardiomyopathy, constrictive pericarditis and normal controls.[55] They did not find significant difference between patients with restrictive physiology versus normal controls. Some patients with restrictive cardiomyopathy had a reduced rate of diastolic filling, producing a more gradual slope of the diastolic compared to the systolic limb of the three-volume curve. However, this was not seen in more than half of the patients. Patients with constrictive pericarditis had a faster rate of early diastolic filling compared to patients with restrictive cardiomyopathy and control subjects, but overlap prevented accurate separation between the two groups. The diagnostic distinction between constriction and restriction is discussed in another section of this chapter (vide infra). Interestingly, in cardiac amyloidosis, there is a marked and diffuse technetium-99m-pyrophosphate myocardial uptake.[56] These authors found 100% positive scans in 10 patients with amyloidosis (nine 4+ and one 3±). However, other authors have reported a low sensitivity of technetium pyrophosphate scintigraphy for documented cases of cardiac amyloidosis.[39,57] Simons and Isner reported a sensitivity of only 23% in 13 patients with proven diagnosis of cardiac amyloidosis.[39]

Computed tomography and magnetic resonance imaging

These imaging techniques are useful in differentiating restrictive cardiomyopathy from constrictive pericarditis (as discussed below), since pericardial thickening is not seen in

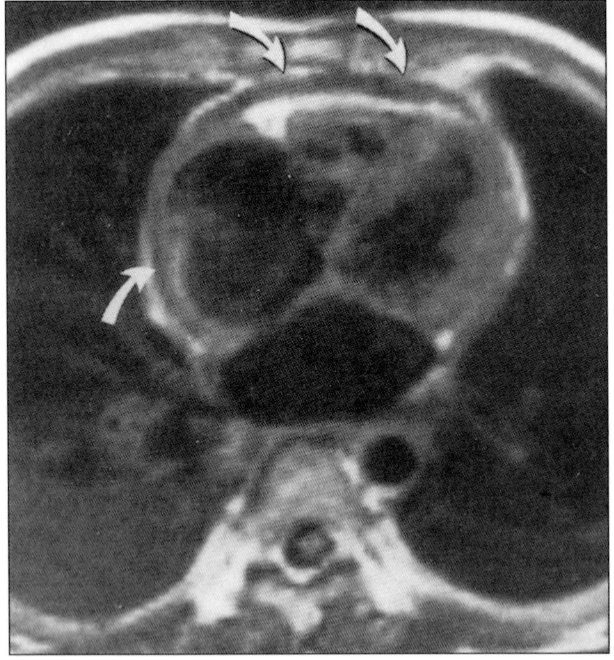
a

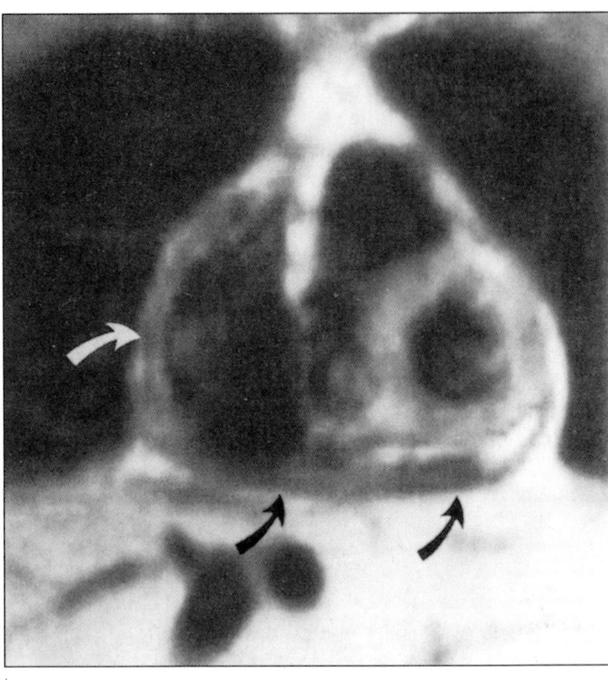
b

Figure 12.7
Computed tomography (a) and magnetic resonance imaging (b) in patients with constrictive pericarditis.

patients with restrictive cardiomyopathy but has been reported in more than 90% of constriction patients (Fig. 12.7).[3] Conventional computed tomography has been said to demonstrate the thickened pericardium in the great majority of patients with constrictive pericarditis, and in one patient with restrictive cardiomyopathy.[58–60] Cine computed tomography is a relatively new imaging technique that provides a very high resolution tomographic cardiac image. It has been reported to be very accurate in the diagnosis of constrictive pericarditis. It simultaneously provides both anatomic and physiologic data (right and left ventricular systolic and diastolic function), and clearly distinguishes constrictive pericarditis from normals and from patients with cardiomyopathy.[61]

Indirect findings of impaired right ventricular diastolic filling (e.g. dilatation of the inferior vena cava and right atrium) are common in both pathologies.[62] A prominent signal within the atria at all phases of the cardiac cycle, consistent with stasis of atrial blood as a consequence of elevated ventricular diastolic pressures, has been reported with magnetic resonance imaging (MRI).[62–64]

Furthermore, MRI may reveal linear calcifications and/or a smooth, isointense, soft tissue mass obliterating the ventricular cavity in endomyocardial fibrosis.[63,65]

The differential diagnosis of restrictive cardiomyopathy and constrictive pericarditis

The most important and difficult differential diagnosis of restrictive cardiomyopathy is constrictive pericarditis. It is necessary to distinguish between these two conditions because constrictive pericarditis can be cured surgically, whereas restrictive cardiomyopathy cannot, except in the case of endomyocardial fibrosis. The symptoms and the clinical presentation are essentially the same. A history of tuberculosis, mediastinal irradiation or cardiac surgery may, at most, suggest the diagnosis of pericardial constriction,[66] and, on the other hand, multiple myeloma is frequently associated with amyloidosis. In many cases, even hemodynamic data from cardiac catheterization may be insufficient in providing the diagnosis. Some clinical clues to the differentiation: pulsus paradoxus and Kussmaul's sign may suggest pericardial constriction, but are, in fact, nonspecific; murmurs of mitral and/or tricuspid regurgitation are common in restrictive cardiomyopathy (e.g. endomyocardial fibrosis) and uncommon in constrictive pericarditis; a pericardial knock (earlier and higher-pitched diastolic third heart sound) when present, is strongly suggestive of constriction. The electrocardiogram has been disappointing in the diagnosis of these diseases. Pericardial calcification in a chest radiograph, on the other hand, is virtually diagnostic of constriction, but, unfortunately, is an infrequent finding (20–50% of cases).[67] It is important to look carefully for this sign on the chest X-ray whenever a constrictive/restrictive condition is suspected, especially in a lateral view (calcifications are often only seen in this projection).

The new cardiovascular noninvasive imaging, such as Doppler echocardiography (transthoracic and transesophageal), computed tomography and magnetic resonance can distinguish these two conditions, obviating in many cases the necessity of endomyocardial biopsy and cardiac catheterization. Doppler echocardiography is the most widely available of these methods, and is usually the first to be performed, as a screening examination. Frequently, it defines the diagnosis, particularly when combined with the clinical and radiological data. Although M-mode and two-dimensional echocardiograms may demonstrate consistent findings of cardiac amyloidosis or endomyocardial fibrosis, and, in a patient with intense pericardial calcification may confirm the diagnosis of constriction, there are many cases where it is not possible to distinguish between these two conditions. For example, in patients with idiopathic restrictive cardiomyopathy, or in patients with constrictive pericarditis without pericardial calcification, the definitive diagnosis is not made by echocardiography alone. There are many signs reported in patients with constrictive pericarditis: the thickened pericardium may present as a single or multiple parallel echo-dense lines on M-mode or an abnormally bright and thick pericardial echo on the 2D echocardiogram, but unfortunately has been seen in less than half of the patients.[53,68] Moreover, a diastolic notch of the interventricular septum on M-mode, and a bouncing motion on 2-D echocardiogram, exacerbated and bulging into the left ventricular side during inspiration, can be frequently detected.

However, findings by Doppler have been described as more definitive to the differential diagnosis. Hatle and coworkers described significant differences in the respiratory variation of mitral and tricuspid peak E waves, and also isovolumic relaxation time (IVRT), between patients with restriction and constriction.[29] The variation from expiration to inspiration in left ventricular isovolumic relaxation time and early flow velocity (E wave) appeared to best separate the patients with restrictive cardiomyopathy from those with constrictive pericarditis. Among those with restrictive cardiomyopathy, no individual patient had more than a 15% respiratory variation of these variables (usually much less), while, all patients with constrictive pericarditis had a greater than 25% increase of E wave and decrease of IVRT on the first beat after the onset of expiration (Fig. 12.8). These measurements were performed during end-tidal volume apnea and on the first beat after the onset of inspiration and expiration. Variation of the sample position during respiratory movements may sometimes influence the peak velocity of E wave, but usually not the IVRT.

The analysis of hepatic vein and superior vena cava flows may help to distinguish restriction from constriction: while a clear Y wave (diastolic forward) predominance is observed in restriction, there may be two patterns in constriction, one with a predominant Y wave (similar to restriction) and another with a predominant systolic forward flow (X wave).[31,53,69] A 'W' aspect of the venous flow has been reported as suggestive of constrictive physiology.[31] In those patients with atrial fibrillation, the expected finding is a predominant Y wave. While the analysis of Doppler flow patterns at baseline provide clues to the differential diagnosis between restrictive cardiomyopathy and constrictive pericarditis, the most important evidence is provided by the analysis during inspiration and expiration: an inspiratory increase of diastolic flow reversals usually increase during expiration (Figs 12.5 and 12.9).[30,53]

Respiratory variation in pulmonary venous flow, measured by transesophageal echocardiography, can also be a useful parameter to distinguish constrictive pericarditis from restrictive cardiomyopathy. A predominant diastolic flow wave (Y>X) is seen throughout the respiratory cycle in restrictive cardiomyopathy, and is accentuated in expiration.[32,54] In constrictive pericarditis there is a relatively larger pulmonary venous systolic/diastolic flow ratio (X/Y) and greater respiratory variation in pulmonary venous systolic, and especially diastolic, flow velocities. The combination of a X/Y ≥0.65 in inspiration and a percent change from expiration to inspiration for peak diastolic flow ≥40% was reported to correctly classify 86% of patients with constrictive pericarditis.[32] Transeosophageal echocardiography may also be more accurate than the transthoracic window to evaluate pericardial thickening, but this needs to be proved.

A fibrous or calcific thickening of the pericardium is the anatomical hallmark of constrictive pericarditis. The finding of a thickened pericardium in the setting of an appropriate clinical/hemodynamic profile is presumptive evidence in favor of this pathology. Both computed tomography (CT) and magnetic resonance imaging (MRI), have been shown to identify thickened pericardium (Fig. 12.7). The diagnostic criteria for both methods is ≥3 mm thickness. However, Suchet and Horwitz reported two children with proven constriction in which the pericardium measured between 2 and 3 mm.[60] In the few studies published in the literature, using CT or MRI, all of the patients with restrictive cardiomyopathy had a normal pericardial appearance, while more than 90% of the patients with constrictive pericarditis had pericardial thickening, which was frequently localized instead of generalized.[58–60]

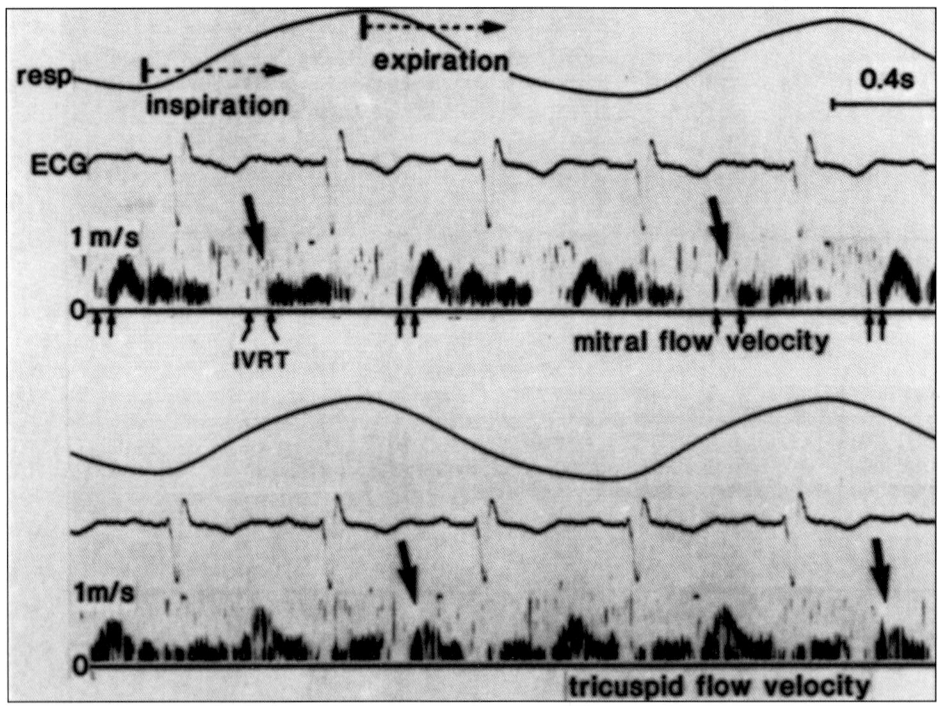

a

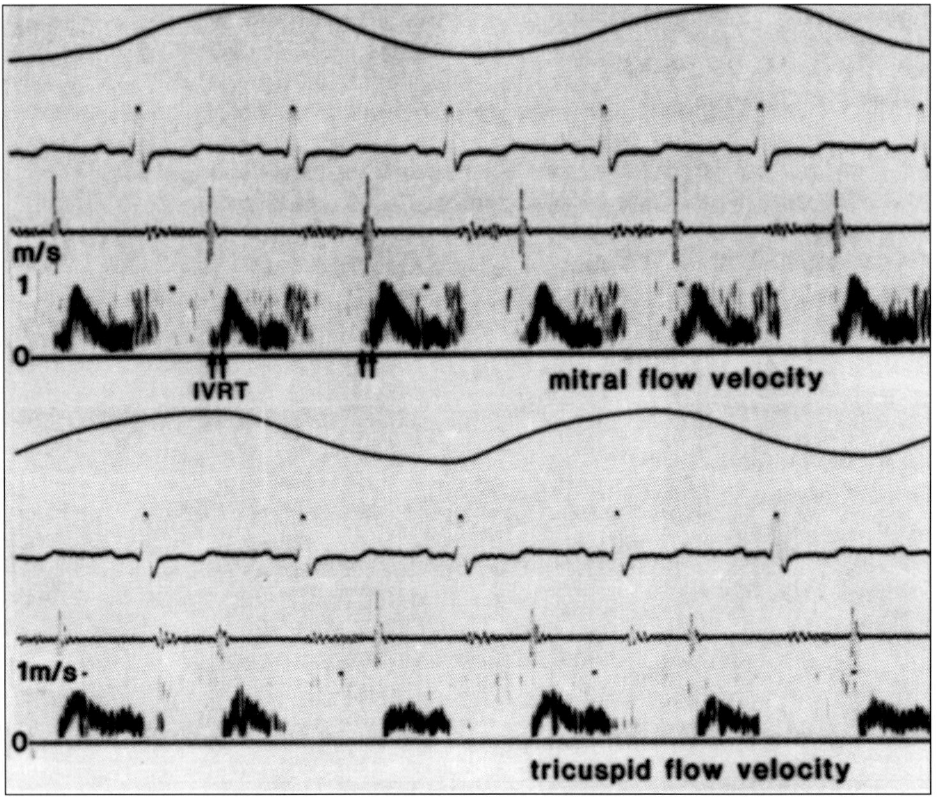

b

Figure 12.8
(a): Tracing of mitral and tricuspid flow velocities recorded together with respiration (resp) in a patient with constrictive pericarditis. Note the marked decrease in early mitral flow velocity (beats 2 and 5, large black arrows) and the increase in left ventricular isovolumic relaxation time (IVRT, pairs of small arrows) on the first beat after the onset of inspiration compared with the other beats. The timing of aortic closure was verified by a simultaneous phonocardiogram not included in the figure. On the first beat after the onset of expiration (beats 3 and 6), an increase in mitral flow velocity and shortening of the IVRT is seen when compared with both inspiration and the intermediate beats. The tricuspid flow velocity shows reciprocal changes, with an increase on the first beat of inspiration (beats 2 and 5) and a decrease on the first beat of expiration (beats 3 and 6, arrows) compared with intermediate beats (1 and 4). The velocity recorded in systole in the tricuspid recording represents systolic flow in the right ventricular inflow tract and should not be confused with transvalvular flow.
(b): Tracing recorded from the same patient 1 week after pericardiectomy; there is minimal respiratory variation in early mitral flow velocity and IVRT with respiration, and the tricuspid flow velocity on the first beats after the onset of expiration (beats 2 and 5) is larger than the next expiratory beat (beats 3 and 6).

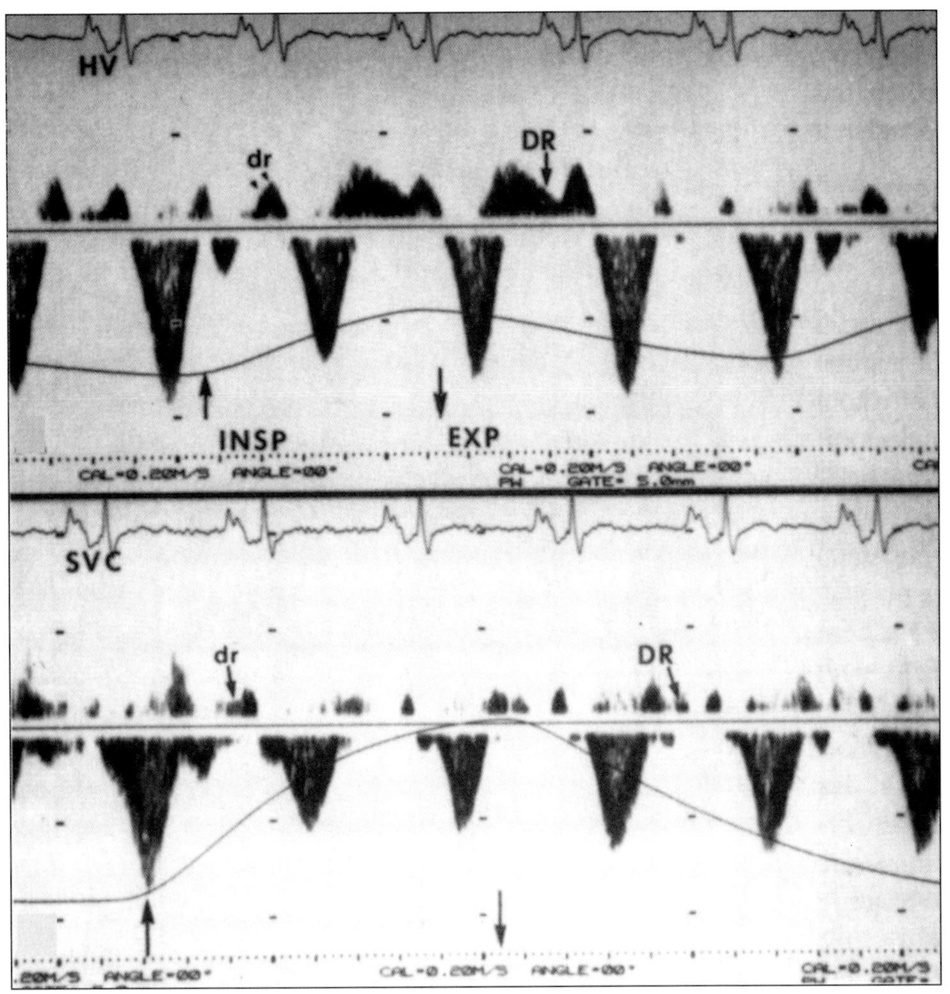

Figure 12.9
Case 7. Typical hepatic venous and superior vena cava Doppler flow pattern of constrictive pericarditis. A, Hepatic venous (HV) flow shows a marked increase in diastolic reversal (DR) during expiration (EXP) compared with diastolic reversal (dr) during inspiration (INSP) (small arrowheads). Note that the predominant hepatic forward flow is during systole. B, Superior vena cavan (SVC) Doppler flow velocity from the same patient. Diastolic flow reversal during inspiration (dr) and expiration (DR) are less prominent than those recorded from the hepatic veing.

Recently, cine computed tomography has been reported to be very accurate in the diagnosis of constrictive pericarditis and in distinguishing it from normal and from patients with cardiomyopathy.[61] Cine computed tomography simultaneously provides both anatomic and physiologic data of constrictive pericarditis. Many studies, however, reported the visualization of the thickened pericardium using conventional computed tomography.[58–60] Comparing cine magnetic resonance angiography (MRA) and spin-echo MRI, Hartnell et al have shown that MRA has a sensitivity of 86% and a very low specificity (63%), with considerable overlap of thickness measurements in patients with and without pericardial constriction, while spin-echo MRI has a sensitivity of 100% and specificity of 96%.[70] These authors referred that MR angiography cannot be used alone to diagnose pericardial thickening.

Therefore, the finding of a thickened pericardium virtually excludes the diagnosis of restrictive cardiomyopathy and a normal pericardial appearance makes the suspicion of constriction unlikely. The principal data used to distinguish these two pathologies are given in Table 12.2.

Recently, a new method using Doppler tissue imaging has been shown to differentiate constrictive pericarditis from restrictive cardiomyopathy. Intrinsic myocardial disease influences elastic recoil forces of the myocardium but should be preserved when diastole is impaired as a result of extrinsic causes. Peak early velocity of longitudinal axis expansion (Ea) was measured in 8 patients with constrictive pericarditis, 7 patients with restriction and 15 normal volunteers. The Ea value was significantly higher in normal subjects (14.5 + 4.7 cm/s) and in patients with constrictions (14.8 + 4.8 cm/s) than in those with restriction (5.1 + 1.4 cm/s, $p<0.001$ – constriction vs restriction).[71] In this study, the measurement of longitudinal axis expansion velocities provided a clinically useful distinction between constrictive pericarditis and restrictive cardiomyopathy.

Table 12.2 Features that distinguish restrictive cardiomyopathy from constrictive pericarditis

	Restrictive cardiomyopathy	*Constrictive pericarditis*
Clinical		
History of tuberculosis, mediastinal irradiation or cardiac surgery	Usually absent	May be present
Kussmaul's sign	Absent	Present
Third heart sound	Rare	Absent
Pericardial knock	Absent	Present
Mitral/Tricuspid murmur	Often present	Usually absent
Electrocardiogram		
Low ECG voltage	May be present	May be present
Electrical alternans	Absent	Absent
Chest X-ray		
Pericardial calcification	Absent	May be present
Echocardiography		
Thickened/calcific pericardium	Absent	Often present
Myocardial thickness and brightness	Usually increased	Normal
LV and/or RV apex obliteration	Endomyocardial fibrosis	Absent
Exaggerated respiratory variation in flow velocity (mitral >25%)	Absent	Present
Exaggerated respiratory variation in LV isovolumic relaxation time (>25%)	Absent	Present
Hepatic vein flow:		
increase in diastolic reversal	Inspiratory	Expiratory
Pulmonary vein flow:		
exaggerated respiratory variation of peak diastolic (Y) flow (%)	Absent	Present
Computed Tomography/Magnetic Resonance		
Thickened/calcific pericardium	Absent	Present
Cardiac Catheterization		
Equalization of diastolic pressures	Usually absent	Usually present

The differential diagnosis of constrictive pericarditis from restrictive cardiomyopathy is a challenge to the clinician. Even the hemodynamic studies have many limitations. To address the lack of a quantitative assessment of the utility of hemodynamic criteria, Vaitkus and Kussmaul undertook an analysis of all published cases of constriction or restriction in which right and left ventricular pressure recordings were reported. They found that about 26% of the patients would not be classifiable by the hemodynamics criteria, and 8% of the remainder would be incorrectly classified.[3]

Some authors believe that transvenous endomyocardial biopsy is a useful method of distinguishing restrictive cardiomyopathies from constrictive pericarditis in patients with symptoms of heat failure and constrictive-restrictive physiology.[23,66,72–74] Schoenfeld et al identified a specific source of restrictive cardiomyopathy in 15 of 38 patients (39%) (11 amyloid, 4 myocarditis) in whom the clinical and noninvasive or hemodynamic features were not able to distinguish it from constrictive pericarditis and diagnostic/therapeutic thoracotomy was contemplated. Of the 23 remaining patients with either normal biopsy findings or nonspecific abnormalities on biopsy, 18 had intraoperative or autopsy evaluation of their pericardium, and constriction was found in 14 (77%).[66] A specific condition such as amyloidosis, endomyocardial fibrosis, iron storage disease, Fabry's disease, sarcoidosis, or glycogen storage disease may be diagnosed. Therefore, in patients with profound symptoms and either normal biopsy results or nondiagnostic abnormalities on biopsy, exploratory thoracotomy should be considered since there is a high likelihood of finding pericardial constriction in such patients.

The data from Doppler echocardiography, computed tomography and MR imaging show a very good sensibility and specificity to the diagnosis of constrictive pericarditis. For this reason we propose a noninvasive approach to the differential diagnosis of these two pathologies.

References

1 Child JS, Perlof JK: The restrictive cardiomyopathies. *Cardiol Clin* 1988; **6**: 289–316.

2 Dolara A, Cecchi F, Ciaccheri M: Cardiomyopathy in Italy today: extent of the problem. *G Ital Cardiol* 1989; **19**: 1074–79.

3 Vaitkus PT, Kussmaul MD: Constrictive pericarditis versus restrictive cardiomyopathy: a reappraisal and update of diagnostic criteria. *Am Heart J* 1991; **122**: 1431–41.

4 Report of the WHO/ISFC. Task Force on the definition and classification of cardiomyopathies. *Br Heart J* 1980; **44**: 672–73.

5 Richardson P, McKenna W, Bristow M et al: Report of the 1995 World Health Organization/International Society and Federation of Cardiology task force on the definition and classification of cardiomyopathies. *Circulation* 1996; **93**: 841–42.

6 Andrade ZA, Guimaraes AC: Endomyocardial fibrosis in Bahia, Brazil. *Br Heart J* 1964; **26**: 813–20.

7 Guimaraes AC, Esteves JP, Filho AS, Macedo V: Clinical aspects of endomyocardial fibrosis in Bahia, Brazil. *Am Heart J* 1982; **103**: 202–3.

8 Guimaraes AC, Santos Filho A, Esteves JP et al: Hemodynamics in endomyocardial fibrosis. *Am Heart J* 1980; **88**: 294–303.

9 Martinez EE, Venturi M, Buffolo E et al: Operative results in endomyocardial fibrosis. *Am J Cardiol* 1989; **1**: 627–29.

10 Connor DH, Somers K, Hutt MSR et al: Endomyocardial fibrosis in Uganda. Part I: An epidemiologic, clinical and pathologic study. *Am Heart J* 1967; **74**: 687–709.

11 Brockington IF, Edington GM: Adult heart disease in Western Nigeria. *Am Heart J* 1972; **83**: 27–40.

12 Vijayaraghavan G, Cherian G, Krishnaswami S, Sukumar IP: Left ventricular endomyocardial fibrosis in India. *Br Heart J* 1977; **39**: 563–68.

13 Nair DV: Endomyocardial fibrosis in Kerala. *Ind Heart J* 1982; **34**: 412–17.

14 Fawzy ME, Ziady G, Halim M et al: Endomyocardial fibrosis: report of eight cases. *J Am Coll Cardiol* 1985; **5**: 983–88.

15 Rashwan MA, Ayman M, Ashour S et al: Endomyocardial fibrosis in Egypt: an illustrated review. *Br Heart J* 1995; **73**: 284–89.

16 Hess OM, Turina M, Senning A et al: Pre- and postoperative findings in patients with endomyocardial fibrosis. *Br Heart J* 1978; **40**: 406–15.

17 Chew CYC, Ziady GM, Raphael MH et al: Primary restrictive cardiomyopathy. Non-tropical endomyocardial fibrosis and hypereosinophilic heart disease. *Br Heart J* 1977; **39**: 399–413.

18 Wiseman MN, Giles MS, Camm AJ: Unusual echocardiographic appearance of intracardiac thrombi in a patient with endomyocardial fibrosis. *Br Heart J* 1986; **56**: 179–81.

19 Wilensky RL, Bourdillon PDV, O'Donnell JA et al: Restrictive hemodynamic patterns after cardiac transplantation: relationship to histologic signs of rejection. *Am Heart J* 1991; **122**: 1079–87.

20 Bouchard A, Sanz N, Botvinick EH et al: Noninvasive assessment of cardiomyopathy in normotensive diabetic patients between 20 and 50 years old. *Am J Med* 1989; **87**: 160–66.

21 Wynne J, Braunwald E: The cardiomyopathies and myocarditides. In: Braunwald E (ed) *Heart Disease. A Textbook of Cardiovascular Medicine*. Philadelphia: W.B. Saunders Company. 1997: 1404–63.

22 Siegel RJ, Shah PK, Fishbein MC: Idiopathic restrictive cardiomyopathy. *Circulation* 1984; **70**: 165–69.

23 Wilmhurst PT, Katritsis D: Restrictive cardiomyopathy. *Br Heart J* 1990; **63**: 323–24.

24 Lengyel M, Arvay A, Palik I: Massive endocardial calcification associated with endomyocardial fibrosis. *Am J Cardiol* 1985; **56**: 815–16.

25 Hesse A, Altland K, Linke RP et al: Cardiac amyloidosis: a review and report of a new transthyretin (prealbumin) variant. *Br Heart J* 1993; **70**: 111–15.

26 Laraki R: Cardiac amyloidosis. General review. *Rev Med Interne* 1994; **15**: 257–67.

27 Meaney E, Shabetai R, Bhargava V et al: Cardiac amyloidosis, constrictive pericarditis and restrictive cardiomyopathy. *Am J Cardiol* 1976; **38**: 547–56.

28 Seward JB: Restrictive cardiomyopathy: reassessment of definitions and diagnosis. *Current Opinion in Cardiology* 1988; **3**: 391–95.

29 Hatle LK, Appleton CP, Popp RL: Differentiation of constrictive pericarditis and restrictive cardiomyopathy by Doppler echocardiography. *Circulation* 1989; **86**: 1099–107.

30 Appleton CP, Hatle LK, Popp RL: Demonstration of restrictive ventricular physiology by Doppler echocardiography. *J Am Coll Cardiol* 1988; **11**: 757–68.

31 Borganelli M, Byrd III B: Doppler echocardiography in pericardial disease. *Cardiol Clin* 1990; **8**: 333–48.

32 Klein AI, Cohen GI, Pietrolungo JF et al: Differentiation of constrictive pericarditis from restrictive cardiomyopathy by Doppler transesophageal echocardiographic measurements of respiratory variations in pulmonary venous flow. *J Am Coll Cardiol* 1993; **22**: 1935–43.

33 Weston LT, Raybuck BD, Robinowitz M et al: Primary amyloid heart disease presenting as hypertrophic obstructive cardiomyopathy. *Cathet Cardiovasc Diagn* 1986; **12**: 176–81.

34 Presti CF, Waller BF, Armstrong WF: Cardiac amyloidosis mimicking the echocardiographic appearance of obstructive hypertrophic myopathy. *Chest* 1988; **93**: 881–83.

35 Mehta AV, Ferre PL, Pickoff AS et al: M-mode echocardiographic findings in children with idiopathic restrictive cardiomyopathy. *Pediatr Cardiol* 1984; **5**: 273–80.

36 Morgan JM, Raposo L, Clague JC et al: Restrictive cardiomyopathy and constrictive pericarditis: noninvasive distinction by digitised M-mode echocardiography. *Br Heart J* 1989; **61**: 29–37.

37 Tyberg TI, Goodyer AVN, Hurst VW et al: Left ventricular filling in differentiating restrictive amyloid cardiomyopathy and constrictive pericarditis. *Am J Cardiol* 1981; **47**: 791–96.

38 Haertel JC, Castro I: Avaliacao ecocardiografica da fibrose endomiocardica. *Arq Bras Cardiol* 1980; **35**: 475–80.

39 Simons M, Isner JM: Assessment of relative sensitivities of noninvasive tests for cardiac amyloidosis in documented cardiac amyloidosis. *Am J Cardiol* 1992; **69**: 425–27.

40 Siqueira-Filho GA, Cunha CLP, Tajik AJ et al: M-mode and two-dimensional echocardiographic features of cardiac amyloidosis. *Circulation* 1981; **63**: 188–96.

41 Chgild JS, Krivokapich J, Abbasi AS: Increased right ventricular wall thickness on echocardiography in amyloid infiltrative cardiomyopathy. *Am J Cardiol* 1979; **44**: 1391–95.

42 Child JS, Levisman JA, Abbasi AS et al: Echocardiographic manifestations of infiltrative cardiomyopathy: a report of seven cases due to amyloid. *Chest* 1976; **70**: 726–31.

43 Sedlis SP, Saffitz JE, Schwob VS et al: Cardiac amyloidosis simulating hypertrophic cardiomyopathy. *Am J Cardiol* 1984; **53**: 969–70.

44 Noma S, Akaishi M, Murayama A et al: Echocardiographic findings of a patient with cardiac amyloidosis and left ventricular outflow obstruction. *J Cardiography* 1982; **12**: 267–78.

45 Carroll JD, Gaasch WH, McAdam KPW: Amyloid cardiomyopathy: characterization by a distinct voltage/mass relation. *Am J Cardiol* 1982; **49**: 9–13.

46 Patel AR, Dubrey S, Mendes LA et al: Discordant geometric response of right and left ventricles in cardiac amyloidosis a potent predictor of survival. *Circulation* 1995; **92**: I–470. Abstract.

47 Acquatella H, Schiller NB, Puigbo JJ et al: Value of two-dimensional echocardiography in endomyocardial disease with and without eosinophilia. A clinical and pathologic study. *Circulation* 1983; **67**: 1219–26.

48 Camara EJN, Guimaraes AC, Godinho AGL: Avaliacao da endomiocardiofibrose pelo ecocardiograma bidimensional. Analise de gravidade e correlacao com a angiocardiografia. *Arq Bras Cardiol* 1991; **57**: 307–12.

49 Xie G-Y, Berk MR, Smith MD et al: Prognostic value of Doppler transmitral flow patterns in patients with congestive heart failure. *J Am Coll Cardiol* 1994; **24**: 132–39.

50 Pinamonti B, Zecchin M, De Lenarda A et al: Persistence of restrictive left ventricular filling pattern in dilated cardiomyopathy: an ominous prognostic sign. *Circulation* 1995; **92**: I–336. Abstract.

51 Traversi E, Pozzoli M, Cioffi G et al: Changes in mitral flow velocity patterns after chronic optimized therapy provide important prognostic information in patients with chronic heart failure. *Circulation* 1995; **92**: I–724. Abstract.

52 Appleton CP, Hatle LK, Popp RL: Superior vena cava and hepatic vein Doppler echocardiography in healthy adults. *J Am Coll Cardiol* 1987; **10**: 1032–39.

53 Oh JK, Hatle LK, Seward JB et al: Diagnostic role of Doppler echocardiography in constrictive pericarditis. *J Am Coll Cardiol* 1994; **23**: 154–62.

54 Schiavone WA, Calafiore PA, Salcedo EE: Transesophageal Doppler echocardiographic demonstration of pulmonary venous flow velocity in restrictive cardiomyopathy and constrictive pericarditis. *Am J Cardiol* 1989; **63**: 1286–88.

55 Gerson MC, Colthar MS, Fowler NO: Differentiation of constrictive pericarditis and restrictive cardiomyopathy by radionuclide ventriculography. *Am Heart J* 1989; **118**: 114–21.

56 Wizenberg TA, Muz J, Sohn YH et al: Value of positive myocardial technetium-99-pyrophosphate scintigraphy in the noninvasive diagnosis of cardiac amyloidosis. *Am Heart J* 1982; **103**: 202–3.

57 Gertz MA, Brown ML, Hauser MF et al: Utility of technetium 99m pyrophosphate scanning in cardiac amyloidosis. *Arch Intern Med* 1987; **147**: 1039–44.

58 Isner MI, Carter BL, Bankoff MS: Differentiation of constrictive pericarditis from restrictive cardiomyopathy by computed tomographic imaging. *Am Heart J* 1983; **105**: 1019–23.

59 Sutton FJ, Whittley NO, Applefield MM: The role of echocardiography and computed tomography in the evaluation of constrictive pericarditis. *Am Heart J* 1985; **109**: 350–55.

60 Suchet IB, Horwitz TA: CT in tuberculous constrictive pericarditis. *J Comput Assist Tomogr* 1992; **16**: 391–400.

61 Oren RM, Grover-McKay M, Stanford W, Weiss RM: Accurate preoperative diagnosis of pericardial constriction using cine computed tomography. *J Am Coll Cardiol* 1993; **22**: 832–38.

62 Masui T, Finck S, Higgins CB: Constrictive pericarditis and restrictive cardiomyopathy: evaluation with MR imaging. *Radiology* 1992; **182**: 369–73.

63 D'Silva SA, Kohli A, Dalvi BV et al: MRI in right ventricular endomyocardial fibrosis. *Am Heart J* 1992; **123**: 1390–92.

64 Sechtem U, Higgins CB, Sommerhoff BA et al: Magnetic resonance imaging of restrictive cardiomyopathy. *Am J Cardiol* 1987; **59**: 480–82.

65 Mousseaux E, Hernigou A, Azencot M et al: Endomyocardial fibrosis: electron-beam CT features. *Radiology* 1996; **198**: 755–60.

66 Schoenfeld MH, Supple EW, Dec GW Jr et al: Restrictive cardiomyopathy versus constrictive pericarditis: role of endomyocardial biopsy in avoiding unnecessary thoracotomy. *Circulation* 1987; **75**: 1012–17.

67 Brockington GM, Zebede J, Pandian NG: Constrictive pericarditis. *Cardiology Clinics* 1990; **8**: 645–61.

68 Mancuso L, D'Agostino A, Pitrolo F et al: Constrictive pericarditis versus restrictive cardiomyopathy: the role of Doppler echocardiography in differential diagnosis. *Int J Cardiol* 1991; **31**: 319–28.

69 Acquatella H, Rodriguez-Salas LA, Gomez-Mancebo JR: Doppler echocardiography in dilated and restrictive cardiomyopathies. *Cardiol Clin* 1990; **8**: 349–68.

70 Hartnell GG, Hughes LA, KO JP et al: Magnetic resonance imaging of pericardial constriction: comparison of cine MR angiography and spin-echo techniques. *Clin Radiol* 1996; **51**: 268–72.

71 Garcia MJ, Rodriguez L, Ares M et al: Differentiation of constrictive pericarditis from restrictive cardiomyopathy: assessment of left ventricular diastolic velocities in longitudinal axis by Doppler tissue imaging. *J Am Coll Cardiol* 1996; **27**: 108–14.

72 Schoenfeld MH: The differentiation of restrictive cardiomyopathy from constrictive pericarditis. *Cardiology Clinics* 1990; **8**: 663–71.

73 Talwar KK, Varma S, Chopra P et al: Endomyocardial biopsy–technical aspects experience and current status. An Indian perspective. *Int J Cardiol* 1994; **43**: 327–34.

74 Fowler NO: Constrictive pericarditis: its history and current status. *Clin Radiol* 1995; **18**: 341–50.

13

Pericardial diseases: effusion, tamponade and constriction. Clinical and imaging perspectives

Henry H Chong and Gary D Plotnick

The pericardium is composed of two distinct components: (1) the visceral pericardium, a smooth serous inner membrane composed of a single layer of mesothelial cells that is the external surface of the heart itself; and (2) the parietal pericardium, a 1-mm layer of dense collagenous fibrous tissue with interspersed elastic fibrils lined with a layer of mesothelial cells.[1] The two layers of pericardium join at their attachment points, which creates a small potential space between them, the pericardial sac. The pericardial space normally contains 15–50 cm^3 of fluid that serves as a lubricant between the two layers of the pericardium. The visceral pericardium is thought to be the source of the pericardial fluid, which is an ultrafiltrate of the plasma. The drainage of the pericardial fluid is through the right lymphatic duct via the right pleural space, and by the thoracic duct via the parietal pericardium.

The two most prominent disorders of the pericardium are pericardial effusion with its complications, and constrictive pericarditis. These two disorders will be discussed in detail in this chapter.

Pericardial effusion (PE)

The pericardium reacts to injury by production of effusion, fibrin formation, and cellular proliferation. PE may or may not be hemodynamically significant, but the presence of an effusion indicates underlying pathology. The causes of PE include malignancy, infection, autoimmune disorders, renal failure, heart failure, acute myocardial infarction, trauma, complication of invasive procedures, radiation exposure, inflammatory disorders, chylopericardium, dissecting aortic aneurysm, myxedema, drug-induced and idiopathic causes.[2]

Clinical diagnosis

Patients with PE, even if this is large, may not have any symptoms if the effusion develops slowly. However, if accumulation is rapid, even small volumes may lead to cardiac tamponade (discussed later). Patients with large effusion occasionally describe chest pressure or aching as well as symptoms that result from compression of adjacent structures such as dysphagia, cough, dyspnea, hiccups, or hoarseness. Patients with small PE may be entirely normal on physical examination, whereas patients with large PE may have distant heart sounds or cardiac dullness extending beyond the area of the apical impulse. Ewart's sign (an area of dullness on percussion, bronchial breathing, and bronchophony beneath the angle of the left scapula), which is caused by compression of the base of the left lung by pericardial fluid, may be present. Electrocardiographic changes tend to be nonspecific, but a large effusion may result in low QRS voltage or electrical alternans if there is a swinging motion of the heart within the pericardium.

Imaging modalities

Several different imaging techniques are available for diagnosis of PE. These include chest radiography, echocardiography (ECHO), computed tomography (CT), and magnetic resonance imaging (MRI).

Chest radiography may suggest PE with an enlarged cardiac silhouette or an unexplained increase in transverse cardiac diameter compared to previous chest radiographs, particularly if a pericardial fat stripe is seen within the cardiac silhouette. Differentiation between four-chamber

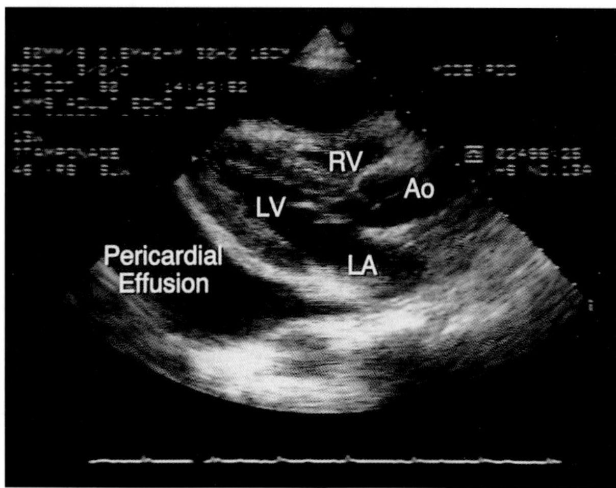

Figure 13.1
Two-dimensional echocardiography parasternal long-axis view shows a large pericardial effusion. Ao, aorta; LA, left atrium; LV, left ventricle; RV, right ventricle.

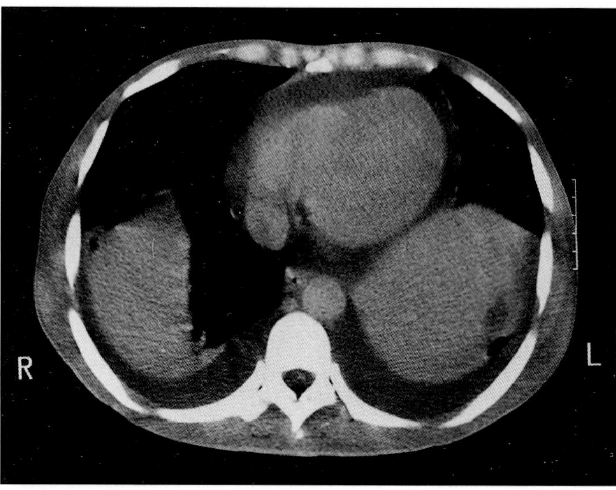

Figure 13.2
Two-dimensional echocardiography short-axis view by computed tomography shows pericardial and pleural effusions. (Courtesy of Dr Charles White.)

dilatation and a large effusion is difficult, while small PE may be inapparent. In 87 patients with ECHO-confirmed PE and 17 controls without PE, Eisenberg et al found that chest radiographic signs were unreliable in either confirming or excluding the presence of a PE.[3]

ECHO has become the imaging technique of choice for detecting a PE with technically good studies yielding very high sensitivity and specificity.[4] A major advantage of ECHO over other imaging modalities is its ability to be brought to the bedside of critically ill patients. On M-mode ECHO, an echo-free space between parietal and visceral pericardium that persists throughout the cardiac cycle is the diagnostic feature.[5] False-positive PE on M-mode ECHO may occur if attention is not paid to technique and angulation of the imaging probe. Two-dimensional (2-D) ECHO has the advantage of showing the size and distribution of the effusion while it enables the operator to distinguish other causes of echo-free spaces such as pleural effusion, enlarged coronary sinus, mitral annular calcification, and descending thoracic aorta. Figure 13.1 illustrates the presence of a large PE on 2-D ECHO. A semiquantitative approach in describing the size of an effusion is frequently used. An echo-free space located posteriorly and <1 cm at its greatest width is designated small, while PE with both anterior and posterior echo-free space but <1 cm is considered moderate. A large PE is defined as an echo-free space that surrounds the heart and is at least 1 cm in width. Eisenberg and others found this method of quantifying the effusion to offer better prognostic information in hospitalized patients than ECHO signs of tamponade.[6] Tamponade and its diagnosis are discussed below.

Following cardiac surgery or pericarditis, localized adhesions may give rise to loculated PE. In such cases, transesophageal echocardiography (TEE) may be necessary to adequately image the effusion. Use of TEE is particularly helpful when proper positioning of the ECHO transducer on the patient is difficult.

In some circumstances, echocardiographic findings may be misinterpreted or nondiagnostic in detecting PE. False-positive interpretations may occur owing to pleural effusions, atelectasis, or mediastinal lesions appearing as effusions, epicardial fat, or pericardial thickening. False-negative interpretations may occur with loculated effusion or hemopericardium.[7] An additional shortcoming of ECHO is that pericardial thickening cannot be reliably determined.

CT can detect as little as 50 cm^3 of pericardial effusion.[8] Effusion is easily seen with CT scan because of the different X-ray absorption coefficients of pericardial fluid and the pericardium.[9] Figure 13.2 shows a CT scan of a patient with a large pericardial effusion. The false-positive rate is less with CT than ECHO reflecting better resolution of boundaries between cardiac, pleural, pericardial, and mediastinal structures. In addition, the composition of the

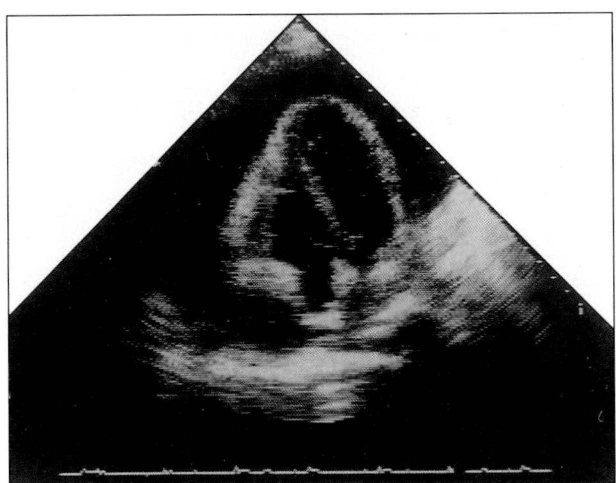

Figure 13.3
Two-dimensional echocardiography apical four-chamber view in late diastole shows right atrial collapse in a patient with tamponade.

effusion may be determined by CT since attenuation coefficients for exudate, chyle, and serous fluid may be sufficiently different to allow identification.[9] Hemopericardium, however, may be difficult to identify because of similar radiodensity of blood and myocardium. The obvious disadvantage of the CT is the need for patient travel to the CT scanner.

MRI can detect PE with high sensitivity, identifying fluid collections as little as 30 cm^3,[10] and size estimation by MRI correlates well with ECHO findings. MRI can accurately define loculated effusion and pericardial thickening. Comparing MRI and 2-D ECHO for PE diagnosis, Mulvagh et al found that the MRI's ability to easily visualize epicardial borders and pericardial fat pad enabled detection of small pericardial effusions that were not detected by ECHO, and that MRI was clearly superior in distinguishing PE from pleural effusion.[11] MRI, as with CT, can image other abnormalities including pericardial inflammation or cysts. With both CT and MRI, pericardial thickness of >4 mm is considered abnormal, and if present, may give a clue as to the cause of the effusion. MRI has the potential to characterize the nature of the PE and has been shown to distinguish hemorrhagic and nonhemorrhagic exudative effusions from transudative effusions in an experimental canine model.[12] The disadvantage of requiring patient transport to the scanner, however, is also present with MRI.

Tamponade

In 1689, Richard Lower, a Cornish physiologist, beautifully described tamponade: 'It sometimes happens that a profuse effusion oppresses and inundates the heart. The envelope becomes filled... The walls of the heart are compressed by the fluid circling everywhere, so that the heart cannot dilate sufficiently to receive the blood... then the pulse becomes exceedingly small, until finally it becomes utterly suppressed by the great inundation of fluid, thence succeed syncope and death itself.'[13]

Cardiac tamponade is best defined as hemodynamic abnormalities that result from accumulation of pericardial effusion *under pressure*. The hemodynamic abnormalities span a spectrum from mild to severe, potentially leading to death.[14] The hemodynamic effects depend on the volume of pericardial fluid and the rapidity with which the fluid accumulates.[15] As aforementioned, rapid accumulation of even a small to moderate amount of PE (as occurs postoperatively or from a traumatic stab wound) may result in full blown tamponade, whereas chronic accumulation of a large amount of PE may be reasonably well tolerated.

The physiology of tamponade may be best explained by reviewing a dog laboratory experiment where increasing amounts of fluid are placed into the pericardial space.[16] Initially, the pericardial pressure rises from the normal (approximately 0 mmHg) to the level of the right atrial or right ventricular diastolic pressure (approximately 5 mmHg). With further accumulation of fluid, pericardial pressure rises to more than the higher level of left atrial or left ventricular diastolic pressure (approximately 10 mmHg). Because these chambers are unable to relax to a lower pressure than that of the surrounding PE, there is the classic *equilibration of diastolic pressures* throughout the heart and pericardium. This increased diastolic pressure reduces venous return (decreased preload), leading to decreased stroke volume which eventually may result in a progressive decrease in cardiac output with hypotension and death.

The sine qua non of tamponade, the presence of a PE, may be confirmed by ECHO, CT or MRI, but detection of tamponade itself depends on specific clinical, hemodynamic, and ECHO findings.

Clinical diagnosis

Symptoms and signs of tamponade include dyspnea, tachypnea, tachycardia, hypotension, jugular venous distention and pulsus paradoxus.[17] The frequency of these features depends on the degree of tamponade. Some or all may be absent in early tamponade, but most will be present in hemodynamically significant or advanced tamponade.

Increased pericardial pressure results in elevated right atrial and jugular venous pressure with characteristic jugular venous wave forms. Instead of the normal systolic X and diastolic Y descents, patients with tamponade have a jugular venous pattern with only an X descent. An absent Y descent is highly suggestive of hemodynamically significant tamponade and occurs because the only time the heart can fill is when blood leaves the heart (during systole). Another hallmark of tamponade is *pulsus paradoxus*, an accentuation of normal drop in systolic blood pressure with inspiration (≥10 mmHg, or >10% decrease). To measure the degree of paradox, a blood pressure cuff is inflated above systolic pressure, then slowly deflated while carefully noting the point at which Korotkoff sounds are heard at first during expiration only. As the cuff is further deflated, sounds are heard during both inspiration and expiration. When this difference exceeds 10 mmHg, pulsus paradoxus is present. The term 'pulsus' originated in 1873 with the description by Kussmaul noting the disappearance of a patient's palpable pulse during inspiration (due to the marked decrease in systolic pressure).[18] There are various conditions where pulsus paradoxus cannot be reliably measured or interpreted. Pulsus paradoxus cannot be determined in patients with irregular rhythms, may be present in conditions such as asthma or chronic obstructive lung disease (where there are marked shifts in intrapleural pressure), and may be absent in patients with tamponade who have left ventricular hypertrophy, severe left ventricular failure, severe hypovolemia, a large atrial septal defect, or severe aortic regurgitation.

Clinical suspicion should be high for patients who present with dyspnea, fatigue, increased jugular venous pressure, and increased cardiac silhouette with clear lung fields on the chest roentgenogram. Further evaluation is imperative in patients with clinical conditions known to be associated with tamponade, such as neoplasm, renal failure, or following penetrating cardiac injury. A high index of suspicion is important in making the diagnosis of tamponade.

Hemodynamic criteria

The diagnosis of tamponade is best confirmed by hemodynamic measurements. In hemodynamically significant tamponade, there is equalization of diastolic pressure in all chambers of the heart that approximates to the intrapericardial pressure. Simultaneously, cardiac output is decreased, but increases substantially (often by more than 50%) when the pericardial fluid is drained. Obviously, lesser degrees of hemodynamic compromise may be present in milder forms of tamponade. Whenever the diagnosis is in doubt and the clinical situation allows, hemodynamic measurements are indicated.

Table 13.1 Echocardiographic clues of tamponade.

Swinging heart
Right atrial collapse
Right ventricular diastolic collapse
Left atrial collapse
Left ventricular diastolic collapse
Marked inspiratory changes in ventricular dimensions
Marked respiratory variation in Doppler velocities (flow velocity paradoxus)
Inferior vena cava plethora

Echocardiographic clues

A number of ECHO signs have been proposed as clues of tamponade (Table 13.1).

A swinging heart within the ECHO-free pericardial sac may be seen, particularly in large effusions, but this is neither sensitive nor specific for tamponade. Right atrial and right ventricular collapse are the most commonly used ECHO clues for tamponade.[19–23] Right atrial collapse, which occurs in late diastole or early systole, reflects increased pericardial pressure inverting the right atrial wall inward when the right atrial pressure is lowest (Fig. 13.3). This is best recorded in the apical four-chamber or parasternal short-axis view and is a relatively early sign of increased pericardial pressure. Of 127 patients with moderate or large pericardial effusion studied by Gilliam et al, right atrial collapse was seen in all patients with cardiac tamponade, but it was also seen in 19 of 104 patients without hemodynamic compromise.[19] In the literature, ECHO evidence of right atrial collapse has a sensitivity of approximately 55–60% and specificity in the range of 50–68%.[19–20] Right ventricular collapse, which occurs in early diastole when the right ventricular diastolic pressure is lowest, is believed to be a sign of a somewhat more advanced degree of increased pericardial pressure (Fig. 13.4). Singh and colleagues found that right ventricular collapse was associated with a significant decrease in cardiac output and blood pressure in patients with hemodynamic evidence of tamponade.[21] With pericardial drainage, hemodynamic improvement continued to occur even after resolution of the right ventricular diastolic collapse in these patients, suggesting that right ventricular collapse is a relatively late sign of tamponade. Volume status of the patient, however, may affect this finding. Klopfenstein et al showed that hypovolemic experimental animals can show right ventricular diastolic collapse at lower intrapericardial

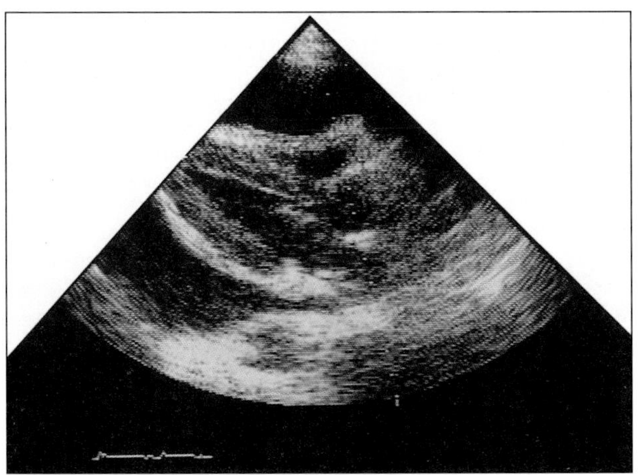

Figure 13.4
Two-dimensional echocardiography parasternal long-axis view in early diastole shows right ventricular collapse in a patient with tamponade.

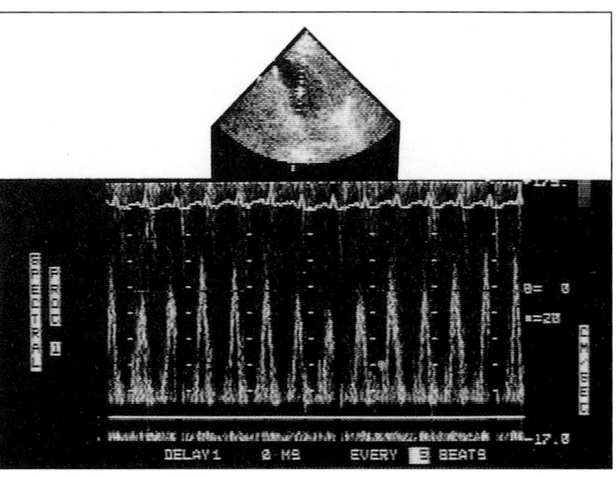

Figure 13.5
Doppler transmitral velocities with pulse wave sample volume placed at tips of mitral valve leaflets show marked respiratory variation (decreases during inspiration).

pressures than during euvolemia or hypervolemia.[22] In the literature, right ventricular diastolic collapse has a sensitivity for detecting tamponade of 38–48% and specificity in the range of 84–100%.[21–23] The key point is that *neither* right atrial nor right ventricular collapse is 100% sensitive or specific for tamponade. Right-sided collapse may not occur if there is right ventricular hypertrophy or pulmonary hypertension. Presence of right atrial or right ventricular diastolic collapse does not automatically necessitate therapeutic intervention, and clinical status should guide the need for intervention.

Left atrial and left ventricular collapse have also been described with tamponade, particularly in perioperative patients with loculated effusions, but both have a low sensitivity.

Doppler *flow velocity paradoxus*, a reciprocal respiratory variation in transvalvular right- and left-sided flow velocities, has been recently described and thought to be a sensitive sign of hemodynamically significant tamponade.[24] Normally, there is no substantial respiratory variation in early diastolic filling velocities. With tamponade, there may be exaggerated increases in right-sided flow velocities and exaggerated decreases in left-sided flow velocities during inspiration (Fig. 13.5). Appleton et al reported an inspiratory decrease in early mitral flow velocity of 43 ± 9% in seven patients with tamponade compared with <10% in normal subjects.[24] With tamponade, the inspiratory decrease in intrapleural pressure is not reflected in intracardiac pressure change due to the surrounding PE, leading to a fall in pulmonary venous pressure but without a corresponding decrease in left ventricular diastolic pressure. Hence, pressure gradient between pulmonary veins and left ventricle declines during inspiration, resulting in reduced early transmitral velocity.[8] While a similar phenomenon may occur with chronic obstructive pulmonary disease, the maximum decrease in this condition tends to occur later during inspiration. In tamponade, maximum decrease occurs on the first beat after the onset of inspiration. Thus, an immediate substantial decrease in Doppler transmitral flow velocity with inspiration or flow velocity paradoxus suggests tamponade physiology.

Recently, Plotnick and colleagues reported an evaluation of ECHO clues in 17 patients with hemodynamically significant tamponade versus 15 patients with large PE without tamponade. The predictive accuracy of right atrial collapse, right ventricular collapse and flow velocity paradoxus were 72%, 72%, and 78%, respectively.[25] In their study, the most accurate sign of tamponade appeared to be inferior vena cava plethora. Normally, the proximal inferior vena cava imaged from the subcostal view decreases by >50% in diameter after a deep inspiration or a sniff.[26] When right atrial pressure is elevated (as occurs with tamponade), the inferior vena cava will not decrease in diameter with these maneuvers. The absence of inferior vena cava plethora makes the presence of tamponade very unlikely (since it suggests normal right atrial pressure). Unfortunately, inferior vena cava plethora may be present in any cause of increased right atrial pressure.

Management of the patient with a pericardial effusion

Need for intervention

If the patient is not hemodynamically compromised, intervention is directed toward management of the underlying etiology if known (such as treatment of heart failure or renal failure) and pericardial drainage is considered only if the diagnosis is unknown. Prompt diagnostic pericardiocentesis is indicated if infection is thought to be playing a role in the etiology of the PE. Hemodynamically significant cardiac tamponade is an indication for urgent intervention to reduce the intrapericardial pressure and improve the hemodynamic situation. Rapid intravenous administration of fluid may help sustain the patient's cardiac output until definitive therapy is available.

Intervention

There are nonsurgical and surgical methods of managing pericardial effusions. Nonsurgical methods include pericardiocentesis with or without catheter drainage, percutaneous balloon pericardiotomy, and sclerotherapy. Surgical management includes pericardial window placement via the subxiphoid or left thoracotomy approach, and pericardiectomy after median sternotomy.

In the absence of continuous bleeding into the pericardium, simple pericardiocentesis may be sufficient as initial treatment. Performed with local anesthesia through a subxyphoid approach, especially with echocardiographic guidance, pericardiocentesis can be a safe procedure. Possible complications include ventricular puncture, cardiac arrhythmia, and pneumothorax. In addition to removing the effusion from the pericardial space, pericardiocentesis allows for analysis of the composition of the fluid. Hemodynamic improvement generally occurs with removal of 50–100 cm^3 of fluid, and once pericardial pressure is below the right atrial pressure, no further hemodynamic improvement may be seen even with further drainage.[27] Continuous drainage can be achieved by placing an indwelling drainage catheter with multiple side holes in the pericardial space. Analysis of the fluid may be useful in diagnosing the cause of the effusion. In patients with malignant pericardial effusion, the cytology may be positive in up to 87% of the cases,[28] but for patients without malignancy the yield is much lower. Ziskind et al have advocated the use of pericardial biopsy using a biotome at the time of the pericardiocentesis to increase the diagnostic yield.[29] In a study of 27 patients, Ziskind et al reported that biopsy increased the chance of obtaining a specific diagnosis from 46% to 62% in patients with malignancy, and from 7% to 29% in patients without malignancy.[29] Because limited pericardial tissue is obtained with this approach, it should not be expected to equal surgical approaches. However, it may have a useful role in patients who cannot tolerate a surgical procedure.

Recurrent pericardial effusions

Although pericardiocentesis is good initial treatment, it can be anticipated that up to 50% of patients will have a recurrence of PE, with the highest frequency occurring with malignancy.[30] Unfortunately, patients with malignant pericardial involvement tend to be in poor general condition and, therefore, are not ideal candidates for surgical intervention. For these patients a newer catheter-based technique termed 'percutaneous balloon pericardiotomy' may be a suitable option (Fig. 13.6).[31] This technique begins with a pericardiocentesis under fluoroscopic guidance in a cardiac catheterization laboratory. Once the pericardial space is entered, a guidewire is placed in the pericardial sac and a balloon catheter is passed over the guidewire and positioned with the balloon straddling the parietal pericardium. Inflation of the balloon then creates an opening in the pericardium that allows internal drainage of the effusion into the pleural space where the reabsorption capacity is much greater. This procedure can be performed

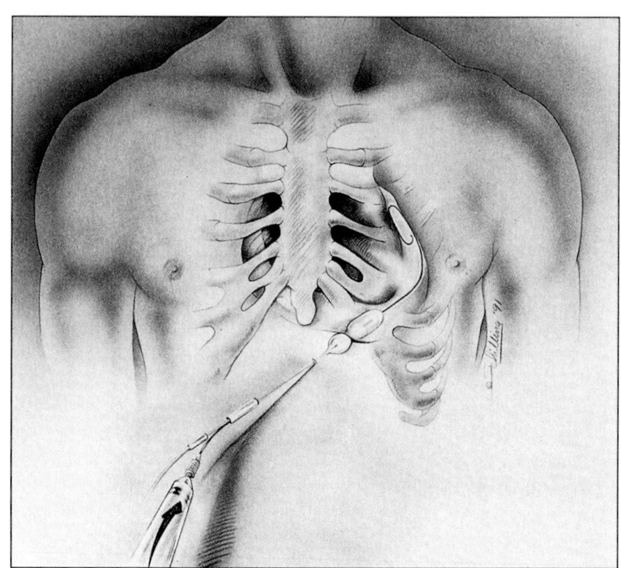

Figure 13.6
Percutaneous balloon pericardiotomy technique. The dilating balloon is advanced over a guidewire to straddle the pericardial margin; it is then inflated to create a pericardial window. (Courtesy of Dr Andrew Ziskind.)

under local anesthesia with minimal sedation. However, it does require a cardiac catheterization laboratory and an experienced operator. In their experience of 50 cases of balloon pericardiotomy for malignant effusions, Ziskind et al reported a success rate of 92%.[32] During the follow-up period of 3.6 ± 3.3 months, 30 of the 50 patients died with a mean survival of 3.3 ± 3.1 months. This high mortality was thought to be due to the primary malignancy itself as opposed to the effusive aspect of the disease or the procedure. Complications of this approach occurred in a minority of patients and included pleural effusions requiring thoracentesis or chest tube drainage, transient fever, and small pneumothorax.

For patients with recurrent effusion, a number of agents have been instilled into the pericardial space. Specific guidelines for use of these agents, however, have not been established. These agents have been selected because of their antitumor activity in cases of malignant effusion, or specific irritant properties intended to cause inflammatory reaction that will sclerose the pericardial space. Agents used have included tetracycline, bleomycin, OK-432, cisplatin, mitomycin C, nitrogen mustard, teniposide, fluorouracil, thiotepa, quinacrine, gold, radionuclides, and ^{131}I-HMFG2 (radioactive iodine coupled to a tumor-associated monoclonal antibody).[33] Varying success rates have been reported with an overall intrapericardial sclerosis success rate of about 80%.[33] Surgical interventions are more invasive, generally have a higher rate of complication, and necessitate longer hospitalization. However, there are several situations when surgery is indicated. In particular, when other modes of therapy fail to control recurrent effusion, surgery is imperative, especially if fluid reaccumulation is rapid. Surgery is indicated for diagnosis of persistent PE of unknown etiology. In properly selected patients, pericardial window via subxiphoid approach is approximately 90% effective in controlling pericardial effusion. In most cases, this procedure can be performed with local anesthesia, thereby avoiding the hemodynamic changes associated with general anesthesia. This approach offers the additional advantage of providing a larger and more optimal pericardial biopsy specimen. In a relatively large series of >100 patients undergoing subxiphoid pericardial window placement, intraoperative mortality associated with the procedure was 1.7% and recurrence rate was 4–11%.[34–35] Patients who fail this procedure usually require total pericardiectomy.

Summary of pericardial effusion

Pericardial effusions may be present in a variety of clinical situations, often presenting challenging clinical diagnostic and therapeutic problems. Although several imaging modalities are available, ECHO has become the diagnostic method of choice due to its portability and wide availability. CT and MRI may also be employed and may be more accurate. A PE under pressure may result in hemodynamic compromise and tamponade. Although there are several echocardiographic clues to tamponade (including diastolic chamber collapse, Doppler flow velocity paradoxus, and inferior vena cava plethora), the diagnosis remains a clinical and hemodynamic one. The clinical signs include elevated jugular venous pressure, hypotension, tachycardia, and pulsus paradoxus. Hemodynamic measurements include equalization of diastolic pressures and decreased cardiac output. Treatment of tamponade involves drainage of the effusion and prevention of reaccumulation. Needle pericardiocentesis via the subxiphoid approach is a reasonable initial treatment. However, this may need to be accompanied by catheter drainage or surgical pericardial window. A new catheter-based technique — percutaneous balloon pericardiotomy — appears useful in select patients with malignancy in order to avoid more invasive surgical procedures. Occasionally, in patients with recurrent effusions, instillation of sclerosing agents into the pericardial space or even total pericardiectomy may be necessary.

Constrictive pericarditis

Historical perspective and etiologies

The condition of constrictive pericarditis has been recognized for a long time. Pericardial knock was described by Corrigan in 1842, paradoxical arterial pulse in mediastinopericarditis was described by Kussmaul in 1873, and ascites and hepatomegaly attributed to constrictive pericarditis was noted by Pick in 1879. In 1935 White described constrictive pericarditis as a chronic fibrous thickening of the wall of the pericardial sac which is so contracted that normal diastolic filling of the heart is prevented.[36] Despite the recognition of its existence, Osler noted 'No serious disease so frequently overlooked by the practitioner' as is pericardial disease.[37]

Historically tuberculous pericarditis had been a frequent cause of pericardial disease, but a decline in the incidence of tuberculosis (TB) has been paralleled by a decrease in TB pericarditis. Causes of constrictive pericarditis are many, and include all the causes of pericardial effusion already noted. In large series, the most common causes were noted to be idiopathic or viral, post-surgical, and post-radiation treatment.[38–39]

The diagnosis of constrictive pericarditis has been, and continues to be, a challenge to the physician because its symptoms may overlap with many other clinical conditions and because of the difficulty in differentiating it from restrictive cardiomyopathy. The importance of correct diagnosis cannot be overstated, however, since the treatment of constrictive pericarditis is surgical, namely pericardiectomy, whereas the treatment of restrictive cardiomyopathy and many other causes of heart failure are often medical.

Clinical presentations

Patients can present with a variety of clinical symptoms. These include edema, dyspnea on exertion, fatigue, increasing abdominal girth, abdominal pain, and fever. Physical examination may reveal jugular venous distention, hepatomegaly, ascites, peripheral edema, Kussmaul's sign, pericardial rub, pericardial knock, and rarely, pulsus paradoxus. Because symptoms and signs overlap with other clinical causes of congestive heart failure, the physician must have a high index of suspicion to consider constrictive pericarditis.

Hemodynamics

Hemodynamic parameters measured during right and left heart catheterization have been used to diagnose constrictive pericarditis, and to differentiate between constrictive pericarditis and restrictive cardiomyopathy as outlined in Table 13.2. Hemodynamic characteristics of constrictive

Table 13.2 Differentiating features of constrictive pericarditis and restrictive cardiomyopathy.

Constrictive pericarditis	*Restrictive cardiomyopathy*
Hemodynamics	
RVEDP approximately equal to LVEDP	RVEDP and LVEDP differ by >5 mmHg
RV systolic pressure ≤50 mmHg	RV systolic pressure ≥50 mmHg
RVEDP >1/3 RV systolic pressure	RVEDP <1/3 RV systolic pressure
Two-dimensional echocardiography	
Thickened pericardium	Normal pericardium
Pericardial effusion	
Diastolic septal bounce	
M-mode echocardiography	
Major filling period of the LV is shorter than normal	Major filling period of the LV is longer than normal
Time from minimal LV dimension to peak filling is shorter than normal	Time from minimal LV dimension to peak filling is longer than normal
Maximal thinning rate of LV posterior wall is greater than normal	
Peak rate of thickening of the posterior wall is greater than normal	
Per cent thickening of the posterior wall is greater than normal	
Doppler echocardiography	
Decreased transmitral Doppler velocity at the onset of inspiration, and increased velocity at the onset of expiration	Little respiratory changes in Doppler velocities
Increased tricuspid inflow velocity at the onset of inspiration, and decreased velocity at the onset of expiration	
Decreased venous diastolic forward flow velocity of pulmonary veins with inspiration	
Expiratory augmentation of diastolic hepatic vein flow reversal	
CT and MRI	
Pericardial thickness of >4 mm	Pericardial thickness of <4 mm
Tubular appearance of right ventricle	Normal right ventricle

pericarditis include: near equalization of increased diastolic pressures between right and left side of the heart, prominent X and Y descents in the right atrial pressure tracings, and 'dip and plateau sign' of right ventricular end-diastolic pressure.[40] Other specific hemodynamic criteria to differentiate constrictive from restrictive disorders have been described. Wood found that equalization (≤5 mmHg) of right ventricular end-diastolic pressure (RVEDP) with left ventricular end-diastolic pressure (LVEDP) favors constriction.[41] Modest elevation of right ventricular (RV) systolic pressure to ≤50 mmHg is more suggestive of constriction, whereas RV systolic pressure >50 mmHg favors restrictive cardiomyopathy.[42] In constriction, RVEDP tends to be greater than a third of RV systolic pressure, whereas in restrictive cardiomyopathy RVEDP tends to be less than a third of RV systolic pressure.[42] In 1991 Vaitkus and Kussmaul[43] reviewed hemodynamics data of 82 cases of constrictive pericarditis and 37 cases of restrictive cardiomyopathy. They found the overall predictive accuracy of the difference between RVEDP and LVEDP, RV systolic pressure, and the ratio of RVEDP to RV systolic pressure to be 85%, 70%, and 76%, respectively. If all were concordant, the probability of correct classification was >90%. However, of those patients studied, 25% could not be classified.

Volume infusion and exercise while RVEDP and LVEDP are monitored have been used in an attempt to differentiate these two conditions. Both maneuvers are thought to raise RVEDP and LVEDP equally in constrictive pericarditis, but show a greater rise in LVEDP than RVEDP in restrictive cardiomyopathy. The reason for this pressure behavior is that in constrictive pericarditis the filling of both right and left sides of the heart is unimpaired initially until the combined volume reaches the limit set by the poorly compliant, fibrotic pericardium. After this point both RV pressure and LV pressure will go up in parallel as filling continues. In restrictive cardiomyopathy there is impairment of the LV to fill; however, the RV is not impaired as much due to its thinner wall. Thus with increased filling in this latter condition, the LVEDP will rise more than the RVEDP. The volume infusion is based on work by Bush et al who reported on 19 patients with symptoms compatible with constrictive pericarditis and normal LV function.[44] In these patients, normal baseline hemodynamics were first noted, then after a rapid infusion of isotonic saline, an increase in both LVEDP and RVEDP was noted. Eleven of 19 patients underwent pericardiectomy with good clinical result; 12 patients with 'myocardial disease' served as controls, but no restrictive cardiomyopathy patients were used as controls. Vaitkus and Kussmaul, in their work of reappraising the diagnostic criteria for restriction and constriction, have pointed out that neither exercise nor volume infusion hemodynamics have undergone controlled prospective evaluation, and that the usefulness of these maneuvers is not yet fully defined.[43]

Imaging modalities

Other ways to further characterize constrictive pericarditis, thereby differentiating it from restrictive cardiomyopathy, include measuring the thickness of the pericardium using a variety of different imaging modalities or measuring diastolic filling parameters using Doppler echocardiography, or high resolution radionuclide ventriculography.

The primary imaging modalities for evidence of pericardial disease include echocardiography, CT, and MRI. The ability to accurately demonstrate thickened and calcified pericardium in a patient with clinical and hemodynamic parameters suggestive of constrictive pericarditis is sufficient to make the diagnosis. CT and MRI are especially useful in this regard since they can best evaluate the pericardial thickness. The normal pericardium is <3-mm thick. Pericardial thickness in normal subjects by MRI is reported to be 1.2 ± 0.5 mm in diastole and 1.7 ± 0.5 mm in systole.[45]

Chest roentgenography may identify diffuse calcification of the pericardium, which in the appropriate clinical setting may strongly suggest constrictive pericarditis. However, chest roentgenography cannot be used to directly measure the thickness of the pericardium. In patients with constrictive pericarditis a typical chest X-ray shows clear lung fields and heart of normal size. The cardiac silhouette may be enlarged in a patient with effusive–constrictive pericarditis.

Echocardiography

There are a number of echocardiographic clues of constrictive pericarditis. These can be categorized as two-dimensional, M-mode, and Doppler findings.

Two-dimensional features:

The 2-D ECHO features include thickened pericardium (with or without calcification), presence of PE, diastolic septal bounce, inferior vena cava plethora, presence of tubular right ventricle, and right atrial enlargement in the setting of normal LV size and function. All these features are suggestive but not diagnostic of constrictive pericarditis. Unfortunately, measurement of pericardial thickness is not reliable using echocardiography. Hutchinson and colleagues suggested that TEE can offer better resolution of the pericardium than TTE.[46] In their study of 13 patients with constrictive pericarditis TEE demonstrated pericardial thickening in 11 whereas only 5 were detected using TTE. Despite the potential of detecting pericardial thickening with ECHO, CT and MRI are clearly better for measurement of pericardial thickness.

M-mode features

M-mode ECHO comparison of constrictive pericarditis and restrictive cardiomyopathy has been carried out by

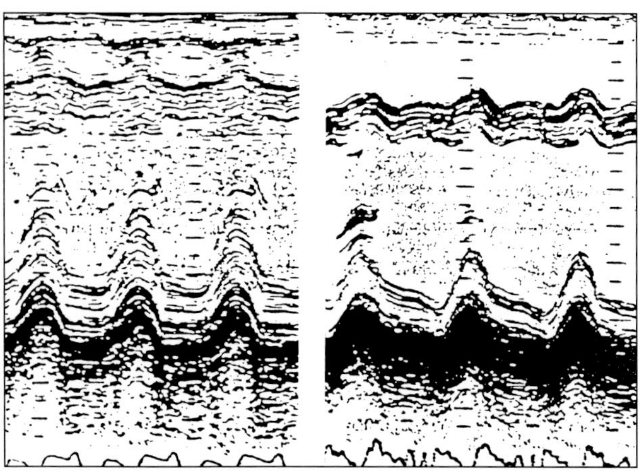

Figure 13.7
M-mode example of left ventricular posterior wall motion in a patient with constrictive pericarditis. Left, an echo prior to pericardiectomy; right, the repeated echo after surgery. See text for details. Courtesy of Dr Alfred Parisi.

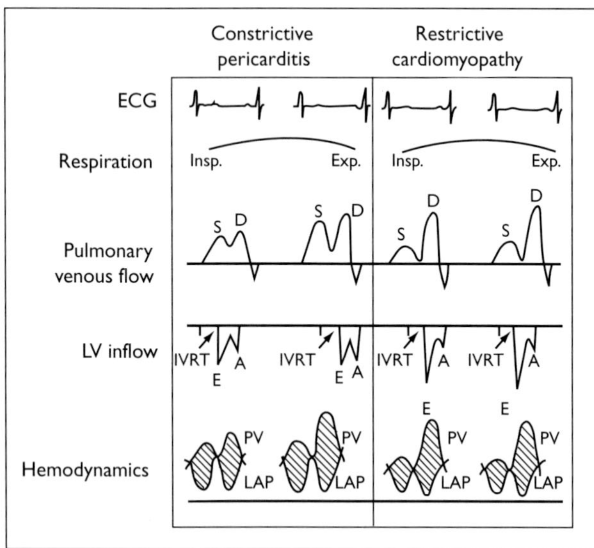

Figure 13.8
The diagram illustrates the respiratory variation of pulmonary venous flow and left ventricular (LV) inflow patterns and their hemodynamics in constrictive pericarditis and restrictive cardiomyopathy. Left, in constrictive pericarditis, the driving pressure from the pulmonary vein (PV) to the left atrium in systole and especially diastole is lower during inspiration (Insp.) than during expiration (Exp.). This results in the large respiratory variation in the pulmonary venous systolic (S) and diastolic (D) flows from expiration to inspiration. The lower transmitral gradient during inspiration should result in a lower peak early (E) filling velocity and a longer isovolumic relaxation time (IVRT) during inspiration. Right, in restrictive cardiomyopathy, the driving pressure from the pulmonary vein to the left atrium is markedly lower during systole than during diastole. The similar gradient during inspiration and expiration results in a markedly decreased pulmonary venous systolic/diastolic flow ratio and no significant variation during the respiratory cycle. There is no significant change in the transmitral gradient and therefore little change in the peak early filling velocity and isovolumic relaxation time from expiration to inspiration. A, late filling velocity; ECG, electrocardiogram; LAP, left atrial pressure. Reproduced with permission from Klein et al.[51]

several investigators. Janos and colleagues in 1983 studied four patients with constriction and three patients with restriction using digitized M-mode ECHO.[47] They found: (1) major filling period of the left ventricle to be significantly shorter than normal in constrictive pericarditis, and significantly longer than normal in restrictive cardiomyopathy; (2) time from minimum left ventricular dimension to peak filling was significantly shorter in constrictive pericarditis; and (3) maximal thinning rate of the left ventricular posterior wall was significantly greater in constrictive pericarditis. In 1989, Morgan and others evaluated digitized M-mode echoes in 13 patients with constrictive pericarditis and 18 patients with restrictive cardiomyopathy.[48] They also found peak rate of thinning of the LV posterior wall to be greater in constrictive pericarditis, but the maximal filling rate did not differ in the two groups. Some notable findings during systole included: (1) peak emptying rate greater in restrictive cardiomyopathy; (2) peak rate of thickening of the posterior wall greater in constrictive pericarditis; and (3) per cent thickening of the posterior wall greater in constrictive pericarditis. However, there was significant overlap of these systolic findings between the two groups. These M-mode features are demonstrated in Figure 13.7 where left ventricular posterior wall motion is shown in a patient with constrictive pericarditis, before and after pericardiectomy.

Doppler features

The classic Doppler flow pattern in constrictive pericarditis is characterized by marked respiratory changes in peak left and right inflow and outflow velocities. This pattern is also seen in cardiac tamponade. An explanation for the respiratory change in transmitral flow velocity follows.

In constrictive pericarditis the presence of thickened and fibrotic pericardium acts to isolate the intracardiac chambers from the normal pressure changes of the intrathoracic cavity during respiration. With inspiration, pulmonary venous pressure drops as intrathoracic pressure decreases. However, the usual drop in left ventricular diastolic pressure seen with inspiration is blunted by the surrounding thickened pericardium. Thus the pulmonary vein to left ventricular diastolic pressure gradient is reduced during inspiration in the presence of a thickened pericardium seen in constrictive pericarditis. This reduced pressure gradient leads to a decrease in transmitral filling gradient with inspiration, and resulting decrease in transmitral Doppler velocity at the onset of inspiration. At the pulmonary veins, the decrease in left-side filling pressure gradient results in a decrease in venous diastolic forward flow velocity. The changes in the pulmonary venous flow and the left ventricular inflow pattern are illustrated in Figure 13.8. The relatively fixed cardiac volume as limited by the pericardium in constrictive pericarditis results in ventricular coupling, and a reciprocal relation between the right and left heart filling. Therefore, decreased filling of the left side during inspiration causes the ventricular septum to shift to the left, and allows for increased filling of the right side. This increased right-sided filling results in an increase in tricuspid inflow velocity during inspiration. The opposite changes occur during expiration. Due to an increase in the left ventricular filling, the septum shifts to the right, with a resulting decrease in right ventricular filling. During expiration there is a decrease in tricuspid inflow velocity, and increased diastolic hepatic vein flow reversal. This is shown graphically in Figure 13.9, and Figure 13.10 schematically illustrates the ventricular coupling as imposed by the poorly compliant pericardium in constrictive pericarditis.

Hatle et al used Doppler ECHO to evaluate mitral and tricuspid inflow pattern with respiratory variation in 7 patients with constrictive pericarditis and 12 patients with restrictive cardiomyopathy.[49] Patients with constrictive pericarditis showed marked inspiratory decrease in early mitral flow velocity and marked inspiratory increase in early

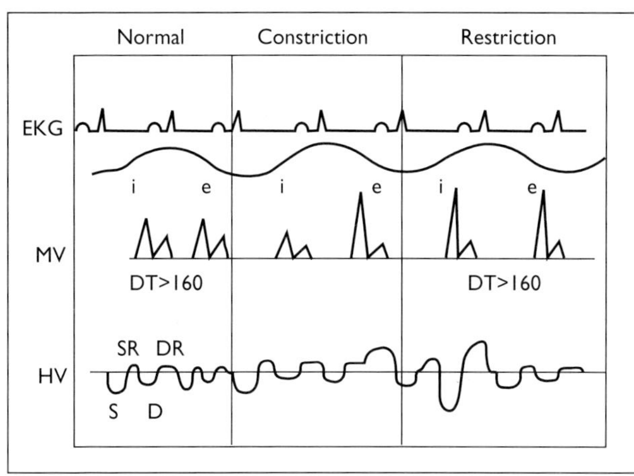

Figure 13.9
Schematic diagram showing the typical Doppler velocity pattern of the mitral inflow (MV) and hepatic vein (HV) in various hemodynamic conditions. Electrocardiogram (EKG) and respitometer tracings are also depicted. See text for details. D, diastolic forward flow; DR, diastolic reversal; DT, deceleration time (ms); e, expiration; i, inspiration; S, systolic forward flow; SR, systolic reversal. Reproduced with permission from Oh et al.[59]

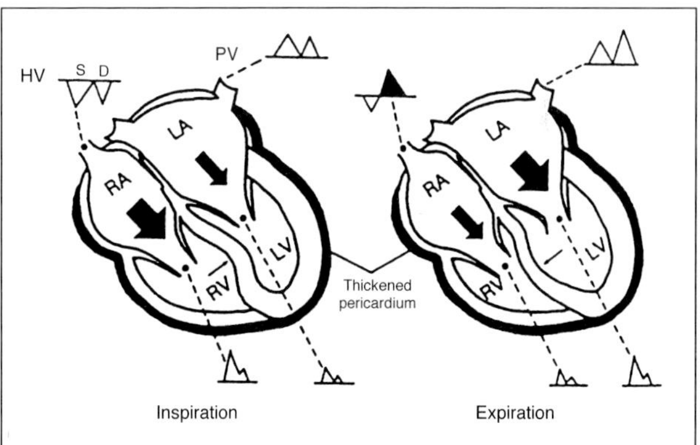

Figure 13.10
Schematic diagram showing the respiratory variation in transvalvular and central venous flow velocities in constrictive pericarditis. With inspiration, the driving pressure gradient from the pulmonary capillaries to the left cardiac chambers decreases, resulting in a decrease in mitral inflow and diastolic pulmonary venous (PV) flow velocity. The decreased left ventricular filling results in ventricular septal shift to the left (small arrow), allowing augmented flow to the right-sided chambers (shown as increased tricuspid inflow and diastolic hepatic venous (HV) flow velocity) because the cardiac volume is relatively fixed as a result of the thickened shell of pericardium. The opposite changes occur during inspiration. D, diastole; LA, left atrium; LV, left ventricle; RA, right atrium; RV, right ventricle; S, systole. Reproduced with permission from Oh et al.[59]

tricuspid flow velocity compared with normal controls and with patients with restrictive cardiomyopathy. Mancuso et al studied 7 patients with constrictive pericarditis and 6 patients with restrictive cardiomyopathy using Doppler ECHO.[50] In patients with constrictive pericarditis they found higher peak diastolic velocities of mitral inflow, and marked increase in velocity of flow at the onset of expiration along with decrease at the onset of inspiration. Reciprocal respiratory variation of the tricuspid inflow velocities were seen. They further demonstrated reversal of hepatic venous flow during systole with accentuated reversal during inspiration. Patients with restricted cardiomyopathy showed little changes in transvalvular velocities with respiration, but had moderate to severe mitral and tricuspid regurgitation. Klein et al studied 14 patients with constrictive pericarditis and 17 with restrictive cardiomyopathy using transesophageal Doppler.[51] They found pulmonary venous peak systolic flow in both inspiration and expiration to be greater and pulmonary venous diastolic flow during inspiration to be lower in the constrictive pericarditis group as compared with the restrictive cardiomyopathy group. During inspiration the pulmonary venous systolic/diastolic flow velocity ratio fell to below 0.65 in constrictive pericarditis patients, and peak diastolic velocity decreased ≥40% on average in the same patients. These features were able to distinguish the two groups of patients. Oh et al also studied Doppler flow characteristics in a study of 28 patients, 25 of whom had constrictive pericarditis documented at surgery.[59] These investigators found ≥25% increase in transmitral early diastolic velocity with expiration compared to inspiration in patients with constrictive pericarditis. In the same series <10% respiratory variation was seen in transmitral velocity in 2 normal and 1 restrictive cardiomyopathy patients. In addition, they noted ≥25% expiratory augmentation of diastolic hepatic vein flow reversal in constrictive pericarditis patients. These Doppler criteria showed a sensitivity of 88% in the 25 patients studied. In a follow-up study of 19 patients who had undergone surgical correction of the constrictive pericarditis, these investigators showed normal findings in 14 and restriction patterns in 5. Twelve of the 14 patients with normal findings became asymptomatic, whereas all 5 patients with a restrictive pattern remained symptomatic. These findings suggest Doppler ECHO to be fairly sensitive in diagnosing constrictive pericarditis, and also in predicting the functional response to pericardiectomy. These Doppler findings, however, may also be present in patients with pulmonary disease and patients with cardiac tamponade.

By combining a strong clinical index of suspicion with careful attention to two-dimensional, M-mode, and Doppler characteristics, one can go a long way in confirming or excluding the diagnosis of constrictive pericarditis. Definitive evaluation of pericardial thickening, however, is dependent upon other imaging modalities.

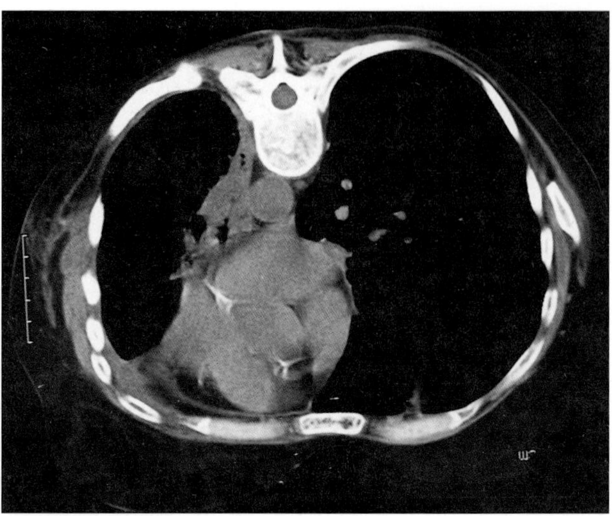

Figure 13.11
Computed tomography of a patient illustrating pericardial effusion and a thickened pericardium. (Courtesy of Dr Charles White.)

Computed tomography

CT and MRI have become established standards in measuring pericardial thickness. Figure 13.11 shows a CT scan of a patient with pericardial effusion and a thickened pericardium. In a study of 100 patients in 1982, Moncada et al established normal pericardial anatomy using CT.[52] In their group, thickness of normal fibrous parietal pericardium was 1–2 mm in 70% of cases. Caudal insertion of the normal pericardium was thicker, sometimes up to 3–4 mm. Patchy areas of thickening were normally found in 30% of the patients. In all 9 patients with surgically proven constrictive pericarditis, CT-detected thickened pericardium was seen as a 5–20 mm thick curvilinear dense structure surrounding the heart. In 1982 Isner et al studied 53 patients with pericardial disease; of these patients, 9 had thickened pericardium, and of these, 4 had surgical confirmation.[53] In 1985, McCaughan et al reported 13 (81%) of 16 patients with constrictive pericarditis to have CT-documented pericardial thickening.[60] In 1989, Killian et al found CT to be helpful in documenting pericardial thickness of 3–19 mm in 23 (79%) of 29 patients with postoperative constrictive pericarditis.[54] In 1992, Suchet and Horwitz reported detection of pericardial thickening in 157 (84%) of 186 patients with constrictive pericarditis caused by TB.[55] In 1994, Oh et al reported finding thickened pericardium by CT in all 21 patients with constrictive pericarditis.[59] Oren et al studied 3 patients with constrictive pericarditis using cine CT.[56] They documented both pericardial thickening and abnormal left ventricular filling fraction as compared to controls. In these studies other CT findings included pericardial calcification, loculated pericardial effusion, inferior vena cava dilatation, deviation of the interventricular septum, and fibrotic changes. These studies all demonstrate the relative high sensitivity of CT to detect thickened pericardium which correlated with constrictive pericarditis.

Magnetic resonance imaging

MRI has shown superior delineation of intracardiac and pericardial structures with the potential to define further tissue characteristics. Sechtem et al demonstrated documentation of thickened pericardium (>4 mm) in 6 of 8 patients with confirmed constrictive pericarditis.[10] They also found a small, tubular-shaped right ventricle to be an additional morphologic sign of constrictive pericarditis. An enlarged right atrium and dilated inferior vena cava were noted, but these were also seen in patients with restrictive cardiomyopathy. Masui et al found sensitivity, specificity, and accuracy of MRI in the diagnosis of constrictive pericarditis to be 88%, 100%, and 93%, respectively in a series of 17 patients with constrictive pericarditis.[57] Pericardial thickening of >4 mm was seen in 88% of the patients with constrictive pericarditis, but not seen in 4 patients with restrictive cardiomyopathy. The most frequent site of pericardial thickening was over the right ventricle. These studies illustrate the high sensitivity of MRI to show thickened pericardium in constrictive pericarditis.

Endomyocardial biopsy

Endomyocardial biopsy remains as the last resort in distinguishing between constrictive pericarditis and restrictive cardiomyopathy in difficult cases. Biopsy is useful if histological diagnosis of infiltrative disease can be made.

Treatment

Treatment of symptomatic constrictive pericarditis is largely surgical. Occasional cases of constrictive pericarditis treated with steroids appear to respond, but only if treatment begins prior to fibrosis of the pericardium. Most patients with symptomatic constrictive pericarditis require pericardiectomy. Cameron et al studied 95 consecutive patients who underwent pericardial resection for constrictive pericarditis.[39] Overall mortality was 12%, with higher mortality (21%) associated with the post-radiation group.[39] DeValeria et al showed overall mortality of 5.6% in a series of 36 patients undergoing pericardiectomy for constrictive pericarditis.[38] In a review of patients who underwent pericardiectomy, Seifert et al showed that 80–90% of hospital survivors had NYHA class I or II functional status.[58]

Summary of constrictive pericarditis

Constrictive pericarditis is a condition of impaired diastolic function of the heart due to physical limitations imposed by a thickened, fibrotic, and poorly compliant pericardium. Constrictive pericarditis can arise from a variety of causes, but the most common etiologies appear to be idiopathic or viral, post-surgical, and post-radiation treatment. Patients may present with signs and symptoms that overlap with heart failure, especially right-sided heart failure. Diagnosis of this condition and differentiation from restrictive cardiomyopathy has been a challenge in the past, and continues to be one today. Hemodynamic studies can be carried out as well as imaging studies including ECHO, CT, and MRI. Unfortunately none of the studies are perfect, and a high clinical index of suspicion is of paramount importance.

ECHO can help in suggesting or excluding the diagnosis, but one must pay careful attention to details of the study including diastolic wall motion in two-dimensional and M-mode, and respiratory variations in transmitral flow velocity as seen in Doppler ECHO. CT and MRI can be used to noninvasively evaluate the thickness of the pericardium. In the appropriate clinical setting pericardial thickness of >4 mm is highly suggestive of constrictive pericarditis. Hemodynamic studies are valuable in confirming the diagnosis. Characteristics of the constrictive pericarditis include near equalization of increased diastolic pressures between right and left side of the heart, prominent X and Y descents in the right atrial pressure tracings, 'dip and plateau sign' of right ventricular end-diastolic pressure, right ventricular systolic pressure <50 mmHg, and RVEDP greater than one-third RV systolic pressure. In difficult cases, endomyocardial biopsy may be necessary to make the correct diagnosis.

In patients with symptomatic constrictive pericarditis, the treatment is surgical pericardiectomy. Patients who successfully undergo the surgery can expect a high chance of symptomatic relief.

Acknowledgement

The discussion of pericardial effusion, tamponade, and management of the patient along with Figures 13.1–13.6 are reproduced from the article: Chong HH, Plotnick GD. Pericardial effusion and tamponade: evaluation, imaging modalities, and management. *Comprehensive Therapy* 1995; **21**: 378–85 with permission of the editors.

The authors express their appreciation to Michael Fisher MD and Andrew Ziskind MD for their critical review of the manuscript, and to Millie Bileck for her excellent secretarial support.

References

1. Lorell BH, Braunwald E: Pericardial disease. In: Braunwald E, ed., *Heart Disease: A Textbook of Cardiovascular Medicine* (WB Saunders: Philadelphia, PA, 1992); 1465.

2. Lorell BH, Braunwald E: Pericardial disease. In: Braunwald E, ed., *Heart Disease. A Textbook of Cardiovascular Medicine* (WB Saunders: Philadelphia, PA, 1992); 1468–9.

3 Eisenberg MJ, Dunn MM, Kanth N et al: Diagnostic value of chest radiography for pericardial effusion. *J Am Coll Cardiol* 1993; **22**: 588–93.

4 Horowitz MS, Schultz CS, Stinson EB et al: Sensitivity and specificity of echocardiographic diagnosis of pericardial effusion. *Circulation* 1974; **50:** 239–47.

5 Feigenbaum H, Waldhausen JA, Hyde LP: Ultrasound diagnosis of pericardial effusion. *JAMA* 1965; **191**: 107–11.

6 Eisenberg MJ, Oken K, Guerrero S et al: Prognostic value of echocardiography in hospitalized patients with pericardial effusion. *Am J Cardiol* 1992; **70**: 934–9.

7 Come PC, Riley MF, Fortuin NJ: Echocardiography mimicry of pericardial effusion. *Am J Cardiol* 1981; **47**: 365–70.

8 Wong BYS, Lee KR, MacArthur RI: Diagnosis of pericardial effusion by computed tomography. *Chest* 1982; **81**: 177–81.

9 Tomoda H, Hoshiai M, Furuya H et al: Evaluation of pericardial effusion with computed tomography. *Am Heart J* 1980; **99**: 701–6.

10 Schectem U, Tscholakoff D, Higgins CB: MRI of the abnormal pericardium. *Am J Radiol* 1986; **147**: 245–52.

11 Mulvagh SL, Rokey R, Vick III GW et al: Usefulness of nuclear magnetic resonance imaging for evaluation of pericardial effusion, and comparison with two-dimensional echocardiography. *Am J Cardiol* 1989; **64**: 1002–9.

12 Rokey R, Vick III W, Bolli R et al: Assessment of experimental pericardial effusion using nuclear magnetic resonance imaging techniques. *Am Heart J* 1991; **121**: 1161–9.

13 Lower R: Tractatus de Corde: Item de Motu et Colare Sanguinis et Chyli in Sum Transitir. *Allestry, London, 1669.*

14 Reddy PS, Curtiss EI, Uresky BF: Spectrum of hemodynamic changes in cardiac tamponade. *Am J Cardiol* 1990; **98**: 627–36.

15 Reddy PS, Curtiss EI. Cardiac tamponade. *Cardiol Clin* 1990; **66**: 1487–91.

16 Savitt MA, Tyson GS, Elbeery JR et al: Physiology of cardiac tamponade and paradoxical pulse in conscious dogs. *Am J Physiol* 1993; **265** (Heart Circ Physiol **24**): H1996–H2008.

17 Kuhn LA: Acute and chronic tamponade. In: Spodick DH, ed., *Pericardial Diseases* (FA Davis Company: Philadelphia, PA, 1976); 177–95.

18 Kussmaul A. Pericarditis and the paradox pulse. *Berl Klin Wochenschr* 1873; **10**: 433–5.

19 Gillam LD, Guyer DE, Gibson TC et al: Hydrodynamic compression of the right atrium: a new echocardiographic sign of cardiac tamponade. *Circulation* 1983; **68**: 294–301.

20 Rifkin RD, Pandian NL, Funai JT et al: Sensitivity of right atrial collapse and right ventricular diastolic collapse in the diagnosis of graded cardiac tamponade. *Am J Noninvas Cardiol* 1987; **1**: 73–80.

21 Singh S, Wann LS, Schuchard GH et al: Right ventricular and right atrial collapse in patients with cardiac tamponade: a combined echocardiographic and hemodynamic study. *Circulation* 1984; **70**: 966–71.

22 Klopfenstein HS, Cogswell TL, Bernarth GA et al: Alterations in intravascular diastolic collapse and the hemodynamic severity of cardiac tamponade. *J Am Coll Cardiol* 1985; **6**: 1057–63.

23 Armstrong WF, Schilt BF, Helper DJ et al: Diastolic collapse of the right ventricle with tamponade: an echocardiographic study. *Circulation* 1982; **65**: 1391–496.

24 Appleton CP, Hatle LK, Popp RL: Cardiac tamponade and pericardial effusion: respiratory variation in transvalvular flow velocities studied by Doppler echocardiography. *J Am Coll Cardiol* 1988; **11**: 1029–30.

25 Plotnick GD, Rubin DC, Feliciano Z et al: Pulmonary hypertension decreases the predictive accuracy of echocardiographic clues for cardiac tamponade. *Chest* 1995; **107**: 919–21.

26 Schiller NB, Botvinick EH: Right ventricular compression as a sign of tamponade: an analysis of echocardiographic

ventricular dimensions and their clinical implications. *Circulation* 1977; **56**: 772–9.

27 Ameli S, Shah PK: Cardiac tamponade: pathophysiology, diagnosis, and management. *Cardiol Clin* 1991; **9**: 665–70.

28 Meyers DG, Bouska DJ: Diagnostic usefulness of pericardial fluid cytology. *Chest* 1989; **95**: 1142–3.

29 Ziskind AA, Rodriguez S, Lemmon C: Percutaneous pericardial biopsy as an adjunctive technique for the diagnosis of pericardial disease. *Am J Cardiol* 1994; **74**: 288–91.

30 Markiewicz W, Borovik R, Ecker S: Cardiac tamponade in medical patients: treatment and prognosis in the echocardiographic era. *Am Heart J* 1986; **111**: 1138–42.

31 Palacios IF, Tuzcu EM, Ziskind AA et al: Percutaneous balloon pericardial window for patients with malignant pericardial effusion and tamponade. *Cathet Cardiovasc Diagn* 1991; **22**: 244–9.

32 Ziskind AA, Pearce AC, Lemmon C et al: Percutaneous balloon pericardiotomy for the treatment of cardiac tamponade and large pericardial effusions: description of technique and report of the first 50 cases. *J Am Coll Cardiol* 1993; **21**: 1–5.

33 Vatikus PT, Herrmann HC, LeWinter MM: Treatment of malignant pericardial effusion. *JAMA* 1994; **272**: 59–64.

34 Ghosh SC, Larrieu AJ, Ablaza SG et al: Clinical experience with subxiphoid pericardial decompression. *Int Surg* 1985; **70**: 5–7.

35 Mills SA, Julian S, Holliday RH et al: Subxiphoid pericardial window for pericardial effusive disease. *J Cardiovasc Surg* 1989; **30**: 768–73.

36 White PD: Chronic constrictive pericarditis (Pick's disease). Treated by pericardial resection. *Lancet* 1935; **2**: 539–48, 597–603.

37 Osler W: *The Principles and Practice of Medicine* (D Appleton Co: New York, 1892).

38 DeValeria PA, Baumgartner WA, Casale AS et al: Current indications, risks, and outcome after pericardiectomy. *Ann Thorac Surg* 1991; **52**: 219–24.

39 Cameron J, Oesterle SN, Baldwin JC et al: The etiologic spectrum of constrictive pericarditis. *Am Heart J* 1987; **113**: 354–60.

40 Hansen AT, Eskildsen P, Gotzsche H: Pressure curves from the right auricle and the right ventricle in chronic constrictive pericarditis. *Circulation* 1951; **3**: 881–8.

41 Wood P. Chronic constrictive pericarditis. *Am J Cardiol* 1961; **7**: 48–61.

42 Yu PN, Lovejoy FW, Joos HA et al: Right auricular and ventricular pressure patterns in constrictive pericarditis. *Circulation* 1953; **7**: 102–7.

43 Vaitkus PT, Kussmaul WG: Constrictive pericarditis versus restrictive cardiomyopathy: a reappraisal and update of diagnostic criteria. *Am Heart J* 1991; **122**: 1431–41.

44 Bush CA, Stang JM, Wooley CF et al: Occult constrictive pericardial disease. Diagnosis by rapid volume expansion and correction by pericardiectomy. *Circulation* 1977; **56**: 924–30.

45 Sechtem U, Tscholakoff D, Higgins CB: MRI of the normal pericardium. *Am J Radiol* 1986; **147**: 239–44.

46 Hutchinson SJ, Smalliing RG, Albornoz A et al: Comparison of transthoracic and transesophageal echocardiography in clinically overt or suspected pericardial heart disease. *Am J Cardiol* 1994; **74**: 962–5.

47 Janos GG, Arjunan K, Meyer RA et al: Differentiation of constrictive pericarditis and restrictive cardiomyopathy using digitized echocardiography. *J Am Coll Cardiol* 1983; **1**: 541–9.

48 Morgan JM, Raposo L, Clague JC et al: Restrictive cardiomyopathy and constrictive pericarditis: non-invasive distinction by digitised M-mode echocardiography. *Br Heart J* 1989; **61**: 29–37.

49 Hatle LK, Appleton CP, Popp RL: Differentiation of constrictive pericarditis and restrictive cardiomyopathy by Doppler echocardiography. *Circulation* 1989; **79**: 357–70.

50 Mancuso L, D'Agosto A, Pitrolo F et al: Constrictive pericarditis versus restrictive cardiomyopathy: the role of Doppler echocardiography in differential diagnosis. *Int J Cardiol* 1991; **31**: 319–28.

51 Klein AL, Cohen GI, Pietrolungo JF et al: Differentiation of constrictive pericarditis from restrictive cardiomyopathy by Doppler transesophageal echocardiographic measurements of respiratory variations in pulmonary venous flow. *J Am Coll Cardiol* 1993; **22**: 1935–43.

52 Moncada R, Baker M, Salinas M et al: Diagnostic role of computed tomography in pericardial heart disease: congenital defects, thickening, neoplasms, and effusions. *Am Heart J* 1982; **103**: 263–82.

53 Isner JM, Carter LB, Banff MS et al: Computed tomography in the diagnosis of pericardial heart disease. *Ann Intern Med* 1982; **97**: 473–9.

54 Killian DM, Furiasse JG, Scanlon PJ et al: Constrictive pericarditis after cardiac surgery. *Am Heart J* 1989; **118**: 563–8.

55 Suchet IB, Horwitz TA: CT in tuberculous constrictive pericarditis. *J Comp Assist Tomogr* 1992; **16**: 391–400.

56 Oren RM, Grover-McKay M, Stanford W et al: Accurate preoperative diagnosis of pericardial constriction using cine computed tomography. *J Am Coll Cardiol* 1993; **22**: 832–8.

57 Masui T, Finck S, Higgins CB: Constrictive pericarditis and restrictive cardiomyopathy: evaluation with MR imaging. *Radiology* 1992; **182**: 369–73.

58 Seifert FC, Miller DC, Oesterle SN et al: Surgical treatment of constrictive pericarditis; analysis of outcome and diagnostic error. *Circulation* 1985; **72** (suppl II): 264–73.

59 Oh JK, Hatle LK, Seward JB et al: Diagnostic role of Doppler echocardiography in constrictive pericarditis. *J Am Coll Cardiol* 1994; **23**: 154–62.

60 McCaughan BC, Schaff HV, Piehler JM et al: Early and late results of pericardiectomy for constrictive pericarditis. *J Thorac Cardiovasc Surg* 1985; **89**: 340–50.

14

Imaging of adults with congenital heart disease

Philip Kilner

Surgical treatment of children born with congenital heart disease has resulted in a growing population of adolescents and adults requiring continued expert management. They are an exceptionally varied and challenging group of patients in whom the effects of congenital disease, surgical intervention and acquired disease may be combined.[1–5] A case has been made for the management of such patients by experienced teams in tertiary referral centers with close links to pediatric cardiac centers. Appropriate imaging facilities represent a key aspect of such centers. Costs of imaging should be weighed against potential costs of inappropriate management, which might involve difficult repeat surgery and extended hospitalization.

The main imaging modalities used in assessment of adult congenital heart disease are summarized in Table 14.1. The role of plain film radiography has become less crucial than in the past, but retains an important place, providing inexpensive overviews of the chest giving diagnostic information, pointers for further investigation and comparison of changes over the years. Other modalities and their roles are in a process of change. Imaging is now inseparably linked with functional measurement, and indications for invasive and high dose radiographic imaging are diminishing with advances in echocardiographic and magnetic resonance investigation. This is particularly true in patients with congenital heart disease modified by surgery, who may need repeated investigation throughout life. Transthoracic echocardiography (TTE) has a primary role in noninvasive evaluation, with magnetic resonance imaging (MRI) and transesophageal echocardiography (TEE) performed when required. Transesophageal and epicardial echocardiography have gained a place in the operating theater, providing windows into the heart during and immediately after surgery.[6] Cardiac catheterization, while still providing high resolution angiograms of coronary and collateral lung arteries, is increasingly used as a route for therapeutic intervention after diagnosis has been established noninvasively.[7] Each investigation should be performed by operators with knowledge of congenital heart disease and surgical management, and their potential complications.

There is little objective information about the comparative clinical value of the noninvasive modalities.[8] Hirsch et al undertook a careful comparative study of TEE and MRI,[9] but it must be remembered that equipment used and operator expertise vary, and evolve with time. When choosing which modality to use, it may be necessary to ask: Who will do it? How? With what equipment? Expertise is necessary for investigation of adult congenital heart patients; it is not enough to have advanced technology. An ideal may be for cardiologists to perform and interpret investigations, with the patient's clinical picture and management in mind. Given time constraints and the history of diagnostic practice, this tends to favor echocardiographic and catheter investigation rather than, say, MRI. But one purpose of this book is to give guidance to clinicians on where to extend their expertise and resources, and to foster informed collaboration. In this chapter I give prominence to MRI, which is my own specialty. Other modalities are described more fully elsewhere in the book.

Although relatively slow and cumbersome, MRI is versatile and has much to offer in diagnosis and follow-up of adults with congenital heart disease.[8–10] It has potential for further development, but remains relatively unfamiliar to many cardiologists. The images serve as illustrations of the abnormal anatomy encountered in adults with congenital heart disease. Each diagnostic technique has its own strengths and limitations, and different approaches tend to be complementary.

Table 14.1 Survey of imaging modalities.

Chest X-ray

Inexpensive overview of chest structures
Gives *pointers for further investigation*
Allows *serial comparison* of *heart size, vascularity, calcification*
Lateral view valuable for sizing and locating chambers, vessels, calcification

TTE

Portable, high-resolution, real-time imaging of *structure-flow* relationships
Safe, convenient and acceptable for repeated study
May be good for *intracardiac structures: septal defects, patch leaks, valve structure and function, stenotic and regurgitant jet velocities, ventricular function* and *flow through coarctation*
Suitable for stress studies; may be used epicardially during surgery
BUT: less good for great vessels and conduits; acoustic windows may be limited after surgery
Searches across volumes by real-time sweep of plane
Operator dependent

TEE

Even *better resolution* of *more posterior cardiovascular structures*
Excellent for visualization of *valves, vegetations, thrombus, septal defects and patch leaks*
Generally less good for vessels and conduits outside the heart
Images parts of thoracic aorta clearly, but coverage is less comprehensive than MRI
Useful intra-operatively
BUT: occasionally distressing. Local or general anesthetic or sedation may be needed
Operator dependent

MRI

Extensive access; entire chest volume can be imaged by multislice acquisitions in all standard and oblique orientations
Good for extracardiac vessels, including *conduits, pulmonary arteries, Fontan* connections, *coarctation* and *entire aorta*
Versatile; cine imaging and *flow velocity mapping* (in-plane or through-plane) supplement anatomic information
Movements and flows shown by cine imaging in oblique planes – sequential cuts can home in on a point of interest
Ventricular function, shunt and *regurgitant flow volumes* and *post-stenotic jet velocities* can be measured
BUT: *slow, expensive*, and, for a few patients, *claustrophobic*
Contraindications: pacemakers, cerebral clips, metallic eye injury
Not real time. Underlying principles and image appearances may be unfamiliar.
There are many choices to be made, from magnet field strength to sequences and planes used
There is scope for progress, with improvement of speed and resolution, and even more versatility
Acquisition of standard planes is straightforward, but oblique imaging of anatomic/surgical connections and functional measurements require skill; they are operator- and equipment-dependent

Catheterization and angiography

High resolution angiography of *coronary* and *pulmonary collateral* arteries
Catheterization also allows *oxygen saturation* and *pressure measurements*, and gives views of ventricular function and flow connections, but there may be alternative noninvasive approaches
Invasiveness and radiation limit repeated use
Previous noninvasive diagnosis makes for swift, informed catheter investigation and intervention

Computed X-ray tomography

High resolution tomographic imaging of *lung* and medastinum. Localization of cardiovascular *calcification*
Radiation dose may limit repeated use
Used, with contrast injection, for imaging of aorta and pulmonary arteries (3-D reconstructions possible), particularly where cardiovascular MRI is unavailable or unfamiliar

Radionuclide scintigraphy

Investigation of myocardial perfusion changes due to *ischaemic heart disease*, at rest and stress. Lung perfusion imaging and measurement, for investigation of effects of pulmonary emboli and shunts

The diagnostic challenge

In assessing an adult with congenital heart disease, it may be necessary to address a series of questions:

1. How are the heart chambers and vessels connected (sequential anatomy, surgical modification, collateral vessels)?
2. How are the components functioning (e.g. ventricular contraction, stenosis, regurgitation, pulmonary resistance)?
3. Is there intra- or perivascular pathology (e.g. thrombus, vegetation, atheroma, aneurysm, abscess)?
4. Is there non-cardiac disease (beyond the scope of this chapter)?

Description of anatomy

In adults with congenital heart disease, underlying cardiac anatomy has probably been described previously. While it is important to understand descriptions, they should not necessarily be assumed to be correct, and should be reviewed in the light of new information.

Abnormal cardiovascular anatomy is described by a systematic sequential approach. This requires determination of the *morphology* of atrial and ventricular cavities, and knowledge of their *connections* (Fig. 14.1). Connections between chambers and vessels are of greater functional significance than locations, although, if surgery is contemplated, locations also need to be clarified.

Atrial and ventricular cavities are characterized as 'right' or 'left' according to structural features rather than location. For determination of atrial morphology, appendage shape is a reliable feature: a right atrial appendage has a broad-based triangular shape, whereas a left atrial appendage is narrow and finger-like (Fig. 14.2). Atrial arrangement is described as usual (situs solitus) or inverted (situs inversus), depending on whether or not right and left atria are located appropriately. If both atria are morphologically similar, the arrangement is called atrial isomerism (right- or left-) depending on which type of appendage appears bilaterally. Atrial appendage type can generally be determined by TEE or MRI in adults. Abnormal atrial arrangement has importance for associated malformations. Bronchial situs, determined from plain film chest X-ray or MRI, is also a useful guide to atrial situs.

The presence or absence of coarse apical trabeculations is important for the determination of ventricular morphology. A right ventricle has coarse apical trabeculations, a moderator band, trabeculations arising from the septum, and is usually located in an anterosuperior position. A right ventricle usually has muscle encircling its outlet portion, known as an infundibulum, whereas the outlet of a left ventricle is partly formed by fibrous tissue continuous with the mitral valve. A left ventricle is said to have a mitral valve, a right ventricle, a tricuspid. The morphology of a ventricle has functional importance: if a morphologically right ventricle has to sustain systemic pressure, it is prone to premature failure and regurgitation of its tricuspid valve.

It is important to define all pulmonary and systemic venous pathways, atrioventricular and ventriculo-arterial connections, and presence of shunting at atrial, atrioventricular, ventricular or arterial level. Atrioventricular connections can be concordant (e.g. LA–LV), discordant (e.g. LA–RV), absent (e.g. tricuspid atresia), or either ventricle can have a double inlet.

Ventriculo-arterial connections can be concordant (e.g. LV–Ao), discordant (e.g. LV–PA), or one ventricle can have a double outlet. A single outlet heart can occur, as in pulmonary atresia or truncus arteriosus.

Different modalities establish cardiovascular connections in various ways. At catheter angiography, the catheter itself, and contrast medium injected from it, may be followed from one region to another. Use of contrast injections with computed X-ray tomography and echocardiography also allows flow connections to be deduced. But the mainstay of anatomic diagnosis is sequential noninvasive imaging of local structure–flow relationships. Echocardiography can establish intracardiac connections, presence and size of septal defects, and structural abnormalities of valves such as overriding or straddling (Figs 14.3 and 14.4). MRI offers wide fields of view in multislice and cine acquisitions which allow both extracardiac and intracardiac connections to be traced (Fig. 14.1). Abnormal connections, such as anomalous venous drainage or a patent arterial duct, are easily missed if not specifically looked for with appropriate acquisitions.

Catheter angiography remains unrivaled for visualization of systemic–pulmonary collateral arteries (Fig. 14.5). It allows the identification of stenoses which may develop in collaterals (Fig. 14.6), with a view to balloon dilatation if this is clinically indicated. After collaterals have been visualized, it is useful to draw them for convenient future reference.

When acquired coronary occlusive disease is suspected, coronary artery branches are still best visualized by invasive catheter angiography, which may also be valuable for detection of coronary fistulae and coronary-pulmonary collaterals. The origins and proximal course of anomalous coronary arteries may be determined by MRI if fat-suppression and breath-hold imaging techniques are available.[11,12]

Functional assessments

Assessment of function is achieved differently by different modalities. Whereas catheterization allows relatively direct measurements of pressures, pressure differences

a

b

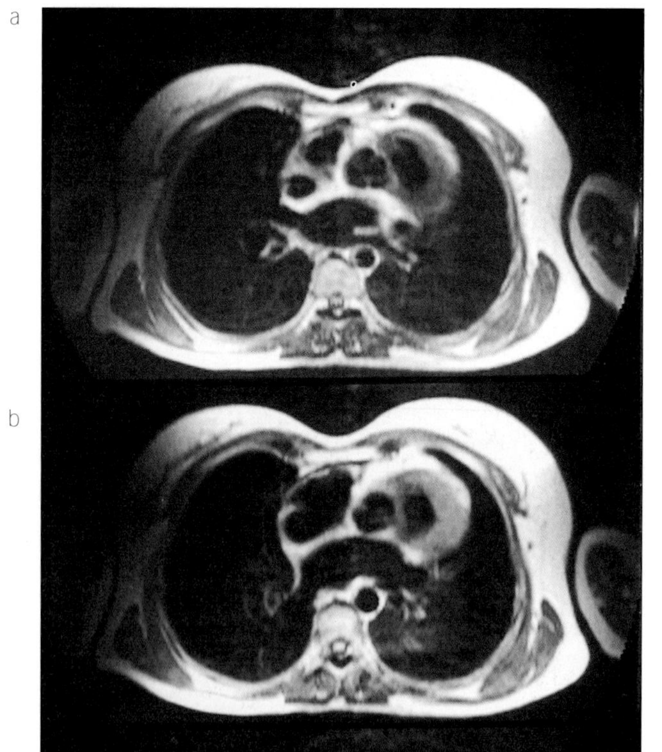

c

d

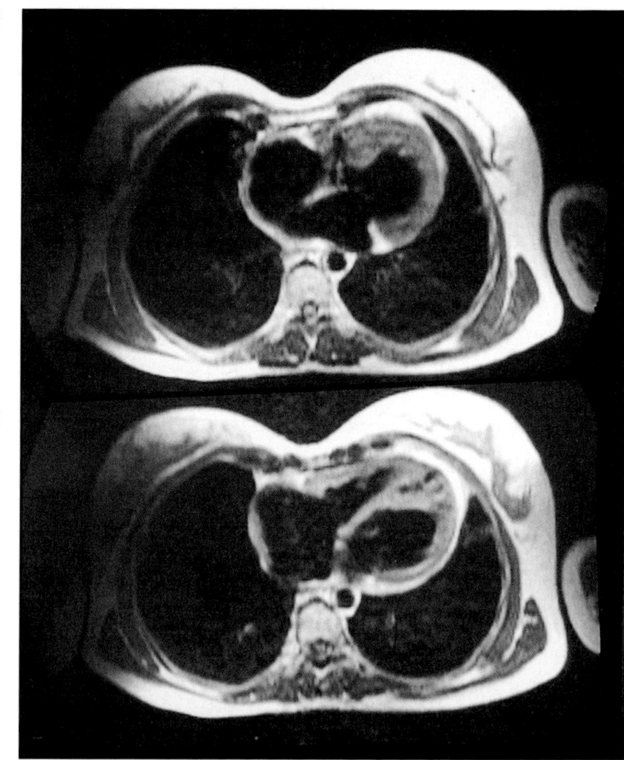

Figure 14.1
Anatomy of congenitally corrected transposition by MRI. Selected TE40 spin echo (a–d,c–k,m), gradient echo (e,f) and velocity map (l) images show features of unoperated congenitally corrected transposition of the great arteries in a young woman. *There is usual atrial arrangement, atrioventricular discordance and ventriculo-arterial discordance.* Pulmonary veins drain normally to the left atrium (a and b), and the systemic caval veins to the right atrium (i and j). The broad base of the right atrial appendage is visible behind the sternum in a. In images d, e, c and m, it can be seen that the more posterior ventricle, which gives rise to the aorta, has coarse apical trabeculations; it is morphologically *right.* Discordant atrioventricular connections can therefore be seen in c,d,e and f, and discordant ventriculo-arterial connections, in k–m. The posterior, *right* ventricle has to deliver systemic pressure, and is hypertrophied (c–f). Its tricuspid valve is regurgitant (e). There is a narrow, high velocity systolic jet above a fibrous subpulmonary shelf (l and k). Aortic outflow is unobstructed (l and m).

e

f

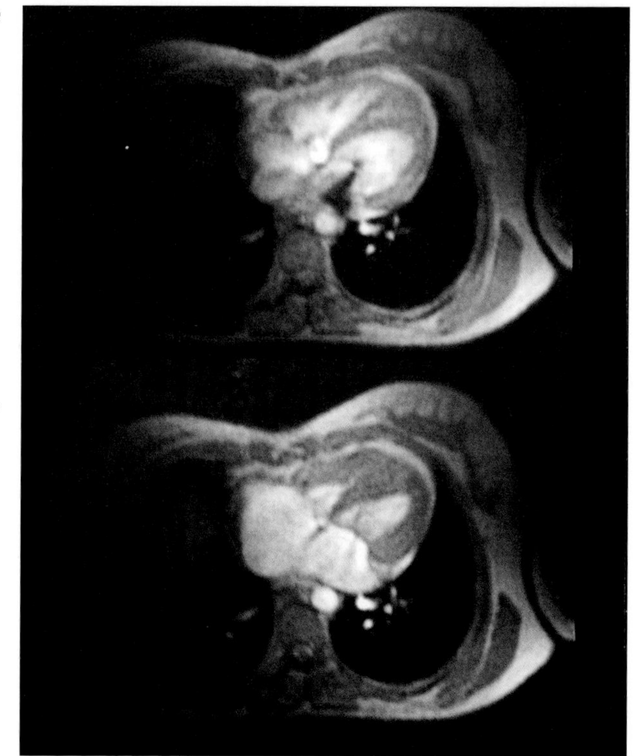

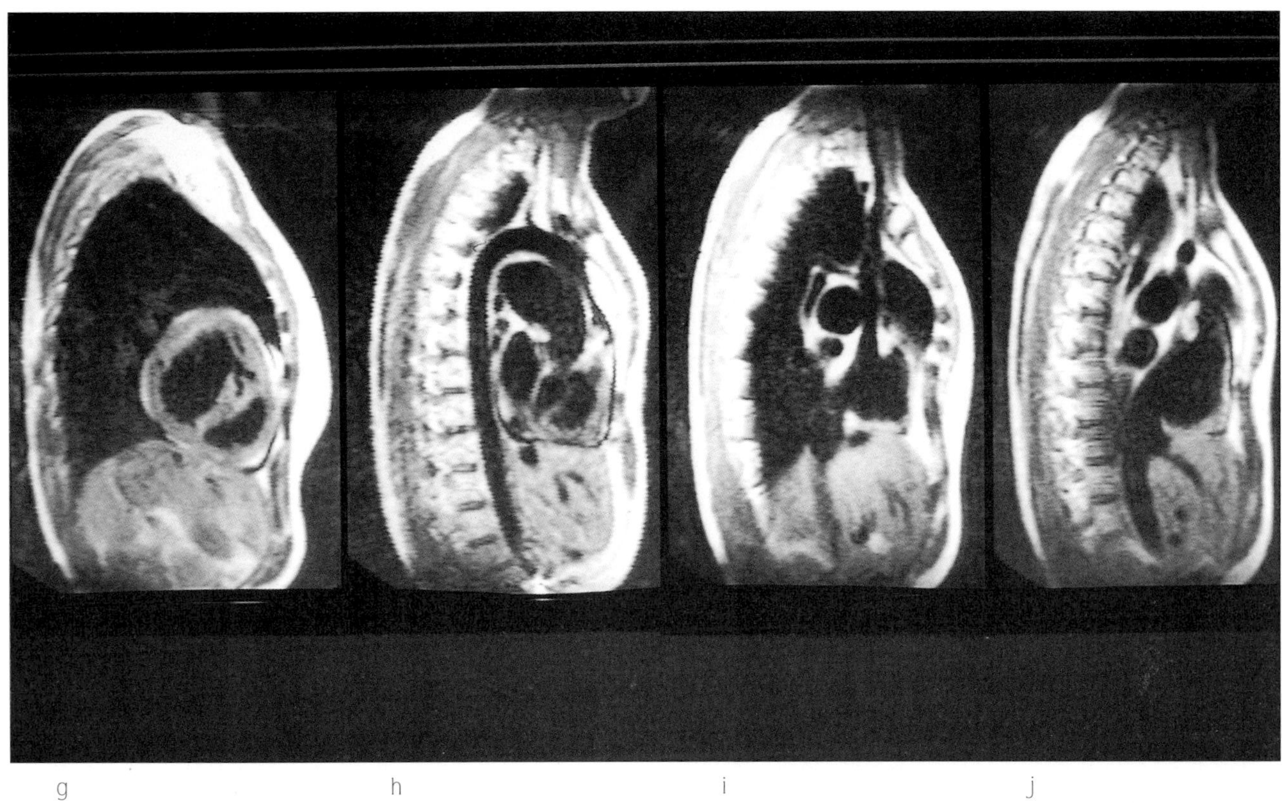

g h i j

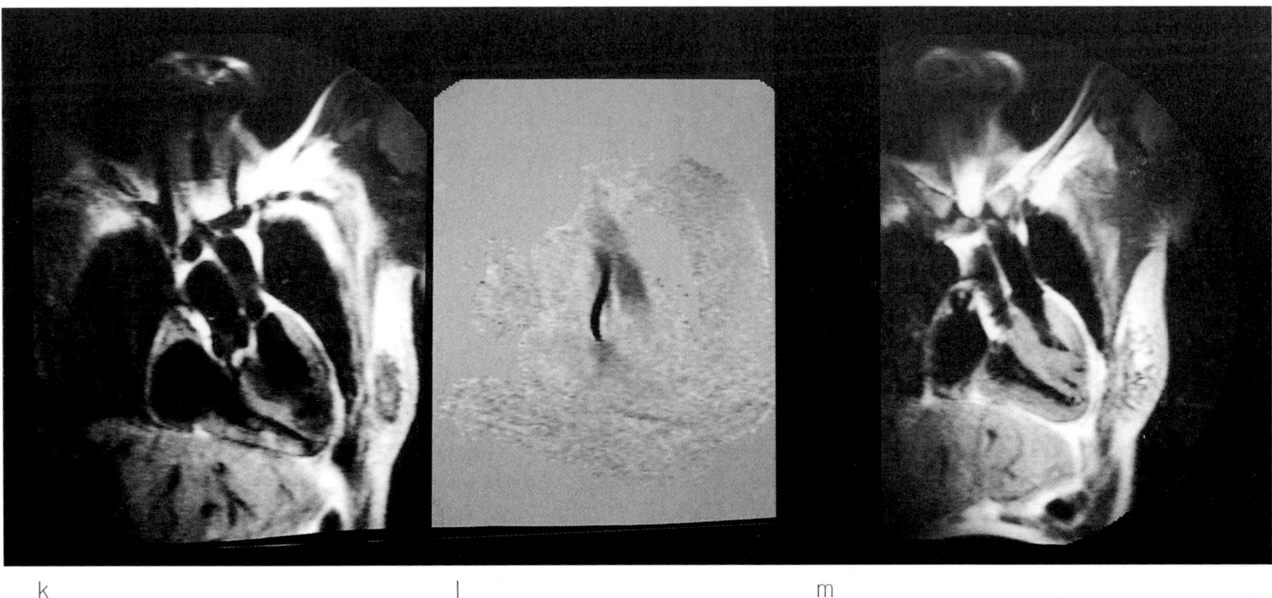

k l m

('gradients') and oxygen saturations, and represents three-dimensional volumes by projection onto two-dimensions, both echocardiography and MRI approach functional questions by different means. Echocardiography and MRI allow visualization of myocardial walls and intracavity flow in cross-sectional slices (Figs 14.3 and 14.4), and they allow measurement of velocities, from which gradients are often deduced by application of the modified Bernoulli equation. Stenosis, regurgitation and ventricular function are considered further below. In choosing which modality to use, it is worth asking what kind of functional information is needed for decisions on patient management.

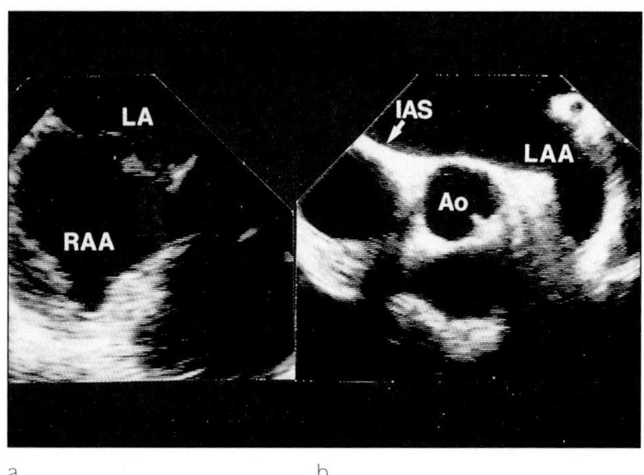

a b

Figure 14.2
Right and left atrial appendages shown by TEE. a. shows the broad-based, triangular right atrial appendage (RAA). LA, left atrium; b. shows the narrow, finger-like cavity of the left atrial appendage (LAA). Ao = aorta, IAS = intra-atrial septum.

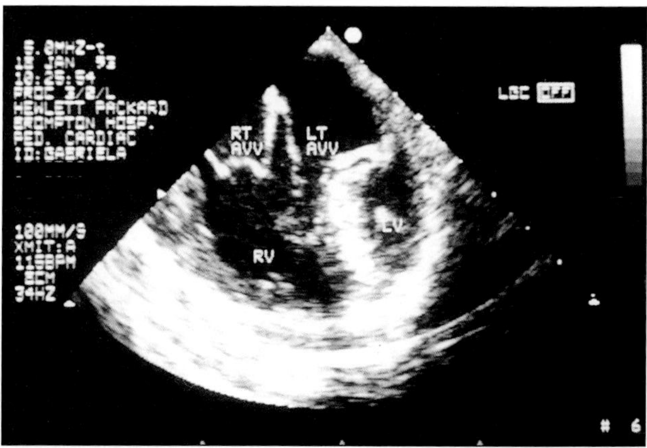

Figure 14.3
Straddling mitral valve leaflet shown by TEE. One leaflet of the left atrioventricular valve (LT AVV) straddles to the right of the ventricular septum. LV, left ventricle; RV, right ventricle; RT AVV, right atrioventricular valve.

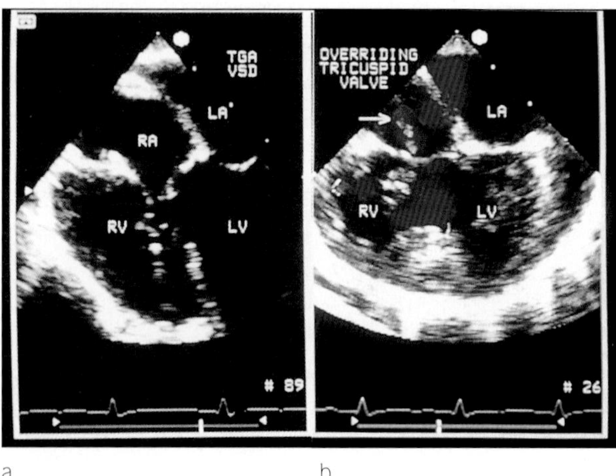

a b

Figure 14.4
Overriding tricuspid valve shown by TEE. a. The tricuspid valve between right atrium (RA) and right ventricle (RV) overrides a defect in the ventricular septum in a patient with transposition of the great arteries (TGA) and ventricular septal defect (VSD). b. Color Doppler shows a red jet of tricuspid regurgitation during systole (arrowed).

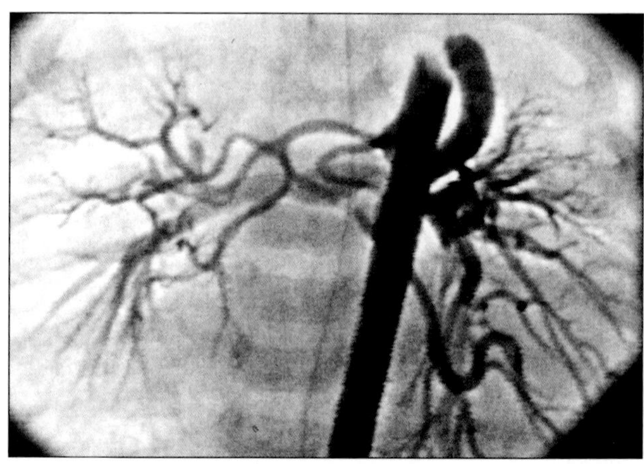

Figure 14.5
Aortopulmonary collateral arteries shown by X-ray angiography. Contrast medium in the descending aorta and aortopulmonary collateral arteries in a child with pulmonary atresia. Contrast also fills the lumen of a curved, surgically placed shunt to the central pulmonary arteries, which can be seen faintly.

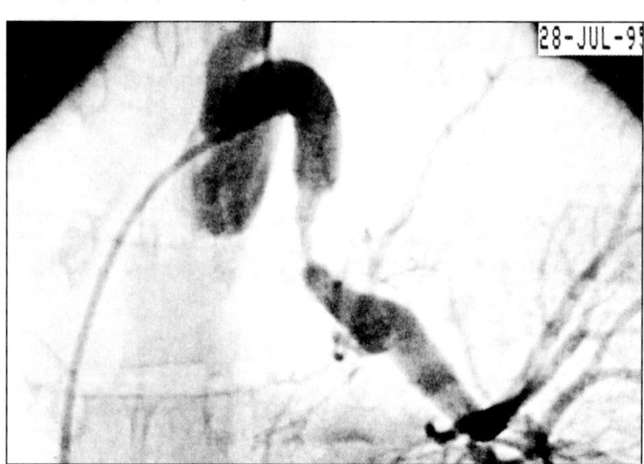

Figure 14.6
Stenosis of an aortopulmonary collateral artery shown by X-ray angiography. Large collateral with tight stenosis, prior to balloon dilatation to restore adequate perfusion of the region of lung supplied.

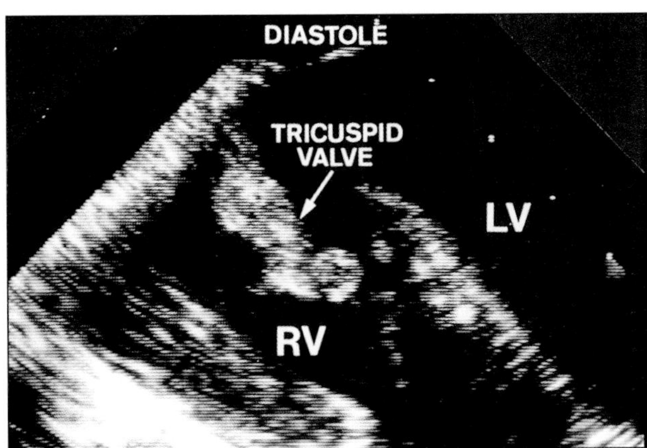

Figure 14.7
Vegetation of infective endocarditis shown by TEE. A leaflet of the tricuspid valve, which had been subjected to jet flow from a ventricular septal defect, is grossly thickened by a bacterial vegetation. LV, left ventricle; RV, right ventricle.

Thrombus, vegetations and perivascular lesions

For establishing the presence or absence of intracardiac thrombus or bacterial vegetation, TTE followed by TEE, are unrivaled (Fig. 14.7).[13] For perivascular lesions outside the heart, such as false aneurysm, MRI is most likely to be suitable.

If all modalities are available, it is wise to start with the one most likely to give the information required, proceeding to another if the information is inadequate.

Chest X-ray, echocardiography and MRI

Plain film chest X-ray

Plain film chest X-rays provide cost-effective images from which physiological as well as anatomic information can be derived. The nature of the technique, with superimposition of multiple structures, makes interpretation challenging. A rational and thorough approach such as that described by Larry Elliott[14,15] is recommended. Plain film radiology is important because many adults with congenital heart disease will have had a series of chest X-rays documenting the changing shapes and proportions of thoracic structures through life. Comparison of serial, technically comparable images is informative, and chest X-rays, with the structures of the whole chest represented on single images, are particularly suitable. Cardiac and vascular shadows can be compared between images. Changes suggestive of atrial enlargement, ventricular enlargement, altered vascularity and aneurysmal dilatation can be compared from year to year, as can calcifications of valves, conduits, arterial walls and pericardium. A normal chest X-ray does not, however, exclude important valve disease, small shunts or ischemic heat disease.

Lateral, and in some cases, oblique views make important contributions.[15,16] The lateral view provides information on atrial and ventricular enlargement, the anatomy of vessels, and calcification, especially of valves in aortic and pulmonary positions.

Figure 14.8 summarizes various features of congenital cardiovascular disease recognizable on plain film chest X-ray,

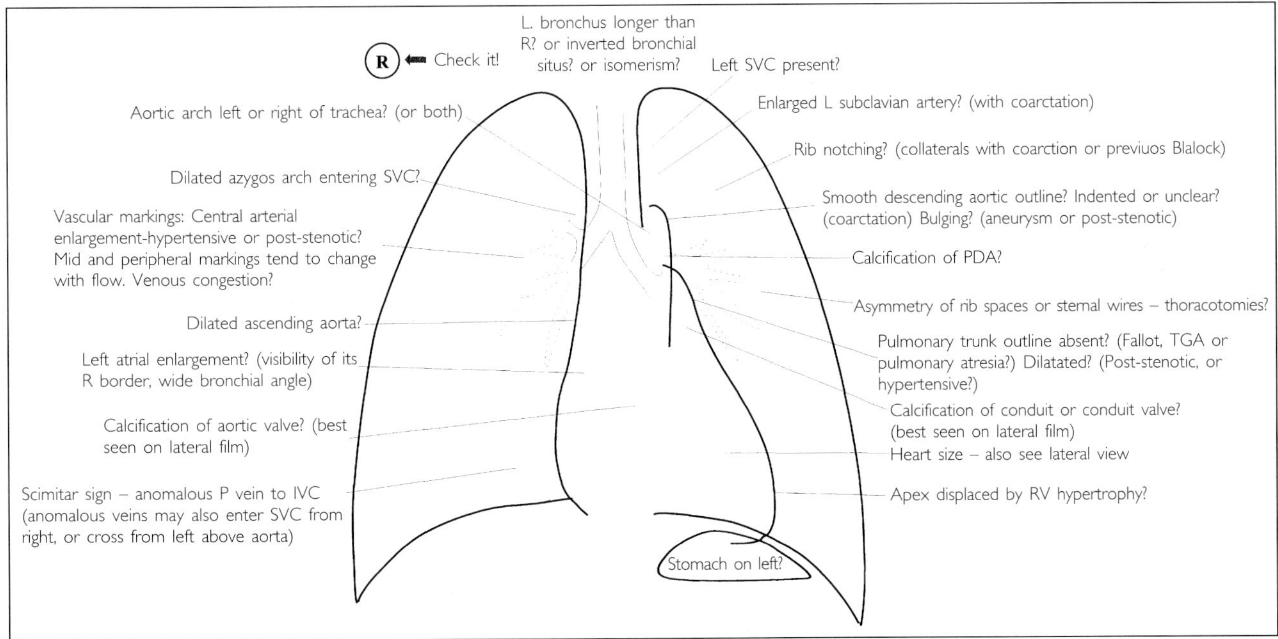

Figure 14.8
Adult congenital heart disease: features to look for on chest X-ray.

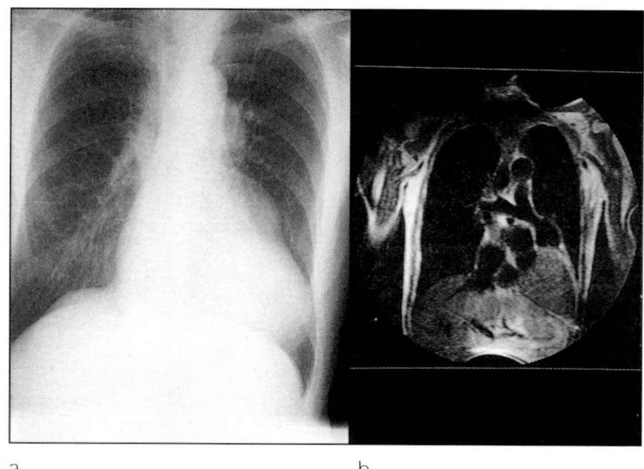

Figure 14.9
Chest X-ray and coronal MRI. This patient with tetralogy of Fallot was unusual in that he survived to the age of 70 without surgery. a. The chest X-ray shows a bulge, upper left heart border, apparently in the region of the pulmonary trunk. b. Coronal spin echo MRI (together with other acquisitions) confirmed that the bulge was the pulmonary trunk, locally enlarged due to post-stenotic dilatation above a hypertrophied and stenotic infundibulum.

although interpretation of actual films is not as simple as the sketch suggests. Abnormalities may be subtle, varied, and sometimes gross. Experience is needed for interpretation. For learning as well as diagnosis, it can be helpful to compare plain films with corresponding magnetic resonance images: posteroanterior with coronal (Fig. 14.9), and lateral with sagittal.

Transthoracic echocardiography

TTE provides high-resolution, real-time imaging of intracardiac structure and flow relationships, particularly in children. It is used routinely in adults with congenital heart disease, but the information it gives may be limited by problems of acoustic penetration, especially in patients who have undergone surgery. It rarely provides high quality images of the great vessels in adults; retrosternally located ventriculopulmonary conduits and Fontan connections are rarely visualized completely. For investigation of aortic coarctation, the extent of two-dimensional visualization, via a suprasternal window, is limited in adults, but color and continuous wave Doppler provide information on flow (see Fig. 14.23) which can complement anatomic images gained from MRI or computed X-ray tomography. TTE also has the advantage that it can be used during or after exercise.

Although transthoracic access can be limited in this patient group, safety, acceptability, immediacy and repeatability all give TTE a routine role in the investigation of adults with congenital heart disease.

Transesophageal echocardiography and MRI

Transthoracic access effectively recedes as children grow, whereas increasing size and willingness to cooperate favor both MRI and TEE. These two different modalities occupy comparable diagnostic ground. Both provide second-line investigations, usually after plain film radiology and TTE. Both may be time consuming and technically challenging in adult congenital heart patients. They may cause distress, and are not without risk to certain individuals. MRI is costly, but both investigations offer significant diagnostic contributions which can avoid the need, or give useful guidance, for subsequent catheter investigation and therapeutic intervention.

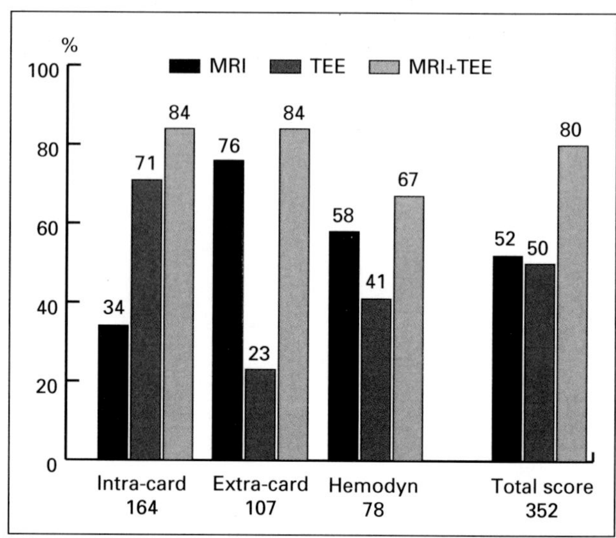

Figure 14.10
Comparison of diagnostic contributions of MRI and TEE in adult congenital heart disease. Chart summarizing findings of a prospective study of patients, mostly operated, aged 12–57 years. Percentages represent the proportion of previously unanswered diagnostic questions answered by each modality, or by both combined. The numbers of questions asked, prior to investigation, are shown beneath each group of bars. They are divided into groups relating to intracardiac regions, extracardiac regions and hemodynamics, which refers to diagnostic measurements of velocity and flow.

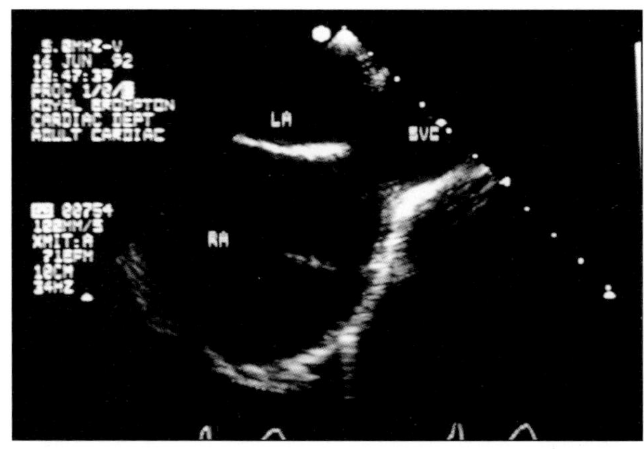

a

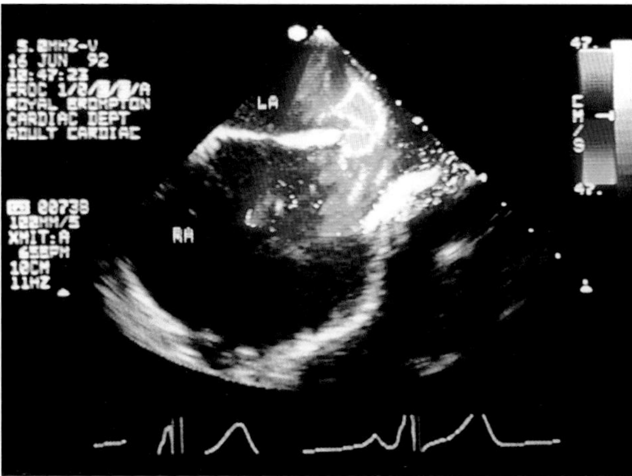

b

Figure 14.11
Atrial septal defect shown by TEE.

Information from MRI and TEE is complementary. Rafael Hirsch undertook a prospective study of the additional diagnostic contributions made by the two modalities in adult congenital heart patients in a tertiary referral center.[9]

For each patient, a list of unanswered diagnostic questions was made after reviewing all previous investigations, including TTE and often earlier catheter studies. MRI and TEE were performed to try to answer the questions, and each was interpreted independently. Answered questions scored one point, so that the number of points divided by the number of questions gave a score representing diagnostic contribution overall, or in a number of subcategories.

Overall, MRI and TEE achieved similar diagnostic scores, each answering about 50% of the previously unanswered diagnostic questions, but when combined, 80% of questions were answered (Fig. 14.10). MRI made its best contribution in diagnoses relating to extracardiac structures, for example obstructions of great vessels and extracardiac conduits, which are frequently out of reach of echocardiographic studies. TEE was most useful in assessment of intracardiac structures, notably the heart valves and the interatrial septum (Fig. 14.11). MRI, acquiring data over many cardiac cycles, depicted these thin, mobile structures less clearly.

It was concluded from the study that MRI should generally be used to answer remaining diagnostic questions about extracardiac structures, that TEE should generally be used for mobile intracardiac structures, and that both may be required if there are questions about both intra- and extracardiac regions. If these techniques are used, diagnostic angiography is rarely needed in this complex patient group, except for visualization of coronary, peripheral pulmonary and pulmonary collateral arteries (Figs 14.5 and 14.6) and sometimes for measurement of pulmonary artery pressure and resistance. This conclusion is important, given the cost and invasiveness of catheterization.

The study was performed over a particular period (1990–3), on particular equipment, by particular investigators. MRI included measurements using velocity mapping techniques, which made important diagnostic contributions. With advancing technology and experience, both TEE and MRI would now achieve higher separate scores. Multiplane TTE probes are now used, and experience has been gained with transgastric views; MRI acquisition times have shortened, and expertise has developed.

MRI: basic principles, versatility and choices

The following sections offer an outline of principles, and some practical guidelines on MRI techniques, particularly flow velocity mapping. Topics of more general interest are returned to later in the chapter.

For MRI, the patient's body is placed in a strong magnetic field which brings the precession frequencies of hydrogen nuclei, which consist of single protons, into the radio frequency range. The precession frequencies of nuclei change with magnetic field strength, and also, to a lesser extent, with local physicochemical surroundings. Applications of magnetic field gradients differentially tune nuclei across spatial regions. Differential tuning is used for selective excitation of nuclei (nuclear magnetic resonance occurs where precession frequency coincides with that of input radio signal) and then for further manipulation of nuclear spins through a sequence of magnetic gradient

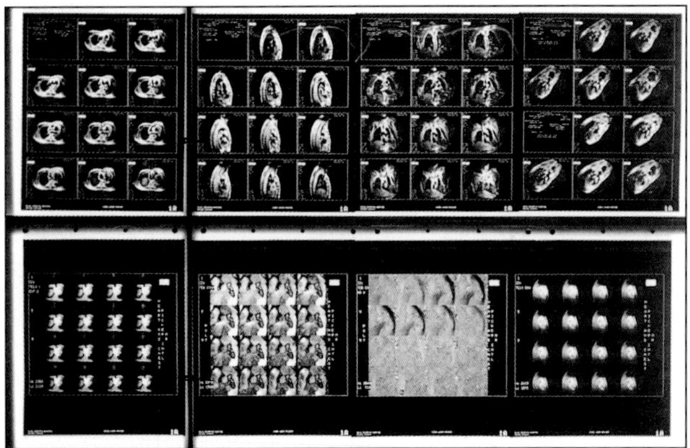

Figure 14.12
Comprehensiveness of cardiac MRI. Transaxial, sagittal, coronal and oblique spin echo images (upper row), and frames of cine acquisitions and velocity maps (lower row), all acquired in about 1 hour in a 0.5 T magnet. Structures throughout the chest are imaged, and areas of interest studied specifically.

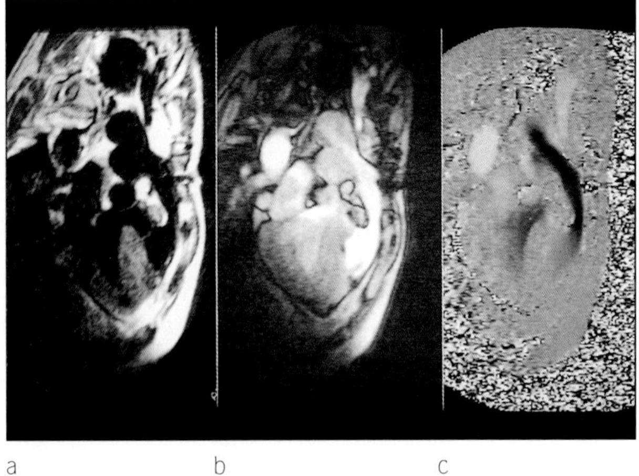

a b c

Figure 14.13
Ventriculopulmonary conduit shown by MRI with velocity mapping. Selected from the images of Figure 14.11, the *spin echo* (a), *TE6 gradient echo* (b) and *velocity map* (c) images all show an oblique sagittal slice aligned with a right ventricle to pulmonary artery conduit, viewed from the right. The plane also passes through the left ventricle and a subaortic VSD, closed from the right ventricular side with a patch, visible in a. The patient had a double outlet left ventricle, with pulmonary stenosis and VSD. After corrective surgery, the patient had palpitations shortness of breath and limb swelling. Conduit obstruction was suspected, but although MRI shows some flattening of the conduit retrosternally, cine imaging and velocity mapping did not show significant stenosis or regurgitation. Peak systolic velocity was under 2 ms. Symptoms may be explained by inadequate right ventricular stroke volume, limited by the patch over the VSD and by patching of the anterior wall of the right ventricle, beneath the conduit. This region was thin and immobile on cine imaging.

changes. In spin echo sequences, a second radio frequency pulse is also applied. The sequence is designed to encode positional and other information into the complex radio signal re-emitted from the body at the culmination of the sequence (read-out). This signal is picked up by a receiver. From the spectra of received radio signal, analysed in relation to the manipulations performed (repeatedly, over many heartbeats) anatomic and functional images are reconstructed.

So, as with other imaging techniques, MRI requires an energy input (radio energy), interaction with the tissues, and reception of the energy that comes out again. What is unique about MRI is the extent to which the energy–tissue interaction can be controlled and modified at tissue level, without contrast injection. Protons are effectively 'played' by radio pulse and magnetic gradient sequences. A sequence is like a short musical score, composed by physicists with certain aims in mind. Information on spatial distributions, physicochemical surroundings and movements of hydrogen nuclei can be obtained. The comprehensiveness and versatility of cardiothoracic MRI is illustrated by the images of Figures 14.12 and 14.13.

The complex nature of MRI means that many choices have to be made, from the field strength of the magnet, which has implications for hardware and software, to the choices of sequence and imaging strategy.

Magnetic field strength

For most users, magnet field strength is given and not chosen. Images and velocity maps shown in this chapter were all acquired on a mid-field, 0.5 T system. Although it recovers less signal-to-noise than a higher-field (1.5 T) magnet, the 0.5 T system has certain advantages. It is less subject to artefacts caused by movement and 'chemical shift', and gives a setting in which ECG gating is straightforward. But on the whole, 1.5 T may prove to be the field strength of choice for cardiovascular MRI. Its higher signal-to-noise ratio facilitates rapid and 3-dimensional acquisition techniques. But direct comparison of different field strengths is hardly feasible. Each system has its own range of hardware, software and capabilities. Choice of equipment must involve an attempt to match capabilities to needs. Different MRI systems may have very different imaging and image processing capabilities.

Range of MRI techniques

The repertoire of possible MRI sequences is extensive. Spin echo and gradient echo sequences are, at present, the most widely used techniques. Gradient echo imaging is itself versatile, providing a basis for rapid FLASH sequences, and for velocity mapping, as discussed below. I will not attempt to deal with variants used for MR angiography, which can be effective for investigation of more peripheral and pulmonary vasculature.[17] Also, I will not discuss echoplanar or spiral imaging techniques, or the use of fat suppression, tissue tagging, magnetization transfer techniques or contrast agents, although each of these are taking on roles in cardiovascular imaging.

Basic cardiovascular MRI

Caution: patients with *pacemakers* should not be allowed near the magnet without careful consideration. The electromechanical switching devices of earlier pacemakers can be damaged by the field; there may be electromagnetic interference from radio frequency fields and there is a possibility of induction of voltage in the wire. MRI is generally regarded as contraindicated in patients with pacemakers, also in patients with metal fragments in the eye following injury, and in patients with intracranial ligation clips. Presence of an intravascular stent, occlusion device or metal valve ring does not usually contraindicate MRI, but these objects cause localized image defects due to magnetic field distortion.

Force exerted by the magnetic field on metal equipment brought near the magnet represents a serious potential hazard: anything from scissors to gas cylinders, infusion pumps, wheel-chairs and patient trolleys can become missiles towards the centre of the magnet. It is essential not only to ensure that necessary equipment is suitably non-ferromagnetic, but also to maintain vigilance for anyone who might bring in metal equipment. These and other MRI safety considerations are discussed in detail in a book by Frank Shellock and Emanuel Kanel.[18]

Cardiac gating from the R wave of the ECG is necessary for imaging the mobile structures of heart and great vessels. Arrhythmia, as in atrial fibrillation, degrades gated images. With cardiac gating, the chosen sequence is applied briefly only at a given phase of the cardiac cycle over many heartbeats, contributing to an averaged image of that cardiac phase. For this reason, atrial fibrillation, or other arrhythmias, cause degradation of cardiac images.

A single image is usually one of a set, each representing a slightly different phase. Sets may be distributed across multiple planes to cover a volume (multislice images). Spin echo images are usually acquired in this way, as multislice sets. It is important to be aware that adjacent slices have different gating delays, and may not be directly comparable. One may be systolic, and the next diastolic. Systolic images tend to be clearer because flowing blood loses signal more completely relative to surrounding tissues. For cardiac imaging, spin echo sequences with echo time (TE) of 20 ms (at 1.5 T) or 40 ms (at 0.5 T) are used. This TE is long enough to give good blood–tissue contrast, and short enough to allow repetition in a particular slice with every heartbeat. Recovery of a spin echo signal from blood usually indicates sluggish flow, occasionally thrombus.

Spin echo imaging is not suitable for multiple repetition per heart beat in a single slice, as is required for cine imaging. For this, gradient echo (also known as field echo) sequences are used. They have relatively short echo times (3–14 ms), and generally recover the signal from flowing blood, which then appears bright. The brightness of blood on gradient echo images is variable. Through-plane movement enhances brightness, whereas turbulence tends to cause dark regions through dephasing of spins and cancellation of the net signal (Fig. 14.1e). Cine images therefore give qualitative information on blood flow in relation to cavity and vessel boundaries, but there is no simple relationship between turbulence and signal loss. In addition to various flow considerations, imaging parameters such as slice thickness, flip angle, gradient profile design and, most importantly, echo time all affect the amount of signal lost or recovered from regions of complex flow (see Fig. 14.17).

Magnetic resonance phase-shift velocity mapping

Recovery of the signal from flowing blood is a prerequisite of velocity mapping, so gradient echo sequences, with the refinement of even-echo rephasing, are used. Phase-shift velocity mapping, if correctly implemented, is accurate and versatile. It has unrivalled capacities for measurement of flow at any location and in any direction through the heart and great vessels. It can make valuable contributions to the assessment of adults with congenital heart disease. Phase velocity mapping techniques are based on the frequency changes experienced by nuclei that move relative to applied magnetic gradients.[19,20] The direction, steepness and timing of applied gradients can be chosen, so that a range of flow velocities, from low velocity venous to high velocity post-stenotic flows, can be measured. Clinical uses include measurements of cardiac output, shunt flow, regurgitant flow, and of jet velocities through stenoses. However, for successful clinical application, the operator should have understanding not only of the pathophysiology and anatomy of operated congenital heart disease, but also of technical velocity mapping choices. It is necessary to select a plane, echo time, velocity encoding direction and sensitivity appropriate for a particular investigation.

Although I am aware that users may not have access to the range of velocity mapping options discussed below, it is important that their roles are appreciated, and that manufacturers are called upon to supply hardware and software capable of accurate clinical measurement.

Velocity mapping techniques and applications

Velocity can be encoded in directions that lie either in or through an image plane, and each pixel across a velocity map can carry quantitative velocity information. In these respects, MR velocity mapping is more versatile and comprehensive than Doppler Ultrasound. Cine velocity mapping records multiple phases through the cardiac cycle. We usually acquire 16 frames per cycle, but 30 or more are possible if TE is short.

Mapping of velocities through a plane transecting a vessel (velocity encoded in the direction of the slice select gradient) allows measurement of flow volume. This is done by measuring the cross-sectional area of the lumen and the mean axially directed velocity within that area, for each frame through the heart cycle. From this, a flow curve is plotted, and systolic forward flow and any diastolic reversed flow are computed by integration (Fig. 14.14). Cardiac output,[21] regurgitant flow volume,[22] and shunt flow[23] can all be measured by this approach. To calculate shunt flow, both aortic and pulmonary artery flows are measured. Two separate acquisitions are needed for this, except in cases of transposition where aorta and pulmonary trunk run almost parallel. For aortic flow measurement, a suitable plane is transaxial, cutting the aorta at the level of the right pulmonary artery, whereas for pulmonary flow measurement, a suitable plane cuts the pulmonary trunk before its bifurcation, and is almost coronal.

Through-plane velocity mapping allows delineation of an atrial septal defect (ASD) (Fig. 14.15);[24] this is a valuable approach. It can give information on size, shape, location and shunt capacity of an ASD, allowing an informed decision on when and how to intervene. Through-plane

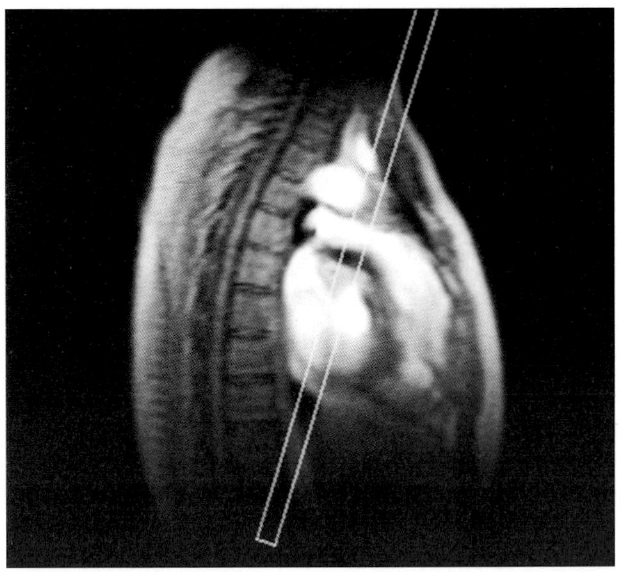

a

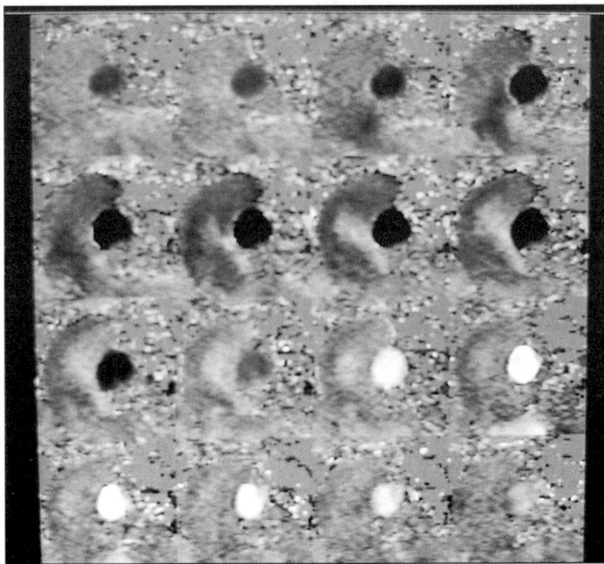

b

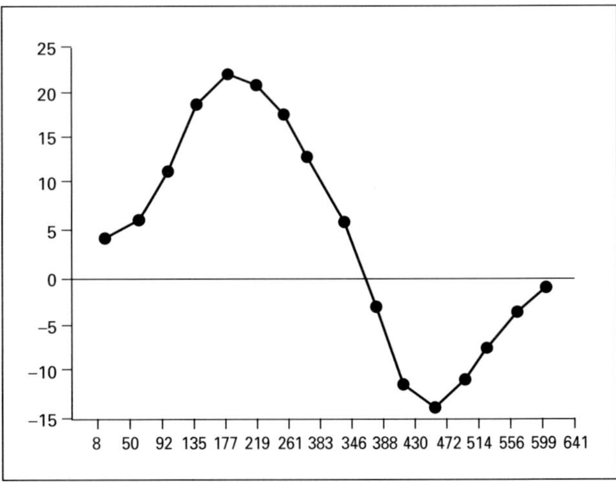

c

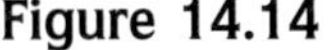

Figure 14.14

Pulmonary regurgitation following repair of tetralogy of Fallot, measured by MRI. a. Gradient echo image in an oblique sagittal plane aligned with the reconstructed right ventricular outflow after repair of tetralogy of Fallot. Cine imaging showed no evidence of an effective pulmonary valve. b. Detail from all 16 frames of a cine velocity map acquisition, TE = 6 ms, velocity encoded through-plane (in direction of the slice select gradient). The plane transects the reconstructed pulmonary trunk, as indicated in a. Systolic forward flow appears black, diastolic reversed flow, white. The frames run from left to right in lines ordered from above downwards. c. Plot showing systolic forward flow (upward curve) and diastolic reversed flow (downward curve) measured by multiplying mean velocity by cross-sectional area of the pulmonary trunk for each frame through the cycle. Integration of areas under the curves allows measurement of forward and reversed flow, and of regurgitant fraction, which was 40% in this case of free pulmonary regurgitation.

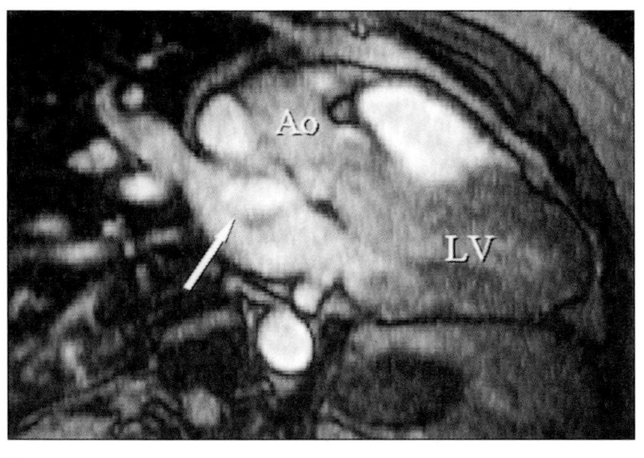

a

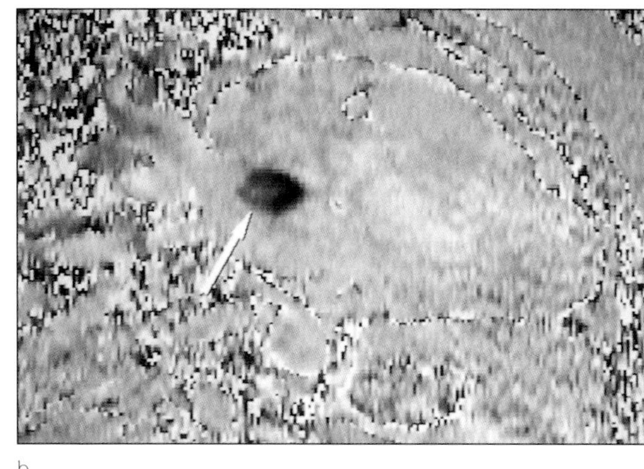

b

Figure 14.15
Atrial septal defect shown by through-plane MRI velocity mapping. a. Gradient echo cine imaging, TE = 8 ms, in a plane parallel to and just on the right atrial side of the atrial septum.[23] Flow through a large ASD can be identified only faintly as a slightly lighter area, indicated by the arrow. Above this area, flow from the SVC appears as a rounded light area, as does flow down the descending aorta, which passes through the lower part of the image. LV, left ventricle; Ao, ascending aorta. b. Corresponding velocity map, velocity encoded through-plane (in the direction of the slice select gradient). The dark area (arrowed) represents flow through the ASD, toward the viewer. Its size and shape are seen clearly: diameters were measured at 27 by 17 mm, cross-sectional area was 3.2 cm^2. MRI measurements of flow through planes transecting pulmonary trunk and ascending aorta[22] indicated a Qp:Qs ratio of 2.5:1.

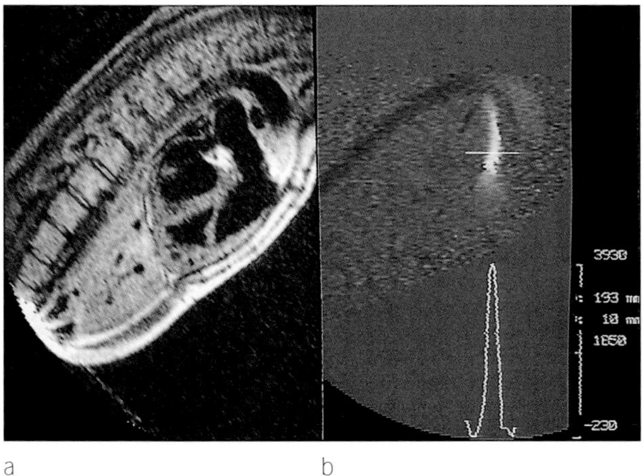

a b

Figure 14.16
Conduit stenosis shown by MRI with velocity mapping. a. On the spin echo image the right ventricle to pulmonary artery conduit appears unobstructed: calcified cusps of the homograft valve are not seen clearly. b. The corresponding velocity map (TE = 3.6 ms) shows significant stenosis, with systolic jet formation, peak velocity 3.9 ms.

velocity mapping has also been used for measurement of velocities and cross-sectional areas of jets through stenotic orifices.[25]

For evaluation of jet flow through stenoses, I generally prefer to map velocities in a plane aligned with the direction of flow, with velocity encoded in the read gradient direction.[26,27] The advantage of this is that the location of stenosis and jet is depicted for upstream and downstream regions (Fig. 14.16). It is necessary, however, to align the image plane carefully, as explained below. Jet velocity mapping can be particularly valuable for assessment of stenoses where ultrasonic access is limited, for example in aortic coarctation[28] (native or repaired), ventriculopulmonary conduits[29] and obstructions at atrial and atriopulmonary level following Mustard, Senning and Fontan operations. Combined cine imaging and velocity mapping can give information on the location, nature and severity of obstruction.

An important consideration when mapping velocities is which sequence (which echo time) to use. In general, the shorter the echo time, the better the recovery of signal from regions of high-velocity turbulent flow (Fig. 14.17).

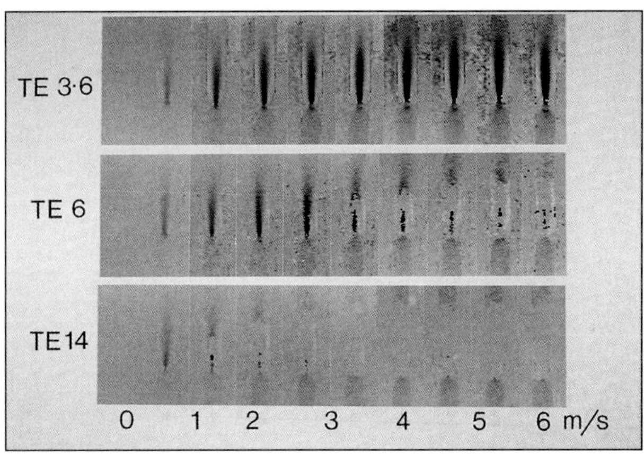

Figure 14.17
In vitro jet velocity mapping. Magnetic resonance velocity maps of continuous jet flow up through a 6 mm orifice. Jet velocities are increased toward the right. Shortening of the echo time from 14 ms (below) to 6 ms and 3.6 ms (above) allows recovery of the signal from increasingly turbulent regions. Only the TE 3.6 sequence allows accurate mapping of high velocity jets, up to a maximum tested velocity of 6 ms. The TE 14 sequence loses signal from jets above 1 ms.[26]

Conversely, the longer the echo time, the better the overall signal-to-noise ratio, and the greater the sensitivity for measurement of low velocity flows. For this reason, some foreknowledge of the velocities likely to be encountered is valuable. If not clinically available, approximate information can be gained from preliminary cine images, which serve to identify the location and orientation of the jet as well as the approximate severity of stenosis. This information also allows the choice of an appropriate velocity window, which is an adjustment of the sensitivity of the phase shift in relation to velocity. Too small a window results in aliasing, whereas too large a window reduces sensitivity.

In this, as in other areas, there is no substitute for experience, but it is important to be aware of and to avoid potential sources of inaccuracy (Table 14.2).

Alignment of plane for jet velocity mapping

Mapping of high-velocity post-stenotic jets is possible if sequences with short echo times are used. Accurate location of a sufficiently thin slice (6–8 mm) in relation to the jet core is essential. The core of the jet is the relatively stable, high-velocity flow region extending immediately downstream of the orifice. In a centrally located free jet, it is surrounded by a turbulent parajet region. If a stenosis is asymmetric, or its vessel angulated, for example at a repaired coarctation, the jet is likely to attach itself to the adjacent outer wall. Planes for velocity mapping, whether they are aligned across or with the jet, should pass through the jet core a few millemeters downstream of the orifice.

Accurate velocity map alignment depends on the use of an oblique imaging strategy, and recognition of the jet core on preliminary cine images. Orthogonal oblique cuts are located in relation to available images. A series of orthogonal cuts can home in with increasing accuracy (as long as the patient remains still) on the area of interest, which is the jet core. Signal loss in preliminary cine gradient acquisitions can be used to visualize jet location. The relative amount of signal loss can be controlled by the choice of the echo time used. It is usually possible to select a cine sequence which, when correctly aligned, will show a signal from the jet core outlined by a signal void in the intensely turbulent parajet region. It is preferable to use a slightly longer echo time for preliminary cine imaging than that chosen for final velocity mapping.

Choice of echo time for velocity mapping

For measurement of jet velocity, the echo time must be short enough to recover the signal from the jet core. To give approximate guidance:

- For low velocity jets, up to 1.5 m/s, which may be obstructive at venous or atrial level, use a longer echo time, TE = 10–14 ms.
- For velocities up to 3 or 4 m/s (mild to moderate obstruction of outflow valves and conduits, or significant coarctation), use TE = 6 ms.
- For higher velocities (severe stenosis of outflow valves or conduits) use the shortest available echo time, e.g. TE = 3 ms.

An outline of cine imaging and velocity mapping strategies is given in Table 14.3. Because shortening of echo time reduces both overall signal-to-noise and velocity sensitivity, use of very short echo time should be reserved for high velocity jets. Longer echo times remain preferable for mapping of low velocity jets. Sequences with short echo times also be associated with unpleasant levels of acoustic noise. Jets of regurgitation and severe aortic stenosis can be so narrow, turbulent and fragmented that they are not suitable for assessment by MR jet velocity mapping; too much signal loss and partial volume effects prevent accurate jet velocity measurement.

Table 14.2 MR velocity mapping: artefacts and how to avoid them.

Signal loss

Gradient echo sequences with even-echo rephasing are designed to recover signal from moving blood. But acceleration and higher orders of motion, particularly in regions of turbulence, still cause phase dispersion and loss of signal at the time of echo. Reduction of echo time is an effective way of minimizing signal loss, but other factors such as reduction of voxel size and optimization of sequence design are also important. In pixels where little or no signal is recovered, background electromagnetic noise causes random phase shifts, appearing as random velocities up to the pre-set aliasing limits. These random pixel readings must not be mistaken for true velocities. If necessary, they can be removed by masking areas with signal below a certain magnitude threshold. Even where signal is recovered, background noise contributes a degree of random phase shift, minimized as signal-to-noise is optimized.

Partial volume averaging

If blood within a single voxel has a range of velocities, then the mean value of phase shift for the voxel will be displayed. The mean vector depends on the relative amplitude as well as phase of signal components contributing to the voxel. Fortunately, the relatively stable jet core contributes a more coherent signal than its turbulent surroundings. Nevertheless, it is important to locate the slice as accurately as possible.

Background phase errors

Factors other than velocity, such as induced electric currents in receiver coils, may result in apparent phase shifts. To correct these, it may be necessary to perform 'background correction'. This requires a program which registers and zeros regions in the chest wall, known to have no velocity, correcting velocities accordingly.

Aliasing

Excessive velocity-related phase shift can lead to aliasing, as in Doppler ultrasound measurements. In MR velocity mapping the problem is avoidable as the sensitivity of velocity encoding can be controlled by adjustment of the gradient profiles used. Ideally a sensitivity giving a total velocity window about 1.5 × the expected maximum velocity is used, so that aliasing may be avoided without undue reduction of sensitivity. This requires prior knowledge of the approximate peak velocity.

Misalignment of velocity encoding

Because only the component of velocity in the chosen direction is encoded, misalignment between the direction of flow and the direction of encoding will introduce an error proportional to the cosine of the angle between the two. Again, this consideration is familiar from Doppler ultrasound studies. As the principal flow direction is usually identifiable, and the direction of encoding can be chosen, this is rarely a problem in velocity mapping.

Misregistration

Signal from nuclei that move during the sequence, with a component of velocity in the image plane, will be displaced slightly in the direction of movement. This misregistration is minimized by reduction of echo time.

Phase shifts caused by higher orders of motion

If velocity is measured where a significant acceleration is also present, the final phase shift may have contributions from both orders of motion. This artefact is negligible in measurements of jet core velocity using sequences with echo times under 6 ms; but it may account for local velocity underestimation where there is high acceleration immediately upstream of a stenotic orifice, and to overestimation where there is abrupt deceleration at the edges of a high velocity jet. The latter may appear as exaggerated spikes of velocity at the edges of a high velocity jet core. The artefact should not affect jet core velocity measurements, and it is minimized by reduction of the echo time.

Image defects caused by ferromagnetic material

Ferromagnetic material such as wire sutures, clips, stents occlusion devices and the metal rings of prosthetic valves all cause local magnetic field distortion, and consequent defects on gradient echo images. These can effect jet velocity mapping. For example, the metal ring of a Hancock valve prosthesis can prevent adequate mapping of flow through the valve. The extent of signal void is minimized by reduction of echo time.

Sequence implementation

Phase velocity mapping depends on appropriate MR hardware and software. Sequences must be implemented, and received signal analyzed, accurately. This is the concern of manufacturers and physicists, but it is advisable for any new user to test velocity map accuracy, for example using rotating disc and flow phantoms.[26]

Table 14.3 MRI velocity mapping strategies.

Type of lesion	Preliminary cine sequences	Velocity mapping: direction, TE of sequence, expected velocity
ASD	TE 14 ms aligned with flow	Encode velocity *through* plane of septum.[24] TE 10–14 ms, up to 1.5 m/s
Obstruction after Fontan, Mustard or Senning	TE 14 ms aligned with flow	(Fontan atriopulmonary flow peaks with atrial systole) Encode in direction of jet, TE 10–14 ms, >1 m/s significant, 2 m/s may be lethal[31]
Obstructed RV–PA conduit	TE 6 ms oblique sagittal	In direction of jet, TE 6 ms (or TE 3 ms), >3 m/s, significant (>4 m/s, severe)[29]
Aortic stenosis	TE 6 ms oblique coronal/sagittal	In direction of jet, TE 3 ms, up to 6 m/s, if severe[27]
Aortic/pulmonary regurgitation	TE 6–10 ms oblique coronal/sagittal	Encode velocity *through* plane transecting artery.[22] TE 6 ms, systole 1–3 m/s, diastole <1 m/s
Shunt: aortic and pulmonary flow	Standard spin echo pilots	*Through* planes transecting ascending aorta and pulmonary trunk.[23] TE 8–12 ms, 1–2 m/s
Aortic coarctation	TE 6 ms, oblique sagittal	In direction of jet, TE 6 ms or TE 3 ms, 3–4 m/s with 'diastolic tail' suggests significant coarct[28]

Surgical and functional considerations

Adults with congenital heart disease may need to be investigated to assess suitability, and need for surgery and outcomes after surgery. After apparently successful surgery, baseline investigation may be valuable for a later assessment of changes. Eventually a decision may have to be made to re-operate. Understanding of operations and their complications is therefore fundamental to investigation.[30] Post-surgical anatomy can vary considerably, depending on the underlying anatomy and the surgical techniques used.

Surgical systemic–pulmonary shunts

These are performed, often as first stage procedures, to increase flow to underperfused lungs. If patent, then turbulent flow through a shunt usually gives rise to an audible murmur, but patency may be uncertain if no murmur is heard. The lumen of a flowing shunt should be identifiable on MRI spin echo images of sufficient resolution. Another useful approach is to look for signal loss from a turbulent jet into the appropriate pulmonary artery using cine imaging (TE 8–14 ms). To do this, it is necessary to know where the shunt is likely to be.

Blalock shunts are from a subclavian artery to the right or the left pulmonary artery, either via the downturned subclavian branch, or via an interposition graft.

There are three types of direct aortopulmonary shunt, each being a hole between vessels sutured side-to-side: a Waterston shunt passes from the back of the ascending aorta to the front of the right pulmonary artery, a central aortopulmonary shunt passes directly from ascending aorta to pulmonary trunk, and a Pott's shunt is from descending aorta to left pulmonary artery.

Pulmonary artery branch stenosis can occur at sites of a previous shunt insertion.

A Glenn shunt is anastomosis of the superior vena cava (SVC) to the right pulmonary artery. Physiologically, it can be considered as a partial Fontan operation (see below).

Ventriculopulmonary conduits and patches

Repairs of tetralogy of Fallot and pulmonary atresia may involve insertion of a valved ventriculopulmonary conduit, or, in certain cases, a transannular patch. Afterwards, the severity of stenosis or regurgitation can be difficult to assess. The connections lie behind the sternum and are poorly visualized by TTE, and sometimes TEE, which gives MRI, with cine imaging and velocity mapping, an important role (Figs 14.13, 14.14 and 14.16).[29]

Corrections of transposition of the great arteries

Surgical 'correction' of transposition of the great arteries (TGA) by rerouting blood at atrial level (Mustard and Senning procedures) was achieved many years before satisfactory correction by arterial switch. Mustard and Senning operations both involve removal of the atrial septum, and rerouting, by means of a baffle of fabric (Mustard) or atrial wall (Senning) of connections between venous returns – systemic and pulmonary – and the two ventricles. In time, complications tend to arise. These include obstruction of either systemic venous or pulmonary venous atrial flow paths, shunting through a baffle suture leak, hypertrophy and eventual failure of the systemic right ventricle, and regurgitation of its tricuspid valve. Both MRI and TEE are valuable for assessing complications, but modified atrial anatomy needs to be understood. Pulmonary venous flow passes forward to the right of the saddle-shaped baffle towards the tricuspid valve. Its passage may be partly obstructed by residual (or regrown) native atrial septum, giving an hour-glass narrowing which can be shown by MRI in an oblique transaxial plane, aligned from sagittal pilots (Fig. 14.18).[31]

To the left of the baffle, flow through a pair of channels – down from the SVC and up from the inferior vena cava (IVC) – converges to pass leftwards through the mitral valve. These systemic venous channels can be traced on oblique coronal cine MRI, aligned from sagittal or transaxial pilots. Flow may be restricted by narrowing of either or both. If one caval channel only is obstructed, azygos veins tend to dilate, relieving the pressure by carrying flow to the other caval system.

The Rastelli operation is used for correction of transposition of the great arteries when there is also a ventricular septal defect (VSD) of sufficient size. Blood from the left ventricle is redirected via the VSD, with an oblique patch, to the aorta. Then an external valved conduit is inserted behind the sternum to carry flow from an incision

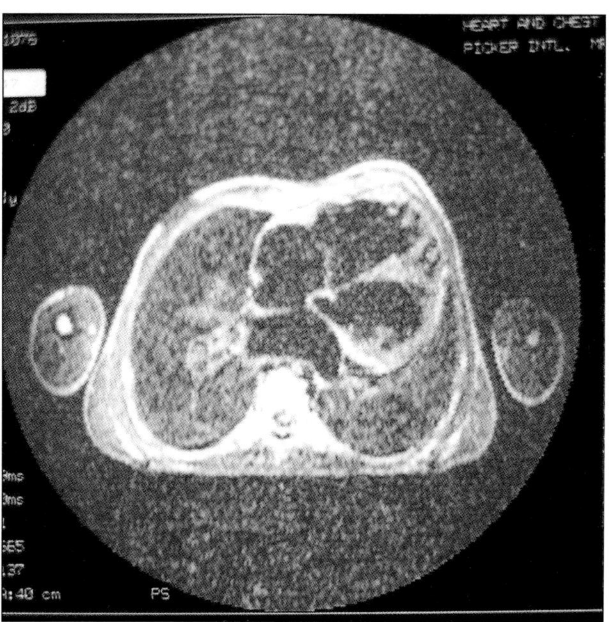

a

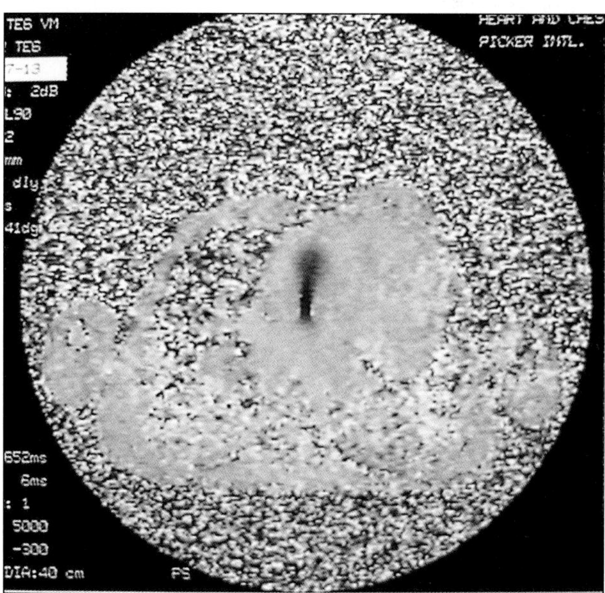

b

Figure 14.18
Mustard operation. Obstruction of pulmonary venous atrial compartment shown by MRI. a. Spin echo image in an oblique transaxial plane aligned with the pulmonary venous atrial flow path. The C-shaped structure in the centre of the heart is part of the surgically placed baffle. To the left of it on the image (to the patient's right) is an hour-glass pulmonary venous atrial compartment, almost divided by what must be residual atrial septal tissue. b. Corresponding velocity map, TE = 6 ms, showing a black jet, peak velocity 2.5 ms, up through the narrow orifice, towards the tricuspid valve. This indicates severe obstruction of the pulmonary venous atrial flow path.

in the front of the right ventricle to the pulmonary trunk, the native pulmonary valve being closed. Either this external conduit, or left ventricular outflow, via the VSD, can become obstructed.

Correction of TGA by arterial switch also has the advantage of allowing the left ventricle to supply aorta and systemic arteries, and does not depend on there being a VSD. It usually involves careful mobilization and reinsertion of coronary artery origins, which is technically challenging. Patency of coronary arteries close to their origins and possible deformations of the re-located great arteries may require investigation.

Fontan operations

Infants born with only one adequately sized ventricle may survive, initially, through mixing of systemic and pulmonary venous blood, but sooner or later their condition is likely to deteriorate due to ventricular volume overload, outflow obstruction, or inadequate or excessive pulmonary flow. The Fontan operation aims to eliminate shunting (usually by ASD closure), routing systemic venous return to pulmonary arteries without passage through an intervening ventricle, so that systemic and pulmonary vasculatures flow in series, propelled by the one ventricle. This results in raised systemic venous pressure, needed to maintain flow through the lungs. Any obstruction of the cavo-atrio-pulmonary flow path easily raises systemic venous pressure to an unsustainable level.

Fontan connection is usually via the right atrium, either by direct connection of the region of the appendage back to the pulmonary arteries, or via a conduit passing round the aorta. More recently total cavopulmonary connection (TCPC) has also come to be used. This results in a cross-like flow path: from above, the SVC is connected into the upper wall of the right pulmonary artery, like a bidirectional Glenn shunt, and from below, flow from the IVC is channeled, by a patch or flap, up one side of the right atrial cavity into the lower end of the transected SVC, which is connected, from below, into the right pulmonary artery. Right and left pulmonary arteries communicate, and the pulmonary trunk is closed.

Whichever variant, it is crucial that cavopulmonary flow paths remain unobstructed. Imaging may be required to look for thrombus in the right atrium, for which TEE is best, or stenosis of connections to pulmonary arteries, for which MRI is likely to be best (Fig 14.19 and 14.20). It is also important to monitor the function and outflow of the one ventricle.

A small residual shunt may be deliberately made at operation, to moderate systemic venous pressure in the postoperative period. This small fenestration in the patch tends to close spontaneously in due course.

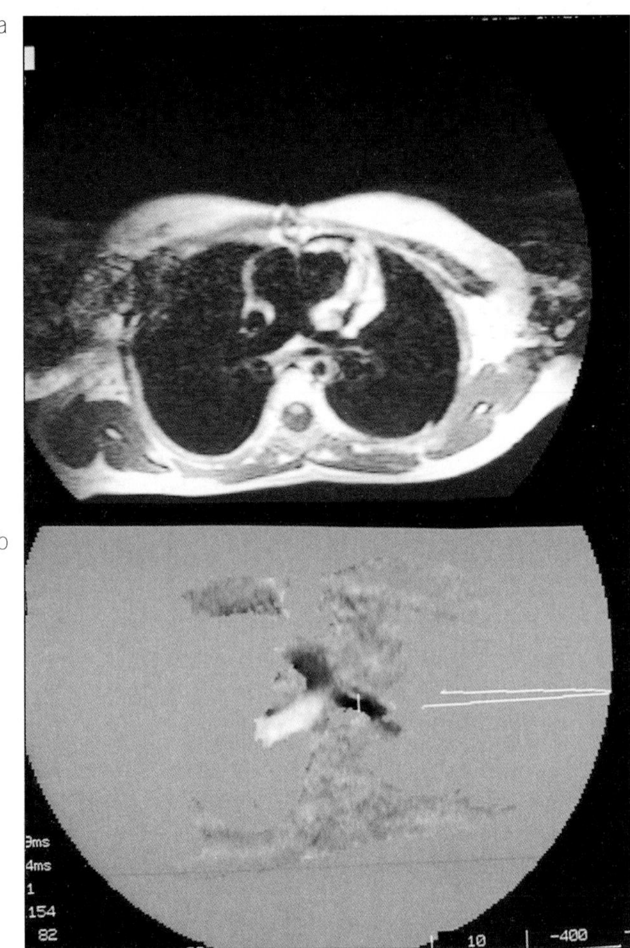

Figure 14.19
Fontan operation – atriopulmonary connection with mild left pulmonary artery stenosis shown by MRI with velocity mapping. a. Spin echo image showing the right atrium connected back to a good-sized right and a narrowed left pulmonary artery. b. Corresponding velocity map, TE = 14 ms. Flow to the left appears dark, to the right, light. It confirms that the lumen of the left pulmonary artery is somewhat narrowed, with a peak recorded of velocity of 0.8 ms with atrial systole. With a regular cardiac cycle and cardiac gating from the R wave of the ECG, this last frame of the sequence is acquired at a gating delay about 50 ms less than the R–R interval.

Stenosis

Obstruction to flow caused by stenosis is the commonest class of lesion requiring re-intervention by catheter or surgery. Stenosis may occur at sites of previous shunt closure, prosthetic valves, suture lines and other regions of reconstruction. Stenosis can also develop spontaneously, notably at subaortic, subpulmonary, and pulmonary artery branch sites.

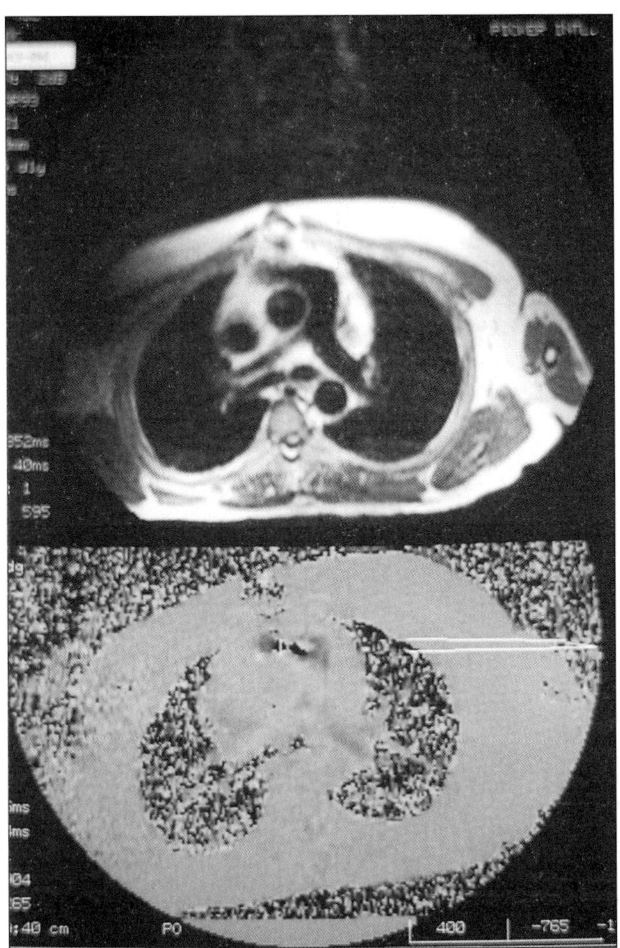

Figure 14.20
Fontan operation – MRI with velocity mapping showing severe obstruction of a valved right atrium to pulmonary artery conduit. a. Spin echo image shows the conduit coming into plane immediately behind the sternum (towards the top of the image). It passes back to the left of the aorta to a good-sized left pulmonary artery. The right pulmonary artery appears narrow, but is slightly out of the image plane. b. Nearly corresponding velocity map (there were intervening pilot cines to determine jet location and direction). There is a narrow black jet, directed towards the patient's left, through the stenosed homograft valve near the inlet of the conduit, peak velocity 1.9 ms coinciding with atrial systole. This represents severe Fontan obstruction. Balloon dilatation was attempted, but the operation was later re-done.

Assessment of the clinical significance of stenosis is a complex issue. Location of stenosis, orifice diameter, lumen geometry, peak jet velocity (or pressure gradient), time course of velocity (or gradient), flow volume, jet size and shape can all be taken into account, but the pathophysiological setting is crucial. Factors such as ventricular function, regurgitation, shunt or collateral flow modify interpretation. There may be discrepancies between gradients measured by catheter and those deduced, using the modified Bernoulli equation, from jet velocity measurements made by Doppler ultrasound or MRI velocity mapping. On the whole, there is a tendency for lower gradients to be recorded at catheterization. Possible explanations include the effect of sedation, fluid dynamic considerations such as 'pressure recovery' distal to stenosis, and the difference between peak to peak and peak instantaneous measurement.

The significance of a stenosis varies greatly with location. Minor obstructions, in terms of jet velocity or pressure gradient, can be serious at venous and atrial levels. Here a gradient of a few millimeters of mercury, or a peak velocity between 1 and 2 m/s, are significant. This applies to obstructions after Mustard, Senning and Fontan operations.

On the outflow side, raised ventricular afterload caused by stenosis at subvalvar, valvar or supravalvar level can lead to ventricular hypertrophy and failure. A morphologically right ventricle is more susceptible than a left, and a resting peak jet velocity of 4 m/s will cause right ventricular deterioration over time. Homograft and allograft valves, in pulmonary or aortic positions, tend to calcify and stenose. Stenosis of ventriculopulmonary valved conduits can be difficult to assess as patients may remain symptom-free while myocardial damage is being caused. Echocardiographic access may be inadequate, and calcified cusps are poorly seen on MRI spin echo images. Cine MRI and velocity mapping therefore have an important role in locating stenosis and measuring jet velocity (Fig. 14.16). Pulmonary artery branch stenosis may also be present, particularly following shunt closure. MRI with cine imaging, or computed tomography with contrast injection, can be used to assess pulmonary branches, which are rarely accessible to TTE or TEE.

Aortic coarctation and recoarctation

In the case of stenosis associated with aortic coarctation, risk is related to systemic hypertension rather than increased ventricular load. In this setting, a resting peak velocity of 3 m/s is considerable, particularly if associated with diastolic prolongation of forward flow (diastolic 'tail'), which is a useful indicator of the obstructive significance of coarctation. The diastolic tail is identifiable by cine MRI velocity mapping (compare Fig. 14.21 and 14.22) and by continuous wave Doppler ultrasound (Fig. 14.23).

When investigating aortic coarctation in adults (unoperated, balloon dilated or operated) there are a number of questions to be considered:

- Is blood pressure high in one or both arms?
- To what extent is it caused by obstruction due to coarctation?

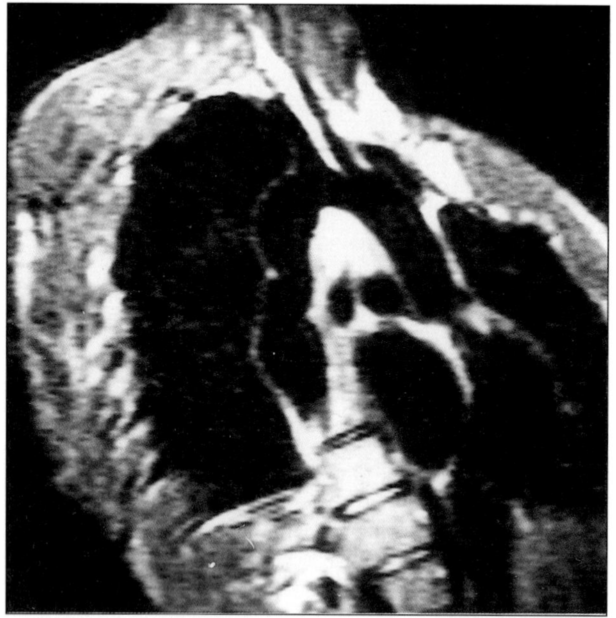

a

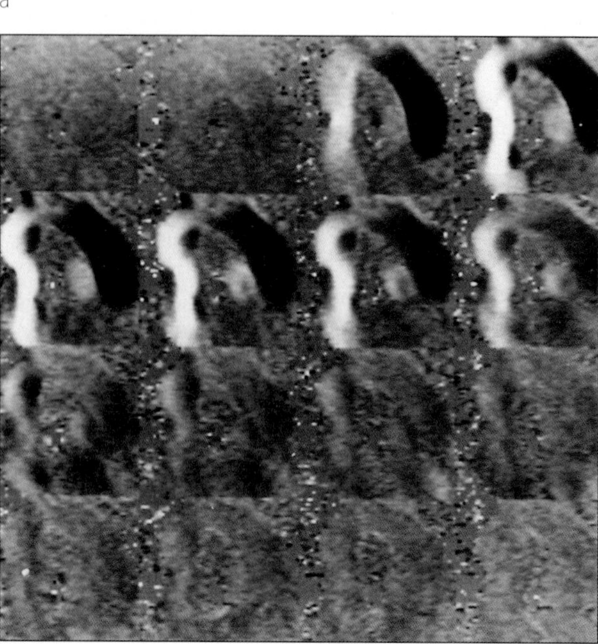

b

Figure 14.21
Mild recoarctation studied by MRI with velocity mapping. a. Spin echo image aligned with the aortic arch and repaired descending aorta, viewed from the right, 12 years after internal mammary artery patch repair of coarctation. b. Detail from all 16 frames of the velocity map acquisition, velocity encoded in the vertical read gradient direction. Downward velocities appear white and upward velocities, dark. The 16 frames run from left to right in lines ordered from above downwards. Systolic forward flow is seen in frames 3–8, after which slight swirling of blood persists for a few frames. The lumen is tortuous, but not severely narrowed. The peak recorded velocity was 2 ms, without significant diastolic prolongation of forward flow.

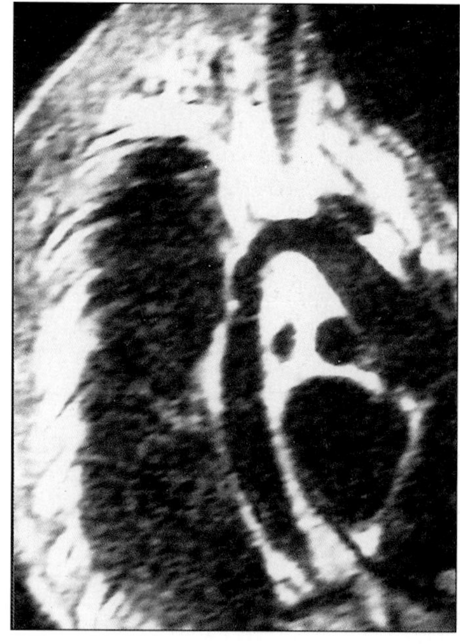

a

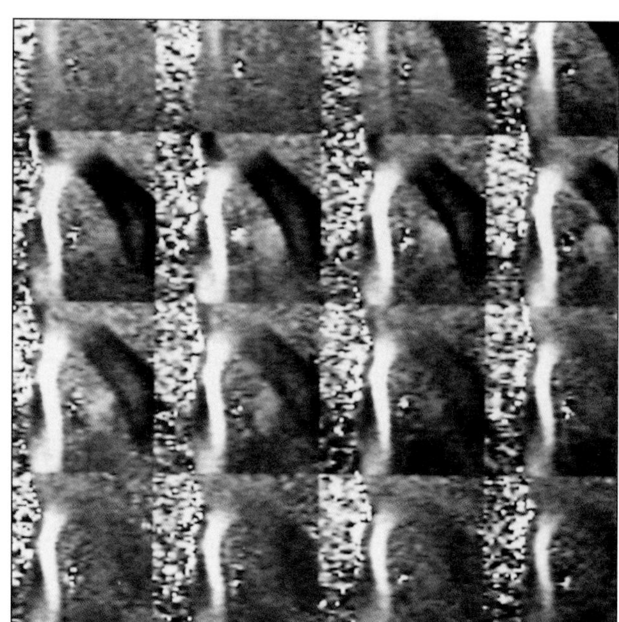

b

Figure 14.22
Significant recoarctation shown by MRI with velocity mapping. a. Spin echo image aligned with the arch and descending aorta 12 years after Dacron tube repair of recoarctation at 4 years of age. The narrowed lumen suggests significant stenosis, which was confirmed by velocity mapping. b. Detail from all 16 velocity map frames in the same patient, encoded and ordered as in Figure 14.16b. A peak jet velocity of 3.4 ms is recorded in frame 6. Forward flow does not cease at the end of systole (frame 10) but continues throughout diastole, showing significant diastolic prolongation of forward flow.

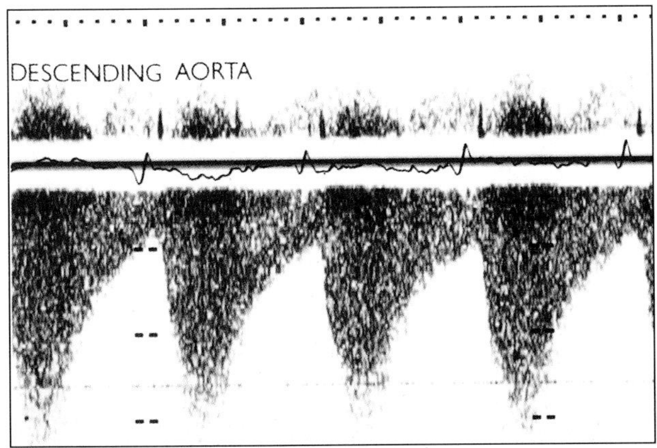

Figure 14.23
Severe coarctation shown by transthoracic ultrasound. Continuous wave Doppler trace of jet flow through severe aortic coarctation, insonated from suprasternal notch. A peak velocity of a least 3 ms and extension of forward flow throughout diastole indicate severe coarctation.

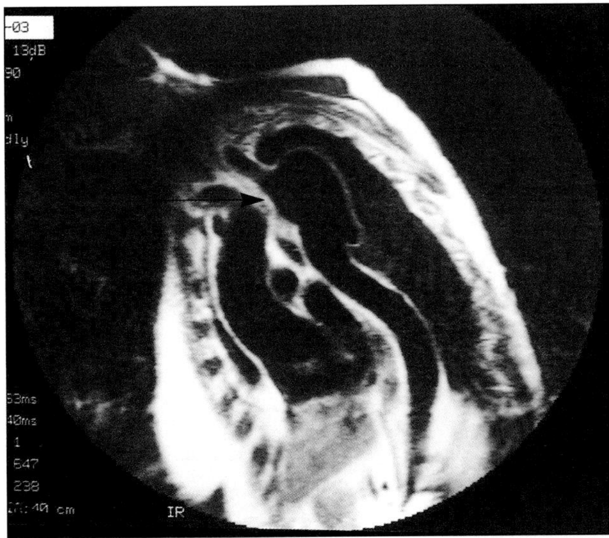

Figure 14.24
Dacron patch aneurysm shown by spin echo MRI. Thin walled aneurysm in the region of a previous Dacron patch repair of aortic coarctation, requiring re-operation (arrow).

- If operated, what type of surgery?
- Is there diastolic prolongation of forward flow?
- Do blood pressure and 'gradient' rise markedly with exercise?
- Is there associated aortic valve disease?
- Is the left ventricle hypertrophied?
- How extensive is collateral flow?
- What is the location and severity of coarctation?
- Of what type is it (e.g. membrane or narrow segment)?
- What is the geometry of aorta and branches in the vicinity of coarctation?
- Is there dissection, aneurysm or false aneurysm?

No single modality answers all questions, but MRI with velocity mapping, in addition to blood pressure measurements and Doppler echocardiography (with stress), should give enough information to proceed to surgery. Invasive angiography should not be needed unless coronary artery disease is suspected. Computed X-ray tomography with three-dimensional reconstruction provides impressive images of aortic arch geometry, but is less effective than MRI for determination of the nature and severity of coarctation, or for diagnosis of dissecting or false aneurysms. Dissecting aneurysm can result from attempted balloon dilatation. True or false aneurysms may complicate repairs, particularly those incorporating patches of incompliant fabric such as Dacron (Fig. 14.24). We recommend that patients with such patches should have annual MRI. Infected false aneurysms can be associated with operated or unoperated coarctation. Post-stenotic dilatation is common, appearing as fusiform dilatation beyond the coarctation, usually distinguishable from aneurysmal dilatation.

Surgery for coarctation or recoarctation in adults may not be straightforward. Imaging has important roles in foreseeing or identifying complications. We have learned to regard hemoptysis, early or late after coarctation repair, as an ominous sign. It may result from blood leaking from aorta to bronchi via a false aneurysm, which can be demonstrated by MRI.[32]

Regurgitation

Valve regurgitation is easier to visualize than to measure. Various imaging features can contribute to evaluation.[33] Echocardiography offers the major advantage that valve cusps, and any infective or subvalvar lesions, can be visualized directly. This is rarely the case with cine MRI, whose contributions rely on visualization and measurement of flow. The Doppler 'proximal isovolumetric surface area' (PISA) approach[34,35] is discussed in Chapter 6. MRI velocity mapping of flow through planes transecting the aorta, pulmonary trunk or conduit above an outflow valve allows measurement of regurgitant fraction,[22] and where only one valve leaks and there is no shunt, regurgitation can be calculated from the difference between right and left ventricular stroke volumes, measured by MRI.

Free pulmonary regurgitation can be an outcome after certain repairs of tetralogy of Fallot or pulmonary atresia. From our MRI measurements, it results in a regurgitant fraction of about 40%; more if exacerbated by pulmonary artery branch stenosis.[36]

Ventricular function

Methods for assessment of ventricular function are discussed in Chapter 1. In patients with congenital heart diseases there are particular considerations. One is that a morphologically right ventricle delivering systemic pressure is prone to hypertrophy and premature failure. Abnormal ventricular shape and orientation can make assessment of function difficult. Cine MRI has the advantage that it can be performed in any oblique plane, chosen to suit the chamber. In many cases, a straight transaxial cine at mid-ventricular level gives a useful comparison of left and right ventricular movement, but it must be remembered that an off-center slice may give a misleading impression of mobility and function.

Right as well as left ventricular stroke volumes and ejection fractions can be measured by MRI. Cine imaging is performed in a stack of slices (e.g. transaxial) to cover the volume of the heart. End-systolic and end-diastolic volumes are calculated by summation of cavity cross-sectional areas (volumes) traced manually. Myocardial mass can also be measured in this way, but the approach is relatively time consuming.

Shunting at any level can result in a discrepancy of volume loading and size between the ventricles. If shunt closure and biventricular surgical repair is being considered, size of the smaller ventricle is important. Restricted stroke volume on one side can be a limiting factor if a ventricle is small.

Finally, surgical repairs of tetralogy of Fallot and pulmonary atresia may involve conduit placement and patching of the anterior wall of the right ventricle. In some cases this leaves a fairly extensive immobile region immediately behind the sternum, not easily seen by TTE, but well demonstrated by transaxial and sagittal cine MRI (Fig. 14.13).

Correlation of clinical information

Diagnostic imaging should not be isolated from findings obtained by history-taking, physical examination and non-imaging investigations such as those of hematology and electrocardiography. Because decision making in adults with congenital heart disease must take many considerations into account, collaborative presentation in the setting of a clinical meeting is particularly valuable. It allows a comprehensive picture to be built up which can clarify questions of management and further the process of learning.

Acknowledgements

This chapter is based on 9 years of rewarding collaboration with Dr Jane Somerville. Thanks also go to Dr Simon Rees, Dr Rafael Hirsch, Dr Michael Rubens, Dr Sara Thorne, to Professor Andrew Redington for providing echocardiographic and angiographic illustrations, and to other colleagues in the Magnetic Resonance and Grown-Up Congenital Heart Units at Royal Brompton Hospital. Philip Kilner is supported by the British Heart Foundation.

References

1 Somerville J: Congenital heart disease in adults and adolescents. *Br Heart J* 1986; **56**: 395–7.

2 Somerville J: The physician's responsibilities: residua and sequelae. *J Am Coll Cardiol* 1991; **18**: 325–7.

3 Perloff JK: Congenital heart disease in adults: a new cardiovascular subspeciality. *Circulation* 1991; **84**: 1881–90.

4 Warnes C: Establishing an adult congenital heart disease clinic. *Am J Card Imag* 1995; **9**: 11–14.

5 Moodie DS: Adult congenital heat disease. *Curr Opinion Cardiol* 1995; **10**: 92–8.

6 Ungerleider RM, Kisslo JA, Greeley WJ et al: Intraoperative echocardiography during congenital heart operations: experience from 1,000 cases. *Ann Thorac Surg* 1995; **60**: S539–S542.

7 Lock JE: The adult with congenital heart disease: cardiac catheter as a therapeutic intervention. *J Am Coll Cardiol* 1991; **18**: 330–1.

8 Simpson IA, Sahn DJ: Adult congenital heart disease: use of transthoracic echocardiography versus magnetic resonance imaging scanning. *Am J Card Imag* 1995; **9**: 29–37.

9 Hirsch R, Kilner PJ, Connelly MS et al: Diagnosis in adolescents and adults with congenital heart disease. Prospective assessment of individual and combined roles of magnetic resonance imaging and transesophageal echocardiography. *Circulation* 1994; **90**: 2937–951.

10 Wexler L, Higgins CB: The use of magnetic resonance imaging in adult congenital heart disease. *Am J Card Imag* 1995; **9**: 15–28.

11 Post JC, van Rossum AC, Bronzwaer JGF, et al: Magnetic resonance angiography of anomalous coronary arteries – a new gold standard for dilineating the proximal course? *Circulation* 1995; **92**: 3163–71.

12 McConnell MV, Ganz P, Selwyn AP et al: Identification of anomalous coronary arteries and their anatomic course by magnetic resonance coronary angiography. *Circulation* 1995; **92**: 3158–62.

13 Shively BK: Transesophageal echocardiography in endocarditis. *Cardiol Clin* 1993; **11**: 437–46.

14 Elliott LP: *Cardiac Imaging in Infants, Children and Adults* (Lippincott: Philadelphia, 1991).

15 Elliott LP, Schiebler GL: *The X-ray Diagnosis of Congenital Heart Disease in Infants, Children and Adults* (Thomas: Springfield, IL, 1979).

16 Steiner RM, Gross GW, Flicker S et al: Congenital heart disease in the adult patient: the value of plain film chest radiology. *J Thorac Imag* 1995; **10**: 1–25.

17 Hartnell GG, Meier RA: MR angiography of congenital heart disease in adults. *Radiographics* 1995; **15**: 781–94.

18 Shellock FE, Kanel E: *Magnetic Resonance Bioeffects, Safety and Patient Management.* (Raven Press: New York, 1994).

19 Firmin DN, Nayler GL, Kilner PJ, Longmore DB: The application of phase shifts in NMR for flow measurement. *Magn Reson Med* 1990; **14**: 230–41.

20 Underwood SR, Firmin DN: *Magnetic Resonance of the Cardiovascular System.* (Blackwell: Oxford, 1990).

21 Hundley WG, Li HF, Hillis LD et al: Quantitation of cardiac output with velocity-encoded, phase-difference magnetic resonance imaging. *Am J Cardiol* 1995; **75**: 1250–5.

22 Rebergen SA, Chin JGJ, Ottenkamp J et al: Pulmonary regurgitation in the late postoperative follow-up of tetraolgy of fallot – volumetric quantitation by nuclear magnetic resonance velocity mapping. *Circulation* 1993; **88**: 2257–66.

23 Hundley WG, Li HF, Lange RA et al: Assessment of left-to-right intracardiac shunting by velocity-encoded, phase-difference magnetic resonance imaging: a comparison with oximetric and indicator dilution techniques. *Circulation* 1995; **91**: 2955–60.

24 Holmvang G, Palacios IF, Vlahakes GJ et al: Imaging and sizing of atrial septal defects by magnetic resonance. *Circulation* 1995; **92**: 3473–80.

25 Sondergard L, Stahlberg F, Thomsen C et al: Accuracy and precision of MR velocity mapping in measurement of stenotic ceross sectional area, flow rate and pressure gradient. *JMRI* 1993; **3**(2): 433–7.

26 Kilner PJ, Firmin DN, Rees RS et al: Valve and great vessel stenosis: assessment with MR jet velocity mapping. *Radiology* 1991; **178**: 229–35.

27 Kilner PJ, Manzara CC, Mohiaddin RH et al: Magnetic resonance jet velocity mapping in mitral and aortic valve stenosis. *Circulation* 1993; **87**: 1239–48.

28 Kilner PJ, Shinohara T, Sampson C et al: Repaired aortic coarctation in adults – MRI with velocity mapping shows distortions of anatomy and flow. *Cardiol Young* 1996; **6**: 20–7.

29 Martinez JE, Mohiaddin RH, Kilner PJ et al: Obstruction in extracardiac ventriculopulmonary conduits: value of nuclear magnetic resonance imaging with velocity mapping and Doppler echocardiography. *J Am Coll Cardiol* 1992; **20**: 338–44.

30 Kirklin JW, Barratt-Boyes BG: *Cardiac Surgery.* (Churchill Livingstone: New York, 1993).

31 Sampson C, Kilner PJ, Hirsch R et al: Venoatrial pathways after the Mustard operation for transposition of the great arteries: anatomic and functional MR imaging. *Radiology* 1994; **193**: 211–17.

32 Holdright DR, Kilner PJ, Somerville J: Haemoptysis from false aneurysm: near fatal complication of repair of coarctation of the aorta using a Dacron patch. *Intl J Cardiol* 1991; **32**: 406–8.

33 Schiller NB, Foster E, Redberg RF. Transesophageal echocardiography in the evaluation of mitral regurgitation: the twenty-four signs of severe mitral regurgitation. *Cardiol Clin* 1993; **11**: 399–408.

34 Simpson IA, de Belder MA, Kenny A et al: How to quantitative valve regurgitation by echo Doppler techniques. British Society of Echocardiography. *Br Heart J* 1995; **73**: 1–9.

35 Simpson IA, Shiota T, Gharib M, Sahn DJ: Current status of flow convergence for clinical applications: is it a leaning tower of "PISA"? *J Am Coll Cardiol* 1996; **27**: 504–50.

36 Chaturved RR, Kilner PJ, White PA et al: Increased airway pressure and simulated branch pulmonary artery stenosis increase pulmonary regurgitation after repair of tetralogy of Fallot: real-time analysis using a conductance catheter technique. *Circulation* 1997; 3: 643–49.

15

Cardiac thrombus and stroke

Mary C Corretti

'The embolus usually enters the carotid, rarely the vertebral artery. In the great majority of cases it comes from the left heart and is either a vegetation or a fresh endocarditis. Less often the embolus is a portion of a clot which has formed in the auricular appendix. Portions of a clot from an aneurysm, thrombi from atheroma of the aorta or from the territory of the pulmonary veins may also cause blocking of branches of the circle of Willis.' W Osler, *Practice of Medicine*, 1892.

Introduction

Stroke is the third leading cause of death in the USA, and a major source of long-term disability and financial burden. Acute stroke has many causes. Approximately 80% of strokes are due to brain ischemia or infarction, and 20% result from intracerebral or subarachnoid hemorrhage. The major cause of ischemic stroke is atherosclerotic thrombotic disease of large arteries such as the extracranial carotid arteries and major intracranial vessels.

Cardioembolic strokes account for approximately 15–20% of ischemic strokes.[1,2] A stroke is considered to have a cardioembolic mechanism if a potential cardioembolic source is present in the absence of cerebrovascular disease in a patient with nonlacunar stroke.[2] Cardiac disease can result in stroke in various ways (Table 15.1).

The link between these clinical entities is the propensity to develop and dislodge thrombotic material. Most cardiac thrombi embolize to the brain (>75%) and the remainder embolize peripherally.[3]

The documentation of a cardioembolic mechanism of ischemic stroke often poses a clinical challenge for the neurologist since multiple causes for stroke often coexist in an individual. Hypertension is considered a predominant risk factor of all types of stroke.[4] Other risk factors for embolic ischemic stroke include heart disease, smoking, coronary artery disease, diabetes, hyperlipidemia, and peripheral vascular disease. The diagnosis of stroke is dependent on a thorough history; physical examination and a constellation of diagnostic tests are often needed to

Table 15.1 Cardiac etiologies of stroke.

- Rhythm disorders
  - Atrial fibrillation
  - Tachybradydysrhythmia
- Myocardial abnormalities
  - Myocardial infarction
  - Myocardial aneurysm
  - Dilated cardiomyopathy
  - Atrial septal defect
    - aneurysm/patent foramen ovale
  - Atrial myxoma/tumors
- Valve disorders
  - Rheumatic valve disease
  - Prosthetic valves
  - Endocarditis (bacterial, nonbacterial thrombotic)
  - Mitral valve prolapse
  - Mitral annular calcification
- Aortic atheroma

determine the causative mechanism. Neurologic and cardiologic features of the clinical presentation can provide clues for a potential cardioembolic mechanism. Clinical characteristics typically associated with cardioembolic stroke include sudden onset of the maximal neurologic deficit, multiple brain infarcts involving several vascular territories and the presence of a potential embolic source. Since a potential embolic source for stroke often coexists with diffuse atherosclerotic disease except in younger patients (<45 years), this finding alone does not necessarily establish cardioembolism as the causative mechanism. Interestingly, the causes of embolic stroke are of unknown etiology in approximately 40% of cases[5,6] despite the accelerated advances in diagnostic modalities. Thromboembolism and its interaction with the vasculature is a complex dynamic process which can exert harmful effects without leaving direct or discernible evidence of its source. Moreover, the timing of diagnostic testing may be critical in determining the underlying stroke mechanism.

Certain laboratory and radiologic features are helpful in the diagnosis of cardiogenic embolism. Embolic strokes appear on computed tomography (CT) as multiple superficial, wedge-shaped, hemorrhagic cortical infarcts, located throughout different vascular territories. CT can readily differentiate ischemia from hemorrhage in the acute lesions. Approximately 5–10% of embolic strokes develop a secondary hemorrhagic infarct seen on an early, initial CT scan. Most hemorrhagic infarcts have evolved and are visible on CT by 48 h. Hemorrhagic infarcts also have a mottled heterogeneous appearance in the cortical area, whereas intracerebral hemorrhages have a rounded homogeneous appearance in the cortical white matter. Occasionally, visualization of a thrombus in an artery can be seen. Compared to CT, magnetic resonance imaging (MRI) has emerged as a more sensitive imaging modality for the detection of brain infarcts and of hemorrhagic infarcts by hemosiderin imaging.

Other diagnostic techniques employed in the evaluation of ischemic stroke include carotid and transcranial ultrasound, magnetic resonance angiography, and intra-arterial angiography. Cardiologic imaging modalities used to detect cardiac sources of embolism include radionuclide angiography, cardiac CT and MRI, and echocardiography (transthoracic and transesophageal).

Since the 1970s, transthoracic echocardiography has been the most widely used cardiac imaging modality in stroke patients to identify an intracardiac source of embolism. In several unselected series of stroke patients, the diagnostic yield in defining a cardiac source of embolism with transthoracic echo has been variable.[7,8] The diagnostic yield of this modality increases when used in individuals with a high prevalence of heart disease and in young stroke patients without risk factors. Limitations of transthoracic echo include acoustic attenuation, limited resolution and inability to fully evaluate the left atrial appendage, interatrial septum and the aorta.

Transesophageal echocardiography (TEE) has emerged as a superior imaging modality in the evaluation of potential cardioembolism,[9–13] the diagnostic yield of TEE being 2- to 10-fold more than transthoracic echo.[9,10,14] TEE has a greater sensitivity in detecting left atrial and appendage thrombus,[15] patent foramen ovale,[13,16] atrial septal aneurysm,[17,18] spontaneous echo contrast[19–21] and aortic atheroma.[22,23]

Ultrafast CT and MRI can define intracardiac thrombus, tumors, valvular and annular calcification as well as septal defects which predispose to paradoxic embolization. Ventricular aneurysms and wall motion abnormalities leading to blood stasis are also visualized. Two-dimensional echo and ultrafast CT are comparable in evaluating intracardiac thrombus in stroke patients.[24,25] These technologies are not as widely available as echocardiography. Ultrafast CT and MRI continue to evolve; but a comparative assessment of diagnostic accuracy of all the above imaging modalities used to determine a cardioembolic etiology of stroke is not yet available.

Etiology of cardioembolism

Often a direct cause and effect relationship cannot be established in the evaluation of cardioembolic stroke. The diagnosis is often made by inference, but with greater certainty when a cardiac disorder which predisposes to embolism is present. Certain conditions are considered high risk or a more direct source of embolism. These include intracardiac thrombus, tumor, vegetation, and aortic atheromas. Other conditions such as valvular disease, septal defects, patent foramen ovale, dilated cardiomyopathy, and spontaneous echo contrast are considered low risk or indirect causes.

Rhythm disorders

Atrial fibrillation in the presence or absence of rheumatic valvular disease is associated with an increased incidence of stroke.[26] The risk of atrial fibrillation varies with the presence and nature of concomitant cardiovascular disease and other risk factors such as age, valvular disease, congestive heart failure, hypertension, and diabetes.[4,26–28] Atrial fibrillation in conjunction with rheumatic valvular heart disease is associated with a 17-fold increased risk of stroke.[27]

Nonvalvular atrial fibrillation has been shown to have a five-fold or greater increase in embolic events.[27] It is the most common cause of cardioembolism accounting for approximately half of cardioembolic strokes in several

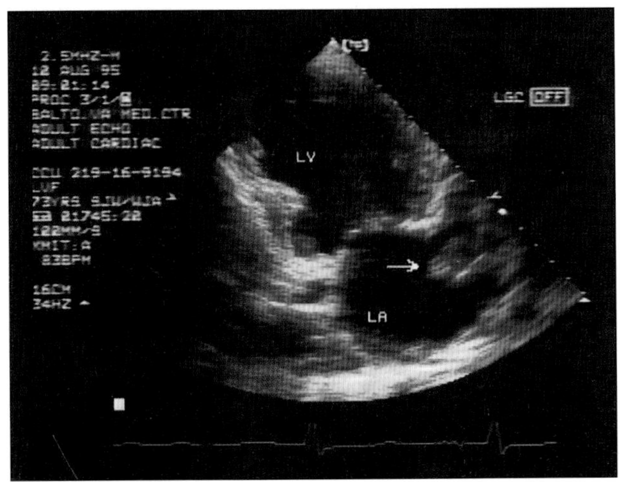

a

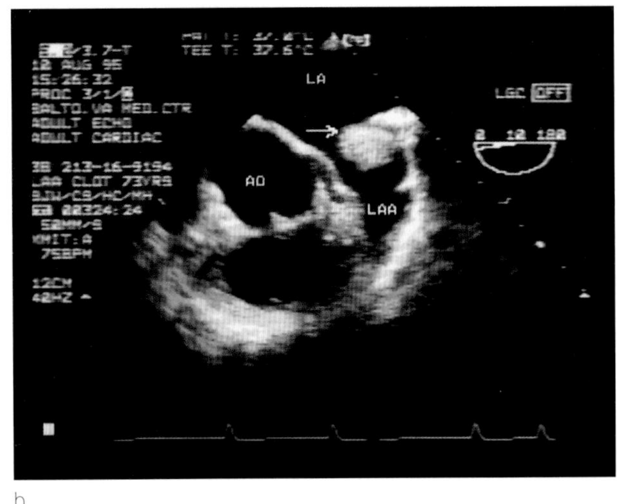

b

Figure 15.1
(a) Transthoracic 2-chamber view of the left ventricle, left atrium, and an amorphous echodensity protruding from the left atrial appendage (arrow). LV, left ventricle; LA, left atrium. (b) Transesophageal short-axis view of the aorta, left atrium and appendage from the same patient illustrating a mobile thrombus (arrow) in the appendage. AO, aorta; LA, left atrium; LAA, left atrial appendage.

series.[29,30] Nonvalvular atrial fibrillation includes a spectrum of diseases from lone atrial fibrillation to dilated cardiomyopathy. 'Lone' atrial fibrillation has a four-fold increased risk of stroke compared with similar age- and sex-matched controls.[31]

The mechanism of atrial fibrillation-associated stroke is multifactorial and complex, but it is generally accepted that it is a predisposition for blood stasis and clot formation in the atria. Rheumatic disease also damages endocardium and valve structures creating a surface for fibrin/clot formation. Atrial fibrillation with spontaneous contrast in the presence or absence of mitral stenosis poses a significant risk for left atrium and appendage thrombus which is best detected by TEE.

Tachybradydysrhythmia, a variant of sick sinus syndrome, consists of intermittent episodes of paroxysmal atrial fibrillation interspersed with periods of bradycardia. Thromboembolism is a complication of this syndrome, with cerebrovascular embolism accounting for an estimated 30–50% of deaths in sick sinus syndrome.[32]

Left atrial thrombus

Left atrial thrombus is a commonly identified cardiac source of embolus documented in 5% of patients following cerebral ischemic events.[9] Approximately 50% of left atrial thrombi are confined to the left atrial appendage. The risk of thromboembolism with left atrial thrombus is considerable and varies widely (5–17%) dependent upon concurrent cardiac conditions.[27] About one-third of patients with concomitant atrial fibrillation and mitral stenosis develop left atrial thrombus.[12,19,20] Other predisposing factors include prosthetic mitral valve, dilatation of the left atrium and appendage, and low cardiac output states. Approximately 5–10% of left atrial thrombus detected by TEE occurs in the absence of mitral valve or rhythm disorder.

Two-dimensional echo detects left atrial masses such as atrial myxomas but not thrombus.[33] Consequently, TEE is the method of choice to evaluate for left atrial thrombus, being close to the relevant structures and having superior resolution. Thrombus appears as a smooth or irregular, sessile or pedunculated echodensity in the left atrium or left atrial appendage (Fig. 15.1). Thrombus may be seen only on one of the atrial walls or noted protruding into the left atrium from the appendage. Thrombi in the appendage must be carefully distinguished from left atrial appendage pectinate muscle ridges which can mimic small thrombi by imaging in more than one plane. Absence of identifiable flow within the left atrial appendage by pulsed wave Doppler has recently been shown to be a predictor of left atrial thrombus.

Spontaneous echo contrast is defined as dynamic echoes that spiral and circulate in a smoke-like fashion in low-flow areas within the cardiovascular system[19] (Fig. 15.2). This finding is seen in a dilated left atrium with mitral stenosis and/or prosthetic valve, a dilated cardiomyopathy,

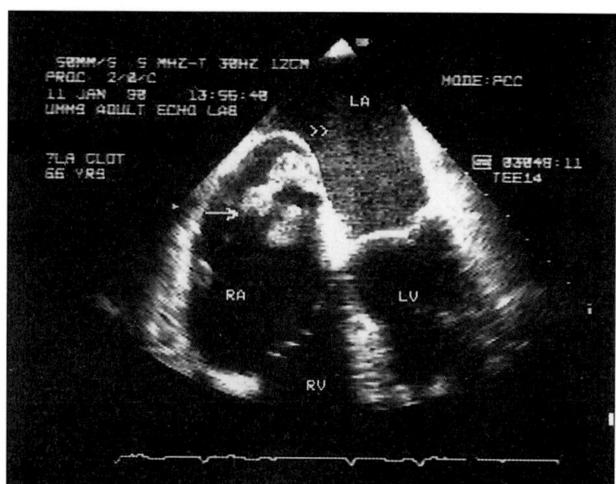

Figure 15.2
Transesophageal transverse 4-chamber view of the left atrium with spontaneous echo contrast (arrowheads) and a long freely mobile thrombus in the right atrium (arrow). LV, left ventricle; RV, right ventricle; RA, right atrium; LA, left atrium.

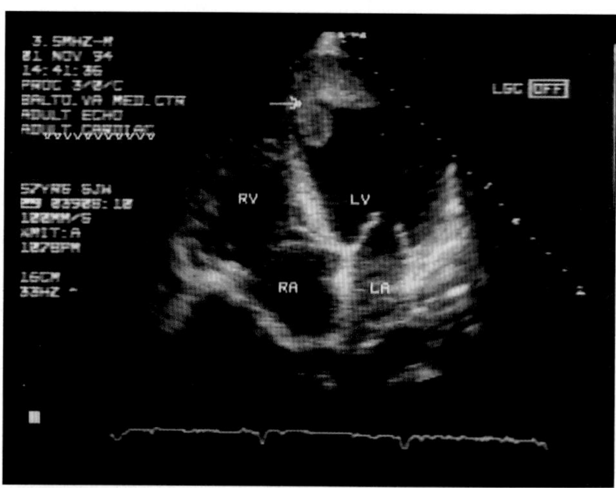

Figure 15.3
Transthoracic 4-chamber view of a large bilobular apical mural thrombus (arrow). RV, right ventricle; LV, left ventricle; RA, right atrium; LA, left atrium.

aneurysms, the false lumen of aortic dissections and the inferior vena cava with constrictive pericarditis. The exact mechanism of spontaneous contrast is unknown, but it appears secondary to blood stasis and rouleaux formation. Spontaneous echo contrast has been described by transthoracic echo; however, the higher frequency and close proximity afforded by TEE markedly improve the diagnostic sensitivity for detection of this entity.[12] It is most commonly associated with atrial fibrillation, mitral valve disease, or both, accounting for 75% of cases of spontaneous echo contrast in the left atrium in one study.[20] Furthermore, spontaneous echo contrast is a precursor to thrombus formation,[34,35] particularly in the left atrium and appendage. This is supported by several studies which demonstrate an association between spontaneous echo contrast and thromboembolic events.[11,19,20,36] It is also positively associated with left atrial enlargement and a history of suspected embolism, while negatively associated with mitral regurgitation.

Myocardial abnormalities

Myocardial infarction/aneurysm

Acute myocardial infarction (MI) accounts for 15% of all embolic events. Approximately 3% of strokes occur within the first 2–4 weeks of the infarct[1,2] especially in the setting of a transmural anterior infarct. Individuals with an anterior MI complicated by left ventricular thrombus, particularly protruding or mobile thrombus, are at significantly higher risk of embolism compared to those without thrombus and anterior MI.[37–39] Anterior MI predisposes to thrombus formation in segments of myocardial dyskinesis, akinesis or aneurysm. Stasis of blood in these areas may form layered organized mural thrombus, or amorphous and pedunculated clot. Morphologic features of left ventricular thrombus such as mobility, protrusion, and texture are predictors of embolic stroke.[40,41] Thrombus can also form within an aneurysm regardless of its location.

Two-dimensional transthoracic echo is relatively sensitive and specific for detection of left ventricular thrombus.[37,39,42,43] The sensitivity of transthoracic echo varies from 77% to 92%, and specificity from 84% to 94%.[43,44] If viewed from multiple tomographic views, transthoracic echo can accurately characterize thrombus location, size, shape, and degree of mobility. The echocardiographic appearance of ventricular thrombus may be laminar along the endocardial surface, or spherical, displaying different acoustic properties than the myocardium (Fig. 15.3). Accurate delineation of thrombus may be limited by inadequate image resolution or acoustic attenuation. Ultrasound reverberations near or at the apex can be misconstrued as thrombus; however, a lack of underlying wall motion abnormality makes thrombus less likely. Whether fixed or freely mobile, ventricular

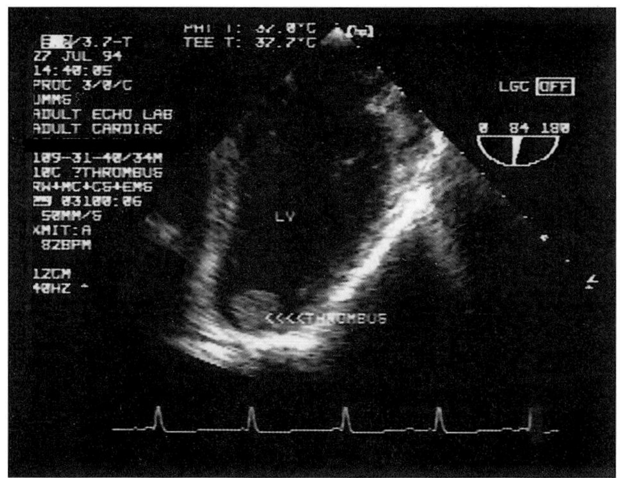

Figure 15.4
Transesophageal longitudinal view of a dilated left ventricle with a round apical thrombus (labeled). LV, left ventricle; LA, left atrium.

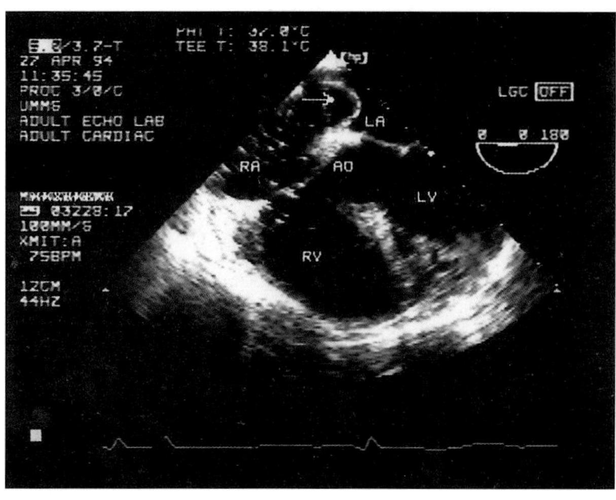

Figure 15.5
Transesophageal transverse 4-chamber view of an interatrial septal aneurysm bulging toward the left atrium (arrow). RA, right atrium; LA, left atrium; AO, aorta; RV, right ventricle; LV, left ventricle.

thrombus moves in concert with the underlying myocardial wall. This differentiates thrombus echodensities from transducer artifact. False tendon, a normal variant, occasionally seen in the distal left ventricle, can also be mistaken for thrombus.

Multiplane TEE, as opposed to single or biplane TEE, allows accurate examination of the cardiac apex. Ventriculography and radionuclide angiography are not as sensitive as echo in detecting left ventricular thrombus.[43,45]

Other modalities which detect and characterize intracardiac thrombus include ultrafast CT,[24,25] MRI,[46] and platelet scintigraphy.[47–49] These technologies continue to evolve and full comparison studies are not yet available.

Dilated cardiomyopathy

Though a less common cause of cardioembolic stroke, nonischemic dilated cardiomyopathy of various etiologies can be complicated by embolism even in the absence of atrial fibrillation. The estimated frequency of embolic complication in dilated cardiomyopathy has ranged from 11% to 18%,[50–52] although some studies suggest no increased risk.[51,53] Mural thrombi are usually the underlying source (Fig. 15.4). The presence of thrombi on noninvasive studies does not always correlate with embolism[51] since mural thrombus may be adherent to the trabeculae carneae of the cardiac apex. Despite controversy, most experts recommend long-term anticoagulation for patients with dilated cardiomyopathy even in the absence of documented thrombus due to the associated risk of thrombus formation.[54]

Atrial septum

The atrial septum may be responsible for a cardioembolic stroke by way of an atrial septal aneurysm with potential for thrombus formation in situ or through a paradoxic embolism through an associated patent foramen ovale. Paradoxic embolus via a patent foramen ovale or septal defect without an aneurysm can also occur. Up to 90% of cases with patent foramen ovale or interatrial communication exhibit shunting with contrast.[55,56]

Echocardiographically, atrial septal aneurysm appears as a redundant thin, mobile outpouching of the interatrial septum localized usually, but not exclusively, around the fossa ovalis (Fig. 15.5). It is defined as a bulging of ≥1.5 cm beyond the plane of the atrial septum with concomitant phasic excursion during the respiratory cycle. Additionally, the aneurysmal base should be ≥1.5 cm in diameter. It is an incidental finding at autopsy in approximately 10% of adults,[57] and its exact etiology is not known.[56] The prevalence of atrial septal aneurysm noted by transthoracic echo is 0.1–0.2%[58] and by TEE is 2–3%.[18] The prevalence of this finding in patients referred for TEE after a cerebral ischemic event is 11–15%.[13,18] Although atrial septal aneurysm is associated with an increased incidence of cerebral thromboembolic events,[55,56,58] a direct cause and effect relationship cannot be drawn conclusively, owing to concomitant factors which have cardioembolic potential.

Patent foramen ovale

Patent foramen ovale (PFO) is an embryologic remnant which results from maldevelopment of the septum primum or incomplete fusion of the septum primum and septum secundum. Whether PFO is a cause of cerebral ischemia is controversial. The prevalence of PFO in the general population is 10–18%,[2,59,60] in patients with an identifiable cause of stroke it is 21%, and among those with cryptogenic (unexplained) stroke it is 40%.[60] There is a particularly high prevalence of PFO in young adults with unexplained stroke.[60–63] Paradoxical embolism via the PFO with venous thrombosis as the main source of embolism is the presumed mechanism.

Transthoracic echo with color flow Doppler and contrast medium injection with provocative maneuvers (e.g. cough, Valsalva) is standardly used to diagnose a PFO and shunt. Recently, TEE has been demonstrated superior to transthoracic echo in visualizing the atrial septum and fossa ovalis membrane.[16,17,55,64] Color flow Doppler imaging helps detect continuous or intermittent uni- or bidirectional flow across the interatrial septum. Contrast medium (microbubbles) injection with provocative maneuvers to increase right atrial blood flow and pressure confirms the presence of a shunt through a PFO (Fig. 15.6). A shunt is diagnosed if constant or intermittent passage of echocontrast bubbles from right to left atrium occurs within three cycles of complete opacification of the right atrium. In individuals with cryptogenic stroke, the size of the PFO directly correlates with the degree of shunt seen by the microbubble technique.[65,66] The number of contrast bubbles correlates with an increased risk of recurrent stroke, suggesting that the size and not just the presence of a PFO may play a causal role.[66] Transcranial contrast Doppler ultrasound has been studied in conjunction with TEE to semiquantitate the degree of shunting, showing a high concordance with larger shunts.[67]

Tumors

The most common benign primary cardiac tumor causing an embolic stroke is atrial myxoma. In 27–55% of affected patients friable tumor fragments from this lesion cause stroke.[2] Emboli can also arise from neoplastic tissue and/or thrombus from other primary or metastic tumors.[2]

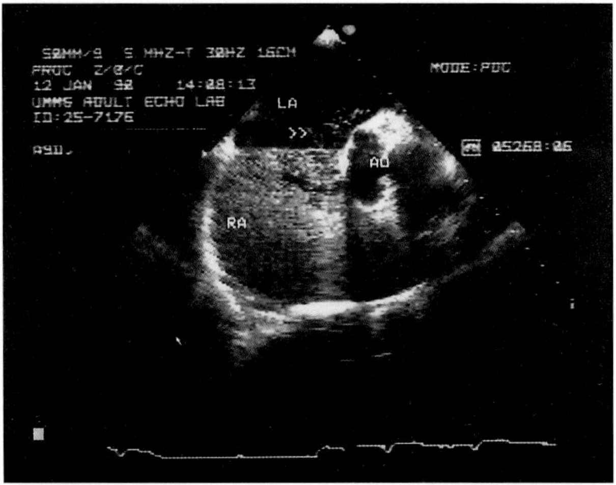

a

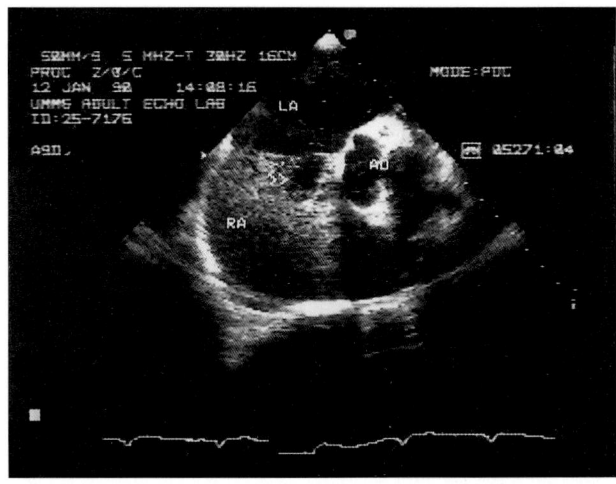

b

Figure 15.6

(a) Transesophageal transverse view of the right atrium, left atrium and aorta illustrating saline contrast injection into the right atrium with bubbles crossing from right to left via a patent foramen ovale. (b) Negative contrast is seen in the right atrium due to left-to-right shunting. RA, right atrium; LA, left atrium; AO, aorta.

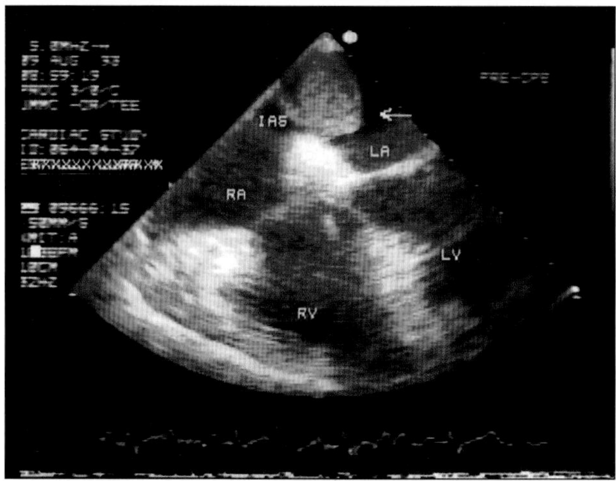

Figure 15.7
Transesophageal transverse 4-chamber view of an atrial myxoma (arrow). RA, right atrium; LA, left atrium; IAS, interatrial septum; RV, right ventricle; LV, left ventricle.

Classically, the myxoma is a mobile mass attached by a stalk at or near the fossa ovalis, and protrudes into the left atrium (Fig. 15.7). These lesions can prolapse into the left ventricle in diastole, mimicking mitral stenosis. Myxomas can arise on the endocardial surface of all cardiac chambers.

The diagnosis of atrial myxoma by transthoracic echo is well established; diagnostic sensitivity is not enhanced by TEE.[12] However, the higher imaging resolution of TEE may help differentiate tumor from thrombus, and detect extracardiac masses.[68]

Ultrafast CT and MRI are also excellent imaging modalities for defining cardiac and extracardiac masses.

Valve disorders

Rheumatic valve disease

Embolism is a significant cause of morbidity and mortality in rheumatic valve disease. The Framingham study demonstrated a 17-fold increase in risk of stroke in individuals with mitral stenosis and atrial fibrillation, compared with a six-fold increase in individuals with nonvalvular atrial fibrillation alone.[27] Pathophysiologic consequences of rheumatic heart disease include mitral stenosis with some degree of mitral regurgitation, atrial dilatation, elevated left atrial pressure, atrial fibrillation, and heart failure. Most emboli originate from the left atrium and appendage thrombus which form as a result of blood stasis. Less often, thrombotic and calcific material from the rheumatic valves embolize.

Spontaneous emboli complicating nonrheumatic calcific aortic stenosis is quite uncommon. Small fragments may embolize to produce a transient retinal ischemic event. Larger emboli have been associated with catheter manipulation of calcific aortic stenosis.[69,70]

Endocarditis

Ischemic stroke and brain hemorrhage are well-known complications of infective endocarditis. The prevalence of ischemic stroke ranges from 15% to 20%, with the majority occurring on presentation or during the initial 48 h after diagnosis.[71,72]

Echocardiography is an integral part of the evaluation of patients with suspected or known endocarditis. Echocardiography detects valve vegetations, and can evaluate the complications and hemodynamic sequelae of endocarditis. Numerous studies have examined the sensitivity and specificity of echocardiography in detecting vegetations in patients with clinical evidence of infective endocarditis.[73–77] Sensitivity for transthoracic echocardiography ranges considerably from 50% to 80%;[73,76,77] with the superior image quality of TEE, sensitivity has greatly increased to 90–100%.[77,78] The enhanced resolution of TEE allows definition of vegetative lesions, periannular abscesses, and valve destruction (Figs 15.8 and 15.9).

The utility of TEE in the evaluation of (infected) prosthetic valves has greatly enhanced the diagnostic yield. Typically, the sewing ring and support structures of prosthetic valves are highly echogenic, creating reverberation artifacts which obscure the presence and extent of valve destruction. Exuberant growth, pannus formation and thrombus may cause valve obstruction. Furthermore, valve dehiscence results from tissue necrosis around the supporting annular structure. This is seen echocardiographically as a rocking or tilting motion of the entire valve apparatus during the cardiac cycle. Excessive rocking occurs with extensive (>40%) dehiscence around the prosthetic annulus.[79] The infectious process can also migrate to the subvalvular structures with resultant rupture, and subsequent flail leaflet segments. Perivalvular abscess is noted echocardiographically as an echodense thickness around the annulus with or without an echolucent center. There is potential for aneurysm formation and rupture with fistulous communications between the abscess and other cardiac chambers.

Although two-dimensional echo is the most sensitive imaging tool to detect valvular vegetations and the complications, endocarditis remains a clinical diagnosis. Furthermore, the clinical significance of vegetations for embolic

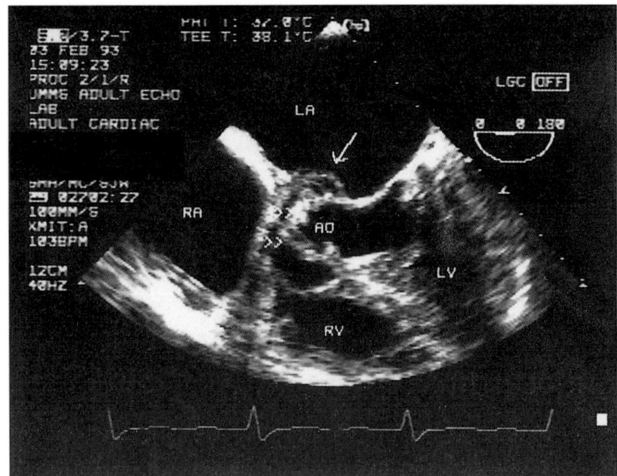

Figure 15.8
Transesophageal transverse 4-chamber view of a diffusely thickened aortic valve (arrowheads) with an echolucent area along the intervalvular fibrosa consistent with aortic root abscess. RA, right atrium; LA, left atrium; AO, aorta; LV, left ventricle; RV, right ventricle.

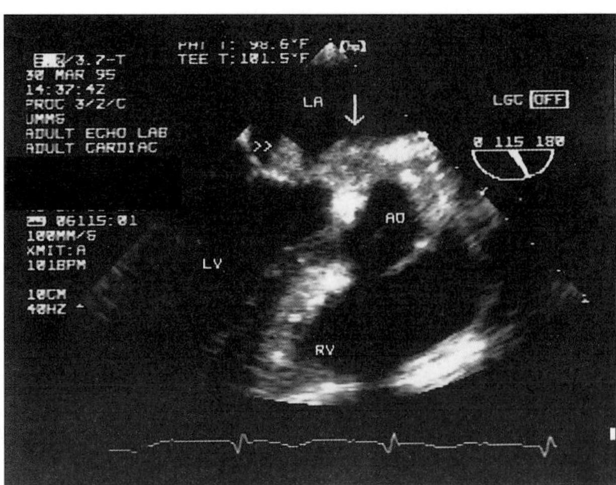

Figure 15.9
Transesophageal oblique longitudinal view of aortic valve vegetation, periannular abscess (arrow) and mitral valve vegetation (arrowheads). LA, left atrium; LV, left ventricle; RV, right ventricle; AO, aorta.

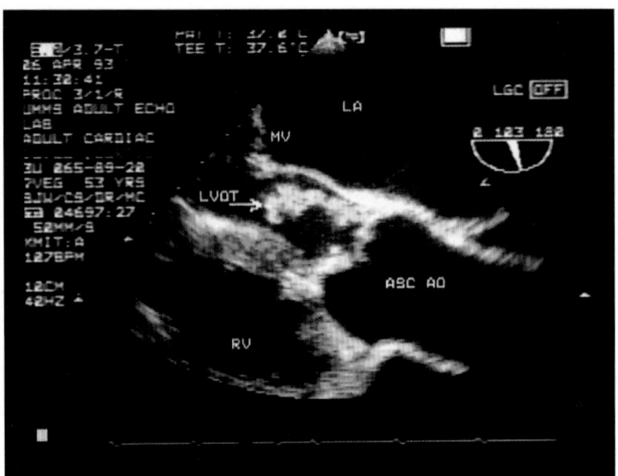

Figure 15.10
Transesophageal longitudinal view of a large vegetation protruding from the aortic valve into the left ventricular outflow tract. LA, left atrium; MV, mitral valve; LVOT, left ventricular outflow tract; RV, right ventricle; ASC AO, ascending aorta.

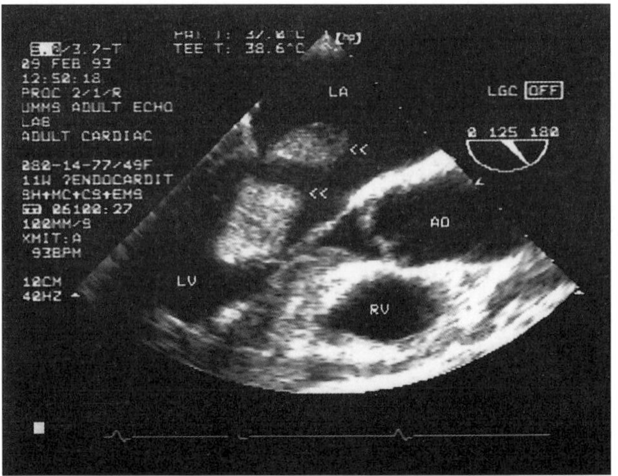

Figure 15.11
Transesophageal longitudinal view of two large vegetations on the mitral valve (arrowheads) and prolapsing into the left ventricle. LA, left atrium; LV, left ventricle; RV, right ventricle; AO, aorta.

events remains controversial due to conflicting data.[73–75,80] Nevertheless, clinical endocarditis with echo evidence of vegetations increases the risk of embolic complications.[73–76,80] Vegetation size (>10 mm), extent, mobility and consistency have been positively associated with embolic risk[73,74,77,80] (Figs 15.10 and 15.11).

About 35% of patients with nonbacterial thrombotic endocarditis, formerly known as marantic endocarditis, develop cardioembolic stroke.[2,81] Nonbacterial thrombotic endocarditis is seen in individuals with malignancies, hypercoagulable conditions, disseminated intravascular coagulation and systemic lupus erythematosus. Embolic arterial occlusion occurs from sterile fibrin/platelet material which adheres to the surface of mitral and/or aortic valves. There are no good imaging techniques to adequately detect small sterile vegetations. TEE may be sensitive enough to detect fine string-like echodensities (strands) hanging off valves which suggest fibrinous/fibrotic material.

Prosthetic valves

Prosthetic cardiac valves account for approximately 10% of all embolic events.[1] The rate of embolism in anticoagulated patients with mechanical valves is about 3%/year for mitral valves, and about 1.5%/year for aortic valves. Embolic rates in non-anticoagulated patients with bioprosthetic valves are approximately 2–4%/year.[2]

Thromboembolism still remains a devastating complication of prosthetic valve implantation despite advances in technology. Thrombi can form on the prosthesis or in the atrial cavity, particularly in the setting of co-existent atrial fibrillation/atrial enlargement. Thrombus can lead to valve obstruction and/or embolism.

Echocardiography with Doppler has been the mainstay of the noninvasive evaluation of native and prosthetic valve structure and function. Thrombus or fibrinous material appear as echodensities on or in the vicinity of the prosthetic valve. Impairment of valve mobility leading to significant obstruction or regurgitation depending on the position and degree of valve fixation by the thrombus can be noted. Transthoracic echo is often limited by the acoustic reverberations from the prosthetic apparatus which obscures valve anatomy and masks more distal structures. TEE obviates these acoustical factors which interfere with the acquisition of high resolution images of prosthetic valves by transthoracic echo.

Mitral valve prolapse

Various clinical studies point to an association of mitral valve prolapse (MVP) with stroke,[82–84] particularly in young individuals with unexplained strokes and transient ischemic attacks. The morphological characteristics of MVP would appear to predispose to fibrin/thrombus deposition. However, despite the common incidence of mitral valve prolapse in the general population (5–15%), the frequency of stroke from this cardiac entity is quite low.[83,85,86] Consequently, a direct link between mitral valve prolapse and stroke is difficult to make.

Two-dimensional echo is the mainstay of diagnosing mitral valve prolapse. This modality displays the morphology, motion, and position of the leaflets and annulus in real-time at rest and under physiologic interventions. Classic MVP is characterized by diffuse leaflet thickening (>5 mm) and redundancy usually at the leaflet tips due to myxomatous degeneration[87] (Fig. 15.12). These findings are more likely to predispose to complications such as endocarditis, severe mitral regurgitation and valve replacement. Prolapse is defined as a >2 mm displacement of one or both mitral leaflets beyond the plane of the mitral annulus as seen in the parasternal long-axis view. Focal prolapse of the medial or lateral scallop of the posterior leaflet in the apical 4- or 2-chamber views is also considered abnormal.[44]

Mitral annular calcification

Mitral annular calcification is a chronic degenerative disorder characterized by calcification and ulceration of the fibrous support structure of the mitral valve.[88] This entity is commonly seen in the elderly and is associated with hypertension, diabetes and chronic renal failure.[89,90] Excessive calcific material can develop and extrude beyond the valve plane, though this rarely causes obstruction. More commonly it immobilizes the basal portion of the leaflets leading to inadequate coaptation and significant mitral regurgitation. Sequelae of mitral annular calcification include conduction system disturbances, atrial fibrillation, mitral regurgitation, embolism and endocarditis.[91]

Echocardiographically, mitral annular calcification appears as a bright highly reflective echodense area usually at the base of the posterior mitral leaflets and subjacent to the left ventricular posterior wall (Fig. 15.13). Calcification can encompass the posterior leaflet and extend to the anterior portion of the annulus and aorta.

The presence of mitral annular calcification as the causative mechanism for cardioembolic stroke is difficult to conclude since it co-exists with other disorders which predispose to stroke, particularly generalized atherosclerosis.[82,92,93]

Aortic atheroma

Aortic atheroma, also known as intra-aortic debris, is a cause of embolic events,[22] and an independent risk factor for systemic embolization.[23] This is particularly true with complex, protruding atherosclerotic plaque that have mobile debris or adherent thrombi (Fig. 15.14).

In a large autopsy series, the prevalence of ulcerated plaques in the aortic arch of individuals with cerebral infarction of unknown etiology was 61% compared to 22% in cases of known etiology.[94] A strong correlation exists between plaque thickness and risk of stroke. Plaque thickness of ≥4 mm in the ascending aorta or proximal arch was found in 28% of individuals with no other identifiable cause of stroke. The risk of stroke increased from 3.3 odds ratio with 1–1.9 mm plaque thickness to 13.8 odds ratio with ≥4 mm plaque thickness. The presence of a mobile component of the plaque or superimposed thrombus is associated with a greater risk of embolic events.[94–96]

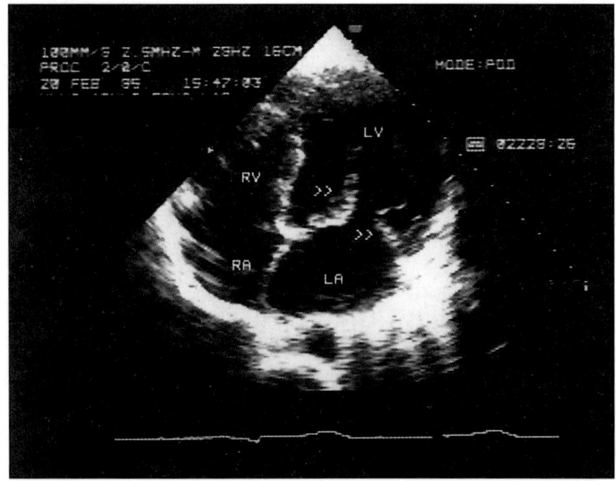

a

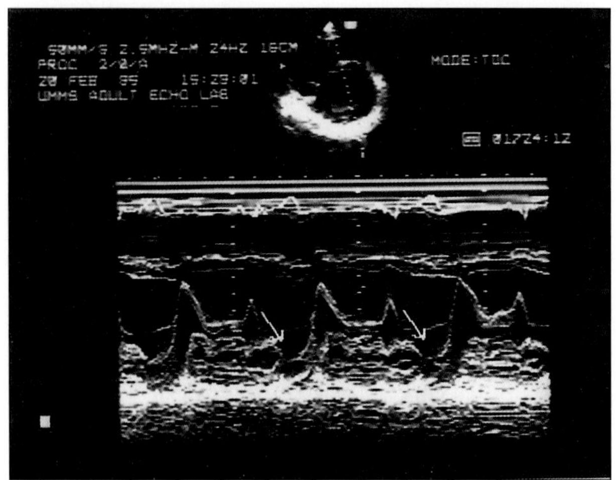

b

Figure 15.12
(a) Transthoracic apical 4-chamber view of a diffusely myxomatous mitral valve (arrowheads). (b) M-mode recording of the same patient illustrating late systolic posterior motion of the mitral valve leaflets (arrows). RV, right ventricle; RA, right atrium; LA, left atrium; LV, left ventricle; AO, aorta.

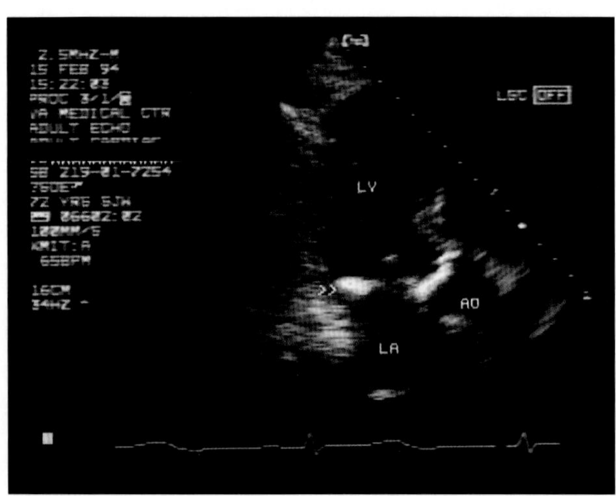

Figure 15.13
Transthoracic apical 2-chamber view illustrating bright hyperreflectile echodensity of the mitral annulus (arrowhead). LV, left ventricle; LA, left atrium; AO, aorta.

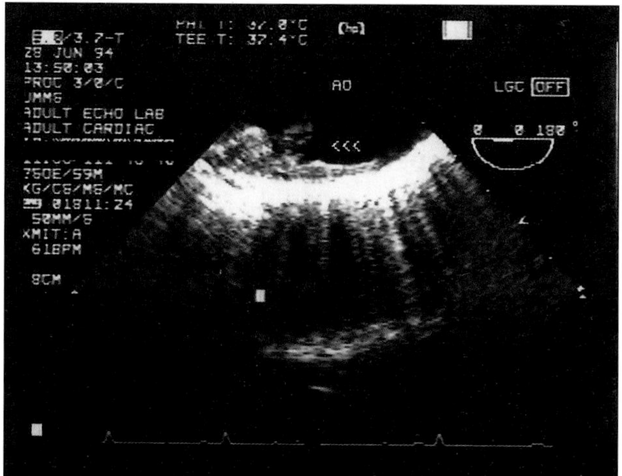

a

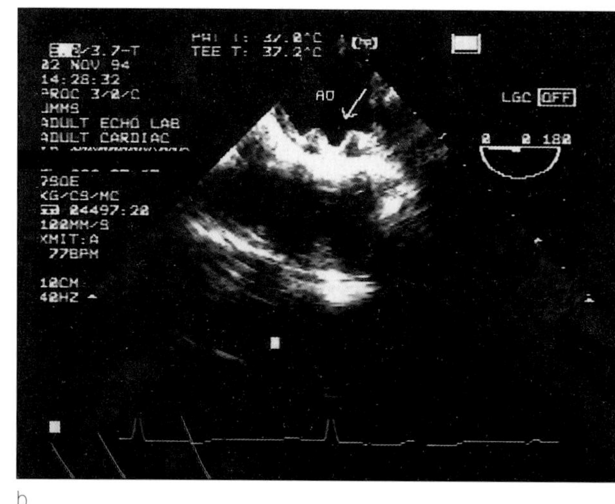

b

Figure 15.14
Transesophageal transverse view of the (a) aortic arch with complex aortic atheroma and mobile thrombus (arrowheads) and (b) descending thoracic aorta with ulcerated plaque (arrow). AO, aorta.

These observations suggest that the thoracic aorta should be evaluated as a potential source of embolism. Aortography, MRI, CT, and TEE are excellent modalities to examine the aorta for dissection and/or aneurysm. TEE has emerged as an excellent tool to inspect the thoracic aorta for atherosclerotic plaque and debris. Attention to this area should be part of a thorough TEE examination. One limitation with regard to evaluating the aorta is the presence of the air-filled trachea and bronchus interposed between the esophagus and upper ascending aorta. This creates a blind area through which the TEE ultrasound cannot penetrate to acquire high-resolution images.

Atherosclerotic atheroma (intra-aortic debris) is defined echocardiographically in the following way:

1. Simple atherosclerotic plaque: discrete zone of thickening and increased echodensity extending <5 mm into the aortic lumen. No overlying echogenic material. No disruption or irregularities of the intimal surface.
2. Complex atherosclerotic plaque: echodense area of intimal thickening with disruption of the intimal surface or marked irregularities of the intimal surface. Presence of overlying or superimposed irregular echogenic material projecting >5 mm into the aortic lumen. Complex plaque may be either layered (broad-based and immobile) or pedunculated (narrow-based and highly mobile).

Summary

The diagnosis of cardioembolic stroke is difficult since the causative mechanism is not always defined. Multiple mechanisms often co-exist in an individual and the presence of a potential source of embolism alone does not confer a diagnosis. Certain cardiac disorders clearly pose a higher risk for thromboembolism than other disorders. Cardiac imaging, particularly echocardiography, defines most of these entities with a high degree of accuracy. The search for a cardiac source of embolism has become the leading indication for TEE in several laboratories. Our approach to the question of a suspected cardiac source of embolism is to obtain a transthoracic echo with saline contrast on all patients prior to performing TEE. In some cases TEE may be omitted if the transthoracic echo adequately demonstrates a source of embolism, or if the transthoracic echo with contrast is entirely normal in an otherwise young, healthy individual with no risk factors for stroke. If the transthoracic echo is of limited quality, a transesophageal echo is obtained in cases where the clinical suspicion for embolism is high. TEE complements the transthoracic echo and is particularly helpful in evaluating the atrial septum, left atrial appendage, prosthetic valves, and the aorta. The utility of TEE in all patients with stroke is controversial, and the cost-effectiveness, impact on patient management and outcome still require careful, prospective study.

References

1 Cerebral Embolism Task Force: Cardiogenic brain embolism. *Arch Neurol* 1986; **43**: 71–84.

2 Cerebral Embolism Task Force: Cardiogenic brain embolism: the second report of the cerebral embolism task force. *Arch Neurol* 1989; **46**: 727–43.

3 Adams RD, Victor M: *Principles of Neurology*, 4th edn. (McGraw-Hill: New York, 1989); 617–92.

4 Kannel WB, Wolf PA, Verter J, McNamara PM: Epidemiologic assessment of the role of blood pressure in stroke: the Framingham Study. *JAMA* 1970; **214**: 301–10.

5 Foulkes MA, Wolf PA, Price TR et al: The Stroke Data Bank: design, methods, baseline characteristics. *Stroke* 1988; **19**: 547–54.

6 Sacco RL, Ellenberg JH, Mohr JP et al: Infarcts of undetermined cause: the NINCDS Stroke Data Bank. *Ann Neurol* 1989; **25**: 382–90.

7 Greenland P, Knopman D, Mikell F et al: Echocardiography in diagnostic assessment of stroke. *Ann Intern Med* 1981; **95**: 51–4.

8 Bergeron GA, Shah PM: Echocardiography unwarranted in patients with cerebral ischemic events. *N Engl J Med* 1981; **304**: 489 (letter).

9 Pop G, Sutherland GR, Koudstaal PJ et al: Transesophageal echocardiography in the detection of intracardiac embolic sources in patients with transient ischemic attacks. *Stroke* 1990; **21**: 560–5.

10 Zenker G, Erbel R, Kramer G et al: Transesophageal two-dimensional echocardiography in young stroke patients with cerebral ischemic events. *Stroke* 1988; **19**: 345–8.

11 Lee RJ, Bartzokis T, Yeoh TK et al: Enhanced detection of intracardiac sources of cerebral emboli by transesophageal echocardiography. *Stroke* 1991; **22**: 734–9.

12 Kronzon I, Tunick PA: Transesophageal echocardiography as a tool in the evaluation of patients with embolic disorders. *Prog Cardiovasc Dis* 1993; **36**: 39–60.

13 Pearson AC, Labovitz AJ, Tatineni S, Gomez CR: Superiority of transesophageal echocardiography in detecting cardiac source of embolism in patients with cerebral ischemia of uncertain etiology. *J Am Coll Cardiol* 1991; **17**: 66–72.

14 Tegeler CH, Downes TR: Cardiac imaging in stroke. *Stroke* 1991; **22**: 1206–10.

15 Mugge A, Kuhn H, Daniel WG: The role of transesophageal echocardiography in the detection of left atrial thrombi. *Echocardiography* 1993; **10**: 405–17.

16 Cujec B, Polasek P, Voll C, Shuaib A: Transesophageal echocardiography in detection of potential cardiac source of embolism in stroke patients. *Stroke* 1991; **22**: 727–33.

17 Pearson AC, Nagelhout D, Castello R et al: Atrial septal aneurysm and stroke: a transesophageal echocardiographic study. *J Am Coll Cardiol* 1991; **18**: 1223–9.

18 Schneider B, Hanrath P, Vogel P, Meinertz T: Improved morphologic characterization of atrial septal aneurysm by transesophageal echocardiography: relation to cerebrovascular events. *J Am Coll Cardiol* 1990; **16**: 1000–9.

19 Daniel WG, Nellessen U, Schroder E et al: Left atrial spontaneous echo contrast in mitral valve disease: an indicator for an increased thromboembolic risk. *J Am Coll Cardiol* 1988; **11**: 1204–11.

20 Black IW, Hopkins AP, Lee LCL, Walsh WF: Left atrial spontaneous echo contrast: a clinical and echocardiographic analysis. *J Am Coll Cardiol* 1991; **18**: 398–404.

21 Castello R, Pearson AC, Labovitz AJ: Prevalence and clinical implications of atrial spontaneous contrast in patients undergoing transesophageal echocardiography. *Am J Cardiol* 1990; **65**: 1149–53.

22 Karalis DG, Chandrasekaran K, Victor MF et al: Recognition and embolic potential of intraaortic atherosclerotic debris. *J Am Coll Cardiol* 1991; **17**: 73–8.

23 Tunick PA, Kronzon J: The improved yield of transesophageal echocardiography over transthoracic echocardiography in patients with neurologic events is largely due to the detection of aorta protruding atheroma echocardiography. *J Cardiovasc Atrial Tech* 1992; **9**: 491–5.

24 Love BB, Struck LK, Stanford W et al: Comparison of two-dimensional echocardiography and ultrafast CT for evaluating intracardiac thrombi in cerebral ischemia stroke. *Stroke* 1990; **21**: 1033–8.

25 Helgason CM, Chomka E, Louie E et al: The potential role for ultrafast cardiac computed tomography in patients with stroke. *Stroke* 1989; **20**: 465–72.

26 Kannel WB, Abbott R, Savage D, McNamara P: Epidemiologic features of chronic atrial fibrillation: the Framingham Study. *N Engl J Med* 1982; **17**: 1018–22.

27 Wolf PA, Dawber TR, Thomas EH, Kannel WB: Epidemiologic assessment of chronic atrial fibrillation and risk of stroke: the Framingham Study. *Neurology* 1978; **28**: 973–7.

28 Davis PH, Dambrosia JM, Schoenberg BS et al: Risk factors for ischemic stroke: a prospective study in Rochester, Minnesota. *Ann Neurol* 1987; **22**: 319–27.

29 Mohr JP, Caplan LR, Melski JW et al: The Harvard Cooperative Stroke Registry. A prospective registry. *Neurology* 1978; **28**: 745–62.

30 Caplan LR, Hier D, D'Cruz I: Cerebral embolism in the Michael Reese Stroke Registry. *Stroke* 1983; **14**: 530–7.

31 Brand FN, Abbott RD, Kannel WB, Wolf PA: Characteristics and prognosis of lone atrial fibrillation: 30 year follow-up in the Framingham study. *JAMA* 1985; **254**: 3449–53.

32 Fairfax AJ, Lambert CD, Leatham A: Systemic embolism in chronic sinoatrial disorder. *N Engl J Med* 1976; **295**: 190–2.

33 Shrestha NK, Moreno FL, Narciso FV et al: Two-dimensional echocardiographic diagnosis of left atrial thrombus in rheumatic heart disease: a clinicopathologic study. *Circulation* 1983; **67**: 341–7.

34 Mikell FL, Asinger RW, Elsperger KJ et al: Regional stasis of blood in dysfunctional left ventricle: echocardiographic detection and differentiation from early thrombosis. *Circulation* 1982; **66**: 755–63.

35 Sigel B, Coelho JC, Spigos DG et al: Ultrasonography of blood during stasis and coagulation. *Invest Radiol* 1981; **16**: 71–6.

36 Chimowitz MI, DeGeorgio MA, Poole M et al: Left atrial spontaneous echo contrast is highly associated with previous stroke in patients with atrial fibrillation or mitral stenosis. *Stroke* 1993; **24**: 1015–19.

37 Domenicucci S, Bellotti P, Chiarella F et al: Spontaneous morphologic changes in left ventricular thrombi: prospective two-dimensional echocardiographic study. *Circulation* 1987; **75**: 737–43.

38 Visser CA, Kan G, Meltzer RS et al: Long-term follow-up of left ventricular thrombus after acute myocardial infarction. *Chest* 1984; **86**: 532–6.

39 Visser CA, Kan G, David GK et al: Two-dimensional echocardiography in the diagnosis of left ventricular thrombus: prospective study in 67 patients with anatomic validation. *Chest* 1983; **83**: 228–32.

40 Visser CA, Kan G, Meltzer RS et al: Embolic potential of left ventricular thrombus after myocardial infarction: a two-dimensional echocardiographic study of 119 patients. *J Am Coll Cardiol* 1985; **5**: 1276–80.

41 Jugdutt BI, Sivaram CA: Prospective two-dimensional echocardiographic evaluation of left ventricular thrombus and embolism after acute myocardial infarction. *J Am Coll Cardiol* 1989; **13**: 554–64.

42 Weinreich DJ, Burke JF, Pauletto FJ: Left ventricular mural thrombi complicating acute myocardial infarction: long-term follow-up with serial echocardiography. *Ann Intern Med* 1984; **100**: 789–94.

43 Stratton JR, Lighty GW, Pearlman AS, Ritchie JL: Detection of left ventricular thrombi by two-dimensional echocardiography: sensitivity, specificity and causes of uncertainty. *Circulation* 1982; **66**: 156–66.

44 Weyman Arthur E: *Principles and Practice of Echocardiography*, 2nd edn. (Lea & Febiger: Philadelphia, 1993).

45 Reeder GS, Lengyle M, Tajik AJ et al: Mural thrombus in left ventricular aneurysm: incidence, role of angiography, and relation between anticoagulation and embolization. *Mayo Clin Proc* 1981; **56**: 77–81.

46 Marcus ML, Skorton DJ, Schelbert HR et al: *Cardiac Imaging: A Companion to Braunwald's Heart Disease* (WB Saunders: Philadelphia, 1990).

47 Ezekowitz M, Wilson DA, Smith EO et al: Comparison of indium-111 platelet scintigraphy and two-dimensional echocardiography in the diagnosis of left ventricular thrombi. *N Engl J Med* 1982; **306**: 1509–13.

48 Kessler C, Henningsen H, Reuther R et al: Identification of intracardiac thrombi in stroke patients with indium-111 platelet scintigraphy. *Stroke* 1987; **18**: 63–7.

49 Seabold JE, Schroder E, Conrad GR et al: Indium-111 platelet scintigraphy and two-dimensional echocardiography for detection of left ventricular thrombus: influence of clot size and age. *J Am Coll Cardiol* 1987; **9**: 1057–66.

50 Fuster V, Gersh BJ, Giuliani ER et al: The natural history of idiopathic dilated cardiomyopathy. *Am J Cardiol* 1981; **47**: 525–31.

51 Gottdiener JS, Gay JA, Van Voorhees L et al: Frequency and embolic potential of left ventricular thrombus in dilated cardiomyopathy: assessment by 2-dimensional echocardiography. *Am J Cardiol* 1983; **52**: 1281–5.

52 Falk RH, Foster E, Coats MH: Ventricular thrombi and thromboembolism in dilated cardiomyopathy: a prospective follow-up study. *Am Heart J* 1991; **123**: 136–42.

53 Ciaccheru M, Castelli G, Cecchi F et al: Lack of correlation between intracavitary thrombus detected by cross-sectional echocardiography and systemic emboli in patients with dilated cardiomyopathy. *Br Heart J* 1989; **62**: 26–9.

54 Gunnar RM, Bourdillon PD, Dixon DW et al: Guidelines for the early management of patients with acute myocardial infarction: a report of the American College of Cardiology/American Heart Association task force on assessment of diagnostic and therapeutic cardiovascular procedures. *J Am Coll Cardiol* 1990; **16**: 249–92.

55 Belkin RN, Hurwitz MB, Kisslo J: Atrial septal aneurysm: association with cerebrovascular and peripheral embolic events. *Stroke* 1987; **18**: 856–62.

56 Hanley P, Tajik AJ, Hynes JK et al: Diagnosis and classification of atrial septal aneurysm by two-dimensional

echocardiography: report of 80 consecutive cases. *J Am Coll Cardiol* 1985; **6**: 1370–82.

57 Silver MD, Dorsey JS: Aneurysm of the septum primum in adults. *Arch Pathol Lab Med* 1978; **102**: 62–5.

58 Gallet B, Malerguw MC, Adams C et al: Atrial septal aneurysm—a potential cause of systemic embolism: an echocardiographic study. *Br Heart J* 1985; **53**: 292–7.

59 Hagen PT, Scholz DG, Edwards WD: Incidence and size of patent foramen ovale during the first 10 decades of life: an autopsy study of 965 normal hearts. *Mayo Clin Proc* 1984; **59**: 17–20.

60 Lechat P, Mas JL, Lascault G et al: Prevalence of patent foramen ovale in patients with stroke. *N Engl J Med* 1988; **318**: 1148–52.

61 Webster MWI, Smith HJ, Sharpe DN et al: Patent foramen ovale in young stroke patients. *Lancet* July 2, 1988; **2**: 11–12.

62 DiTullio M, Sacco RI, Gopal A et al: Patent foramen ovale as a risk factor for cryptogenic stroke. *Ann Intern Med* 1992; **117**: 461–5.

63 Hausmann D, Mugge A, Becht I, Daniel WG: Diagnosis of patent foramen ovale by transesophageal echocardiography and association with cerebral and peripheral embolic events. *Am J Cardiol* 1992; **70**: 668–72.

64 deBelder MA, Tourikis L, Griffith M et al: Transesophageal contrast echocardiography and color flow mapping—methods of choice for the detection of shunts at the atrial level. *Am Heart J* 1992; **124**: 1545–50.

65 Homma S, DeTullio MR, Sacco RL et al: Characteristics of patent foramen ovale associated with cryptogenic stroke. A biplane transesophageal echocardiographic study. *Stroke* 1994; **25**: 582–6.

66 Stone D, Godard J, Corretti MC et al: Patent foramen ovale: an association between the degree of shunt by contrast transesophageal echocardiography and the risk of future ischemic neurologic events. *Am Heart J* (in press).

67 Job FP, Ringlestein B, Grafen Y et al: Comparison of transcranial contrast Doppler sonography and transesophageal contrast echocardiography for the detection of patent foramen ovale in young stroke patients. *Am J Cardiol* 1994; **74**: 381–4.

68 Mugge A, Daniel WG, Haverich A, Lichtlen PR: Diagnosis of noninfective cardiac masses by two-dimensional echocardiography: comparison of the transthoracic and transesophageal approaches. *Circulation* 1991; **83**: 70–8.

69 Davidson CJ, Skelton TN, Kisslo KB et al: The risk of systemic embolization associated with percutaneous balloon valvuloplasty in adults. *Ann Intern Med* 1988; **108**: 557–60.

70 Safian RD, Berman AD, Diver DT et al: Balloon aortic valvuloplasty in 170 consecutive patients. *N Engl J Med* 1988; **319**: 125–30.

71 Salgado AV, Furlan AJ, Keys TF et al: Neurological complications of native and prosthetic valve endocarditis: a 12 year experience. *Neurology* 1989; **39**: 173–8.

72 Hart RG, Foster JW, Luther MF, Kanter MC: Stroke in infective endocarditis. *Stroke* 1990; **21**: 695–700.

73 Stafford WJ, Petch J, Radford DJ: Vegetations in infective endocarditis: clinical relevance and diagnosis by cross-sectional echo. *Br Heart J* 1985; **53**: 310–13.

74 Buda AJ, Zotz RJ, Lemire MS, Bach DS: Prognostic significance of vegetations detected by two-dimensional echocardiography in infective endocarditis. *Am Heart J* 1986; **112**: 1291–6.

75 Lutas EM, Roberts RB, Devereux RB, Prieto LM: Relation between the presence of echocardiographic vegetation and the complication rate in infective endocarditis. *Am Heart J* 1986; **112**: 107–13.

76 Stewart JA, Silimperi D, Harris P et al: Echocardiographic documentation of vegetative lesions in infective endocarditis: clinical implications. *Circulation* 1980; **61**: 374–80.

77 Mugge A, Daniel WG, Frank G, Lichtlen PR: Echocardiography in infective endocarditis: reassessment of prognostic complication of vegetation size determined by the transthoracic and transesophageal approach. *J Am Coll Cardiol* 1989; **14**: 631–8.

78 Erbel R, Rohmann S, Drexler M et al: Improved diagnostic value of echocardiography in patients with infective endocarditis by transesophageal approach: a prospective study. *Eur Heart J* 1988; **9**: 43–53.

79 Effron MK, Popp RR: Two-dimensional echocardiographic assessment of bioprosthetic valve dysfunction and infective endocarditis. *J Am Coll Cardiol* 1983; **2**: 597–606.

80 Sanfilippo AJ, Picard MH, Newell JB et al: Echocardiographic assessment of patients with infectious endocarditis: prediction of risk for complications. *J Am Coll Cardiol* 1991; **18**: 1191–9.

81 Biller J, Challa VR, Toole JF, Howard VJ: Nonbacterial thrombotic endocarditis. A neurologic perspective of clinicopathologic correlations of 99 patients. *Arch Neurol* 1982; **39**: 95–8.

82 Barnett HJM, Jones MW, Boughner DR, Kostuk WJ: Cerebral ischemic events associated with prolapsing mitral valve. *Arch Neurol* 1976; **33**: 777–82.

83 Lauzier S, Barnett HJM: Cerebral ischemia with mitral valve prolapse and mitral annular calcification. In: Furlan AJ, ed. *The Heart and Stroke* (Springer: London, 1987); 63–100.

84 Barletta GA, Gagliardi R, Benvenuti L, Fantini F: Cerebral ischemic attacks as a complication of aortic and mitral valve prolapse. *Stroke* 1985; **16**: 219–23.

85 Boughner DR, Barnett HJM: The enigma of the risk of stroke in mitral valve prolapse. *Stroke* 1985; **16**: 175–7.

86 Jones HR, Naggar CZ, Selyan MP, Downing ZZ: Mitral valve prolapse and cerebral ischemic events. A comparison between a neurology population with stroke and a cardiology population with mitral valve prolapse observed for 5 years. *Stroke* 1982; **13**: 451–3.

87 Marks AR, Choong CY, Sanfilippo AJ et al: Identification of high-risk and low-risk subgroups of patients with mitral-valve prolapse. *N Engl J Med* 1989; **320**: 1031–6.

88 Benjamin EJ, Plehn JF, D'Agostino RB et al: Mitral annular calcification and risk of stroke in an elderly cohort. *N Engl J Med* 1992; **327**: 374–9.

89 Forman MB, Virmani R, Robertson RM, Stone WJ. Mitral annular calcification in chronic renal failure. *Chest* 1984; **85**: 367–71.

90 Furlan AJ, Craciun AR, Salcedo EE, Mellino M: Risk of stroke in patients with mitral annulus calcification. *Stroke* 1984; **15**: 801–3.

91 Fulkerson PK, Beaver BM, Auseon JC, Graber HL: Calcification of the mitral annulus: etiology, clinical associations, complications and therapy. *Am J Med* 1979; **66**: 967–75.

92 Rubin DC, Hawke MW, Plotnick GD: Relation between mitral annular calcium and complex intraaortic debris. *Am J Cardiol* 1992; **71**: 1251–2.

93 Aronow WS, Schoenfeld MR, Gutstein H: Frequency of thromboembolic stroke in persons >60 years of age with extracranial carotid arterial disease and/or mitral annular calcium. *Am J Cardiol* 1992; **70**: 123–4.

94 Amarenco P, Duyckaerts C, Tzourio C et al: The prevalence of ulcerated plaques in the aortic arch in patients with stroke. *N Engl J Med* 1992; **326**: 221–5.

95 Amarenco P, Cohen A, Tzourio C et al: Atherosclerotic disease of the aortic arch and the risk of ischemic stroke. *N Engl J Med* 1994; **331**: 1474–9.

96 Stone DA, Hawke MW, LaMonte M et al: Ulcerated atherosclerotic plaques in the thoracic aorta are associated with cryptogenic stroke: a multiplane transesophageal echocardiographic study. *Am Heart J* 1995 (in press).

16

Cardiac tumors

Norbert Goebel, Markus Hauser, Rolf Jenni and Gustav K von Schulthess

Since the advent of modern cardiopulmonary bypass techniques, many cardiac tumors can be cured by surgery. In malignant disease at least palliative therapy may be possible. The clinical diagnosis, however, is often difficult.

Tumors of the heart can be subdivided into primary tumors (benign or malignant) and secondary or metastatic tumors. Primary tumors of the heart are rare. Based upon the data of 22 large autopsy series, the frequency is approximately 0.02%, corresponding to 200 tumors in one million autopsies.[1] About 75% of primary cardiac tumors are benign and 25% are malignant. Nearly half of the benign tumors are myxomas; about one-tenth each are lipomas, papillary fibroelastomas, and rhabdomyomas. Fibromas, hemangiomas, teratomas and mesotheliomas of the atrioventricular node are found less frequently.[2] In children under 1-year rhabdomyomas comprise 50–60% of cardiac tumors. Up to the age of 15 years, the tumors encountered are—in the order of frequency—myxoma, rhabdomyoma and fibroma. The malignant primary cardiac tumors (25%) are usually sarcomas. Secondary tumors of the heart are 20–40 times more common than primary tumors and are observed in 5–20% of malignant tumors.[3]

Specific cardiac tumors

Benign tumors

Myxoma

Myxomas are the most common type of primary cardiac tumor[4] with 93% reported to occur sporadically.[5] The mean age of patients with sporadic myxomas is 56 years (range 3–83 years), and 70% are females.[6] Approximately 86% of myxomas occur in the left atrium and over 90% are solitary.[6] In the left atrium the usual site of attachment is in the area of the fossa ovalis by either a narrow pedicle or a broad base. Myxomas may also occur in the right atrium, and still less often in the right or left ventricle. Myxomas of the mitral valve have been reported.[7] Multiple tumors may occur in the same chamber or in a combination of chambers.[6] The average tumor size is 4–8 cm in diameter. Most myxomas are gelatinous and polypoid, although they may be smooth and round. Multilobulated friable soft tumors are more prone to embolization.[8] Calcification was observed in 5% of tumors according to one series.[9] Myxomas may be familial. In addition, some patients with myxoma may have a syndrome that involves a complex of abnormalities including myxomas of the skin and similar mammary tumors, lentiginous or pigmented naevi or both, primary nodular adrenal cortical disease with or without Cushing's syndrome and testicular tumors ('Swiss syndrome').[10]

Papillary tumors of heart valves (papillary fibroelastoma)

Papillary tumors of the cardiac valves and adjacent endocardium are found not uncommonly post-mortem or are identified by two-dimensional echocardiography.[11,12] It appears that they may originate from organized mural thrombi.[4,13] They have a characteristic frond-like appearance, may measure 3 or 4 cm in diameter, are single or multiple, and may occur on any valve; most often the ventricular surface of semilunar valves and the atrial surface of AV valves are affected. Rarely, they may be present on papillary muscles, chordae tendineae, or endocardium.[14] The tricuspid valve is most commonly involved in children; the mitral and aortic valves in adults. Papillary tumors are distinguished from Lambl's excrescences, which are ubiquitous acellular deposits of thrombus and connective tissue covered by a single layer of endothelium and are found on heart valves at the site of endothelial damage in many adults, particularly along the closure margins of the aortic valve cusps. In contrast, papillary fibroelastomas are usually found at valvular contact areas. Papillary fibroelastomas may produce symptoms due to embolization or by causing valvular dysfunction.[15]

Rhabdomyoma

Rhabdomyomas are the most common cardiac tumors of infants and children, most occurring in patients younger than 1 year.[16] Rhabdomyomas are strongly associated with tuberous sclerosis, a familial syndrome characterized by hamartomas in several organs, epilepsy, mental deficiency, and adenoma sebaceum. Of patients with cardiac rhabdomyomas, 80% have tuberous sclerosis.[17] Rhabdomyomas invariably involve the ventricles, affecting the left and right sides equally; 90% are multiple, and in 30% there is involvement of at least one of the atria. The size ranges from 1 mm to several centimeters. Approximately 50% of rhabdomyomas are large enough to cause significant obstruction of a cardiac chamber or valvular orifice.[16,18] Nonspecific clinical manifestations—including cardiomegaly, right or left ventricular failure or both, an S_3, S_4 and systolic or diastolic murmurs—may mimic mitral stenosis, mitral atresia, aortic, subaortic, as well as infundibular pulmonic stenosis.[15]

Fibroma

Fibromas occur predominantly in children, most before the age of 10 years, and about 40% are diagnosed in infants of <1 year.[19] They constitute the second most common type of primary cardiac tumor occurring in infants and children.[19] Almost all fibromas occur within the ventricular myocardium, most frequently within the anterior free wall of the left ventricle or the interventricular septum, and relatively seldom in the posterior left ventricular wall or right ventricle. They range in size from 3 to 7 cm. Approximately 70% of fibromas at some time will cause mechanical interference with intracardiac flow or ventricular contraction, or cause conduction disturbances.[4] Clinical manifestations are protean and include murmurs, atypical chest pain, congestive heart failure and signs of subaortic stenosis, valvular or infundibular pulmonic stenosis with right ventricular hypertrophy, tricuspid stenosis, conduction disturbances, ventricular tachycardia, and sudden death.[15]

Lipoma

Lipomas occur at all ages and with equal frequency in both sexes. Most range in diameter from 1 to 15 cm. Most tumors are sessile or polypoid and occur in the subendocardium or subepicardium, although about 25% are completely intramuscular. The most common chambers affected are the left ventricle, right atrium, and interatrial septum. Subendocardial tumors with intracavitary extension produce symptoms that are characteristic of their location, whereas subepicardial tumors may cause compression of the heart and pericardial effusion.[15] The so-called lipomatous hypertrophy of the interatrial septum represents the accumulation of mature adipose tissue within the interatrial septum. These lesions range from 1 to 7 cm, most often protrude into the right atrium, and are more common in obese, elderly or female patients.[20] The problem with this lesion—which can be seen by different imaging methods—is to differentiate it from a true tumor. A variety of atrial arrhythmias have been attributed to these lesions, but a cause-and-effect relationship has been difficult to establish.[21,22]

Angioma

Benign vascular tumors (hemangiomas, lymphangiomas, and angioreticulomas) are extremely rare.[23] They may occur in any part of the heart, are usually intramural, often in the interventricular septum or AV node, where they may cause complete heart block and sudden death. Cardiac tamponade due to hemopericardium may be the presenting clinical symptom. More commonly found in the right heart chambers, hemangiomas are generally sessile or polypoid subendocardial nodules ranging from 2 to 4 cm in diameter.[15]

Teratoma

These tumors, which contain elements of all three germ cell layers, occur within the heart less frequently than in the anterior mediastinum. They are generally observed in children, and when located in the heart, they occur predominantly within the right atrium, right ventricle, or the interatrial or interventricular septum.[24]

Cystic tumor ('mesothelioma') of the atrioventricular node

They are small multicystic lesions, generally <15 mm, that are found in the area of the AV node.[25,26] They occur virtually at any age and frequently cause death by complete heart block, ventricular fibrillation[27] or cardiac tamponade.[28]

Endocrine tumors of the heart

Approximately 2% of paragangliomas are intrathoracic, and of these most are located in the posterior mediastinum. They can also occur in close association with the left atrial or left ventricular epicardium, or, more rarely still, may arise within the interatrial septum.[29] They may secrete catecholamines and therefore can be associated with signs and symptoms of pheochromocytoma. Rarely, benign thyroid tumors arise in the heart, presumably from ectopic rests of thyroid tissue.[30] These tumors most often arise from the interventricular septum and present, not infrequently, as ventricular outflow obstruction.

Malignant cardiac tumors

Of all cardiac tumors, 25% are malignant, and virtually all of these are sarcomas. They occur at any age, but are most common between the third and fifth decades and show no sex preference. In decreasing order of frequency the sites involved are the right atrium, left atrium, right ventricle, left ventricle, and the interventricular septum. Death most often occurs from a few weeks to 2 years after the onset of symptoms. These tumors proliferate rapidly and generally cause death through widespread infiltration of the myocardium, obstruction of flow within the heart, or distant metastases. Of all patients with cardiac sarcoma, 75% have pathological evidence of distant metastases at the time of death[31] and 30% at the time of diagnosis.[32] The most frequent sites are the lungs, thoracic lymph nodes, mediastinum and vertebral column; less often the liver, kidneys, adrenals, pancreas, bone, spleen and bowel are involved. Because the right side of the heart is most commonly affected, sarcomas frequently cause signs of right heart failure as a result of obstruction of the heart cavities or the caval veins. Tumors limited to the myocardium may cause arrhythmias and conduction disturbances. When there is extension into the pericardial space, hemorrhagic pericardial effusion is common and tamponade may occur.

Sarcomas may be subdivided as angiosarcoma, rhabdomyosarcoma, fibrosarcoma and lymphosarcoma.

Angiosarcoma

Included within this category are malignant hemangioendothelioma, angiosarcoma, Kaposi's sarcoma, angioreticuloma and cavernous angiosarcoma.[33,34] This class of lesions forms the most common cardiac malignancy. All 40 patients in one series were adults. In distinction to most other cardiac sarcomas, in which the sex distribution is equal, there appears to be a 2 : 1 male-to-female ratio among patients with angiosarcoma. These tumors have a striking predilection for the right atrium[35] and may be infiltrative or polypoid in nature.

Rhabdomyosarcoma

These tumors often diffusely infiltrate the myocardium but may also, occasionally, form a polypoid extension into the cardiac chamber.[36] There is a high incidence of rhabdomyosarcoma in infants and children, in conjunction with a predilection for the septum in younger as opposed to older patients.

Fibrosarcoma and malignant fibrous histiocytoma

Fibrosarcoma of the heart can extensively infiltrate the heart, often involving more than one cardiac chamber. A thrombus may form in an obstructed pulmonary vein, in the vena cava, or over the mural surface of the tumor.[4]

Lymphosarcoma

Although cardiac involvement of systemic lymphoma has been reported in 25–36% of cases, primary lymphosarcoma involving only the heart or pericardium is much less common.[37] Myocardial infiltration by lymphoma may be nodular or diffuse, and the clinical syndrome of hypertrophic cardiomyopathy has been mimicked. Some of these tumors are predominantly intracavitary.

Pulmonary artery sarcoma

These tumors usually present after the fourth decade and show a 2 : 1 female predominance. They may present as tumor emboli to the lungs or as right ventricular outflow obstruction. Symptoms include dyspnea, chest pain, cough, and hemoptysis, and this type of neoplasm may be associated with radiographic findings of a pulmonary hilar mass or cardiomegaly.[32]

Tumors of the pericardium

Pericardial cysts are the most frequent benign 'tumors' of the pericardium. They occur most frequently in the third or fourth decade of life and are usually located in the right cardiophrenic angle. In general they are found coincidentally on routine chest X-rays: 25–30% of these patients, however, will have chest pain, dyspnea, cough, or paroxysmal tachycardia.[38] Clinically and radiographically, they resemble other tumors of the pericardium such as hemangioma, lymphangioma, or lipoma, as well as retrosternal hernia, a pericardial fat pad, and eventration of the hemidiaphragm.

Teratoma is a rare intrapericardial tumor. Most are found in infants and children with a strong female preponderance. Recurrent non-hemorrhagic pericardial effusion is common in children with this tumor, and intrapericardial teratoma is the most likely diagnosis in this setting.[39]

Mesothelioma ranks third in frequency among malignant tumors of the heart and pericardium.[6] The clinical manifestations resemble those of pericarditis, constrictive pericardial disease, and vena caval obstruction. The prognosis is poor.

Secondary tumors of the heart

Being much more common than primary tumors, they may involve the heart by direct infiltration through lymphatic channels or via the hematogenous route. The most common primary tumor producing cardiac metastases is carcinoma of the lung, with carcinoma of the breast, malignant melanoma, lymphoma and leukemia next in order of frequency. At autopsy, 15–35% of patients dying with lung cancer show cardiac involvement, while 60% of patients with malignant melanoma have cardiac metastases.[40] Hematological malignant tumors, especially lymphomas, account for 15% of all cardiac and pericardial metastases.[41] A unique type of cardiac involvement that occurs most commonly with renal cell carcinoma (and occasionally with adrenal and hepatic neoplasm) consists of venous extension of the tumor via the inferior vena cava, with resultant tumor involvement of the right atrial cavity.

Usually the metastases involve the pericardium and myocardium, and the right side of the heart appears to be affected more frequently than the left.[42] Metastatic nodules in the heart are generally multiple; they even may become diffuse and lead to the manifestations of restrictive cardiomyopathy. Clinically, many metastatic cardiac lesions are silent. The most common clinical manifestations result from pericardial effusion with tamponade, tachyarrhythmias, AV block or congestive heart failure.[43]

Pseudotumors of the heart

Pseudotumors of the heart can be intracavitary (pedunculated or endothelialized thrombi, abscess, foreign body, etc.), intramural (congenital or acquired cysts, abscess, etc.), or epicardial (congenital diverticula, ventricular aneurysms, coronary aneurysms, etc.). Thrombi must always be included in the differential diagnosis of intracavitary masses of the heart. They usually occur in the region of infarctions or in aneurysms, or they may appear in the left atrial appendage in patients with mitral stenosis.

A not so uncommon tumorous mass of the heart is the hydatid cyst which is usually solitary and tends to grow in the myocardium. After 1–5 years, rupture occurs into the ventricle, atrium or pericardium unless the cyst dies. Secondary cysts may then grow in multiple distant sites or locally in the heart or pericardium. Cysts in the left side of the heart may cause death from rupture into the ventricle, massive embolism or anaphylactic shock.[44]

On chest X-ray, any mediastinal tumor abutting the heart, an aneurysm of the left ventricle, or a coronary artery aneurysm, may appear like a heart tumor.

Clinical manifestations of cardiac tumors

Cardiac tumors may produce: (1) hemodynamic disturbances; (2) constitutional symptoms; (3) mechanical hemolysis; and (4) biochemical effects.

Hemodynamic disturbances include: (1) arrhythmias; (2) pericardial effusion; (3) heart failure (low output syndrome); (4) intracavitary obliteration and obstruction; and (5) systemic embolism.

The most common cardiovascular symptoms of cardiac tumors are dyspnea, syncope, chest pain, palpitations, and congestive heart failure. The next most common group of symptoms are those considered 'constitutional'—fever, fatigue, weight loss, night sweats. They are common to many disease states and do not pinpoint which organ system is involved. Of cardiac myxomas, 90% provoke systemic illness (right atrial less often than left atrial myxomas). Some special symptoms and physical findings of patients with primary or secondary cardiac tumors can be grouped according to the anatomic location of the tumor: thus we discern tumors with pericardial, myocardial, and endocardial involvement.[45]

1. *Pericardial involvement:* Pericardial tumors may provoke pericarditis or pericardial effusion resulting in palpitations and dyspnea. Chest pain aggravated by positional or respiratory changes suggests the presence of a tumor around the heart. In patients with cancer of other organs, pericardial friction rub, tachycardia, jugular venous distention, changing electrocardiogram and pulsus paradoxus point at pericardial involvement. Additional features may be cardiac enlargement and hepatomegaly.
2. *Myocardial involvement:* The spectrum of symptoms of patients with myocardial tumors is wide. Patients may

complain about palpitations, tachycardia, even Adams–Stokes' attacks. The ECG may show arrhythmias, primarily atrial fibrillation, and recurrent supraventricular or ventricular tachycardias. Furthermore, the invasion of the ventricular wall by a tumor sometimes gives rise to chest pain and the syndrome of myocardial infarction with electrocardiographic signs of necrosis. Conduction abnormalities and AV-block, especially in younger patients are noted; angiomas and mesotheliomas may produce complete heart block and sudden death. In the presence of extended myocardial infiltration by the tumor, patients may show symptoms of left- or right-sided heart failure, such as dyspnea, peripheral edema, and general fatigue.

3. *Endocardial involvement:* In patients with intracavitary cardiac tumors, dizziness, nonexertional syncope, or palpitations related to changes in position are often observed.[46] This is probably related to tumor obstruction of ventricular outflow or inflow. Myxomas, fibromas or sarcomas may provoke valve obstruction, resulting in valve regurgitation or stenosis. With myxoma, the clinical course is relatively recent in origin, distinguishing myxoma from rheumatic mitral valvular disease;[45] however, the course may occasionally span many years. Intracavitary tumors or tumors with valvular neoplastic implants causing tricuspid and mitral involvement, are usually associated with pathological heart murmurs. These murmurs typically change with position. Left atrial myxomas may mimick the auscultatory signs of mitral stenosis; in addition, there may be a systolic murmur of mitral regurgitation. These murmurs are due to either tumor obstruction to valve flow or tumor interference with valve closure. It is common for the signs of mitral valve disease to be much less impressive than the degree of pulmonary hypertension that accompanies them; this discrepancy is useful in suggesting the presence of a myxoma. Tumors located in the right ventricle may simulate pulmonary stenosis, tricuspid incompetence, or restrictive cardiomyopathy. The constitutional symptoms which are so common in patients with atrial myxomas are usually absent in patients with tumors of the right ventricle.[45] Left ventricular tumors may mimick findings of aortic stenosis, subaortic stenosis, hypertrophic cardiomyopathy, and endocardial fibroelastosis.

Intracardiac tumors may give rise to systemic or pulmonary embolism. The embolism may be due to blood clots which become attached to the tumor, or due to fragments of the tumor itself. In one series, all patients with embolization presented with a highly mobile or pedunculated mass.[47] Tumor fragments originating from right-sided tumors may provoke acute pleuritis with effusion or pulmonary hypertension (in case of multiple emboli). Systemic emboli from left-sided cardiac tumors are rather frequent; they commonly occur with left atrial myxomas.[45] The tumor may embolize to the central nervous system, peripheral arteries, viscera, kidneys, and rarely to the coronary arteries. The neurologic syndrome due to systemic embolization includes transient ischemic attacks, major cerebrovascular accidents, especially in younger patients, and spinal cord or retinal infarction.[48] Sometimes emboli may be multiple and involve many different organs, thus simulating a generalized vascular disease with little, if any, signs of cardiac obstruction or of constitutional features.[49]

A variety of laboratory findings has been reported, particularly with myxomas, including hypergammaglobulinemia, elevated erythrocyte sedimentation rate, thrombocytosis, thrombocytopenia, polycytemia, leukocytosis, and anemia. The association of constitutional symptoms with cardiac myxoma is likely to be due to the tumor's constitutive synthesis and secretion of interleukin-6, an inflammatory cytokine.

Imaging methods

Chest radiography

With many intracavitary and intramural tumors of even moderate size, there are no changes seen on plain films unless hemodynamic alterations are produced, such as functional mitral stenosis due to a left atrial myxoma. When the pericardium is affected, the heart shadow usually is enlarged (Fig. 16.1). Rarely the plain film alone is typical for a special mass (Fig. 16.2). Calcification visible by roentgenographic methods may occur with several types of cardiac tumors, including rhabdomyomas, fibromas, hamartomas, teratomas, myxomas, and angiomas. Visualization of intracardiac calcium in an infant or child should immediately raise the question of an intracardiac tumor. In summary, approximately half of adults had some abnormal findings on their chest X-ray.[9] Clues suggestive of cardiac tumor[50] are: (a) ectopic or peculiar calcification; (b) bizarre cardiac silhouette; (c) unusually clear evidence of pulmonary venous obstruction.

Angiocardiography

For two decades angiocardiography was the main imaging method for cardiac tumors. It can show: (1) compression or displacement of cardiac chambers or large vessels; (2) deformity of cardiac chambers; (3) intracavitary filling defects (Fig. 16.3a,b); (4) marked variation in myocardial thickness; (5) alterations in wall motion; and (6) pericardial

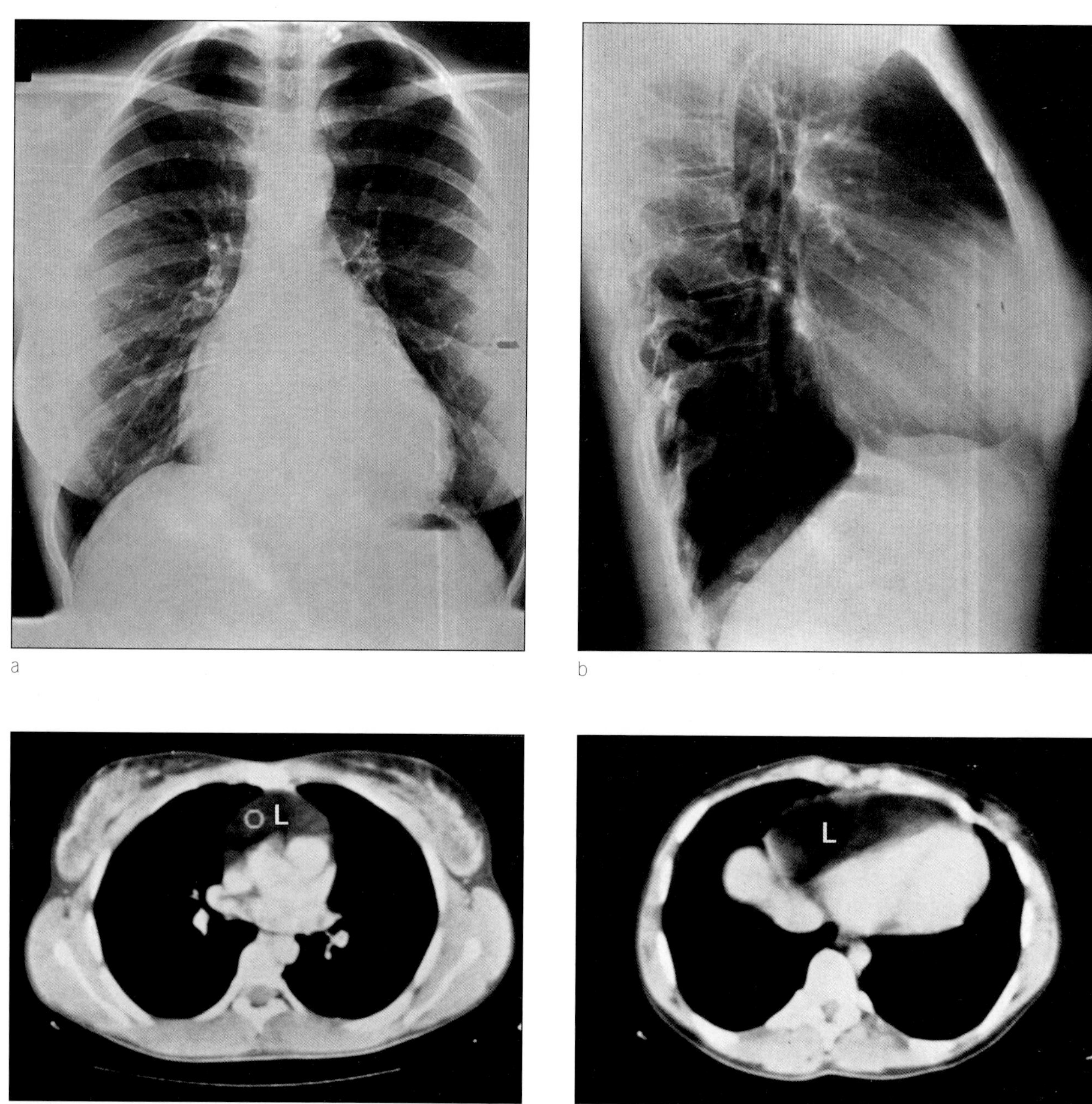

Figure 16.1
Intrapericardial lipoma. Chest X-ray (a, b) showing apparently enlarged right ventricle. CT at the level of the aortic root (c) and at the level of the ventricles (d) showing intrapericardial lipoma (L). Circle for density measurement in (c).

effusion. On angiocardiography, an intracavitary tumor or a cyst may look the same (Figs 16.4 and 16.5). A ventricular thrombus is usually located in an infarcted area (Fig. 16.6). The efficacy of the noninvasive imaging techniques has largely supplanted contrast angiocardiography, and usually permits immediate surgery without additional invasive studies, especially in myxomas. Coronary angiography is required to confirm the clinical suspicion of concomitant coronary artery disease, and can demonstrate the vascular supply of tumors (Fig. 16.3c,d).

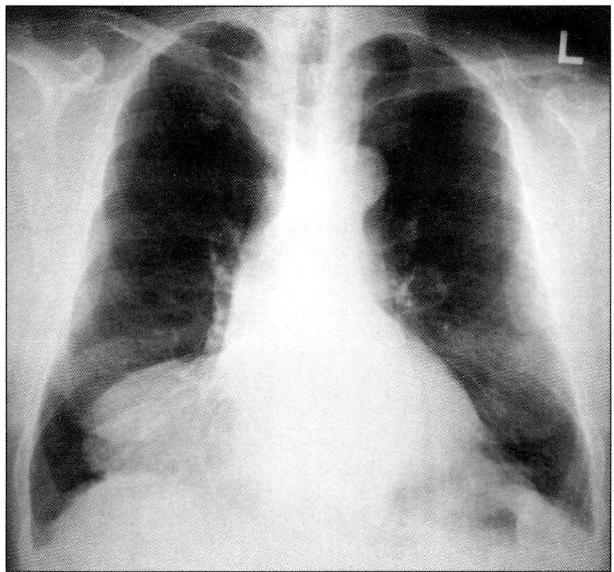

a

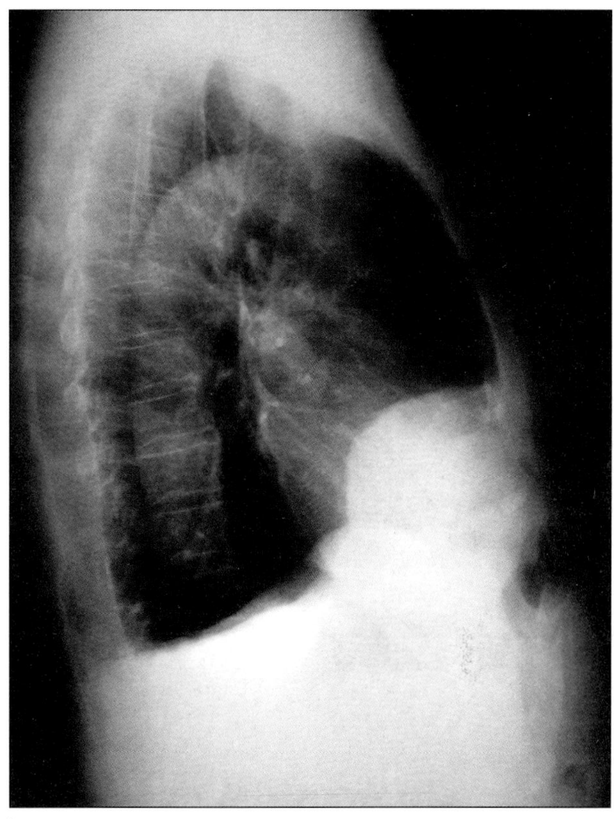

b

Figure 16.2
Lipoma in the right cardiophrenic angle. Chest X-ray showing smooth mass, which is more transparent than the heart (a pericardial cyst would have the same density as the heart). Reprinted with permission from Goebel N, *Prax Klin Pneumol* 1985; 39: 309–314.

Echocardiography

Two-dimensional echocardiography (2-D ECHO) is the preferred method for detection of intracardiac masses. Tumor size, shape, site of attachment, and mobility can be accurately determined, thus allowing resection without preoperative angiocardiography (Fig. 16.7). The method even allows the detection of small tumors, in many cases prior to the onset of clinical signs and symptoms (Figs 16.8 and 16.9). The transthoracic examination may be extended by transesophageal echocardiography (TEE), the latter providing unimpeded visualization of the atria, atrial septum and portion of the ventricles. TEE is therefore particularly helpful in detecting the site of insertion and morphologic features of atrial and ventricular myxomas (compare the image quality in Figs 16.10 and 16.11a). Even cysts, calcifications, necrotic foci, and hemorrhage in atrial myxomas may be easily identified. The TEE view can be used to detect small vegetations and tumors (1–3 mm in diameter). Left atrial myxomas are typically attached to the interatrial septum near the fossa ovalis (Fig. 16.12). Large tumors obstruct the atrioventricular valves or prolapse from the atria into the ventricles in early diastole (Fig. 16.11a).

Doppler echocardiography is useful for evaluating the hemodynamic consequences of valvular obstruction or incompetence caused by cardiac tumors.[51] Follow-up after resection of a cardiac tumor, especially myxoma, is also performed by 2-D ECHO (Fig. 16.11b,c, Fig. 16.13). In malignant cardiac tumors the intracardiac component of the tumor is well seen (Fig. 16.14), but in large pericardial masses the assessment of the extent of the whole tumor may be limited (Fig. 15).

The main differential diagnosis to heart tumors are thrombi (Fig. 16.16). The formation of thrombi usually occurs in patients with regional or global wall motion abnormalities, such as those that develop after myocardial infarction and in association with dilated cardiomyopathy or atrial fibrillation, especially if mitral valve disease and an enlarged atrium are present. Left atrial thrombi usually are localized on the left atrial appendage; if they are pedunculated and mobile, distinguishing them from a myxoma may be difficult. Ventricular thrombi are exceedingly rare in

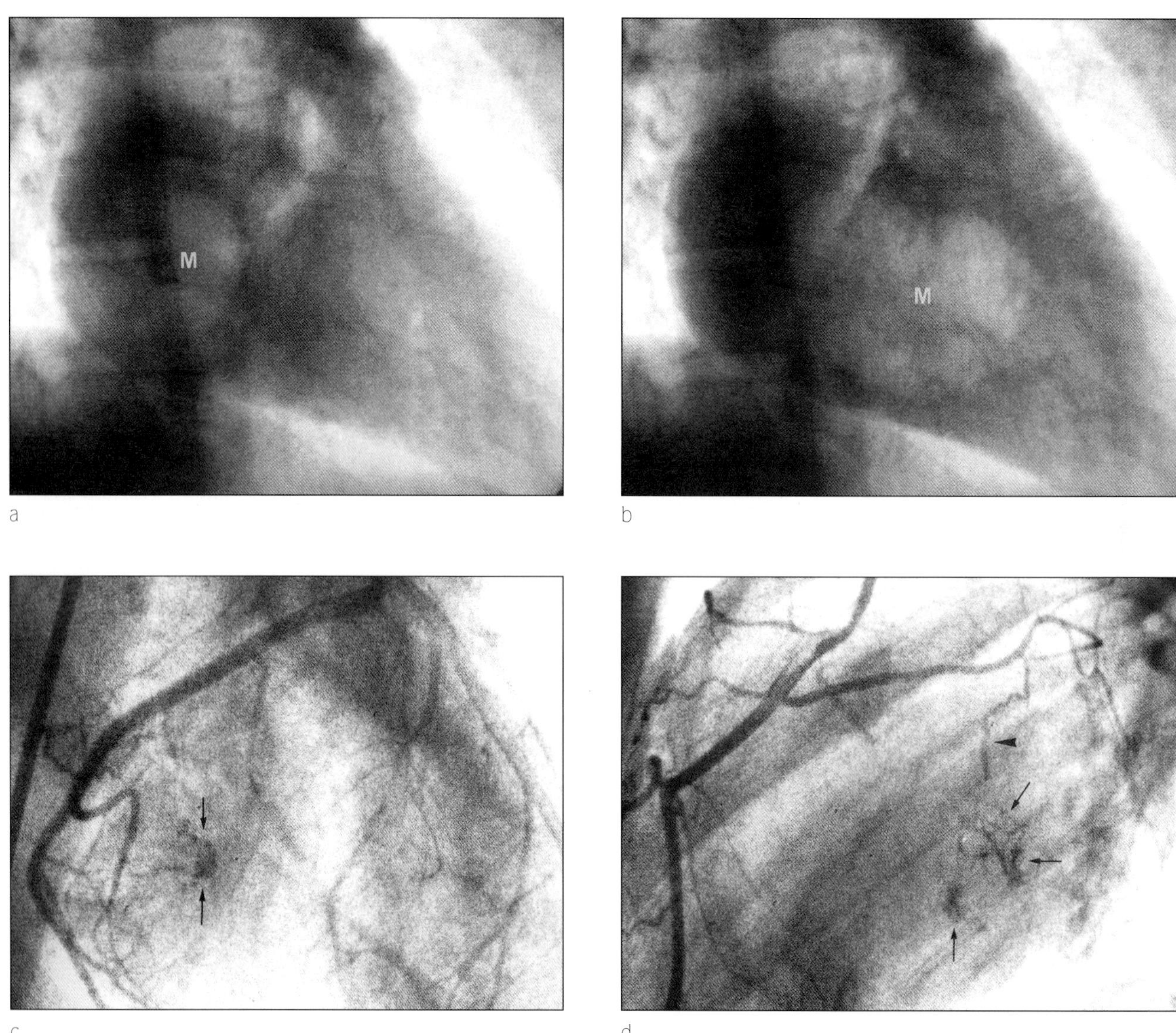

Figure 16.3
Right atrial myxoma (M) in systole (a), in diastole (b) prolapsing into the right ventricle. Tumor vessels (arrows) from the left coronary artery (c) and the right coronary artery (d). Arrowhead: branch of sinus node artery. Reprinted with permission from Hinterauer L, Goebel N, Hess O. *Fortschr Roentgenstr* 1985; 42: 99–101.

patients with normal ventricular function. Valvular vegetations also form an important part of the differential diagnosis. In cases of right atrial masses, a prominent Eustachian valve and aneurysm of the interatrial septum must be considered, in addition to tumors, sessile or mobile thrombi, and vegetations on the mitral valve. In a multicentre study concerning the diagnosis of heart tumors,[47] TEE had the highest detection rate of all imaging modalities for myxomas and intracardiac tumors (100%).

Computed tomography (CT)

Contrast-enhanced CT has gained an important role in the management of patients with tumors in general and is usually applied in the diagnostic work-up of thoracic tumors, where it allows the demonstration of the relationship of the tumor to the heart (Figs 16.17,16.18 and 16.19). Bizarre contours at the heart shadow, caused by pseudotumors, can be clarified by CT examinations (Figs 16.20,

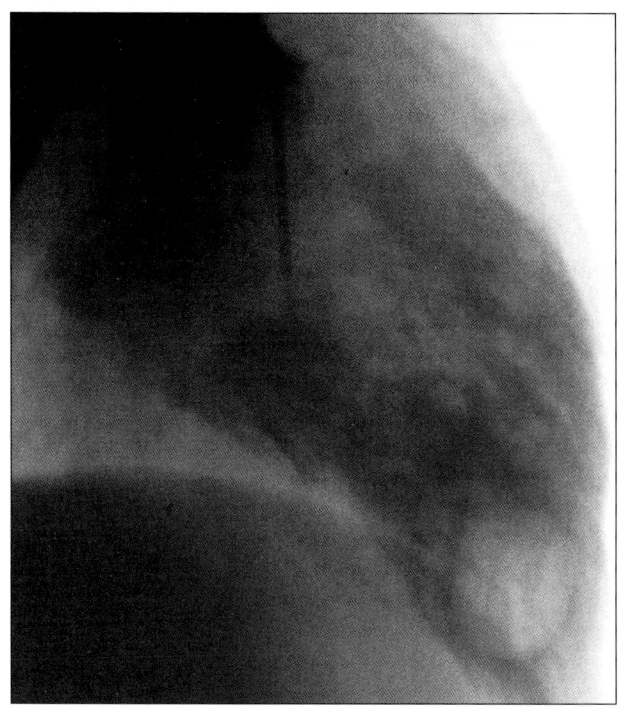

a

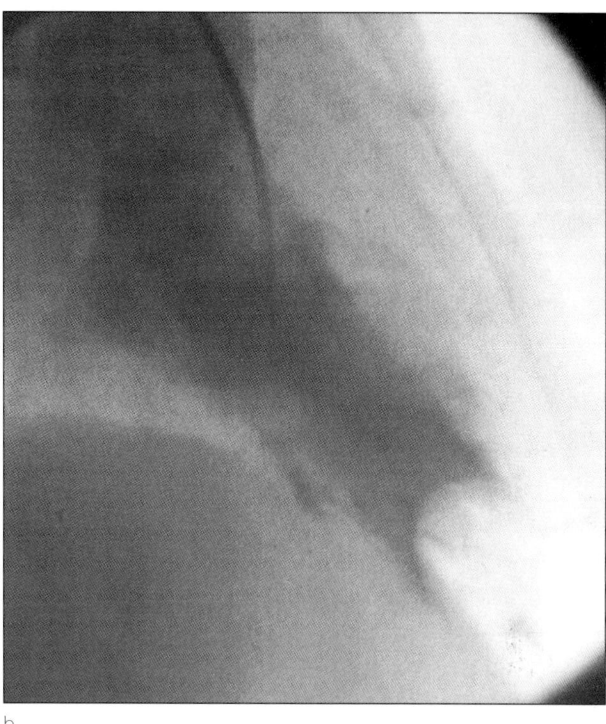

b

Figure 16.4
Left ventricular angiography: spherical tumor in the apex of the left ventricle in diastole (a) and systole (b). Histological diagnosis: leomyofibroma. Reprinted with permission from Goebel N, Gander MP. *Fortschr Roentgenstr* 1977; 126: 591–2.

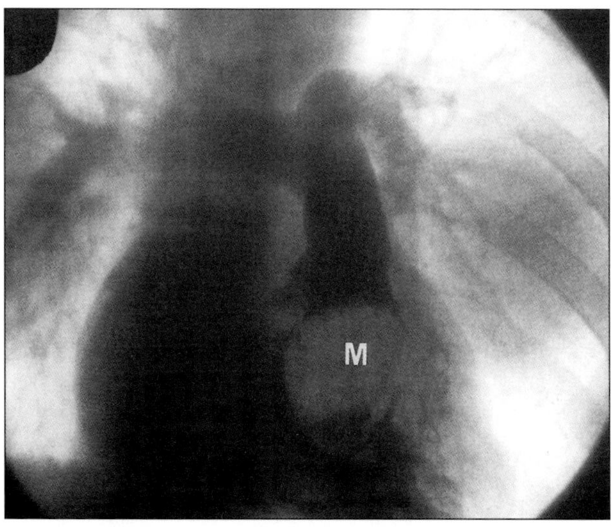

a

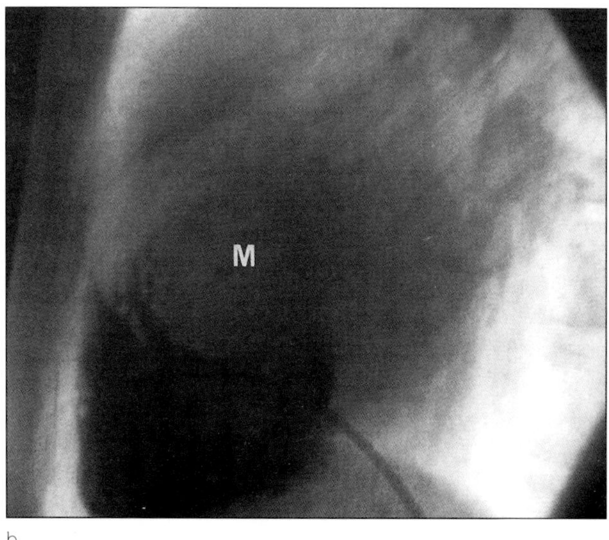

b

Figure 16.5
Right ventricular angiogram: (a) AP-projection; (b) lateral projection: rounded mass (M) protruding from the interventricular septum into the right ventricular outflow tract. Intraoperative diagnosis: hydatid cyst. No recurrence or dissemination. Reprinted with permission from Goebel N, Gander MP. *Fortschr Roentgenstr* 1977; 126: 11–14.

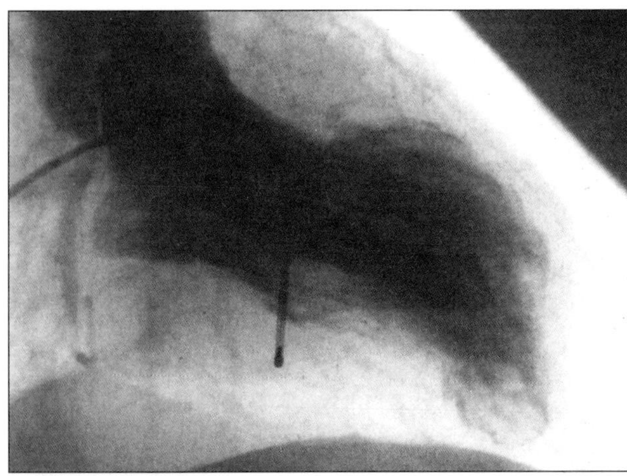

Figure 16.6
Left ventricular angiogram: oval thrombus in the left ventricular apex. Systolic frame showing large infarcted area of anterolateral wall and apex.

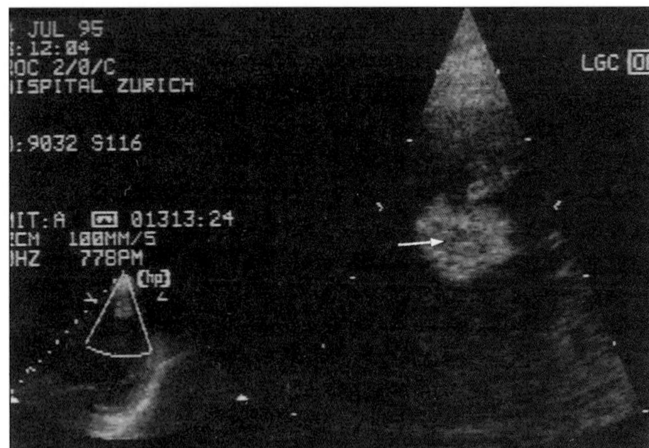

Figure 16.7
Fibroelastoma. Parasternal short-axis view showing a hyperechoic pedunculated tumor (arrow) in the left ventricle, originating from the apical anterior wall. There was no local hypokinesia.

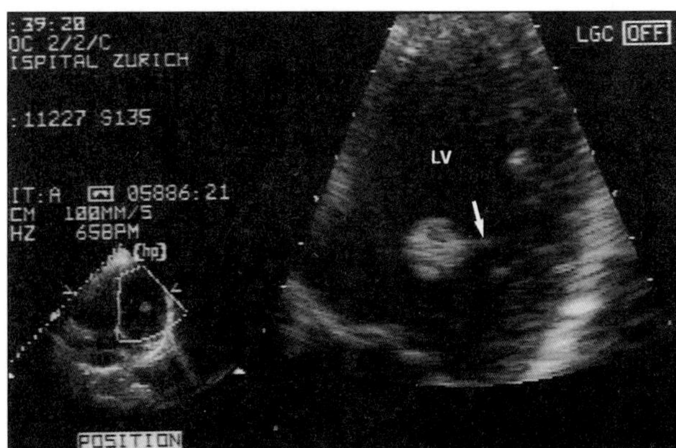

Figure 16.8
Fibroelastoma of the left ventricle (LV). Apical 4-chamber view showing a spherical pedunculated mass originating from the posteromedial papillary muscle (arrow).

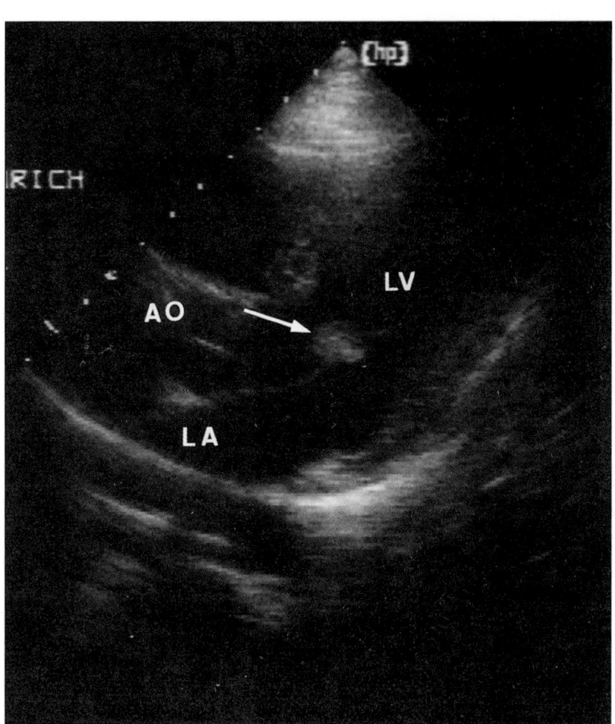

Figure 16.9
Chordal fibroma of the anterior mitral valve leaflet (arrow). Parasternal long-axis view. AO, aorta; LA, left atrium; LV, left ventricle.

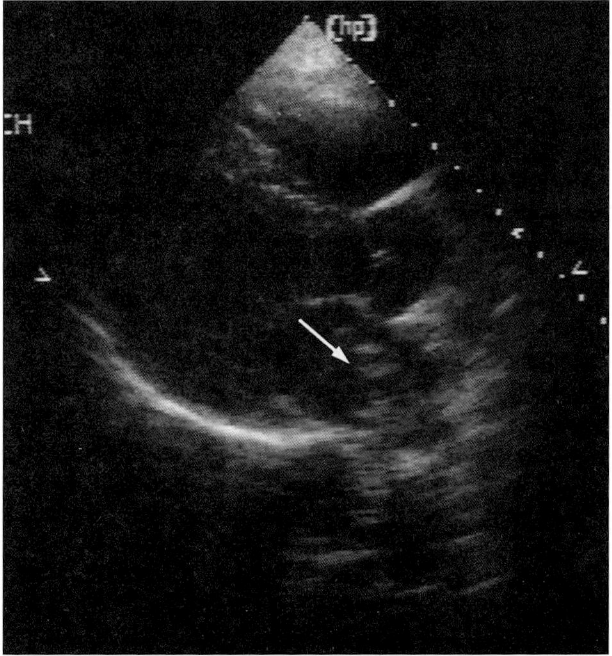

Figure 16.10
Left atrial myxoma. Parasternal long-axis view showing a spherical, smoothly marginated pedunculated mass (arrow).

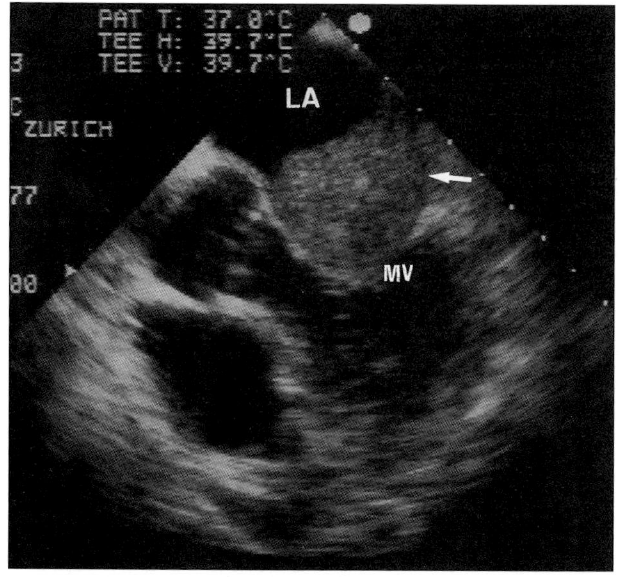

a

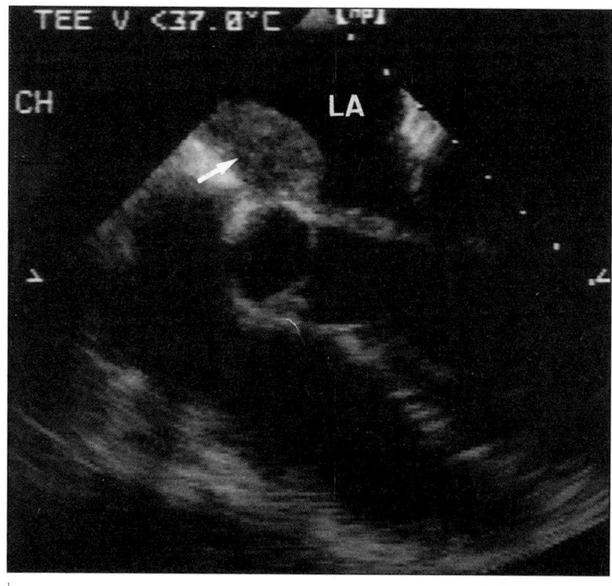

b

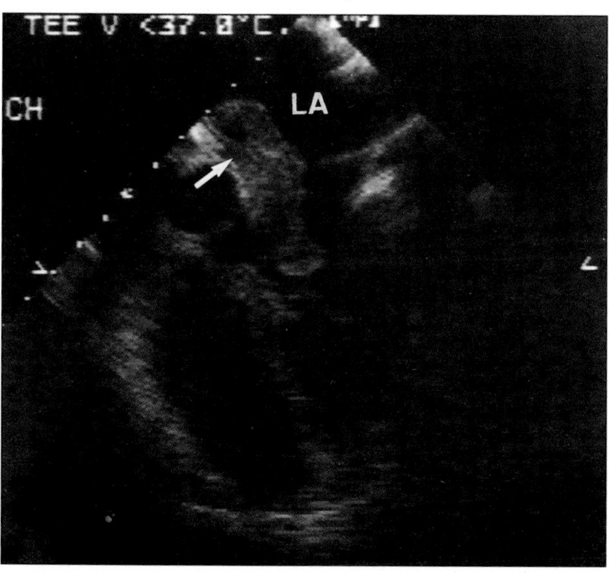

c

Figure 16.11
Malignant myxoma of the left atrium. (a) Transesophageal echocardiogram, horizontal plane: large tumor in the left atrium (LA) with a broad base of attachment in the left atrial appendage (arrow). Note the diastolic occlusion of the mitral valve (MV). (b) Tumor recurrence 3 years following resection. Note the different site of recurrence (arrow) at the opposite wall of left atrium. (c) Two months later there is almost doubling of the left atrial mass (arrow).

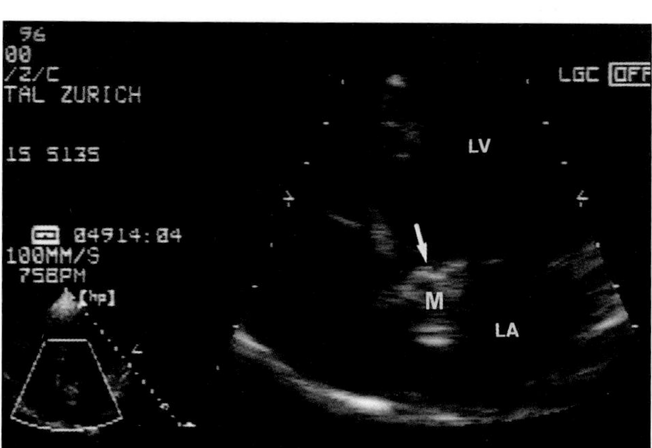

Figure 16.12
Myxoma of the left atrium. Apical 4-chamber view disclosing a spherical mass (M) in the left atrium (LA) with attachment medially and posteriorly next to the mitral annulus (arrow). Laboratory examination revealed an elevated level of interleukin-6. LV, left ventricle.

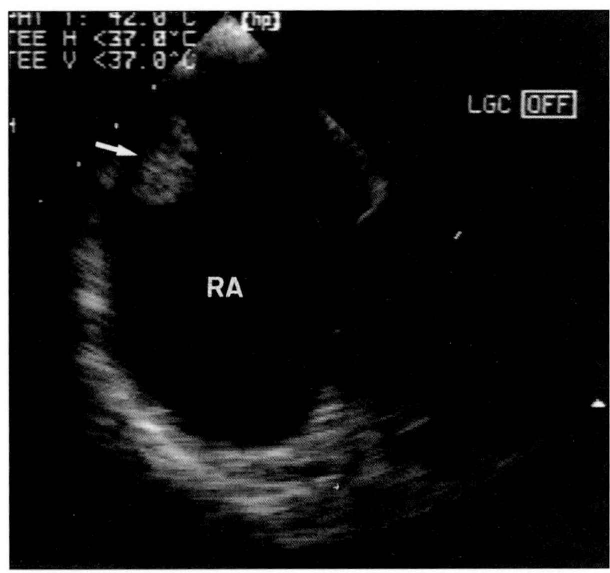

a

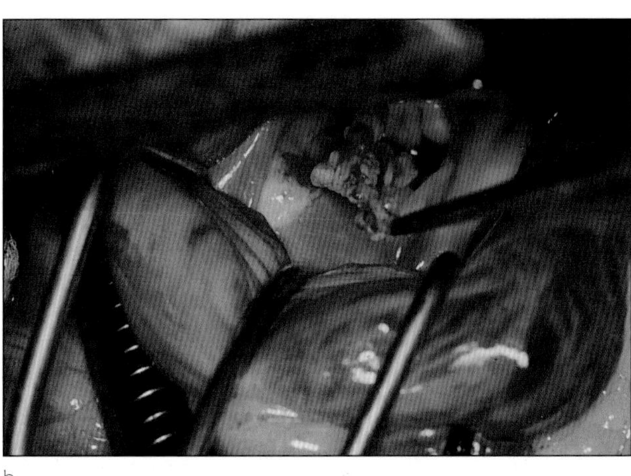

b

Figure 16.13
Patient with 'Swiss syndrome'. (a) Transesophageal echocardiography (horizontal plane). Broad-based recurrent myxoma (arrow) measuring 1.2 × 1.8 cm at the posterior wall of the right atrium (RA). (b) Intraoperative view of the primary right atrial myxoma (situs after atriotomy), showing cauliflower-like irregular surface of the tumor.

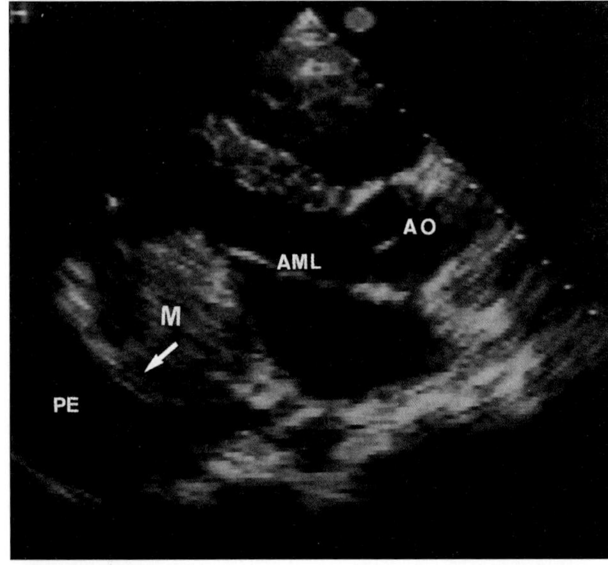

Figure 16.14
Sarcoma of the left ventricle. Parasternal long-axis view disclosing a hyperechoic mass (M) originating from the posterior wall (arrow). Large pericardial effusion (PE). AML, anterior mitral valve leaflet; AO, ascending aorta.

16.21 and 16.22). It has also been used to demonstrate cardiac tumors and thrombi (Fig. 16.23). Because of its ability of tissue discrimination it can differentiate between solid, liquid, hemorrhagic, and fatty masses (Figs 16.1 and 16.24). It appears most useful to determine the degree of myocardial invasion and the involvement of pericardial and extracardial structures (Fig. 16.25). The differentiation of a typically located myxoma from a thrombus may present the same difficulties as in 2-D ECHO (Fig. 16.26). A more angulated appearance of thrombi has been described as an important differentiating characteristic.[52]

Magnetic resonance imaging (MRI)

MRI has a wide variety of applications in the cardiovascular system and, when compared with other noninvasive imaging techniques, offers excellent anatomical resolution, good reproducibility, both static and dynamic information, and lack of ionizing radiation. Recent developments include

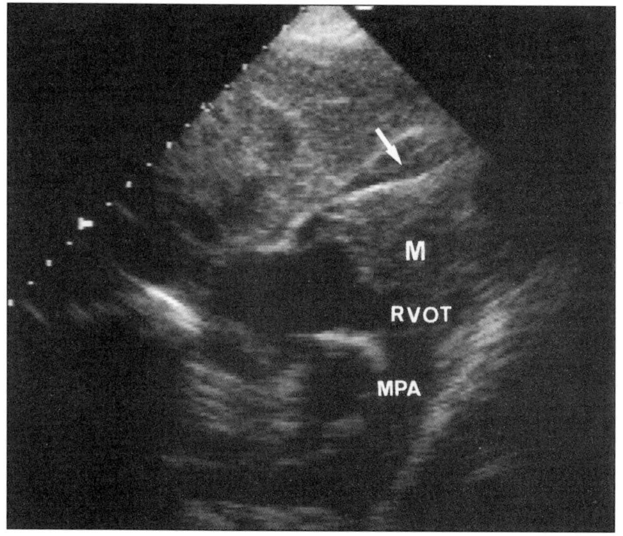

a

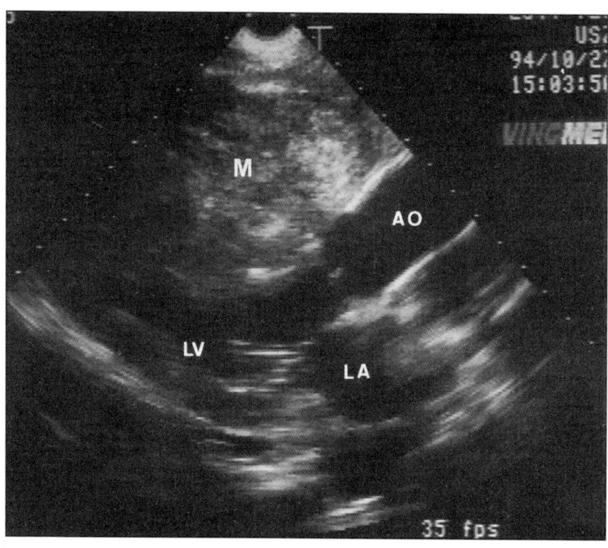

b

Figure 16.15
Malignant mesothelioma of the right ventricle. (a) Subcostal view showing a mass (M) compressing the apex and the right ventricular outflow tract (RVOT). Note also small pericardial effusion (arrow). MPA, main pulmonary artery. (b) Parasternal long-axis view showing the large heterogeneous mass (M) infiltrating the right ventricle. LV, left ventricle; LA, left atrium; AO, aorta.

ultrafast imaging with a single acquisition time of as low as 50 ms, which has opened the door to real-time data acquisition. The versatility of MRI makes the technique a strong competitor to other imaging modalities in the future, and costs will rapidly decrease due to the growing patient throughput resulting from ultrafast techniques.

Gated spin-echo MRI has been effective for demonstrating the presence, location and extent of an intracardiac mass, sometimes also revealing the nature of the mass[53–56] (Figs 16.27–16.30). The larger field of view and the three-dimensional information provide better definition of the tumors, cardiac chambers and the surrounding structures, a feature that is especially important in large or malignant tumors (Fig. 16.28). MRI also provides excellent definition of tumor prolapse and secondary valvular changes. Intracavitary tumors are readily recognized within the low signal intensity of the blood-pool on spin-echo images and within the high signal intensity of the blood-pool on gradient-echo images. With MRI and CT, tumors measuring at least 0.5–1 cm in diameter can be identified.[57] Some tumors have had a characteristic signal intensity: lipomas and lipomatous hypertrophy of the interatrial septum are recognized by high signal intensity on T1-weighted images; fibroma of the

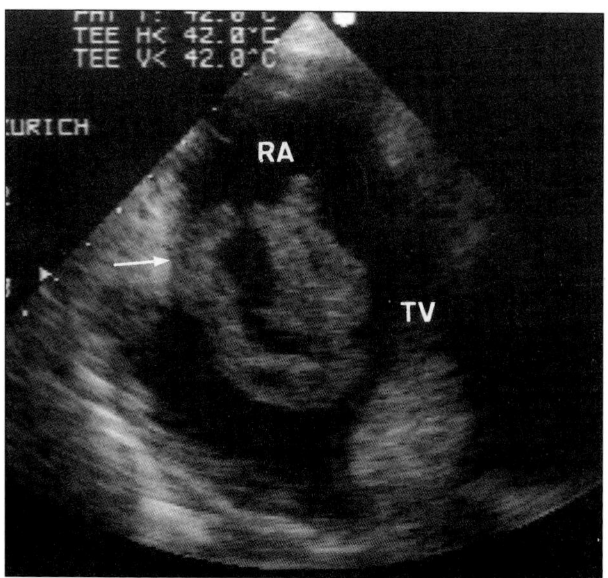

Figure 16.16
Right atrial thrombus. Transesophageal echocardiography (horizontal plane) disclosing a large worm-like mass originating from the lateral wall of the right atrium (arrow). RA, right atrium; TV, tricuspid valve.

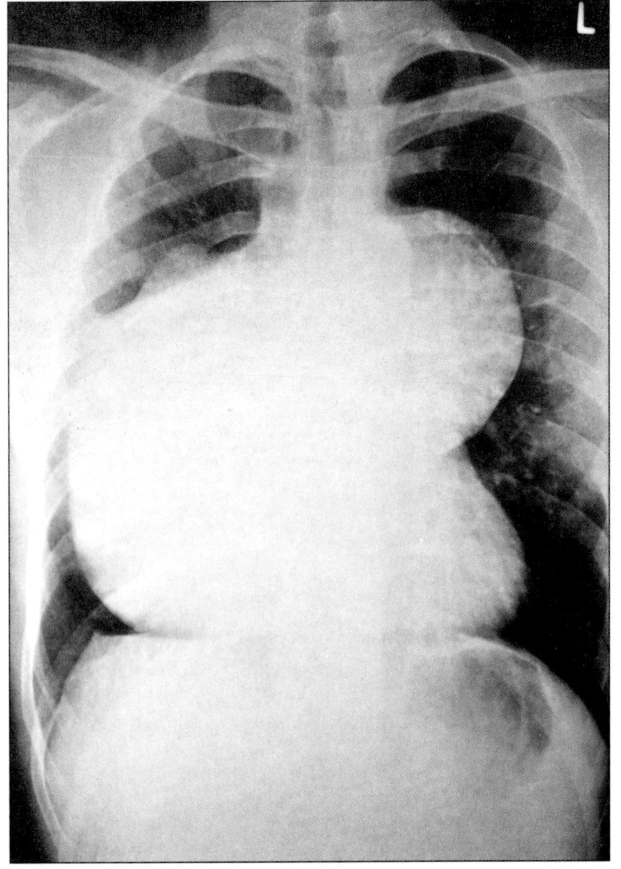

a

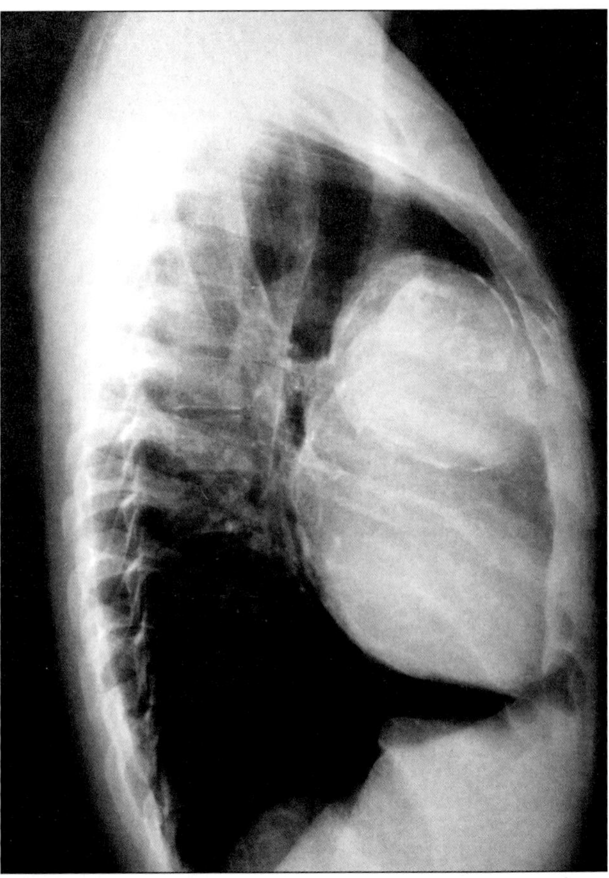

b

c

Figure 16.17
Two dermoid cysts causing bizarre contour of heart and mediastinum in the plain films (a, b). The lower cyst is compressing the right atrium as shown by CT (c). RA, right atrium; LA, left atrium; RV, right ventricle; S, septum; LV, left ventricle. Reprinted with permission from Goebel N, Jenni R, Turina M. *Z Kardiol* 1982; 71: 549–51.

ventricular wall produces a low signal intensity on T2-weighted images,[58] although T2-weighted images may be difficult to acquire in high quality due to cardiac motion. The most frequent intracardiac masses, myxoma and thrombi, can be differentiated by their location, mode of attachment and by application of Gd-DPTA: enhancement of the mass generally excludes the possibility that the mass is a thrombus. Many types of cardiac sarcoma can be found

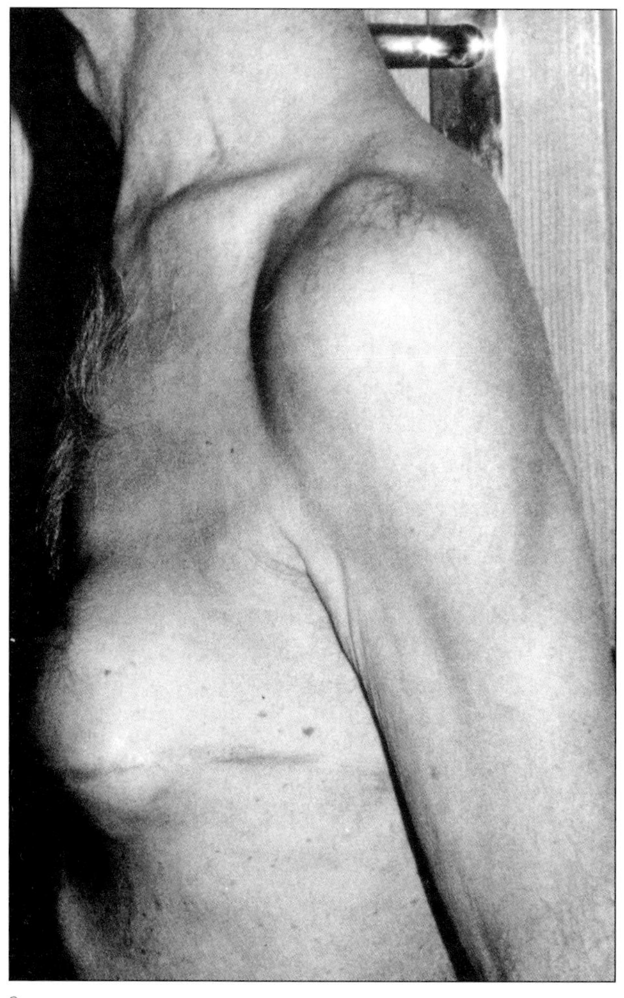

a

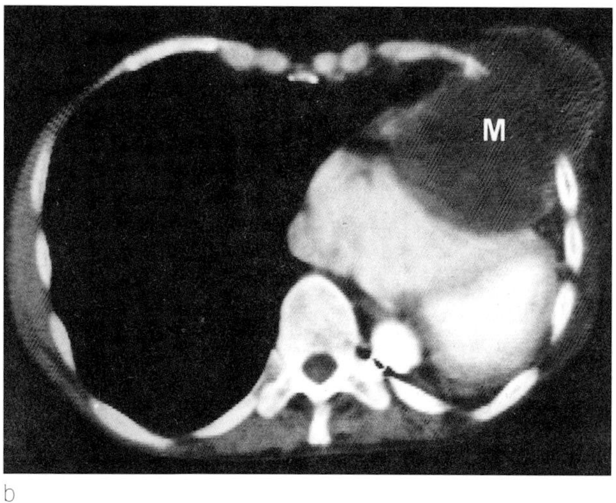

b

Figure 16.18
Patient with lung carcinoma, after pneumonectomy. (a) Pulsating mass in the scar of the thoracotomy. Herniation of the heart ? (b) CT: necrotic intra- and extrathoracic metastasis (M), invading the right ventricle. Reprinted with permission from Goebel N, Hauser J. *Z Kardiol* 1983; 72: 553–5.

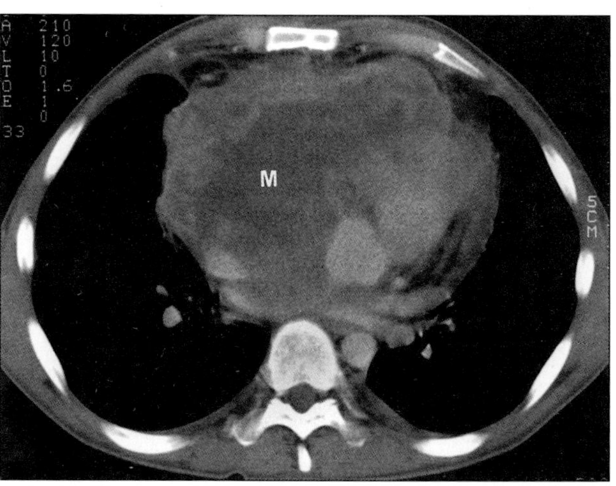

a

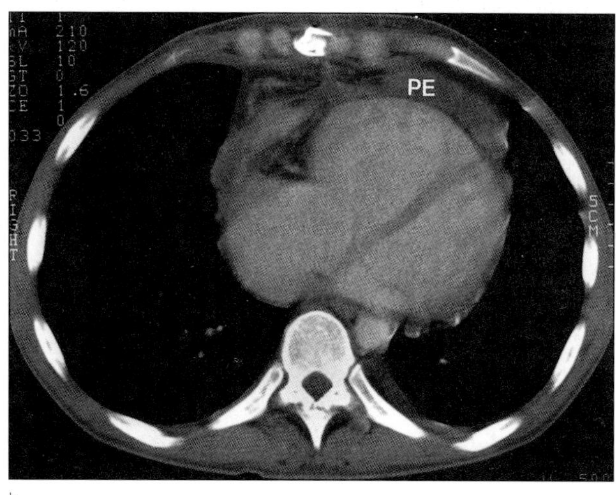

b

Figure 16.19
High-grade non-Hodgkin's lymphoma. Contrast-enhanced CT at the level of the roof of the left atrium (a) and the interventricular septum (b). Large heterogeneous, extensively necrotic mass (M) arising in the anterior mediastinum and infiltrating both atria as well as portions of the right ventricle. Pericardial effusion (PE) in front of the right ventricle.

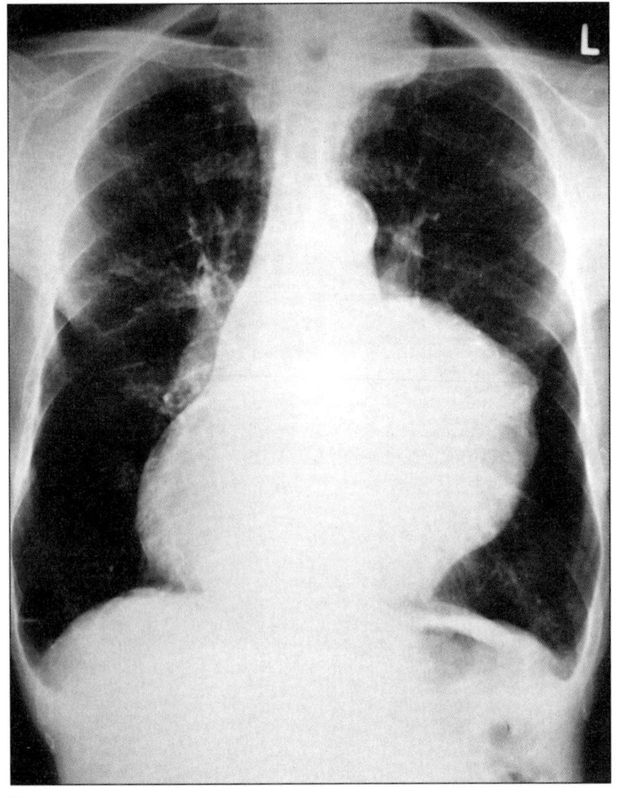

a

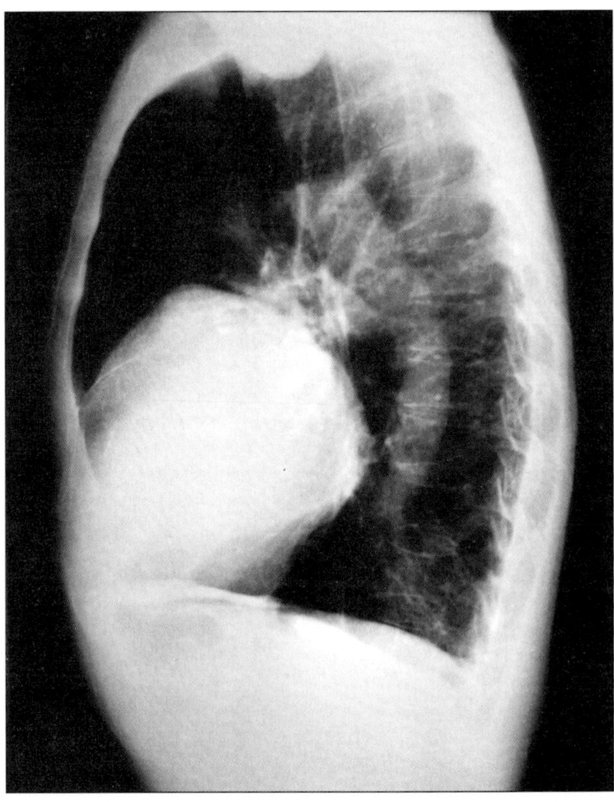

b

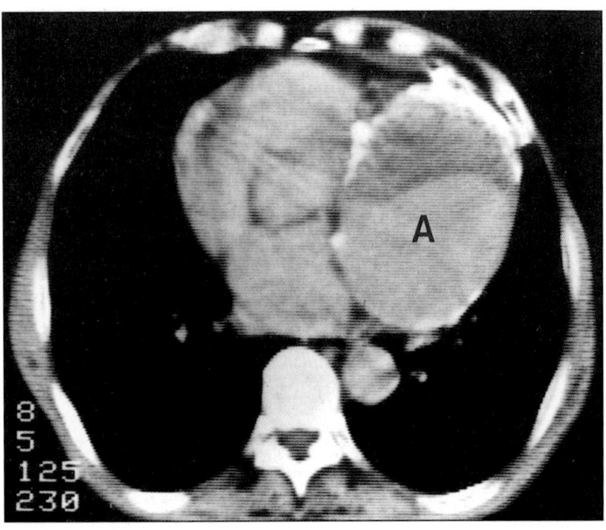

c

Figure 16.20
Rounded prominence at the upper left lateral heart contour in the plain films (a, b), which was caused by a large, partially thrombosed and calcified aneurysm (A) of the left coronary artery, as shown by CT (c). Reprinted with permission from Hinterauer L, Roelli H, Goebel N, et al. *Cardiovasc Intervent Radiol* 1985; 8: 127–30.

in the left atrium, and sarcomas can be attached to the atrial wall by a stalked myxoma. Infiltrative growth is more common in sarcomas than in myxoma. When this feature is identified using MRI or CT, the diagnosis of sarcoma should be favored over myxoma.[32] Rhabdomyomas, the most frequent tumors in children, may be difficult to recognize because of their small size and intramural location. However, many cause a focal distortion of the myocardial wall or project into the chamber, and some have demonstrated higher signal intensity than the myocardium. In one study echocardiography was definitely superior to MRI in the detection of rhabdomyomas in children.[59] The involvement

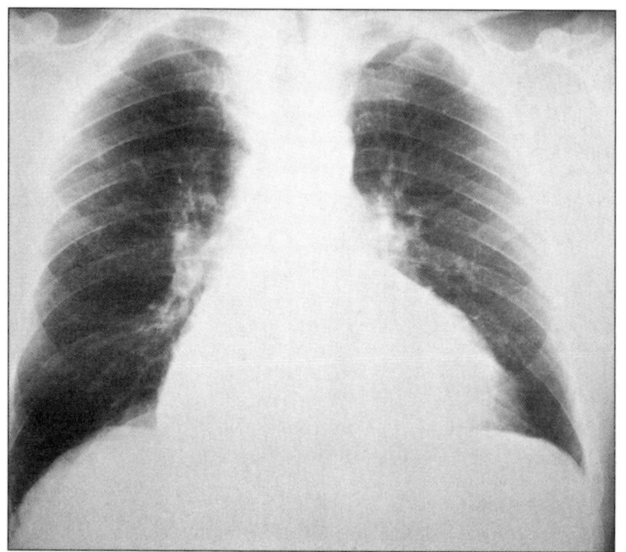

a

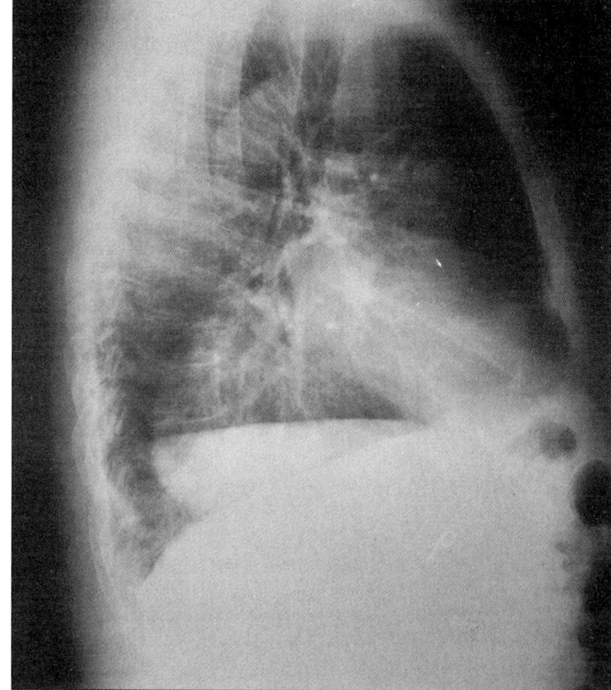

b

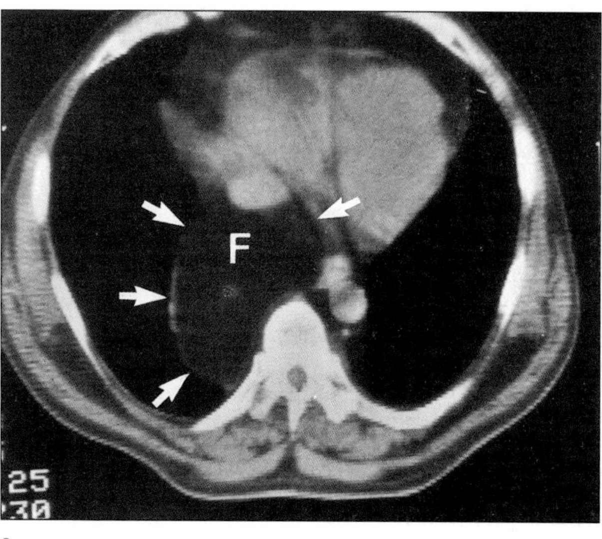

c

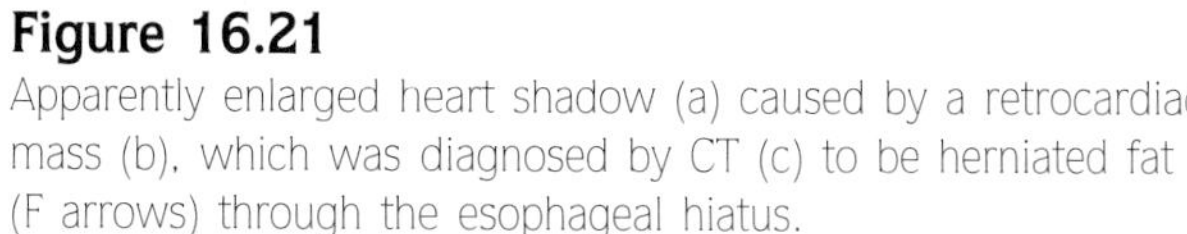

Figure 16.21
Apparently enlarged heart shadow (a) caused by a retrocardiac mass (b), which was diagnosed by CT (c) to be herniated fat (F arrows) through the esophageal hiatus.

of the heart by direct spread from mediastinal and lung tumors, by extension of tumors of the upper abdomen into the inferior vena cava and into the right atrium, and by metastasis to the pericardium, myocardium, or cardiac chambers is effectively demonstrated by MRI, which also displays the extent of the tumor attachment to the cardiac walls. An extracardiac tumor extending to the pericardium, but not through the pericardium, can be recognized by the presence of an intact pericardial line. Tumors that have extended through the pericardium may be recognized by focal obliteration of the pericardial line and the presence of a pericardial effusion.[58]

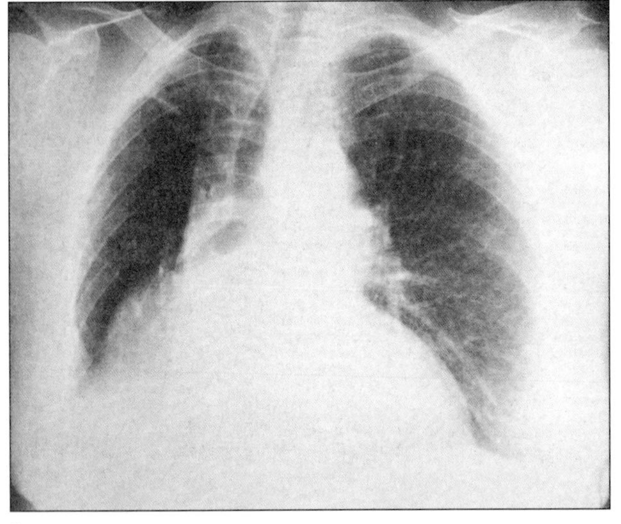
a

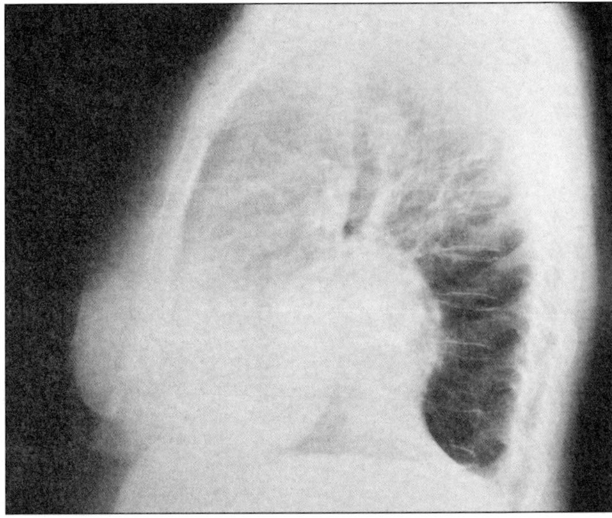
b

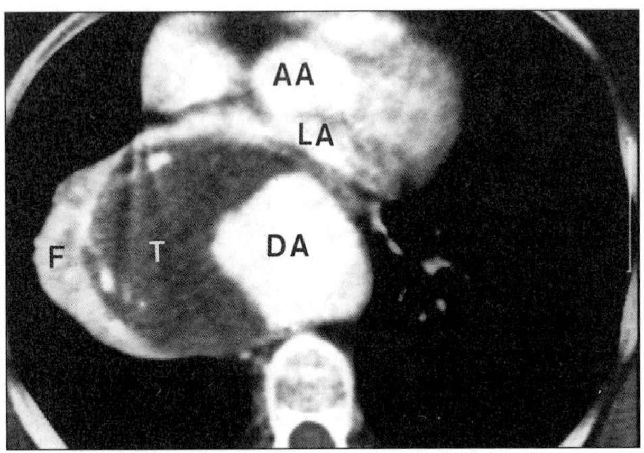

c

Figure 16.22
Apparently enlarged heart shadow (a) caused by a retrocardiac mass (b), which was diagnosed by CT (c) to be a partly thrombosed and calcified aneurysm of the descending aorta. Severe compression of the left atrium (LA). AA, ascending aorta; DA, descending aorta; T, thrombus with some calcifications; F, fibrosis.

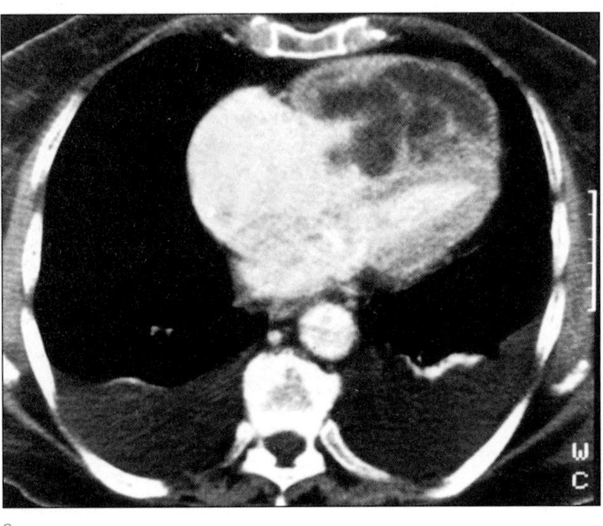

a

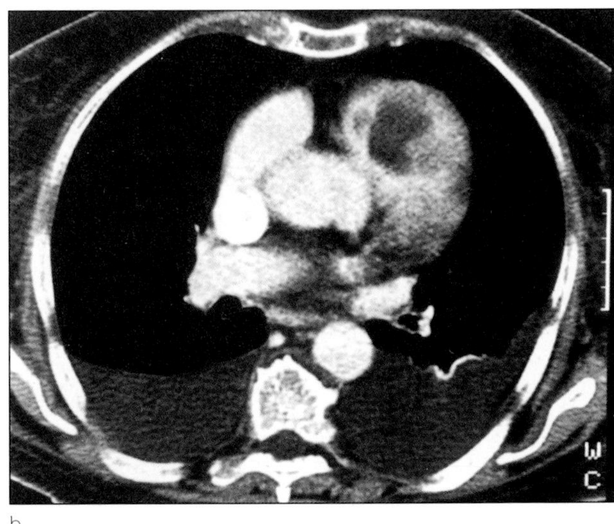

b

Figure 16.23
CT of leiomyosarcoma of the right ventricle, filling a distended right ventricular cavity (a), with propagation of the tumor into the right venticular outflow tract (b). Bilateral pleural effusions.

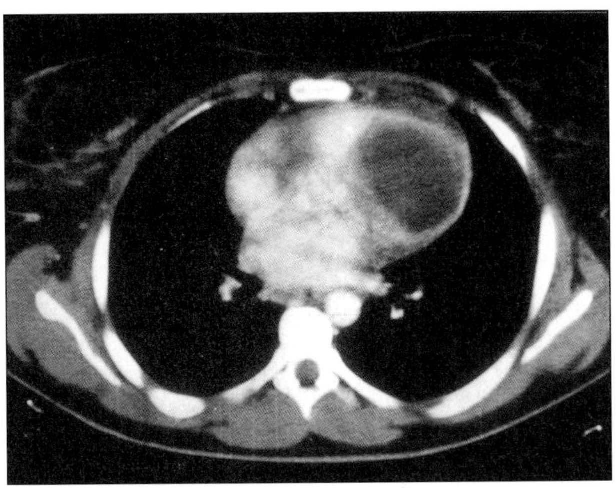

a

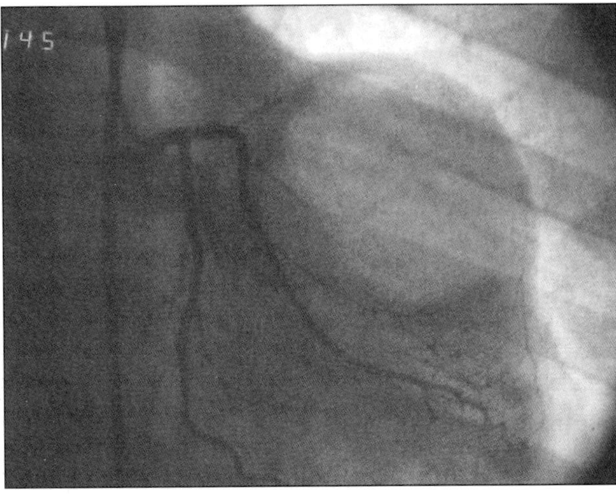

b

Figure 16.24

Hydatid cyst of the heart. (a) CT: large cyst in the free left ventricular wall. (b) Left coronary angiogram: no vessels inside the cyst. Occlusion of the left anterior descending artery by the cyst.

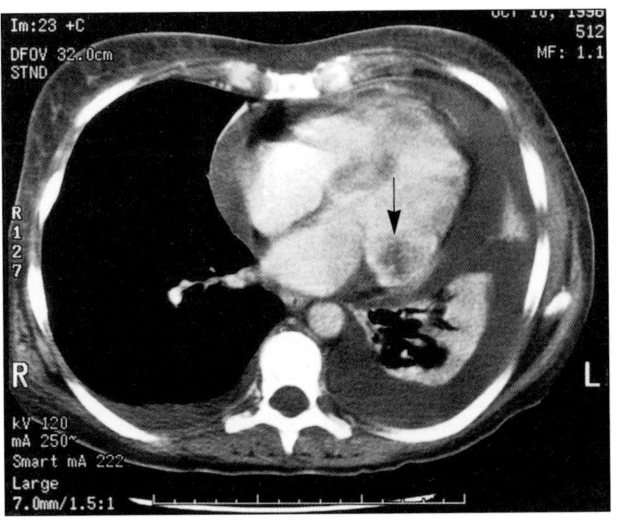

a

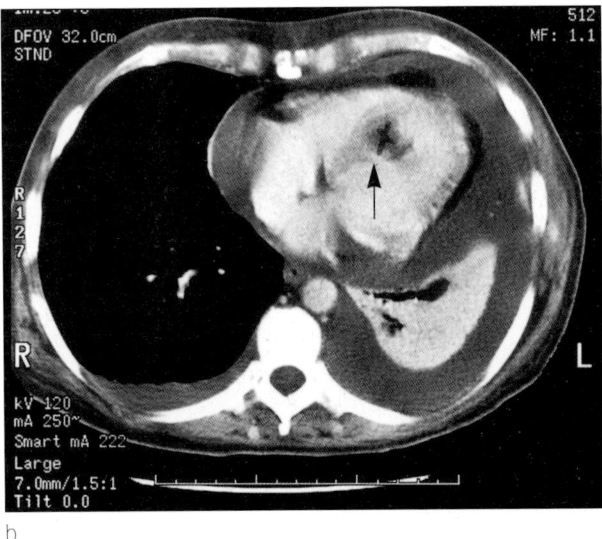

b

Figure 16.25

CT of patient with lung carcinoma. (a) Metastasis in dorsal left ventricular wall (arrow). (b) Metastasis in interventricular septum (arrow). Pericardial effusion (P). Bilateral pleural effusions with atelectasis of left lower lobe and lingula.

Therapy

Surgical resection of a myxoma is the only acceptable therapy and, in view of the dangers of embolization and sudden death, should be performed promptly. In general, operative excision is the treatment of choice for most benign cardiac tumors and is curative in many cases. Effective palliation and local control of the disease can be achieved with extensive resection of malignant primary tumors. Adjuvant chemotherapy and radiation therapy are necessary to improve long-term prognosis. The response to therapy can be assessed by MRI.[60]

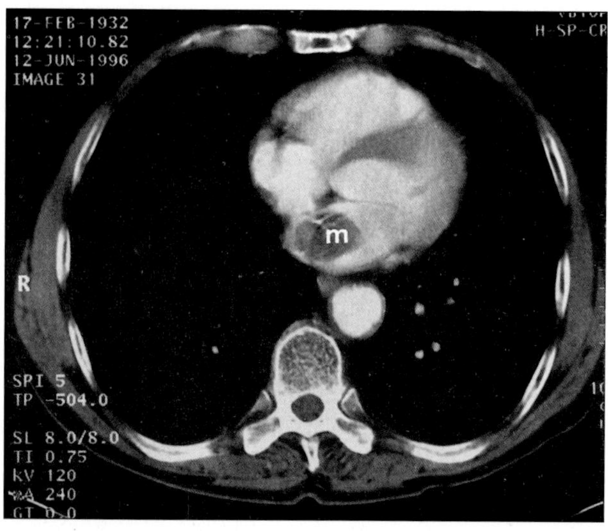

a

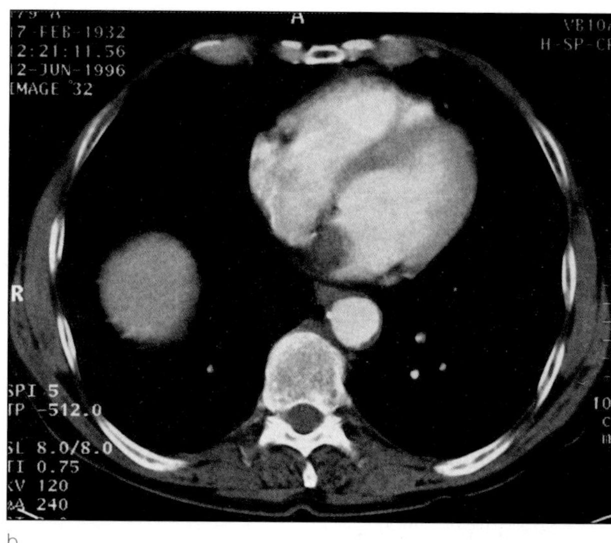

b

Figure 16.26

Left atrial thrombus. Contrast-enhanced spiral CT scan at the level of the left atrium (a, b) disclosing a hypodense, sharply marginated mass (m) originating in the left atrium (LA) and extending near to the mitral valve. Small calcification inside the mass. Patient had paraneoplastic thrombosis.

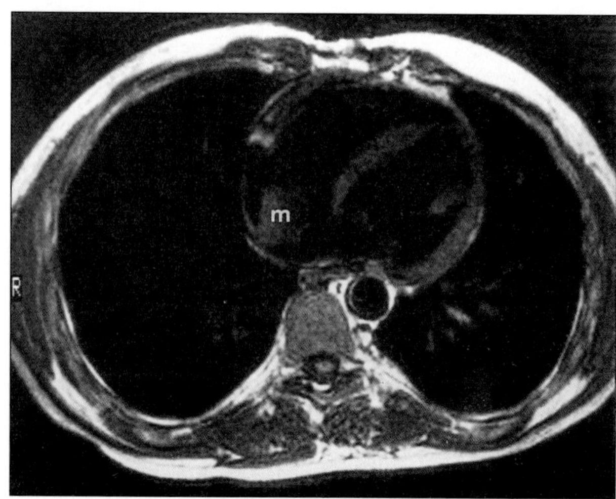

a

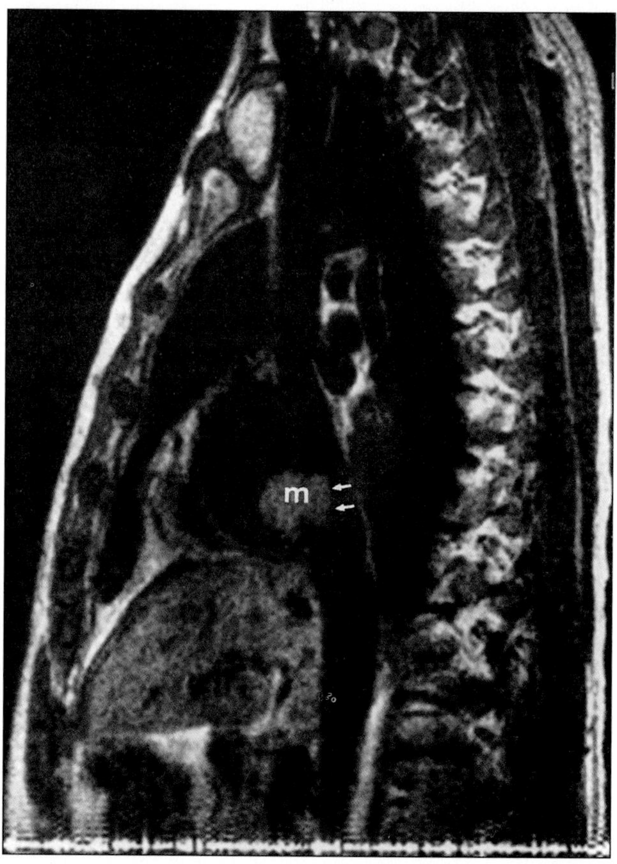

b

Figure 16.27

Right atrial myxoma. (a) Axial plane T1-weighted spin-echo magnetic resonance scan. Pedunculated mass (m) arising from the posterolateral aspect of the right atrial wall. (b) Oblique sagittal plane T1-weighted spin-echo magnetic resonance scan through the level of the venae cavae. Mass (arrow) located just superior to the inflow of the inferior vena cava.

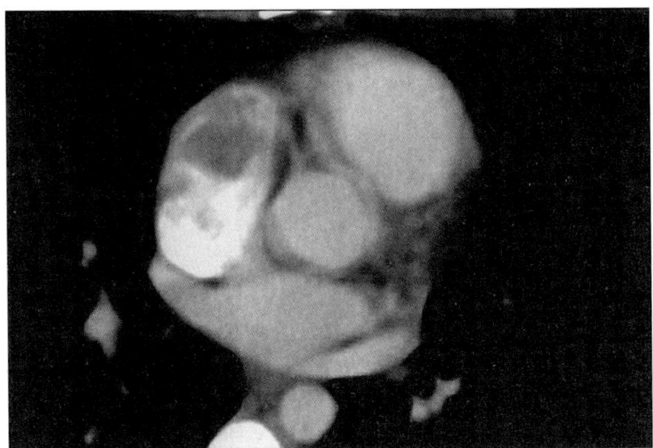

a

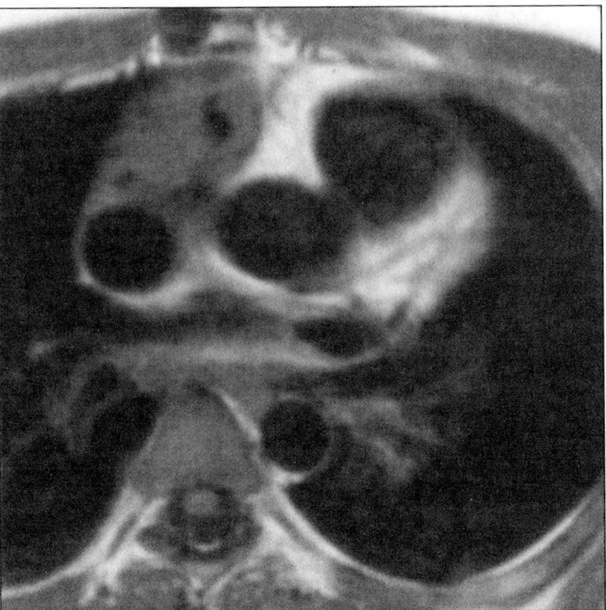

b

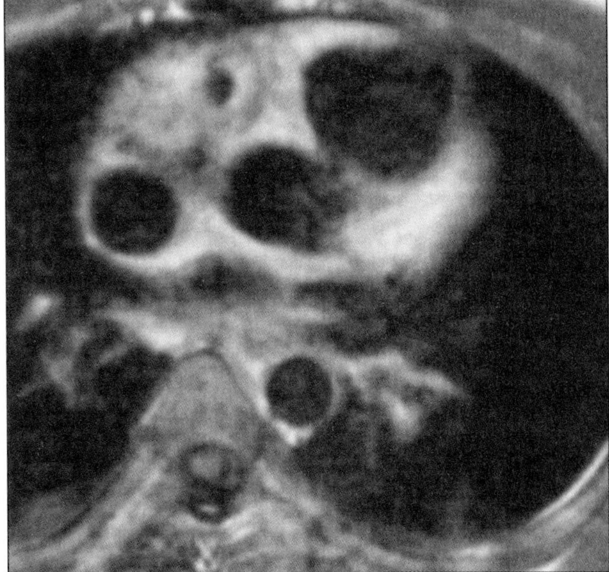

c

Figure 16.28
Atrial myxoma in the right atrium. (a) Contrast-enhanced CT, (b) axial T1-weighted spin-echo before and (c) after intravenous injection of gadolinium. In CT, the application of contrast medium is necessary to discern the mass in the blood; in MR, the application of contrast medium is only necessary to differentiate the tumor from a thrombus by showing its enhancement. (Courtesy of Dr St Duewell, Zurich.)

Cardiac transplantation has been used to completely resect 'inoperable' benign tumors[61] and unresectable malignant primary cardiac neoplasm.[62]

Finally, the imaging modalities of the heart have now reached such an efficiency and the use of echocardiography is so widespread, that the detection of a cardiac mass may be an incidental finding, and the clinician should carefully evaluate whether the patient's symptoms are caused by a more hidden disease process that is not as 'easily' imaged as heart tumors (Fig. 16.31).

Summary

Since the clinical diagnosis of heart tumors is often difficult, imaging is the preferred tool for diagnosis. Echocardiography has proven effective in demonstrating cardiac tumors and thrombi as well as valvular dysfunction, and has thereby substituted angiocardiography. CT and MRI are the methods of choice in the investigation of extracardiac, pericardial and large tumors involving the heart, and also allow limited tissue characterization.

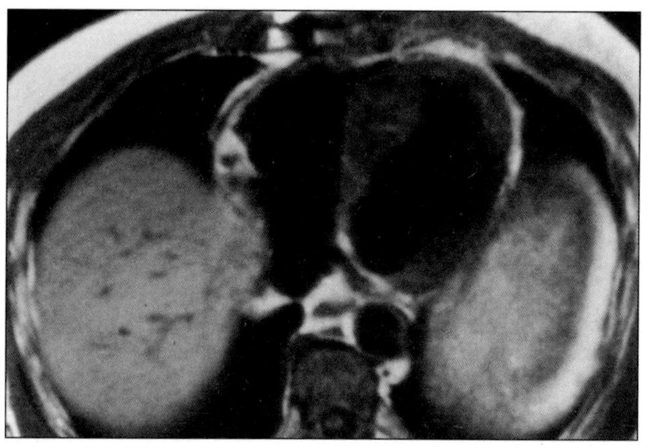

a

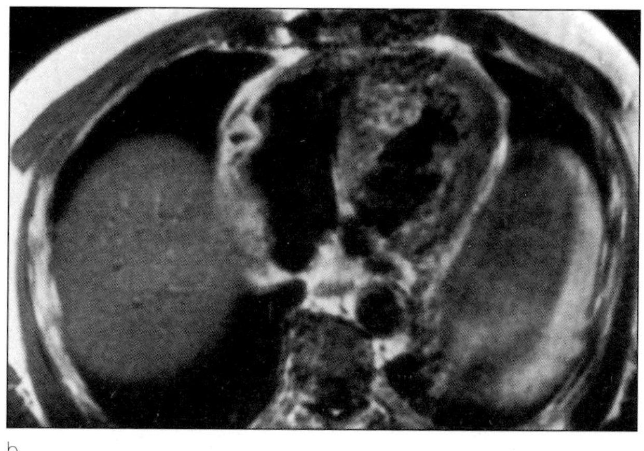

b

Figure 16.29

Rhabdomyosarcoma of the heart. ECG-gated axial T1-weighted spin-echo (a) before and (b) after intravenous injection of gadolinium. Irregular distension of the ventricular septum by the tumor which shows heterogeneously increased signal intensity after the application of contrast medium. (Courtesy of Dr St Duewell, Zurich.)

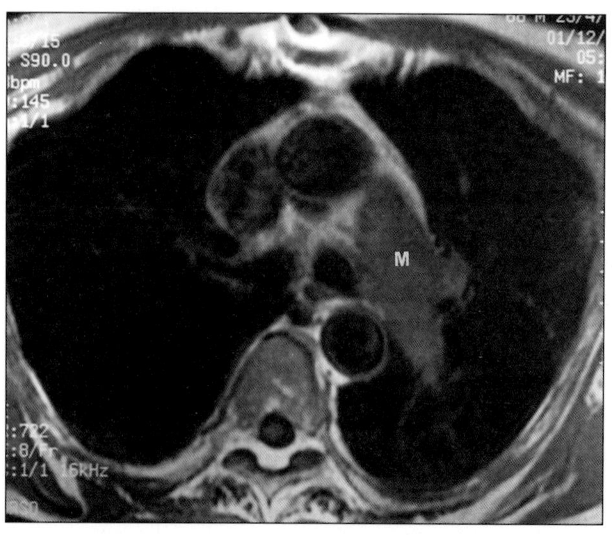

a

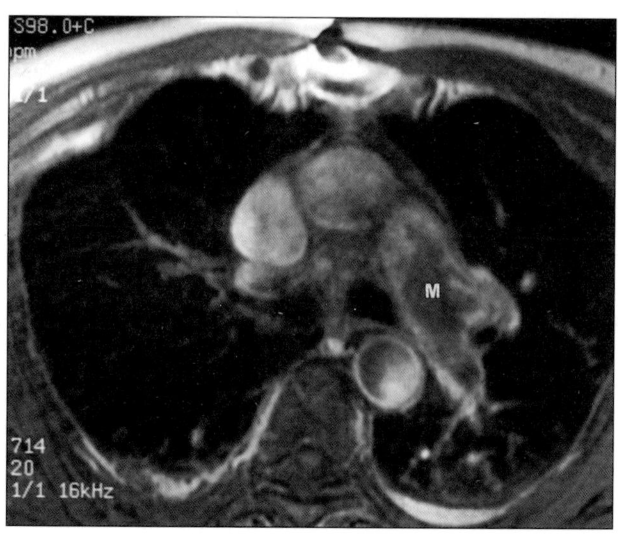

c

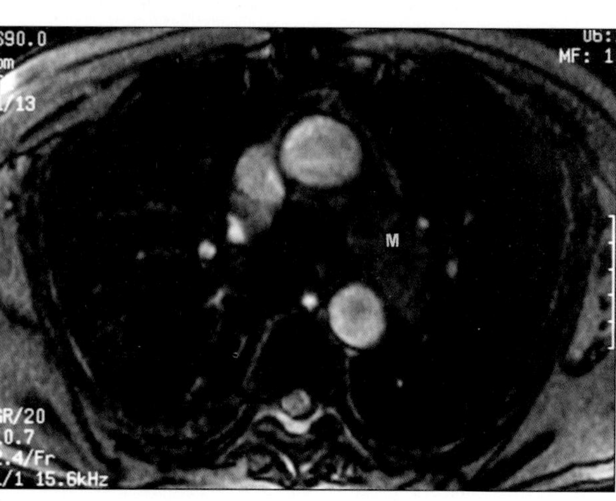

b

Figure 16.30

Angiosarcoma of the left pulmonary artery. (a) T1-weighted axial spin-echo image showing left pulmonary artery filled with a mass (M) infiltrating the adventitial fat. (b) Axial spoiled gradient echo image showing blood-flow in the aorta and the superior vena cava but not in the left pulmonary artery. (c) Axial contrast-enhanced T1-weighted spin-echo image with fat suppression showing peripheral contrast uptake in the tumor and the vessel wall of the left pulmonary artery. Small left-sided pleural effusion. (Courtesy Dr GM Kacl, Zurich.)

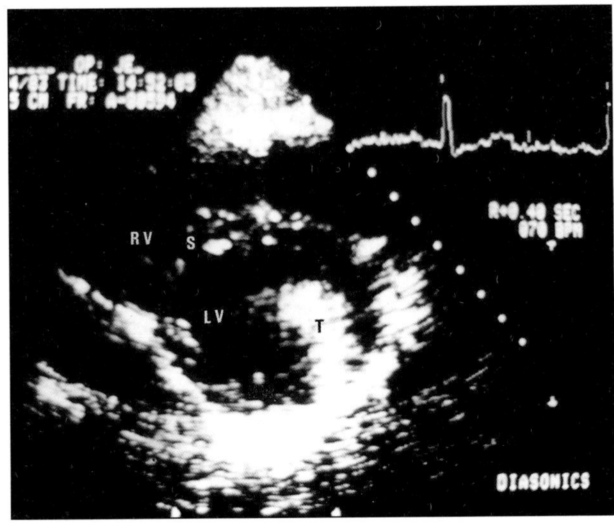

a

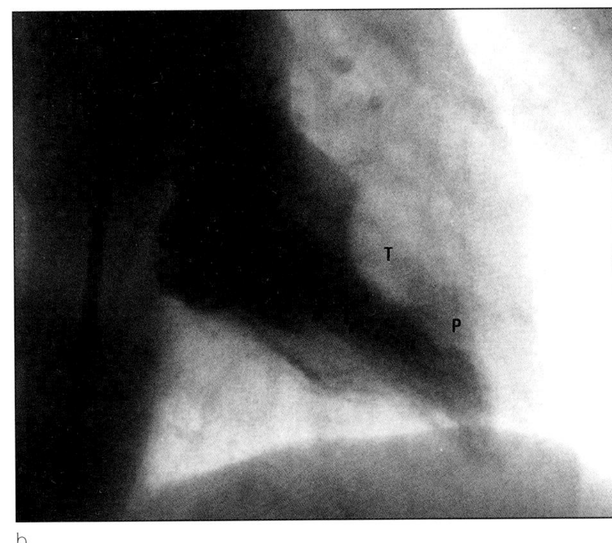

b

Figure 16.31
Patient with spells (caused by emboli?). (a) Echocardiographic diagnosis of a tumor (T) at the posterolateral wall of the left ventricle. (b) Tumor (T) near the papillary muscle (P), proven by angiography. Resection of the tumor (histologically a lipoma) caused a pseudoaneurysm. Spells continued. Final diagnosis was insulinoma of the pancreas. Reprinted with permission from Goebel N, Gander M, Jenni R, et al. *Z Kardiol* 1984; 73: 792–5.S.

References

1 Reynen K: Cardiac myxomas. *New Engl J Med* 1995; **333**: 1610–15.

2 McAllister HA Jr, Fenoglio JJ Jr: Tumors of the cardiovascular system. In: Hartmann WH, Cowan WR, eds, *Atlas of Tumor Pathology*, 2nd edn, fasc 15 (Armed Forces Institute of Pathology: Washington DC, 1978); 1–3.

3 Cohen GU, Peery TM, Evans JM: Neoplastic invasion of the heart and pericardium. *Ann Intern Med* 1955; **42**: 1238–45.

4 Heath D: Pathology of cardiac tumors. *Am J Cardiol* 1968; **21**: 315–27.

5 Carney JA: Differences between non-familial and familial myxomas. *Am J Surg Path* 1985; **9**: 53–5.

6 Davison ET, Mumford D, Zaman Q, Horowitz R: Left atrial myxoma in the elderly. Report of four patients over the age of 70 and review of the literature. *J Am Geriatr Soc* 1986; **34**: 229–33.

7 Gosse P, Herpin D, Roudant R et al: Myxoma of the mitral valve diagnosed by echocardiography. *Am Heart J* 1986; **111**: 803–5.

8 Moggio RA, Pucillo AL, Schechter AG et al: Primary cardiac tumors. Diagnosis and management in 14 cases. *NY State J Med* 1992; **92**: 49–52.

9 St John Sutton MG, Mercier LA, Giuliani ER, Lie IT: Atrial myxoma: a review of clinical experience in 40 patients. *Mayo Clin Proc* 1980; **55**: 371–6.

10 Hedinger C: Kombination von Herzmyxomen mit primärer nodulärer Dysplasie der Nebennierenrinde, fleckförmigen Hautpigmentierungen und myxomartigen Tumoren anderer Lokalisation — ein eigenartiger familiärer Symptomenkomplex ('Swiss syndrome'). *Schweiz Med Wschr* 1987; **117**: 591–4.

11 Shahian DW, Labib SB, Chang G: Cardiac papillary fibroelastoma. *Ann Thorac Surg* 1995; **59**: 538–41.

12 LiMandri G, Homma S, Di Tullio MR et al: Detection of multiple papillary fibroelastomas of the tricuspid valve by transesophageal echocardiography. *J Am Soc Echocardiogr* 1994; **7**: 315–17.

13 Topol EJ, Bierm RO, Reitz BA: Cardiac papillary fibroelastoma and stroke. *Am J Med* 1986; **80**: 129–32.

14 Lichtenstein HL, Lee JCK, Stewart S: Papillary tumor of the heart: incidental finding at surgery. *Hum Pathol* 1979; **10**: 473–5.

15 Colucci WS, Schoen FJ, Braunwald E: Primary tumors of the heart. In: Braunwald E, ed, *Heart Disease* (WB Saunders: Philadelphia, 1997); 1464–77.

16 Fenoglio JJ, McAllister HA, Ferrans VJ: Cardiac rhabdomyoma. A clinicopathologic and electron microscopic study. *Am J Cardiol* 1976; **38**: 241–51.

17 Webb DW, Thomas RD, Osborne JP: Cardiac rhabdomyomas and their association with tuberous serosis. *Arch Dis Child* 1993; **68**: 367–70.

18 Howanitz EP, Teske DW, Qualman SJ et al: Pedunculated left ventricular rhabdomyoma. *Ann Thorac Surg* 1986; **41**: 443–5.

19 Van der Hauwaert LG: Cardiac tumors in infancy and childhood. *Br Heart J* 1971; **33**: 125–32.

20 Prior JT: Lipomatous hypertrophy of cardiac interatrial septum. *Arch Path* 1964; **78**: 11–15.

21 Simons M, Cabin HS, Haffe CC: Lipomatous hypertrophy of the atrial septum: diagnosis by combined echocardiography and computerized tomography. *Am J Cardiol* 1984; **54**: 465–6.

22 Hutter AM Jr, Page DL: Atrial arrhythmias and lipomatous hypertrophy of the cardiac interatrial septum. *Am Heart J* 1971; **82**: 16–21.

23 Chao JC, Reyes CV, Hwang MH: Cardiac hemangioma. *South Med J* 1990; **83**: 44–7.

24 Cox JN, Friedli B, Mechmoche M et al: Teratoma of the heart. *Virchows Arch A Pathol Anat Histopathol* 1983; **402**: 163–74.

25 James TN, Galakhow I: De subitaneis mortibus XXVI. Fatal electrical instability of the heart associated with benign congenital polycystic tumor of the atrioventricular node. *Circulation* 1977; **56**: 667–78.

26 Nishida K, Kamijima G, Nagayama T: Mesothelioma of the atrioventricular node. *Br Heart J* 1985; **53**: 468–70.

27 Balasundaram S, Halees SA, Duran C: Mesothelioma of the atrioventricular node: first successful follow-up after excision. *Eur Heart J* 1992; **13**: 718–19.

28 Meysman M, Noppen M, Demeyer G, Vincken W: Malignant epithelial mesothelioma presenting as cardiac tamponade. *Eur Heart J* 1993; **14**: 1576–7.

29 Hodgson SF, Sheps SG, Subramanian R et al: Catecholamine-secreting paraganglioma of the interatrial septum. *Am J Med* 1984; **77**: 157–61.

30 Shemin RJ, Marsh JD, Schoen FJ: Benign intracardiac thyroid mass causing right ventricular outflow tract obstruction. *Am J Cardiol* 1985; **56**: 828–9.

31 Whorton CM: Primary malignant tumor of the heart. *Cancer* 1949; **2**: 245–60.

32 Burke AP, Virmani R: Tumors of the heart and great vessels. In: Rosai J, Sobin LH, eds, *Atlas of Tumor Pathology*, 3rd edn, fasc 16 (Armed Forces Institute of Pathology: Washington, DC, 1996).; 132

33 Klima G, Wimmer-Greinecker G, Harringer W et al: Cardiac angiosarcoma—a diagnostic dilemma. *Cardiovasc Surg* 1993; **1**: 674–6.

34 Herrmann MA, Shankerman RA, Edwards WD et al: Primary cardiac angiosarcoma: a clinicopathologic study of six cases. *J Thorac Cardiovasc Surg* 1992; **103**: 655–64.

35 Keohane ME, Lazzam C, Halperin JL et al: Angiosarcoma of the left atrium mimicking myxoma. Case report. *Hum Pathol* 1989; **20**: 599–601.

36 Fine G: Neoplasms of the pericardium and heart. In: Gould SE, ed, *Pathology of the Heart and Blood Vessels* (Charles C Thomas: Springfield, IL 1968); 851–83.

37 Proctor MS, Tracy GP, von Koch L: Primary cardiac B-cell lymphoma. *Am Heart J* 1989; **118**: 179–81.

38 Feigin DS, Fenoglio JJ, McAllister HA, Madewell JR: Pericardial cysts: a radiologic–pathologic correlation and review. *Radiology* 1977; **125**: 15–20.

39 Reynolds JL, Donahue JK, Peerce CW: Intrapericardial teratoma: a cause of acute pericardial effusion in infancy. *Pediatrics* 1969; **43**: 71–8.

40 Roberts WC, Glancy DL, De Vita VT: Heart in malignant lymphoma. A study of 196 autopsy cases. *Am J Cardiol* 1968; **22**: 85–107.

41 Petersen CD, Robinson QA, Kurnich JE: Involvement of the heart and pericardium in the malignant lymphomas. *Am J Med Sci* 1976; **272**: 161–5.

42 Kapoor AS: Clinical manifestations of neoplasia of the heart. In: Kapoor AS, ed., *Cancer and the Heart* (Springer: New York, 1968); 21–5.

43 Shulman LN, Braunwald E, Rosenthal SE: Hematological–oncological disorders and heart disease. In: Braunwald E, ed., *Heart Disease* (WB Saunders, Philadelphia, 1997; 1786–808.

44 Jefferson K, Rees S: *Clinical Cardiac Radiology* (Butterworths: London, 1975); 282.

45 Goodwin JF: The spectrum of cardiac tumours. *Am J Cardiol* 1968; **21**: 307–14.

46 Harvey WP: Clinical aspects of cardiac tumors. *Am J Cardiol* 1968; **21**: 328–43.

47 Engberding R, Daniel WG, Erbel R et al: Diagnosis of heart tumours by transesophageal echocardiography: a multicentre study in 154 patients. *Eur Heart J* 1993; **14**: 1223–8.

48 Sandok BA, van Esteroft I, Giuliani TB: CNS embolism due to atrial myxoma. Clinical features and diagnosis. *Arch Neurol* 1980; **37**: 485–8.

49 Bulkley BH, Hutchins GM: Atrial myxomas: a fifty year review. *Am Heart J* 1979; **93**: 639–43.

50 Abbott OA, Warshawski FE, Cobbs BW: Primary tumors and pseudotumors of the heart. *Ann Surg* 1962; **155**: 855–72.

51 Panidis IP, Mintz GS, McAllister M: Hemodynamic consequences of the left atrial myxomas as assessed by Doppler ultrasound. *Am Heart J* 1986; **111**: 927–31.

52 Tsuchiya F, Kohno A, Saitoh R, Shigeta A: CT findings of atrial myxoma. *Radiology* 1984; **151**: 139–43.

53 Brown JJ, Barakos JAA, Higgins CB: Magnetic resonance imaging of cardiac and paracardiac masses. *J Thorac Imag* 1990; **4**: 58–64.

54 Fujita N, Caputo GR, Higgins CB: Diagnosis and characterization of intracardiac masses by magnetic resonance imaging. *Am J Card Imag* 1994; **8**: 69–80.

55 Funari M, Fujita N, Peck WW, Higgins CB: Cardiac tumors: assessment with Gd-DTPA enhanced MR imaging. *J Comput Assist Tomogr* 1992; **15**: 953–8.

56 Semelka RC, Shoenut JP, Wilson ME et al: Cardiac masses: signal intensity features on spin echo, gradient echo, gadolinium enhanced spin echo, and turbo FLASH images. *J Mag Res Imag* 1992; **2**: 415–20.

57 Rienmüller R, Tilings R: MR and CT for detection of cardiac tumors. *Thorac Cardiovasc Surg* 1990; **38**: 168–72.

58 Higgins CB: Acquired heart disease. In: Higgins CB, Hricak H, Helms CA, eds, *Magnetic Resonance Imaging of the Body*, 3rd edn (Lippincott-Raven: Philadelphia, USA,, 1997); 409–60.

59 Rienmüller R, Lloret JL, Tiling R et al: MR imaging of pediatric cardiac tumors previously diagnosed by echocardiography. *J Comput Assist Tomogr* 1989; **13**: 621–6.

60 Szucs RA, Reks RB, Yanovick S, Tatum JL: Magnetic resonance imaging of cardiac rhabdomyosarcoma: quantifying the response to chemotherapy. *Cancer* 1991; **67**: 2066–70.

61 Dein JR, Frist WH, Stinson EB et al: Primary cardiac neoplasms. Early and late results of surgical treatment in 42 patients. *J Thorac Cardiovasc Surg* 1987; **93**: 502–11.

62 Horn M, Phebus C, Blatt J: Cancer chemotherapy after solid organ transplantation. *Cancer* 1990; **66**: 1468–71.

17

Cor pulmonale and pulmonary hypertension

Victor A Ferrari, Zahi A Fayad and Harold I Palevsky

Introduction

A broad variety of etiologies for pulmonary hypertension exist, and in a given patient the history and clinical scenario will generally provide important clues to the diagnosis. Often, noninvasive imaging studies will play a central role in the diagnostic evaluation of these patients, and will frequently direct the course of management toward a specific therapeutic strategy. Current therapeutic practice includes pharmacologic (anticoagulation and/or vasodilator therapy (oral or continuous infusion), mechanical (balloon valvular dilatation), and surgical (valvular repair or replacement, pulmonary thromboendarterectomy, or lung transplantation) approaches. Once treatment is initiated, noninvasive imaging also becomes an important part of the chronic management plan. To follow the response to medical, catheter-based interventional, or surgical therapies, an accurate and reliable imaging method must be used.

This chapter reviews the specific causes and cardiovascular sequelae of pulmonary hypertension, discusses the noninvasive diagnostic imaging techniques available and the factors determining their use in certain disease states, and looks at the role of imaging in the long-term management of pulmonary hypertension.

Pathogenesis of pulmonary hypertension

The pulmonary circulation is a low-pressure, low-resistance system with a high degree of capacitance. It can normally accommodate several times the resting cardiac output with a minimal rise in pulmonary artery pressure, primarily by recruitment of additional capillary beds (known as pulmonary vascular reserve) and by vascular distention. Pulmonary artery pressure (and therefore pulmonary hypertension) is related to pulmonary vascular resistance (PVR) and pulmonary blood flow by the following relationship:

$$\text{PVR} = \frac{\begin{matrix}\text{Mean pulmonary} \\ \text{artery pressure} \\ \text{(mmHg)}\end{matrix} - \begin{matrix}\text{pulmonary capillary} \\ \text{wedge pressure} \\ \text{(mmHg)}\end{matrix}}{\text{pulmonary blood flow (l/min)}}$$

Pulmonary hypertension is defined as a pulmonary artery (PA) systolic pressure of >35 mmHg, a PA diastolic pressure of >15 mmHg, or a mean pulmonary artery pressure (PAP) of >20–25 mmHg. Even with exercise, the mean PA pressure in normal people does not exceed 30 mmHg at sea level.[1]

The main factor leading to the development of pulmonary hypertension is an elevation in the PVR, which in the normal circulation is regulated primarily at the level of the precapillary arterioles and arteries. This regulation is based on a combination of neural, local, and feedback mechanisms which cause vasoconstriction. Chronic vasoconstriction, even for only a few days, is associated with structural changes in the vessel wall leading to narrowing of the vessel lumen.[2] Proliferative changes such as intimal or medial hypertrophy occur as a result of chronic elevations in flow, pressure, or shear stress, and potentiate the vascular obliterative process. These vascular abnormalities decrease the total recruitable capillary area and decrease vessel distensibility, causing a decrease in the pulmonary vascular reserve. The overall effect of these changes is an increase in resting PVR and a significant increase in PAP, first with exertion, and eventually at rest (Fig. 17.1). Pathologic changes in the intima, media, or lumen may be identified on biopsy, and may be reversible early in the course of the process; however, at a certain

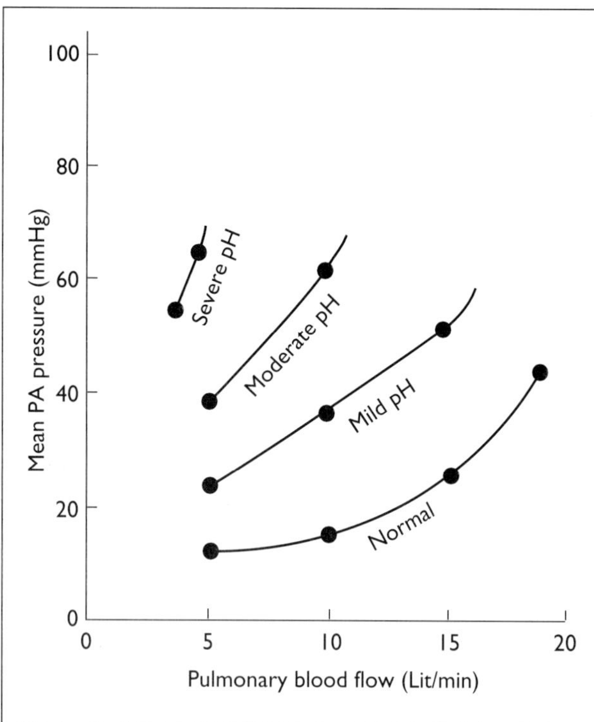

Figure 17.1
Relationship between cardiac output in normal patients and patients with pulmonary vascular disease.

point they will become irreversible.[3] The point of irreversibility is unclear, but is complicated by the state of local hypercoagulability that exists in the microvasculature, due in part to abnormal endothelial function (loss of fibrinolytic and platelet inhibition activity). This leads to the development of in situ thrombosis, which further decreases the size of the microvascular bed.[4–6]

Factors which may trigger pulmonary vasoconstriction include alveolar hypoxia, systemic hypoxemia, acidosis (pH <7.2), pulmonary venous hypertension, hypercapnia, or release of vasoactive mediators. Within the pulmonary vascular endothelium, endothelins have been shown to play an important role in modulating vasoconstriction, particularly in response to hypoxia, while prostacyclin and nitric oxide are important vasodilators with clinically useful properties.[7,8]

Table 17.1 Causes of pulmonary hypertension

- Passive
  - Left ventricular failure
  - Mitral valve disease
    - Stenosis, regurgitation, hypoplasia, atresia
  - Left atrial obstruction
    - Myxoma, tumor, thrombus, cor triatriatum
  - Pulmonary venous obstruction
    - Tumor, fibrosing mediastinitis, adenopathy
- Hyperkinetic
  - Intracardiac shunt lesions
    - ASD, VSD, anomalous venous return (partial and total)
  - Systemic to cardiac shunt
    - Patent ductus arteriosus
  - Pulmonary arteriovenous fistulas
- Obstructive
  - Pulmonary embolism – acute and chronic
    - Venous thromboemboli, tumor emboli
  - Pulmonary arterial thrombosis
    - Sickle cell disease, Eisenmenger syndrome (tetralogy of Fallot, etc.)
- Obliterative
  - Pulmonary arteritis
    - Scleroderma, SLE, vasculitis, other collagen vascular diseases
  - Schistosomiasis
  - Pulmonary parenchymal disease
    - Obstructive (bronchitis, emphysema, bronchiectasis)
    - Restrictive (fibrosis of any etiology, thoracic cage abnormalities)
- Vasoconstrictive
  - Hypoxemia
    - High altitude disease, sleep apnea syndrome
- Idiopathic
  - Primary pulmonary hypertension including pulmonary veno-occlusive disease
  - Dietary related pulmonary hypertension (e.g. aminorex, Phen-Fen)
  - Coexistent portal and pulmonary hypertension (hepatopulmonary syndrome)
  - Human immunodeficiency virus (HIV)

Causes of cor pulmonale and pulmonary hypertension

The potential causes of pulmonary hypertension are quite varied, but often discernible based on a combination of clinical, laboratory, and imaging data. Most disorders can be described as either cardiac or pulmonary in origin, and only a few will ultimately be designated as idiopathic. Cardiac diseases tend to cause pulmonary hypertension via elevations in pulmonary blood flow or in pulmonary venous pressure, while pulmonary disorders cause obliteration of the vascular bed through mechanisms such as parenchymal

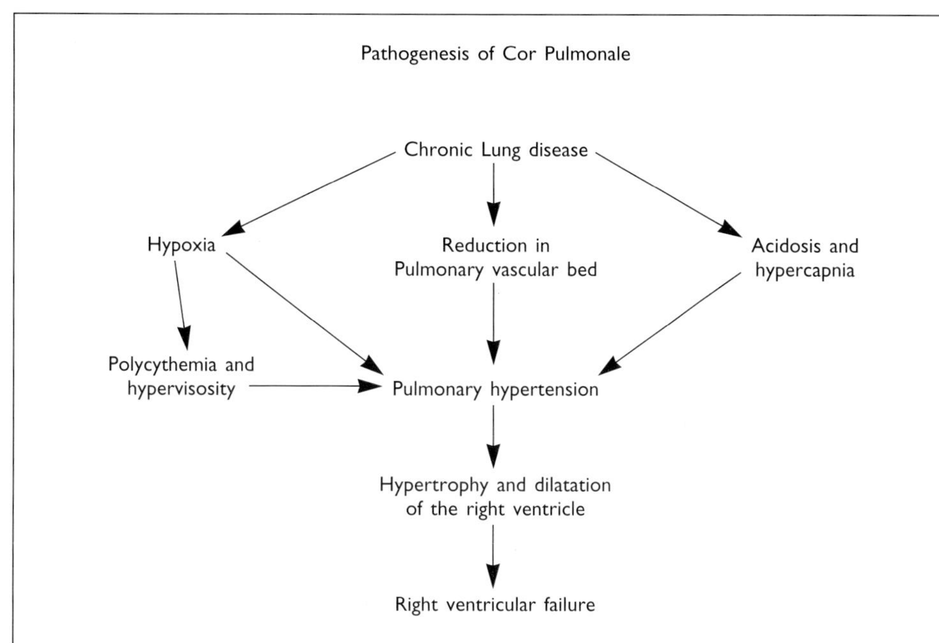

Figure 17.2
Pathogenesis of cor pulmonale.

disease or vascular obstruction. A detailed list of various causes of pulmonary hypertension is contained in Table 17.1.

'Cor pulmonale' is a collective term which refers to disease states which cause right heart dysfunction due to pulmonary hypertension, and which have abnormalities of the pulmonary circulation in common. Acute cor pulmonale causes right heart overload and dilatation because of acute pulmonary hypertension from processes such as decompensation of chronic obstructive pulmonary disease and/or massive pulmonary embolism. Chronic cor pulmonale is a combination of right ventricular (RV) dilatation and hypertrophy owing to diseases of the pulmonary vasculature, extending from the main PA to the pulmonary veins (excluding left heart problems). Specific pathophysiologic mechanisms include direct obliterative (parenchymal disease or arteritis), vascular obstructive (acute or chronic thromboembolic or tumor embolism, or in situ thrombosis), hypoxic vasoconstrictive (sleep apnea or neuromuscular diseases), or idiopathic (primary pulmonary or portal-pulmonary hypertension). The pathogenesis of cor pulmonale is schematically represented in Fig. 17.2.

Cardiac diseases

Pulmonary hypertension owing to cardiac diseases can be caused by hyperkinetic (intra- or extracardiac shunts, pulmonary arteriovenous fistulas) or passive (elevated left ventricular end-diastolic pressure (LVEDP), mitral stenosis, or left atrial obstruction) mechanisms. Extracardiac left-to-right shunts include total or partial anomalous pulmonary venous return, patent ductus arteriosus, aortopulmonary window and a large (or multiple) pulmonary arteriovenous malformation(s). Congenital intracardiac shunts such as atrial or ventricular septal defects (ASD and VSD, respectively) are common causes of increased volume and/or pressure overload, depending on the size of the defect.[9,10] Usually there is a low likelihood of developing progessive pulmonary hypertension provided the left-to-right shunt (or Qp/Qs) is <1.5. Thus, a restrictive VSD will be less likely to cause late problems than a nonrestrictive VSD. Since increased lung blood flow alone (e.g. after pneumonectomy) does not commonly result in pulmonary hypertension, factors other than flow must be operative in shunt states. The duration of elevated flow, shear stress, and reflex pulmonary vasoconstriction due to pulmonary venous distention have all been postulated as potential mechanisms for the development of pulmonary hypertension.[11] Eisenmenger's syndrome is described as chronic pulmonary hypertension that has led to an elevation in PVR to such a degree that a left-to right shunt becomes bidirectional or reverses (i.e. becomes right-to-left). This syndrome is generally associated with congenital cardiac lesions with large left-to-right shunts such as atrial and ventricular septal defects, or a patent ductus arteriosus. The pulmonary hypertension and PVR elevation at this stage is mainly irreversible, and usually requires bilateral lung transplantation with cardiac repair or heart–lung transplantation for curative therapy.[12–14]

Passive causes of pulmonary hypertension are related to chronic increases in left atrial pressure. An elevated LVEDP leads to chronic left atrial (LA) hypertension, and thus increased pulmonary venous pressure. A 'passive' form of pulmonary hypertension develops at first, eventually followed by a reactive or vasoconstrictive form.[15] Initially, the rise in PA pressures parallels the rise in LA pressure; however, the rise in PA pressure accelerates when vasoconstriction begins. The pulmonary hypertension causes structural changes in the microvasculature – first in the pulmonary venous system, then in the pulmonary arterial system. Hypertrophic intimal or medial changes lead to fibrosis of the pulmonary veins and venules, along with interstitial edema (predominantly dependent) which also promotes perivascular fibrosis.[16,17] Treatment of increased LA pressure can potentially allow for regression of any reversible component of this process, before irreversible changes occur.[18] Mitral valve stenosis due to rheumatic heart disease, or mitral regurgitation from myxomatous valvular disease or ischemic papillary muscle dysfunction can significantly raise LA pressure.[19] Rare disorders such as cor triatriatum also lead to elevated pulmonary venous pressures and secondary pulmonary hypertension.[20] Certain cardiac or metastatic tumors may cause inflow obstruction to the mitral valve (e.g. myxoma, lung or breast cancer), as may thrombus. Common causes of elevated LVEDP include left ventricular (LV) systolic dysfunction due to coronary artery disease or dilated cardiomyopathy, or diastolic dysfunction due to disorders such as hypertensive LV hypertrophy and hypertrophic or restrictive cardiomyopathy.[21,22] Diseases of the pericardium such as constrictive pericarditis may also lead to elevated LVEDP.[23] The pulmonary veins may be obstructed from within by tumor or thrombus, or extrinsically by lymphadenopathy, tumor, or fibrosis (e.g. post radiation, idiopathic), leading to chronic pulmonary venous hypertension. Pulmonary veno-occlusive disease, a rare disorder of uncertain etiology, leads to progressive fibrotic obstruction of the veins (particularly the venules) of the lungs.[24]

Pulmonary diseases

Obliterative

Pulmonary hypertension due to diseases of the respiratory system can be described as obliterative, with actual loss of pulmonary parenchyma and vasculature. In chronic obstructive airways diseases (emphysema, chronic bronchitis, chronic obstructive pulmonary disease), pulmonary hypertension develops secondary to a combination of arterial and alveolar hypoxemia resulting from imbalances in ventilation–perfusion (V/Q) matching. Patients with emphysema alone typically do not manifest pulmonary hypertension, as the remaining lung tissue can compensate for the parenchymal loss, and the degree of V/Q mismatch is less. Pulmonary hypertension occurs intermittently in patients with emphysema, typically during exacerbations of the disease, as well as during upper respiratory infections. Chronic bronchitis, however, results in chronic pulmonary hypertension because of alveolar hypoxia, high P_{CO_2}, low P_{O_2}, and low pH (clinically described as the 'blue bloater').

Restrictive physiology, whether owing to interstitial lung disease (ILD), alveolar hypoventilation syndromes, or chest wall abnormalities, also leads to elevated pulmonary pressures. ILD may be secondary to systemic disorders such as collagen vascular diseases or sarcoidosis, or idiopathic in origin. The microvasculature is destroyed by the interstitial inflammatory process, which leads to fibrosis of the lung tissues.[25,26] The PVR becomes elevated owing to the loss of pulmonary vascular reserve, decreased compliance of the remaining vessels, and V/Q mismatch secondary to closure of small airways as a result of the inflammatory process.

Disorders of alveolar hypoventilation include sleep apnea syndromes, neuromuscular syndromes (e.g. Guillain–Barre, myasthenia gravis, muscular dystrophy), and chest cage defects (e.g. ankylosing spondylitis, kyphoscoliosis). Alveolar hypoxia and systemic hypoxemia and hypercapnia in these disorders are the common paths to pulmonary hypertension.[27]

Certain collagen–vascular diseases (e.g. systemic lupus erythematosus (SLE), scleroderma, CREST syndrome) are frequently complicated by pulmonary hypertension. The pulmonary vascular abnormalities which may occur during the course of these disorders lead to pulmonary hypertension through a combination of pulmonary interstitial inflammation, interstitial fibrosis, and pulmonary vasculitis.[25,28] In some patients, however, there is no pulmonary parenchymal involvement and solely vascular involvement. The lesions seen in these cases are indistinguishable from those of primary pulmonary hypertension (PPH), leading to the speculation that some patients with PPH may represent cases of SLE or scleroderma localized to the pulmonary vasculature, or may represent a systemic vasoconstrictive disorder.[29]

Obstructive

Pulmonary hypertension may occur as a result of both acute and chronic (or unresolved) pulmonary embolism. The hemodynamic effects of embolic disease rely on the degree of embolic pulmonary vascular obstruction, the patient's previous cardiopulmonary status, and the chronicity of the embolic disease.[30] Acute pulmonary embolism can cause acute pulmonary hypertension, generally through a combination of pulmonary vascular obstruction, alveolar hypoxia due to splinting from pleuritic chest pain, or direct vasoconstriction from vasoactive substances.[31] Although the degree of pulmonary hypertension tends to be proportional to the extent of vascular obstruction, even massive embolism cannot acutely raise the peak (systolic) PAP to >50–60 mmHg in a normal RV.[32,33] However, in patients with a history of cardiopulmonary disease, the corresponding elevations in PA and right atrial pressures and the decreases in cardiac output are greater than in those without such a history.[32]

Chronic pulmonary embolism occurs in two separate forms – in situ thrombosis and chronic unresolved thromboembolic occlusion of the proximal pulmonary arteries. In situ thrombosis develops because of endothelial dysfunction of the microvasculature by high pulmonary artery pressures and flows, resulting in a local relative hypercoagulable state. These microthrombi may result in a patchy inhomogeneity on lung scanning, but are not detectable on pulmonary angiography. As pulmonary hypertension worsens, these lesions may become more common, prompting some to suggest that all patients be treated with long-term anticoagulation with drugs such as warfarin and/or antiplatelet therapy.[34,35]

The syndrome of chronic unresolved pulmonary embolism occurs because of partial obstruction of the proximal pulmonary vascular bed by organized, but incompletely lysed, thrombotic material. The most likely mechanism is a defective local thrombolytic system, although a systemic coagulation disorder could also be contributory. It remains unclear whether multiple recurrent emboli or a single unresolved embolism occurs. The latter is most probable, with incomplete clot lysis leading to propagation (antegrade and retrograde) and organization of the thrombus with chronic vascular obstruction. Obstruction of the vasculature can be due to luminal blockage by the fibrinous mass itself, or to fibrous webs or rings which can partially occlude the vessels. These obstructions are detectable by both invasive and noninvasive means, and remain visible even after 6 months of anticoagulation therapy. It is important to recognize this entity, as it is surgically remediable, often with dramatic reductions in PA pressures and significant improvement in clinical status.[36–38]

Idiopathic

Primary pulmonary hypertension is the designation given to those patients with no cardiac, pulmonary, or systemic etiology to explain their pulmonary hypertension. It is a rare disease with a female predilection in adults, often of early onset (mean age at diagnosis, 30–36 years), but nearly 10% of cases can occur in patients older than 60.[39] Heterogeneity of the patient population and uncertainty of the age of onset of the disorder make studies of the pathophysiology and the course of the disease difficult. It is known that neither the age at diagnosis nor the severity of pulmonary hypertension correlate with survival in PPH; however, the cardiac output correlates with survival, with low values indicating a poorer prognosis.[40–42] In earlier studies, the precapillary histopathologic lesions in PPH were felt to correlate with a specific mechanism of injury. However, it is now clear that the pulmonary microvasculature can only respond to injury in a limited number of ways, and that several types of lesions may be present in an individual patient. The lesions seem to represent different stages of response to vascular injury, perhaps modulated by the specific type of injury, the rapidity of onset and duration of the stimulus, and differences in the degree and chronicity of the pulmonary hypertension.[3–5]

Other idiopathic disorders leading to elevated PVR include diet-related pulmonary hypertension (aminorex, toxic oil syndrome), the hepato-pulmonary syndrome, and HIV-associated pulmonary hypertension.[43–45]

Cardiovascular sequelae of pulmonary hypertension

The vascular changes which characterize cor pulmonale and pulmonary hypertension result in important changes in right heart configuration, mass, and function as a consequence of ventricular remodeling. In addition, important changes and complications can develop in the main and branch pulmonary arteries as a result of severe chronic pulmonary hypertension.

The response of the RV to acute or chronic pressure or volume overload depends mainly on the presence of antecedent pulmonary disease. Acute cor pulmonale owing to pulmonary embolism may follow various patterns based on the pulmonary vasculature. Right ventricular function is greatly dependent on afterload conditions. If the RV is not accustomed to operating against an increased PVR or elevated PAP, it may be vulnerable to sudden increases in afterload. A massive pulmonary embolism in an otherwise normal patient may cause cardiovascular collapse and result in a dilated RV with an RV ejection fraction of nearly zero.[46] RV hypertrophy (RVH) has been shown to develop quickly in a feline model, with a 71% increase in RV mass just 2 days after PA banding, and a 150% increase by 1 month.[47] Therefore, patients with subacute massive embolism developing over several days will have greater PAPs for the same degree of PA occlusion as patients with acute massive embolism, and are better able to accommodate to the increased afterload.[33]

In chronic pressure overload states the RV at first hypertrophies, then dilates as RV failure develops. In chronic volume overload conditions, the RV first dilates, then hypertrophies as PVR and pulmonary hypertension increase. Several decades may pass until the RV develops dysfunction, and the exact mechanism of the pulmonary hypertension at that time may not be readily apparent. Noninvasive imaging, however, may indicate the most likely etiology for the disorder, as will be discussed in the next section.

In the past, the right ventricle was viewed as simply a passive conduit for delivering blood to the primary pump, the left ventricle.[48] Early investigators reported no detectable impairment of overall cardiac performance with complete destruction of the right ventricular free wall (RVFW) in normal dogs, and therefore viewed the RV as unnecessary for circulatory stability.[48–50] However, recent experiments in dogs involving cauterization of the RVFW have demonstrated severe RV dysfunction and decreased hemodynamic performance, especially when the PAP was abnormal.[51,52] Studies in patients after RV infarction also showed worsened RV performance in the setting of elevated PAPs.[53] It is now well recognized that the function of the RV is critical for the maintenance of efficient overall cardiac performance[54] particularly in the presence of pulmonary vascular disease. RV dysfunction, which often results from chronic pulmonary hypertension, is a known cause of significant morbidity and mortality, and in some studies may account for up to 40% of patients with clinical heart failure.[55] Prior to the onset of RV dysfunction, pulmonary hypertension frequently leads to changes in RV shape, which may include cavity dilatation, wall thickening,[56] and septal flattening.[57] These changes are generally reversible provided the offending influence is removed before chronic changes in myocardial structure, such as fibrosis, occur.

Furthermore, while the acute hemodynamic response to vasodilating agents or surgical therapy may be monitored with a pulmonary artery catheter, the chronic response is often followed by a clinical exam, chest radiographs, and echocardiography . The pathophysiology and mechanisms of RVH and RV failure due to pulmonary hypertension, as well as the changes in myocardial performance during the chronic phase of therapy, have not been well characterized. A major obstacle to the study of this problem has been the lack of a reliable serial noninvasive method for the analysis of RV function and performance with little associated risk for the patient.

Overall, there is incomplete knowledge regarding RV function in the normal state, a lack of understanding of the adaptive changes the RV undergoes in response to disease, as well as the mechanisms responsible for the progression to RV failure. Despite the availability of various invasive and noninvasive imaging techniques, many questions still remain unanswered.

Several important changes and complications may result as a consequence of chronic severe pulmonary hypertension. Severe pulmonary artery dilatation may occur, which can result in paralysis of the recurrent laryngeal nerve (usually the left) and resultant hoarseness (Ortner's syndrome). In rare cases, the left main or left anterior descending coronary artery may be compressed by the dilated left pulmonary artery. Occasionally, a patient with severe pulmonary hypertension who presents with chest pain may be found to have a pulmonary artery dissection (see Case 4 below).

Limitations of current diagnostic methods for RV evaluation

Despite the importance of RV performance, its assessment has had only limited success, owing partly to the complex anatomic configuration of the right heart. The RV is a relatively thin-walled (<5 mm), heavily trabeculated crescent-shaped chamber, with widely separated pulmonary and tricuspid valves. Unlike the relatively thick-walled (up to 11 mm), nearly conical-shaped LV chamber, the RV does not correspond to a simple geometric shape, and therefore is not amenable to simple structural analysis (see Fig. 17.3). The RV has two potential axes of orientation – the inflow axis (from tricuspid valve to apex) and the outflow axis (from apex to RV outflow tract). This complex morphology makes evaluation of the normal RV as well as assessment of the RV in abnormal states challenging.

The differences in LV and RV geometry result in distinctive wall motion patterns. The concentric thick-walled LV cavity contracts predominantly by radial contraction and longitudinal (base to apex) shortening of the chamber.[58,59] RV contraction has been described as a sequence of three distinct events: (1) the trabeculae and the papillary muscles pull the tricuspid valve plane toward the apex,[58,60] resulting in shortening of the longitudinal axis with little net ejection; (2) the RVFW moves toward the septum, with little shortening from apex to base; and (3) the curvature of the already convex interventricular septum increases due to contraction of the circular fibers of the thicker left ventricle. The crista supraventricularis also aids RV emptying by moving the RVFW toward the septum during systole.[61] This combination of complex anatomy and wall motion make it difficult for standard imaging techniques to evaluate RV structure and function.

Conventional imaging methods for evaluating RV function include angiography (contrast or radionuclide),[62,63] echocardiography,[64] and computed tomography (CT).[65] Although these techniques are useful for assessment of LV function, each has limitations that hinder its applicability for serial studies of RV global (e.g. ejection fraction, end-diastolic and end-systolic chamber volumes, mass) and regional function. Direct angiographic approaches require invasive techniques for catheter placement in the RV and subject the patient to X-ray and contrast agent exposure. Often only a single plane of imaging is possible, which limits regional evaluation of RV function. These limitations make standard angiographic techniques impractical for serial RV

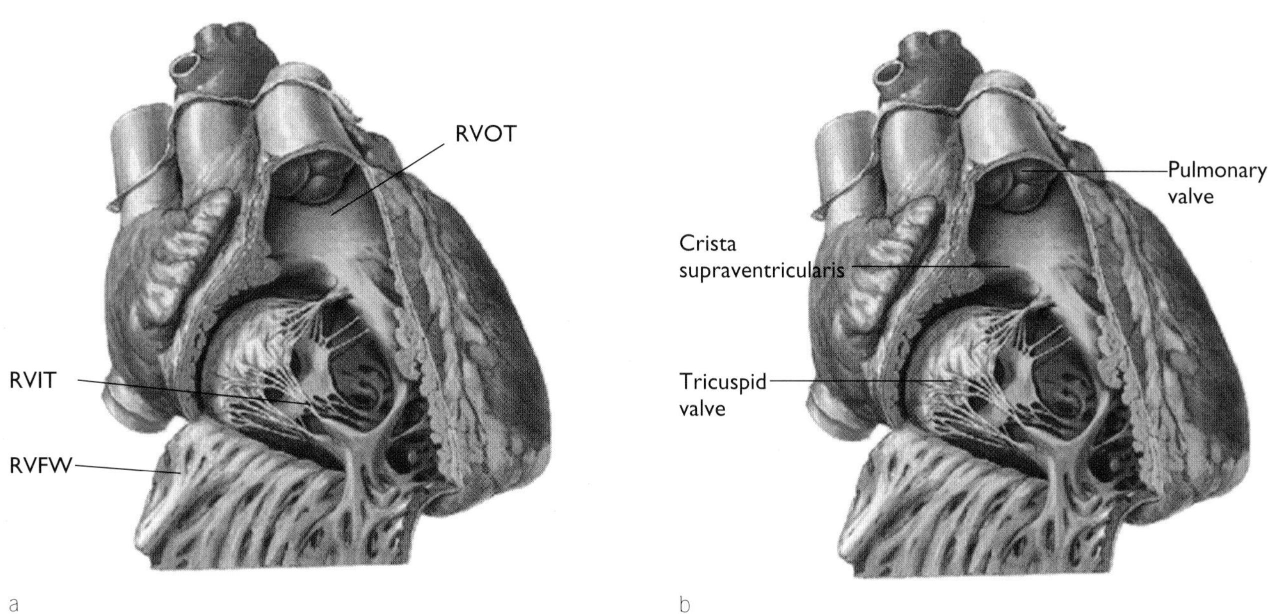

Figure 17.3
(a) and (b) Drawing of the right ventricle opened and viewed from the anterior aspect. The inflow region (RVIT) which is located below the tricuspid valve is heavily trabeculated in contrast to the somewhat smoother left ventricle. The outflow region (RVOT) is located below the pulmonic valve and consists of relatively smooth myocardium. A muscular ridge called the crista supraventricularis separates the RVIT and RVOT regions. The right ventricular free wall (RVFW) is also identified.

assessment. Radionuclide angiography provides useful information regarding relative chamber volume and global RV function, particularly using the first-pass method.[66] However, the low image resolution cannot provide important anatomic detail, and the dependence on the rapid injection of radionuclide during an arrhythmia-free period further limit this approach.

Echocardiography is the most common modality used for evaluation of RV structure and function. It can provide qualitative and quantitative assessment of RV size, ejection fraction, wall thickness, and segmental wall motion. However, certain simplifying assumptions must be made about RV geometry in order to estimate chamber volumes and ejection fraction. The relatively anterior position of the RV in the chest cage results in limited visualization by echo, particularly of the lateral walls. Three-dimensional methods are under development to reduce the need for these assumptions, but they are not currently widely available.[67] In patients with chronic obstructive pulmonary disease, use of the normal imaging windows may be restricted due to hyperinflated lungs or increased anteroposterior chest wall dimension. Ultrafast and spiral CT can be used to demonstrate global and segmental RV function,[65,68] but require ionizing radiation and iodinated intravenous contrast injection. All of the techniques above are limited in their evaluation of regional RV function, particularly for intramural function.

Recently, cardiac magnetic resonance imaging (MRI) techniques have been developed to assess global, regional, and intramural RV function and have several advantages over other modalities.[69,70–74] MRI is a noninvasive technique which uses no ionizing radiation, requires no contrast injection for routine studies, and provides tomographic data that may be registered in three dimensions. There are no limitations for imaging windows, and the free choice of orientation of imaging planes at the time of scanning permits separation of adjacent or overlapping structures. Image resolution is routinely below 1 mm with standard techniques, and improved signal-to-noise benefits may be achieved using a custom cardiac surface coil.[75] In recent studies, MRI is increasingly the standard to which other techniques are now compared for RV volume, mass, and function.[76]

Expanded reviews of all techniques may be found in several recent texts.[77,78]

Diagnostic and imaging approach to pulmonary hypertension

Given the large capillary reserve capacity in the normal pulmonary circulation, extensive changes in the pulmonary

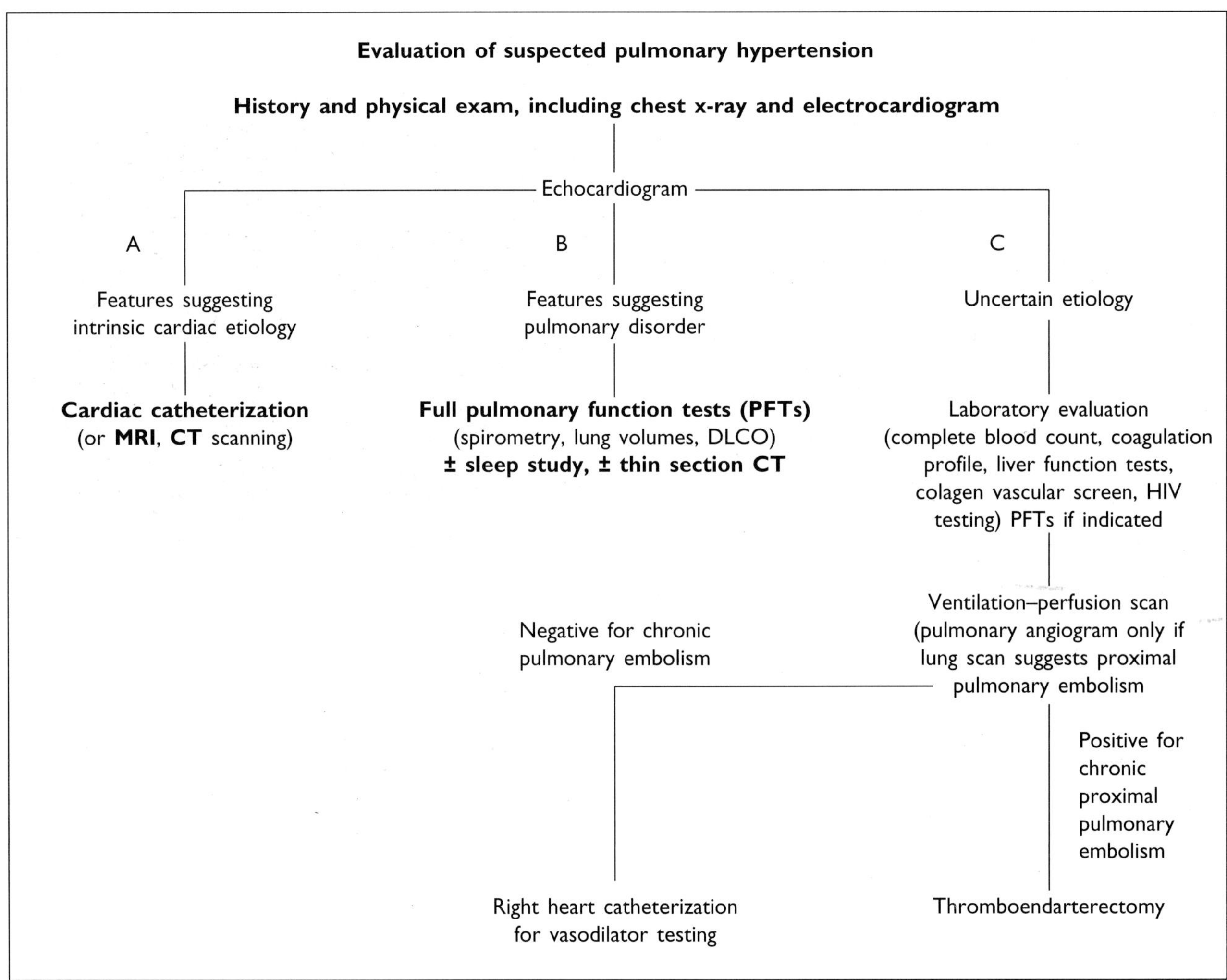

Figure 17.4
Evaluation of suspected pulmonary hypertension.

vasculature must be present before pulmonary hypertension develops. Pulmonary hypertension develops first during periods of exertion in these patients, and later progresses to elevated resting PA pressures. Therefore, symptoms associated with pulmonary hypertension such as dyspnea, easy fatigability, or chest pain may first present during exertion. Since these symptoms are relatively nonspecific or associated with other more common disorders, it may delay the proper diagnosis in some patients.

A general algorithm for the evaluation of patients with suspected pulmonary hypertension is outlined in Fig. 17.4. A detailed history, physical examination, chest X-ray, and electrocardiogram (ECG) are valuable initial steps in the work-up of this group of patients. While it is beyond the scope of this chapter to conduct a detailed discussion of the chest roentgenogram in the differential diagnosis of cor pulmonale, readers are nonetheless urged to pursue further information in appropriate textbooks (e.g. Steiner and Levin).[79] Unfortunately, the chest X-ray, ECG, and physical exam abnormalities seen in chronic pulmonary hypertension may not be specific for the underlying disorder.

A two-dimensional transthoracic echocardiogram with pulse wave, continuous wave, and color Doppler imaging is the best initial screening study for determining potential etiologies for the patient's complaints. A general description of the right and left heart chamber sizes and wall thicknesses can be determined, and estimates of global ventricular function may be assessed. Regional wall motion abnormalities and areas of wall thinning suggestive of ischemic heart disease can also be detected. Doppler imaging can provide accurate measurements of the degree of valvular stenosis or regurgitation, as well as estimates of the pulmonary artery systolic pressures (provided tricuspid regurgitation is present). A transesophageal echocardiogram may be used when a more detailed depiction of the intracardiac structures is desired, such as the interatrial septum (to evaluate for atrial septal defect) and the mitral valve leaflets (e.g. to assess whether valve repair rather than valve replacement may be possible). It is at this first decision point (Fig. 17.4) where echocardiography, in combination with the preceding clinical evaluation, can help distinguish cardiac from pulmonary etiologies in patients with pulmonary hypertension. In patients without a clear etiology for their disorder, the pathway leads to studies which will help identify those with chronic pulmonary emboli from those with PPH. Echo can also provide important prognostic information in patients with PPH. For example, the presence of a pericardial effusion associated with severe pulmonary hypertension is a poor prognostic indicator.[80]

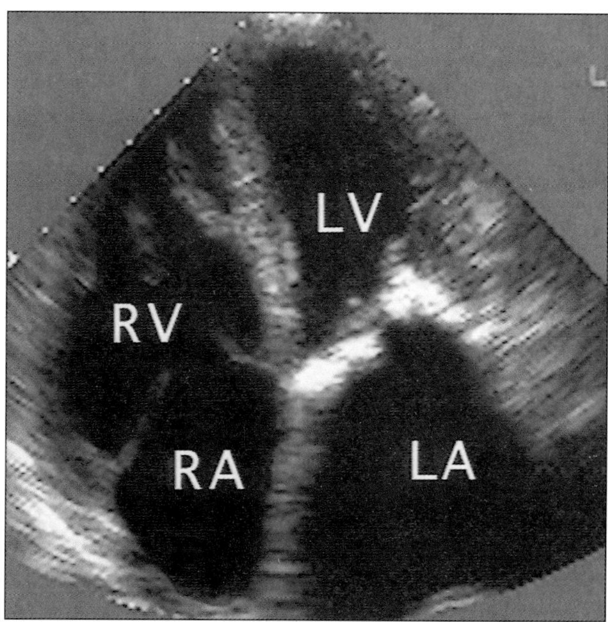

Figure 17.5
Apical four-chamber view demonstrating thickened and calcified mitral valve leaflets with decreased mobility typical of rheumatic disease. Note that the right atrium (RA), right ventricle (RV), and left atrium (LA) are dilated, while the left ventricle is normal in size. There is also mild RV hypertrophy. Echo provides an excellent description of the abnormal motion of the leaflets, including the diastolic bowing characteristic of rheumatic valvular disease.

Features suggesting cardiac etiology for pulmonary hypertension (pathway A, Fig. 17.4)

Echocardiography is very useful in identifying cardiac disorders which may lead to pulmonary hypertension. It can be used to interrogate the interatrial or interventricular septum for defects, and is especially valuable for identifying valvular lesions. In rheumatic mitral stenosis the echocardiographic findings are pathognomonic, and clearly illustrate the mechanism of left ventricular inflow tract obstruction. The leaflets become thickened and commissural fusion restricts their motion, along with shortening and cicatrization of the chordae tendineae (see Case 1).

Case 1

A 46-year-old nonsmoker presented with a 6-month history of dyspnea on exertion for evaluation. The patient had no risk factors for coronary artery disease and the only notable additional symptom was occasional palpitations. On examination, the jugular venous pressure was mildly elevated, the lungs had mild bibasilar rales, and there was 1+ bilateral pedal edema. Cardiac exam was notable for a normal S1, a loud second component of the S2, and an opening snap with diastolic rumble. There was also a harsh grade III/VI holosystolic murmur at the left lower sternal border which radiated to the left anterior axillary line. The point of maximal impulse was normal; however, an RV heave was present. ECG demonstrated normal sinus rhythm with frequent premature atrial contractions, and a biatrial abnormality. A chest X-ray could not be obtained owing to technical reasons; however, an echocardiogram was performed. There was moderate enlargement of the right atrium and ventricle, a moderately enlarged left atrium, and normal left ventricular size. The mitral valve leaflets were moderately thickened and calcified with moderately decreased mobility. Doppler examination demonstrated moderate-to-severe mitral stenosis, as well as moderate mitral regurgitation (Fig. 17.5). There was moderate tricuspid regurgitation with an estimated PA systolic pressure of 50 mmHg, consistent with moderate pulmonary hypertension. The use of echocardiography in this case of suspected mitral stenosis allowed confirmation of the diagnosis as well as quantitation of the severity of the valvular disease. Given its excellent temporal resolution and superiority in characterization of valvular disease, echo was the best imaging option for this patient. The degree of mitral stenosis as well as the severity of mitral regurgitation may be quantitated using pulsed and continuous wave Doppler measurements. The presence of mitral and

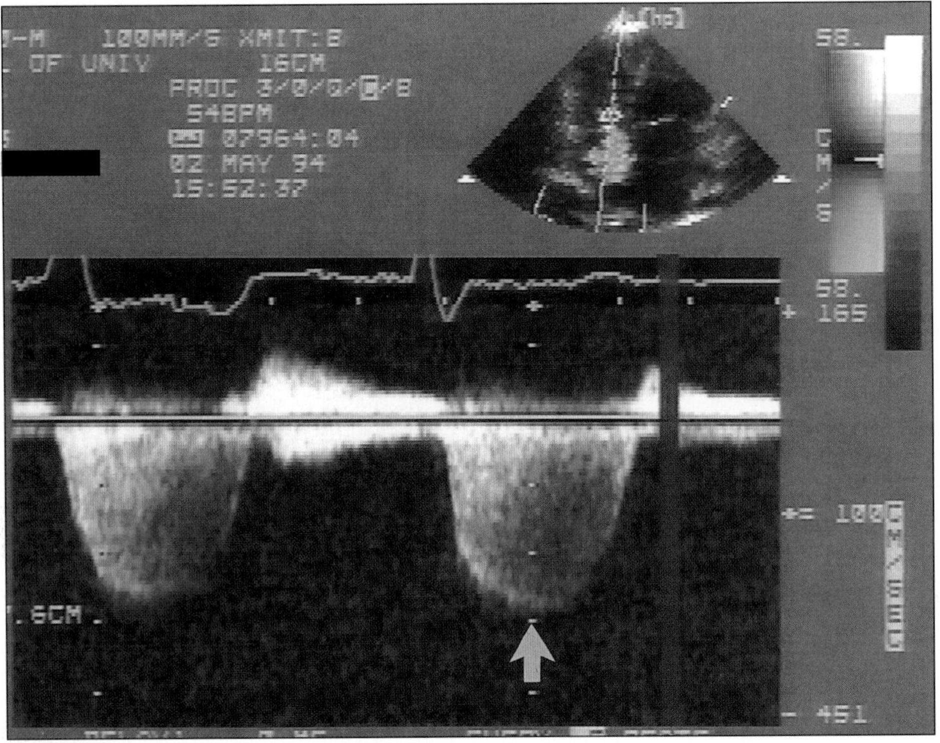

a

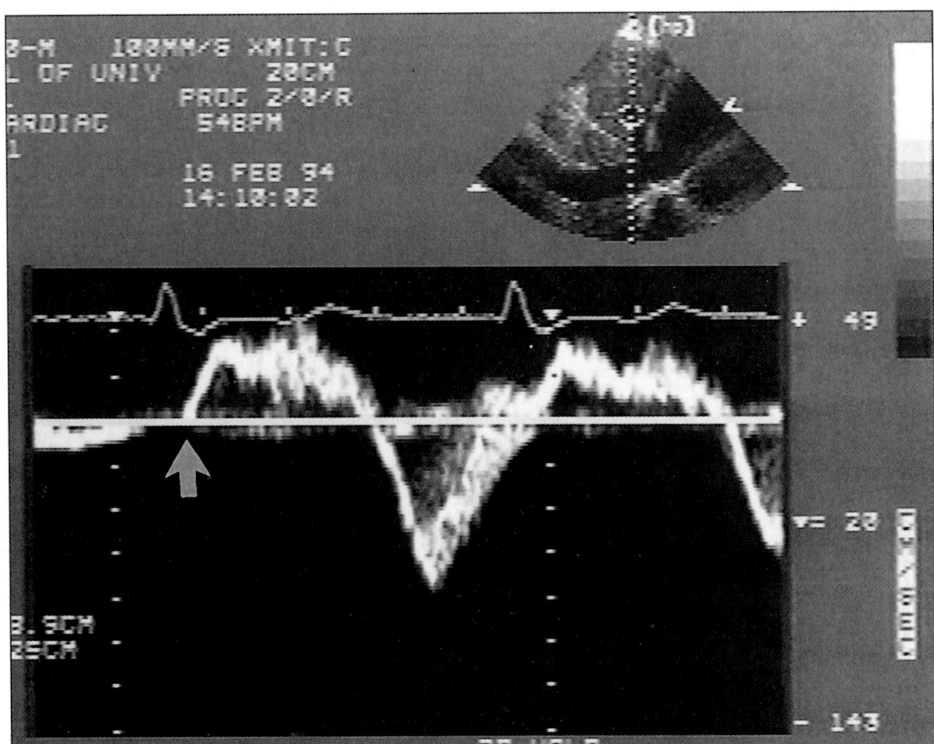

b

Figure 17.6
Continuous wave Doppler velocity signal of a tricuspid regurgitation (TR) jet from the apical four-chamber view. The peak velocity of the jet is nearly 3 m/s (arrow, scale on right), therefore, the estimated pulmonary artery pressure (assuming no pulmonic stenosis) is: PA pressure $= 4\ (3)^2 + 14$ mmHg = 50 mmHg. In patients with very severe TR, there may be flow reversal in the hepatic veins during systole. This may be detected using pulsed wave Doppler sampling in the hepatic vein. (b) Flow velocity is from superior to inferior during diastole as the hepatic vein drains to the inferior vena cava. However, during systole there is reversal of flow velocity in the hepatic vein (arrow) due to the large regurgitant TR jet.

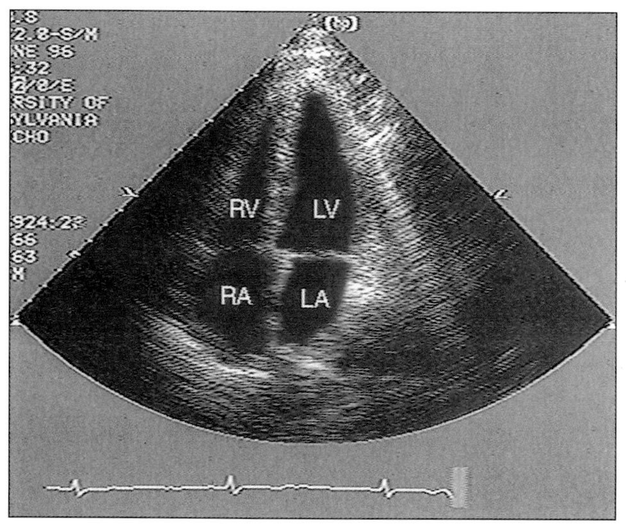

a

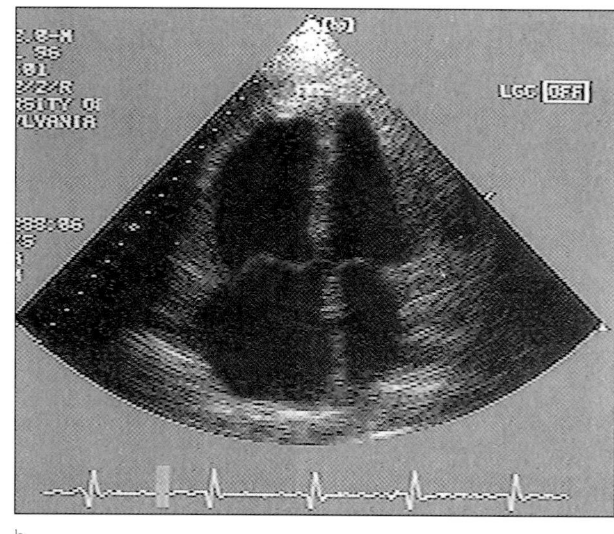

b

Figure 17.7
Two apical four-chamber echocardiographic views from the same patient approximately 1 month apart demonstrate the changes in cardiac shape and contraction pattern after a large acute pulmonary embolism. The right atrium (RA) and ventricle (RV) become acutely dilated and the RV demonstrates global hypokinesis. Of note is the absence of RV hypertrophy. The left ventricle (LV) becomes underfilled and more tachycardic as LV preload decreases. This patient had bilateral deep venous thromboses on further testing.

tricuspid regurgitation are readily appreciated with color Doppler flow mapping. The peak velocity of the tricuspid regurgitant jet is used to estimate the pulmonary artery systolic pressure (Fig. 17.6), which has prognostic value for both medical and surgical management of patients with valvular and myocardial disease. Pulmonary artery pressure can be calculated, providing the pulmonary valve is not stenosed, using the modified Bernoulli equation to assess the pressure difference across the tricuspid valve from the peak velocity of the regurgitant jet ($4V^2$) and adding either a clinical assessment of right atrial pressure from the height of the jugular venous pulse, or by adding 14 mmHg (validated from a regression correction of simultaneous measurements of invasive and Doppler estimates of pulmonary artery systolic pressures). Echocardiographic criteria have important prognostic value in selecting patients as candidates for percutaneous balloon valvuloplasty.[81] This technique permits patients who are candidates for the procedure to undergo an invasive cardiologic procedure rather than an open (or now 'minimally invasive') surgical procedure.

Case 2

A 67-year-old nonsmoker was admitted for urosepsis complicated by adult respiratory distress syndrome and had an echocardiogram to exclude valvular vegetations as part of an evaluation for persistent fever. The study was relatively unremarkable (Fig. 17.7a); however, he had a prolonged period of respiratory insufficiency requiring mechanical ventilation. One month later, a brief episode of acute hypoxemia and hypotension prompted another echo to reassess the patient's ventricular function and chamber sizes. On this study, there was severe dilatation of the RA and RV, with severe RV hypokinesis (Fig. 17.7b). The estimated PA systolic pressure was 50 mmHg, and there was no RV hypertrophy. Vascular Doppler studies of the lower legs demonstrated bilateral deep venous thromboses, and an inferior vena caval filter was placed because of concomitant gastrointestinal bleeding. No further interventions were undertaken owing to a prompt improvement in pulmonary hemodynamics.

The rapid assessment of chamber size, global and regional ventricular function, and vavlular disorders as well as portability to an acutely ill patient's bedside make echo an extremely valuable tool in the intensive care unit setting. A comparison of the two studies described above permitted an efficient determination that acute pulmonary embolism was the leading diagnosis, based on the fact that under acute conditions, the otherwise normal right heart can only respond to a large pulmonary embolism by dilating. Other features on the echo that are typical for an acute embolism include global RV hypokinesis and the ability to generate an estimated PA pressure of only 50 mmHg. Recently, investigators have further refined

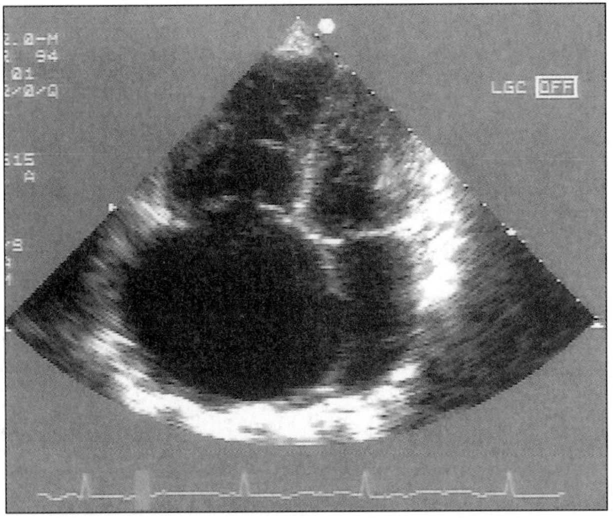

a

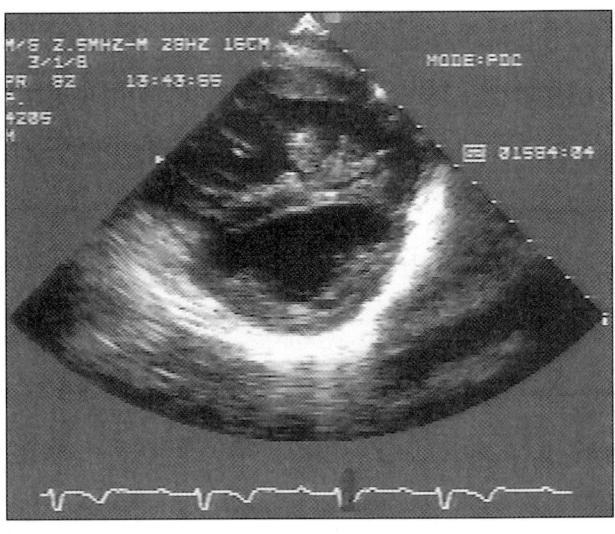

b

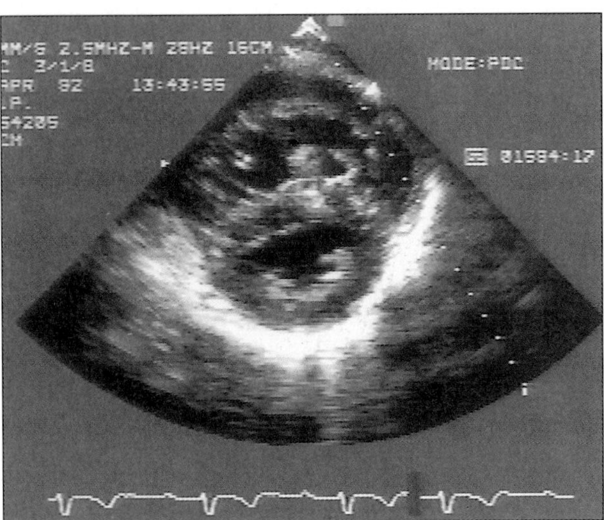

c

Figure 17.8
Apical four-chamber view (a) of a patient with chronic severe pulmonary hypertension demonstrating the characteristic echocardiographic features including a dilated right atrium and right ventricle (RV), severe RVH, and diastolic septal shift toward the left. In the parasternal short-axis view at end-diastole (b), the flattened septum results in a 'D'-shaped, rather than the normally round, LV. The thickened RV wall is easily seen. With systole, the septum shifts further to the left (c), consistent with a severe pulmonary hypertension pattern.

echocardiographic analysis to describe regional RV wall motion abnormalities that appear to correlate with episodes of acute pulmonary embolism.[82,83]

Case 3

A 40-year-old woman with a long history of scleroderma and moderate pulmonary hypertension on chronic anticoagulation and Procardia was admitted with chest pain and severe dyspnea. A chest X-ray demonstrated an enlarged cardiac silhouette, and suggested severe enlargement of the pulmonary artery. An echocardiogram (Figure 17.8a) revealed a massively dilated RA and markedly dilated RV with severe RVH and severe RV dysfunction. The LA and LV were small and the septum moved toward the left ventricle during systole. The estimated PA pressure estimated by the severe tricuspid regurgitation (TR) jet was 115 mmHg. The patient underwent PA catheter placement and evaluation for continuous intravenous (IV) prostacyclin therapy.

Echocardiography in this situation aided in the assessment of the patient's current physiology, identified her as a patient with chronic severe pulmonary hypertension, and directed treatment specifically toward newer vasoactive therapy. The characteristic echocardiographic features of

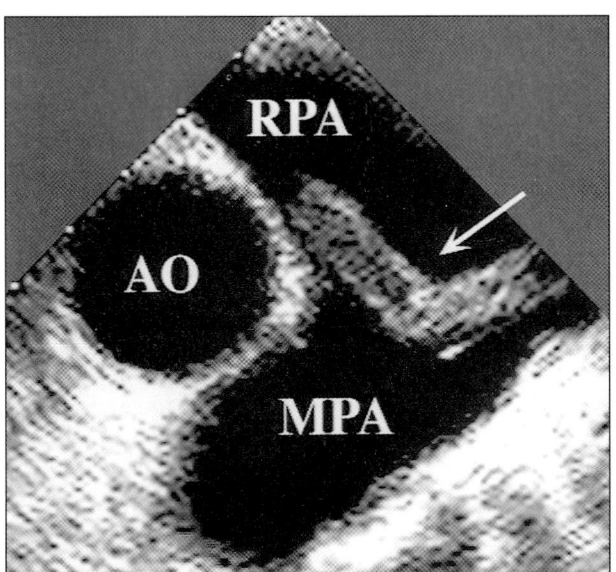

Figure 17.9
In this transesophageal echocardiographic image oriented in the horizontal plane at the pulmonary artery bifurcation, a large mobile thrombus is seen occluding most of the main and left pulmonary arteries. In real-time imaging, the proximal end of the thrombus is very mobile and distinct from the arterial walls. This abnormality was poorly seen using transthoracic echocardiography owing to limited imaging windows.

chronic pulmonary hypertension are demonstrated in the apical four-chamber view in Fig. 17.8a, and in the parasternal short-axis views (from another patient) in Figs 17.8b and 17.8c. The short-axis images demonstrate the severe RVH and end-diastolic shift of the septum toward the LV in diastole (Fig. 17.8b). With systole, there is a further shift of the septum toward the left and generally normal systolic function of the LV otherwise (Fig. 17.8c). Frequently, the pulsed Doppler diastolic filling of the LV will demonstrate a pattern consistent with diastolic dysfunction.[84] The prognosis, given this marked degree of pulmonary hypertension in a patient on vasodilator and anticoagulant therapy, is poor unless agents such as prostacyclin are successful. No long-term data on chronic IV prostacyclin therapy is available in adults; however, studies are ongoing.

Transesophageal echocardiography (TEE) may be useful in certain cases where transthoracic imaging is unsatisfactory or incomplete. Inspection of the atrial or ventricular septum, or examination of pulmonary venous drainage may be aided by this approach. In an unstable patient, TEE may assist in diagnosing a massive pulmonary embolism in the proximal pulmonary arteries (Fig. 17.9). Elsewhere in this text is a more detailed description of the use of TEE in the assessment of valvular disorders, where this technique has a major role.

Structural abnormalities assessed with MRI or CT scanning

Occasionally, echocardiography may not be able to fully characterize the cardiopulmonary anatomy in a definitive manner. Under these circumstances, MRI or CT scanning may provide important diagnostic information to clinicians. The choice between the two techniques must be made on an individual case basis. Patients with contraindications to testing on a certain device (e.g. pacemakers and MRI scanning, contrast allergy and CT) will help direct their study to the alternative modality. In addition, the expertise or equipment available at an institution may importantly influence this decision. Since MRI is a newer noninvasive imaging technique, and may have some potential advantages over CT scanning in certain applications, we will briefly focus on a few basic principles. One major advantage is that MRI does not require the use of iodinated contrast agents as CT does. In addition, dynamic or multiphase scans are only available on the most sophisticated CT scanners (Electron Beam CT), whereas dynamic scanning is an integral part of the MRI methodology.

MRI provides excellent definition of anatomic structure, assessment of cardiac function, and measurement of blood flow velocity and flow direction.[77] The principle underlying MRI is that atoms are excited in a strong magnetic field by radio frequency energy. The MRI scanner detects the signal produced by the atoms of the heart as they relax and return to their equilibrium energy state. Hydrogen atoms, which are ubiquitous in the body, are the most common atoms used for clinical MRI purposes; however, phosphorous or carbon may be used when assessing myocardial metabolism. Differences in tissue composition (muscle, fat, liver, etc.) alter the relaxation properties of the protons and permit differentiation of tissues from one another. In particular, abnormal myocardial tissue (e.g. infarcted, infiltrated by sarcoidosis) can often be detected even before wall thinning or conduction abnormalities occur.

MRI produces images with excellent spatial resolution in any planar orientation, and is the technique which provides the most complete tomographic imaging of the heart. Newer rapid imaging sequences permit faster image acquisition and, together with three-dimensional reconstruction algorithms, enable detailed assessment of the anatomy of the cardiac chambers and great vessels, and their intrathoracic relationships. For this reason MRI is often the diagnostic modality of choice for investigating abnormalities of the pulmonary arterial tree and of the aorta. MRI is particularly useful in evaluating aortic dissections and aneurysms in which precise localization of the dissected intimal flap is critical in diagnosis, treatment and surgical repair. Gating the MRI signals to the electrocardiographic QRS complex permits dynamic (or multiphase) information to be

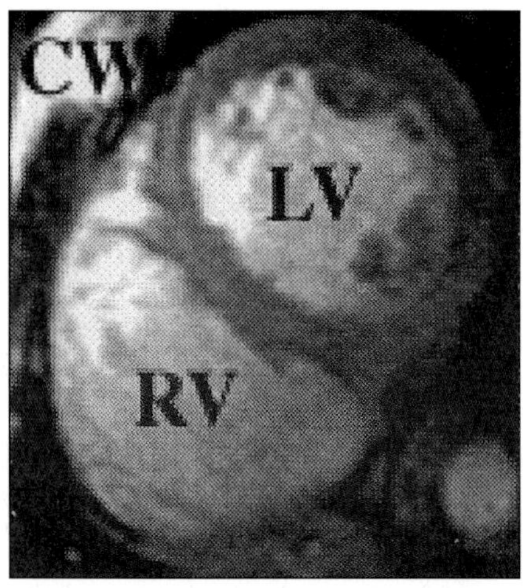

a

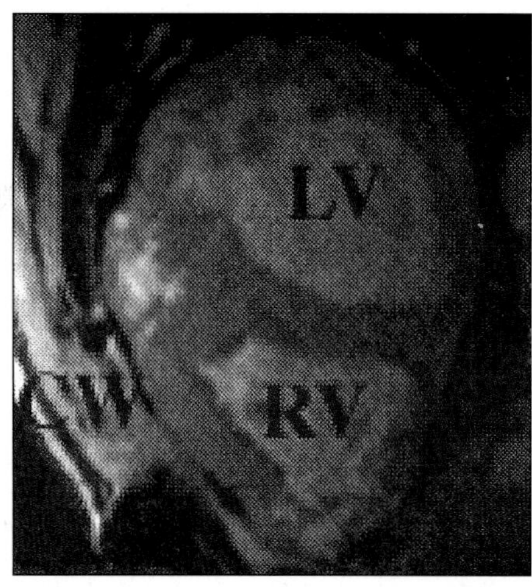

b

Figure 17.10
Short-axis image of the right ventricle (RV) and left ventricle (LV) at end-diastole (ED) in a normal volunteer (a) at the high papillary muscle level using a fast breath-hold technique. This single slice location was acquired in approximately 15 s with 16 phases spanning the cardiac cycle. Note the high spatial resolution and trabecular detail achieved without the use of contrast agents. (b) A short-axis image at ED in a patient with severe pulmonary hypertension and severe RV hypertrophy depicts the diffusely thickened RV wall and the leftward shift of the interventricular septum. CW, chest wall.

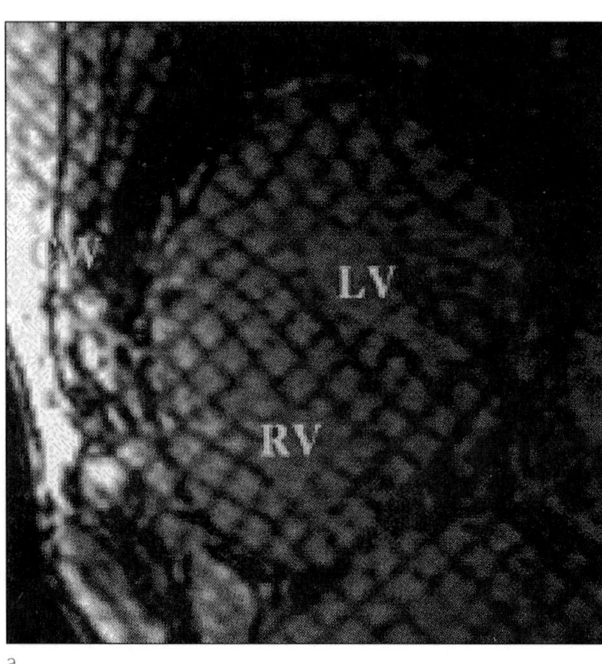

a

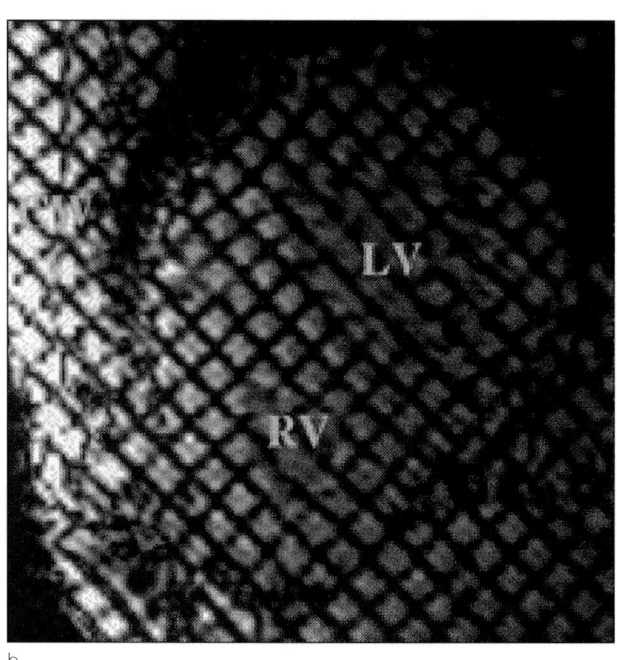

b

Figure 17.11
Short-axis end-diastolic (ED) image (a) at same location as Figure 17.10b demonstrating the myocardial tagging technique. Equally spaced orthogonal sets of tags are placed noninvasively across the image at ED by special preparation pulses. The tags are retained by the myocardium and move and deform with the wall throughout the cardiac cycle. At end-systole (ES), the tags are undeformed in the stationary tissue (chest wall (CW) and liver, inferior to heart), however, the myocardial tag lines are displaced and the square tissue elements have deformed to a more diamond-like or rhomboidal shape. Also note that the tag lines closer to the endocardium have deformed to a greater degree than those at the epicardial surface, consistent with greater endocardial shortening.

obtained during the cardiac cycle. Objective parameters of cardiac function such as wall motion, wall thickening, and change in chamber size and volume can be easily measured due to the high spatial resolution achieved. This makes MRI particularly useful for the RV, given its unusual shape (Figs 17.10a and b). Measurements of RV mass and volume are more easily performed using this new technique. A new technique known as myocardial tissue tagging allows

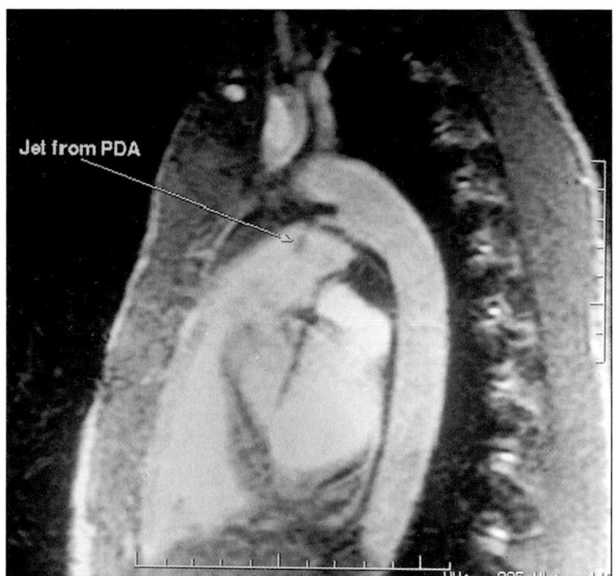

Figure 17.12
Single frame from a multiphase ECG-gated cine MRI acquisition in the coronal plane demonstrating a small patent ductus arteriosus connecting the descending aorta with the left main pulmonary artery (LPA). A systolic jet from the aorta to the LPA is seen as a dark linear flow disturbance in the LPA. MRI permits the precise level of the shunt to be localized for purposes of surgical or percutaneous closure, and can identify other associated abnormalities.

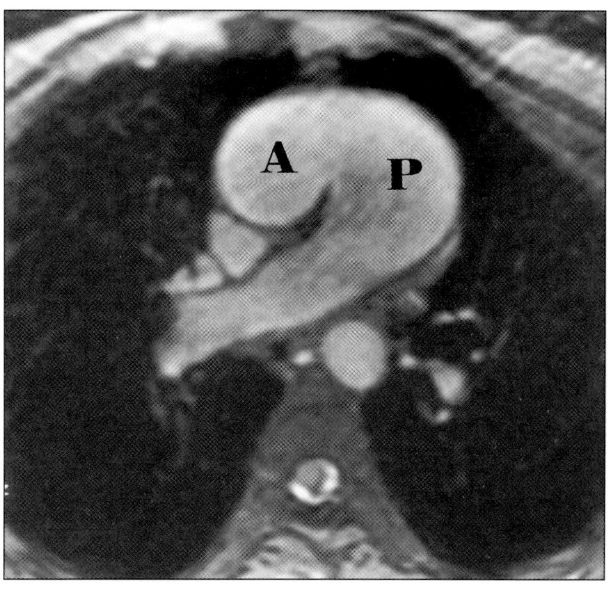

Figure 17.13
Single frame from an axial cardiac-gated cine MRI sequence clearly demonstrating the communication between the aorta (A) and main pulmonary artery (P). The mildly dilated right pulmonary artery is seen coursing to the right lung. Note that no contrast agent was required to acquire this 'bright-blood' image. Using the intrinsic contrast properties of moving blood in a magnetic field, blood was easily seen to move from the aorta to the main PA, and appeared directed more toward the left PA.

measurement of regional contraction within the wall of the heart. This method provides a more detailed understanding of regional right and left ventricular function, and may be useful in long-term management and therapy (Fig. 17.11). Recently, ultrafast three-dimensional angiographic techniques have made it feasible to examine both arterial and venous structures in a large enough field of view to encompass the mediastinum. This has permitted rapid evaluation of the cardiopulmonary anatomy in a single breath-hold and at serial time points during the contrast bolus passage (see Case 6 below).

Case 4

A 17-year-old male was discovered to have a systolic murmur on a screening physical examination for a sports program. His findings were remarkable only for a normal S1 and S2 (with normal second component) and normal splitting. Carotid and peripheral impulses were normal. A soft systolic murmur was heard best at the left upper sternal border, appeared to peak before the second heart sound, and was heard into diastole. An echocardiogram was performed which revealed normal valvular morphology and function but a mildly dilated pulmonary artery and a suggestion of a patent ductus arteriosus (PDA). He refused TEE and underwent cardiac-gated MRI scanning. As seen in Fig. 17.12, a small PDA was demonstrated with only a slightly dilated left pulmonary artery noted, indicating a small shunt. No associated anomalies were detected. The precise localization of the communication by MRI and the detailed depiction of the surrounding anatomy obviated the need for conventional diagnostic angiography, and permitted planning for percutaneous closure of the PDA, should this be recommended.

Case 5

A 39-year-old female presented with complaints of palpitations and fatigue, having had a lifelong history of murmur. On exam, she had a hyperdynamic precordium with a prominent palpable impulse in the left second intercostal space. There was a loud, harsh holosystolic murmur, loudest at the left sternal border but heard throughout the precordium. Chest X-ray demonstrated mildly dilated pulmonary arteries with evidence of shunt flow. An electrocardiogram showed normal sinus rhythm with premature atrial contractions, a rightward axis, and right ventricular hypertrophy. An echocardiogram demonstrated a probable defect between the ascending aorta and main pulmonary artery with apparent left-to-right shunt flow consistent with a diagnosis of aortopulmonary window; however, the sizes of the pulmonary arteries were not measurable. Cardiac-gated MRI scanning was performed which showed a large aortopulmonary window defect and a moderately enlarged main and left pulmonary artery. The right PA was only mildly enlarged (Fig. 17.13).

Case 6

A 21-year-old male was referred because of palpitations without presyncope or true syncope. He notes a remote history of an 'enlarged heart' on chest X-ray for an upper respiratory infection during childhood, but normal development. Recently, he was more fatigued with exercise, but denied dyspnea. Examination was remarkable for an estimated jugular venous pressure of 12 cm, an RV heave, and a palpable P2, and a systolic ejection murmur in the left upper sternal area. The point of maximal impulse was normal, and the lungs were clear. Chest X-ray showed a density in the right hilar area appearing to angle toward the diaphragm. Electrocardiogram showed normal sinus rhythm and a right atrial abnormality. Echo demonstrated a moderately dilated RA and RV with mildly decreased RV function. Left heart chambers were normal, but the inferior vena cava (IVC) was dilated. It was uncertain whether an anomalous pulmonary vein was draining from above the diaphragm into the IVC, and therefore, an ultrafast ungated three-dimensional gadolinium contrast-enhanced acquisition (3-D MR angiography) was performed in the coronal plane. This image set was gathered in approximately 34 s and covered the majority of the mediastinum. The scan demonstrated that the superior and middle pulmonary veins drained to the inferior vena cava, but that the right inferior pulmonary vein drained properly to the left atrium (Fig. 17.14).

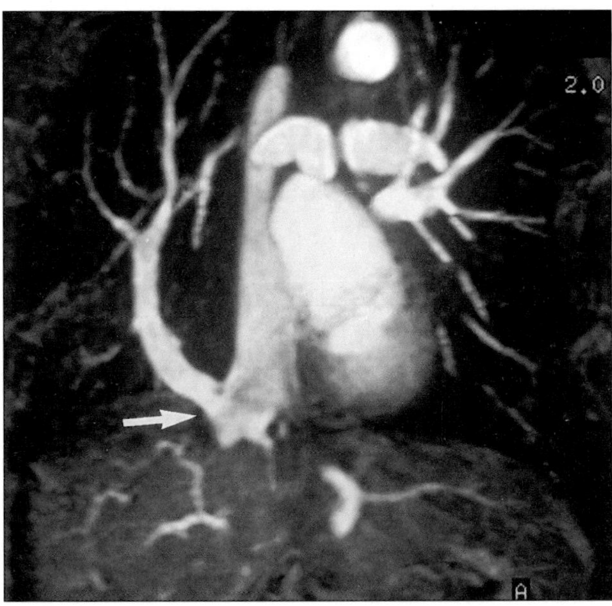

Figure 17.14
Oblique reformatted contrast-enhanced 3-D MR angiogram in the coronal plane demonstrating the anomalous pulmonary vein draining from the superior right lung and joining the inferior vena cava (IVC) below the diaphragm (arrow). Note the dilated segment of IVC at the junction of the vessels.

Pulmonary etiologies of pulmonary hypertension (pathway B, Fig. 17.4)

In patients with a history of chronic bronchitis or sleep apnea symptoms and no other cardiac lesions on echo, a search for pulmonary causes of the pulmonary hypertension is appropriate. This would include a full set of pulmonary function tests (PFTs) and a sleep study if indicated. If interstitial lung disease is suspected, a thin-section CT scan may be useful to confirm the presence of parenchymal changes in the lung.

Uncertain etiology of pulmonary hypertension (pathway C, Fig. 17.4)

A laboratory evaluation should be undertaken to exclude sickle cell disease, collagen vascular disease, hepatopulmonary syndrome, hypercoagulable states, or HIV disease. PFTs may be performed to exclude subclinical pulmonary or interstitial lung disease.

When pulmonary embolism must be excluded, another noninvasive imaging study, the ventilation–perfusion scan, can be an extremely useful screening test. This examination uses two radionuclide tracers, ^{99}Tc and ^{133}Xe, which are the perfusion and ventilation agents, respectively, and a scintillation camera to image the lungs from numerous views. Together, these tracers provide the sensitivity and specificity necessary to suggest a high likelihood of pulmonary embolism, or perhaps as importantly, to assure the clinician that there is a low likelihood of embolism. The clinical use of this study is described in the following sections.

Ventilation–perfusion lung scans

Both acute and chronic (unresolved) pulmonary emboli can result in pulmonary hypertension. In neither condition are the signs or symptoms diagnostic; therefore testing is necessary to establish the diagnosis. The ventilation–perfusion (V/Q) lung scan remains the cornerstone of the diagnosis of both acute and chronic thromboembolic disease.[85]

Acute thromboembolic disease

The fundamental premise underlying the use of ventilation–perfusion lung scans for the diagnosis of pulmonary embolism is that in most pulmonary diseases or disorders other than pulmonary emboli, a perfusion defect is accompanied by a ventilation defect which is at least as large as the perfusion defect; in contrast, pulmonary emboli elicit perfusion defects that are unaccompanied by ventilation defects. Interpretations of ventilation–perfusion scan is based on the presence, size, and correspondence of ventilation and perfusion defects. Scans are classified on these grounds into four categories: normal, high probability, intermediate (indeterminate) probability, or low probability of pulmonary embolism (see Table 17.2).

Table 17.2 Criteria for the interpretation of ventilation–perfusion lung scans*

Normal†
- No perfusion defects
- Perfusion outlines that correspond exactly to the contour of the lungs as seen on the chest radiograph (chest radiograph and/or ventilation scan may be abnormal)

High probability
- ≥2 large (>75% of a segment) segmental perfusion defects either without any abnormalities on the chest radiograph or with abnormalities that are considerably larger than corresponding defects in the ventilation scan or the chest radiograph
- ≥2 moderate (≥25% and ≤75% of a segment) segmental perfusion defects without corresponding defects in the ventilation scan or the chest radiograph plus one large mismatched segmental defect
- ≥4 moderate segmental perfusion defects without corresponding defects in the ventilation scan or the chest radiograph

Intermediate probability (indeterminate)
- Not falling into low- or high-probability categories
- Difficult to categorize as low or high probability

Low probability
- Single moderate mismatched segmental perfusion defect in association with normal chest radiograph
- Small (<25% of a segment) segmental perfusion defects in association with a normal chest radiograph
- Any perfusion defects involving no more than four segments in one lung and no more than three segments in one region of either lung with *matching* defects on the ventilation scan that are either equal to, or larger in, size
- Nonsegmental perfusion defects (e.g. blunting of the costophrenic angle by a pleural effusion; cardiomegaly; enlarged aorta, hilum, and/or mediastinum; or elevated hemidiaphragm)

*Modified after PIOPED criteria (*JAMA* 263, 2753–59, 1990).
†Ventilation scan is not necessary to determine if perfusion scan is normal; all other interpretations are based on a comparison of the perfusion and ventilation scans.
From: Fishman, A. P., *Pulmonary Diseases and Disorders*, 1988.

Normal perfusion scans

Perfusion lung scans, per se (i.e. without accompanying ventilation scans) are sensitive, but not specific, tests for detection of pulmonary emboli. They are sensitive in that the finding of a normal lung scan excludes clinically significant pulmonary emboli.

Abnormal perfusion scans

Lung scans are not specific for the diagnosis of pulmonary embolism. In individuals with abnormal perfusion scans, comparison with ventilation scans improves the accuracy of lung scans for detecting pulmonary embolism. This holds true even for patients with underlying cardiac or pulmonary disease.[86]

High-probability lung scans

The largest (at least 75% of a segment) perfusion defects, particularly when multiple and not matched by ventilation defects, are likely to represent more significant embolic events. Scans of this type are classified as high probability for pulmonary embolism (Fig. 17.15a). However, the Prospective Investigation of Pulmonary Embolism Diagnosis

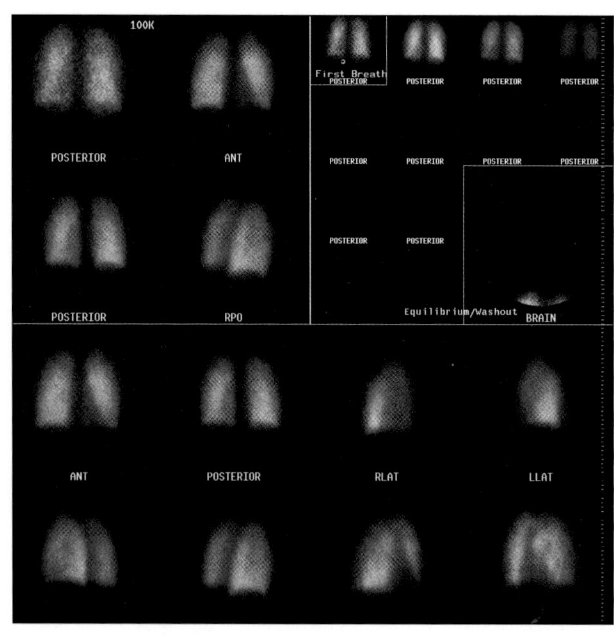

a

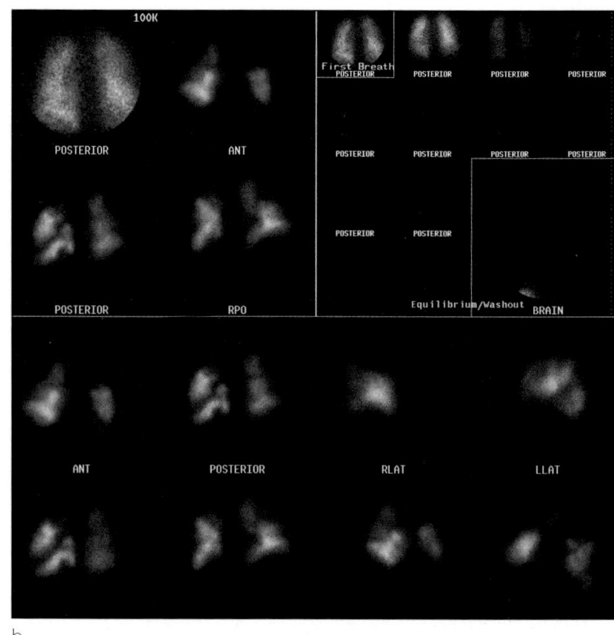

b

Figure 17.15

In the normal scan (a), the ventilation portion of the study is shown in the upper right of the figure following 'first breath'. Note the homogeneous distribution of the inhaled tracer throughout the lung fields. The remainder of the image depicts various orientations of the perfusion portion of the study. Again, note the homogeneous uptake of tracer throughout the lungs, except in those areas which contain the cardiovascular structures. In the high probability scan (b), the ventilation portion of the scan is relatively normal. However, there are numerous segmental defects in the perfusion scans which do not have corresponding ventilation defects in the same territory (unmatched defects). The defects are somewhat rounded or wedge-shaped, and in same regions the entire lobe appears to be missing. These abnormal regions of perfusion most commonly represent vascular obstruction due to pulmonary emboli. Figures courtesy of Darryl Shnier, MD

(PIOPED) study sponsored by the National Institutes of Health (NIH) found high-probability lung scans to be relatively insensitive, that is, they occurred in only 41% of the patients in whom the presence of pulmonary emboli was documented by pulmonary angiography.[87] Despite this lack of sensitivity, the high-probability scan was accurate with the positive predictive value of a high-probability scan of 88%. The positive predictive value of the high-probability lung scan fell to 74% in patients who had a prior history of pulmonary embolism, because of residual perfusion defects due to the previous pulmonary emboli.

Non-high probability lung scans

Intermediate- and low-probability lung scans are often considered together in dealing with patients suspected of pulmonary emboli, since these scan patterns are not diagnostic of pulmonary emboli. In addition, distinguishing between intermediate- and low-probability scan is often difficult. In the PIOPED study, concordance of interpretation among readers of lung scans was only 70–75% for these categories. In both groups, the rationale for subsequent diagnostic evaluations and treatment are similar. In PIOPED, the most frequent scan pattern found in patients confirmed to have pulmonary embolism was an intermediate-probability scan; 42% of all confirmed pulmonary emboli were in this group.

Chronic thromboembolic pulmonary hypertension

The ventilation–perfusion lung scan is the essential test for establishing the diagnosis of unresolved pulmonary thromboembolism.[38] A normal lung scan excludes the diagnosis of both acute or chronic (unresolved) thromboembolism. The typical lung scan pattern in most patients with pulmonary hypertension (of nonthromboembolic origin) is either relatively normal or shows diffuse nonuniform perfusion.[88] When subsegmental or larger perfusion defects are noted on the V/Q scan in patients with pulmonary hypertension, even with matched ventilation defects, pulmonary angiography is appropriate to confirm or exclude thromboembolic disease.

Pulmonary angiography

The pulmonary angiogram continues to be the most accurate diagnostic study for evaluating pulmonary embolism.[89] Two angiographic findings are characteristic of acute pulmonary embolism: an intravascular filling defect, or an abrupt cut-off of the contrast stream (Table 17.3). Of the two, the filling defect is the more frequent and reliable. When properly performed using magnification and selective injections and views, pulmonary angiography can detect clots as small as 0.5 mm. With rare exceptions, a normal angiogram excludes the diagnosis of embolism in all but the most distal vessels of the lungs.

The major limitations of pulmonary angiography are its invasiveness, expense, technical complexity, and limited availability. To reduce these disadvantages, digital subtraction angiography has been developed whereby a bolus of contrast material is injected into a large peripheral vein, and the resultant radiographic image of the pulmonary circulation is enhanced through special computerized techniques. Unfortunately, this method has not proven to be as sensitive as standard pulmonary angiography.

Pulmonary angiography remains the gold standard for the diagnosis of chronic, unresolved thromboemboli. Organized thromboembolic lesions do not resemble the intravascular filling defects seen with acute pulmonary emboli, and experience is essential for proper interpretation of pulmonary angiograms in patients with unresolved, chronic embolic disease.[90] Organized thrombi appear as unusual filling defects, webs, or bands, or completely thrombosed vessels that may resemble the congenital absence of a vessel. Organized material along a vascular wall of a recanalized vessel produces a scalloped or serrated luminal edge. Because of both vessel-wall thickening and dilation of proximal vessels, the contrast-filled lumen may appear relatively normal in diameter. Distal vessels frequently demonstrate the rapid tapering and pruning characteristic of pulmonary hypertension.

Although there was once reluctance to perform angiography in patients with pulmonary hypertension, use of selective and subselective injections with small amounts of contrast material have significantly reduced the risks of this technique.[91] Although some risk remains, the benefit of establishing the presence of a treatable cause of the hypertension far outweighs the small risk; pulmonary angiography should be performed whenever ventilation–perfusion lung scanning suggests that chronic thromboembolism is the probable etiology of pulmonary hypertension.

Computed tomography (CT)

Recent advances in CT scan technology (helical (spiral) CT and electron-beam CT) have improved visualization of the pulmonary arterial tree to at least the level of segmental arteries.[92] Both techniques rapidly acquire images so that opacification of the pulmonary vasculature following bolus administration of intravenous contrast is at its maximum during scan time. CT provides direct visualization of central pulmonary arterial clots, including nonocclusive thrombi (Fig. 17.16). Unlike the ventilation–perfusion scan, the imaging of the chest by CT has the potential of indicating

Table 17.3 Angiographic findings suggesting chronic pulmonary artery thrombus

- Pouching – A concave pattern of contrast seen with complete or nearly complete occlusion of a proximal pulmonary artery
- Webs or bands
- Post-stenotic dilatation (may be aneurysmal)
- Scalloped appearance of the pulmonary arterial wall
- Abrupt narrowing of a major pulmonary vessel
- Discrepancy between the apparent outer edge of the vessel and the column of contrast (MRI may be particularly useful in evaluating this condition)
- Absence of vessels – Owing to obstruction of pulmonary arterial vessels at their origin

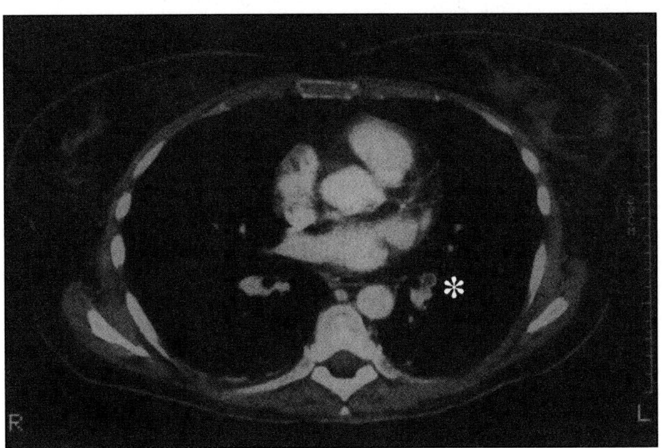

Figure 17.16
Axial images from an ultrafast electron beam CT scan demonstrating partially occlusive thrombus at four slice levels in the left inferior pulmonary artery (*). Note that these images are contrast-enhanced and were acquired closely in time to one another.

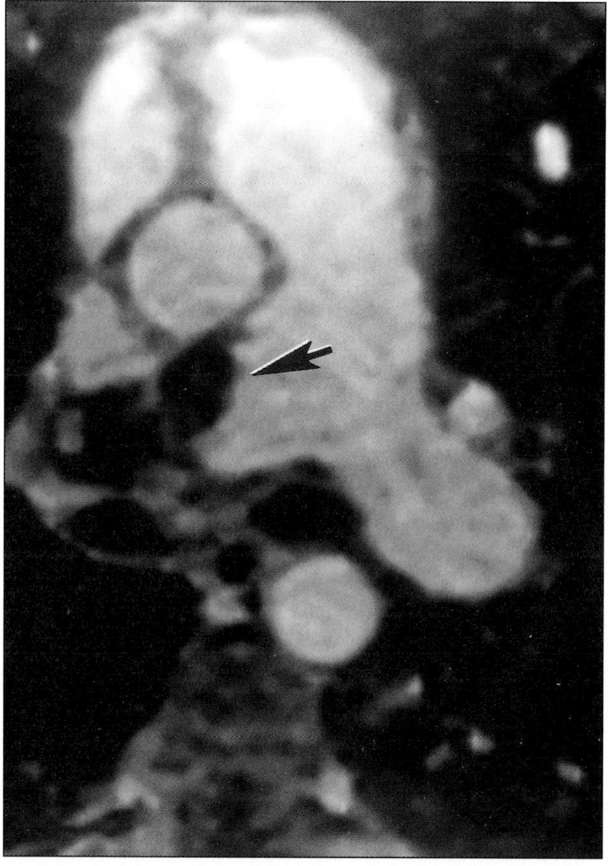

a

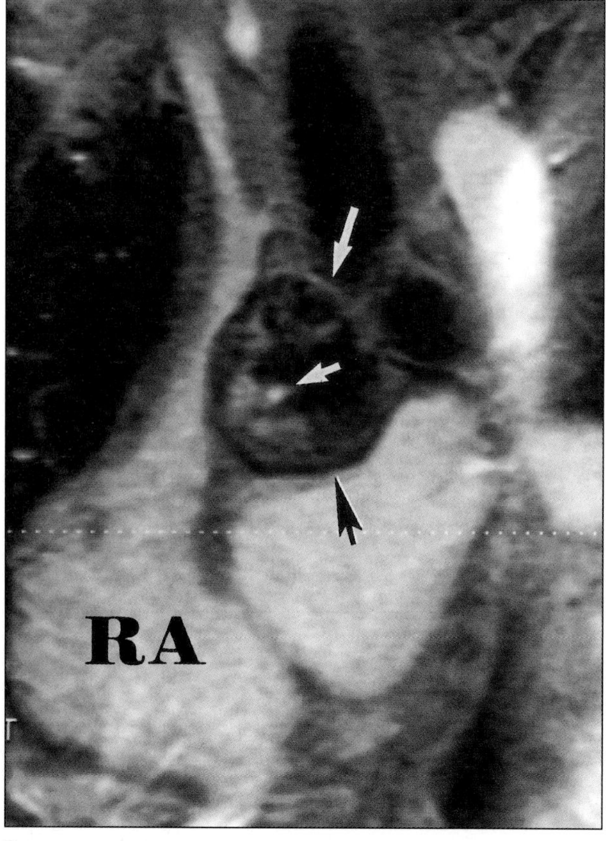

c

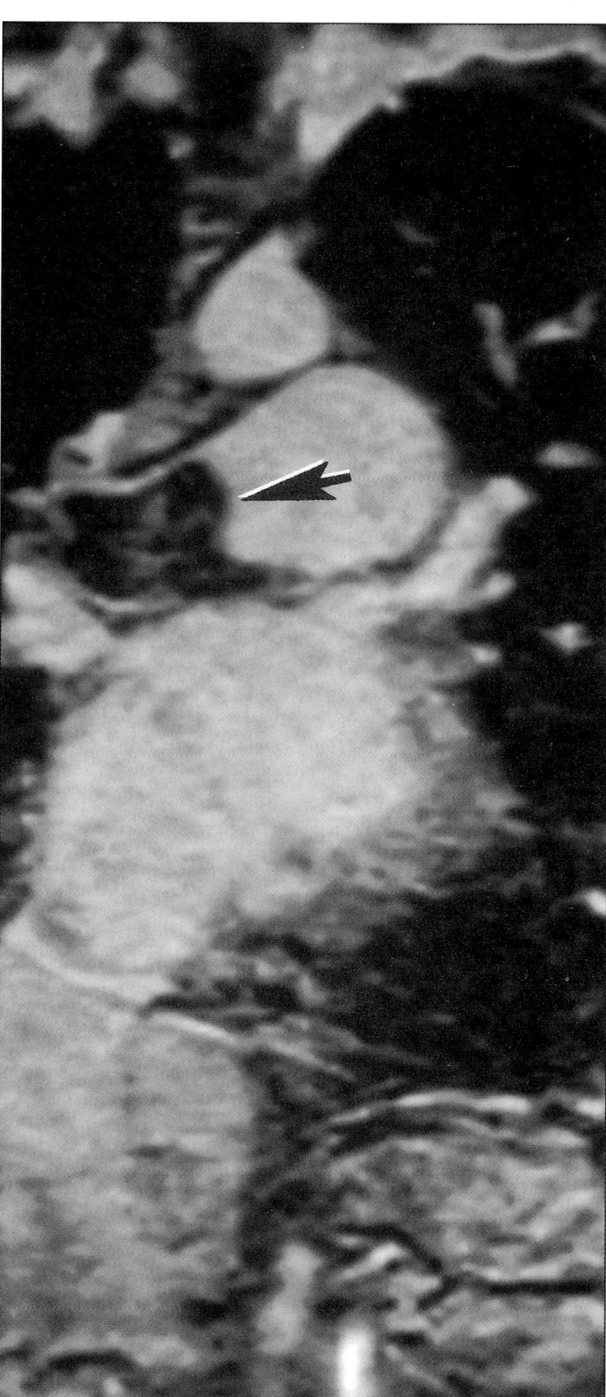

b

Figure 17.17
Reformatted images from an ultrafast 3-D contrast-enhanced MR angiographic sequence demonstrating occlusive thrombus in the right pulmonary artery in the axial plane (a, arrow), coronal plane (b, arrow), and oblique parasagittal plane (c). In (c), the large black and white arrows delineate the original border of the dilated right pulmonary artery, which is now nearly occluded by thrombus. The snall white arrow points to the residual lumen, which is a fraction of the original lumen size.

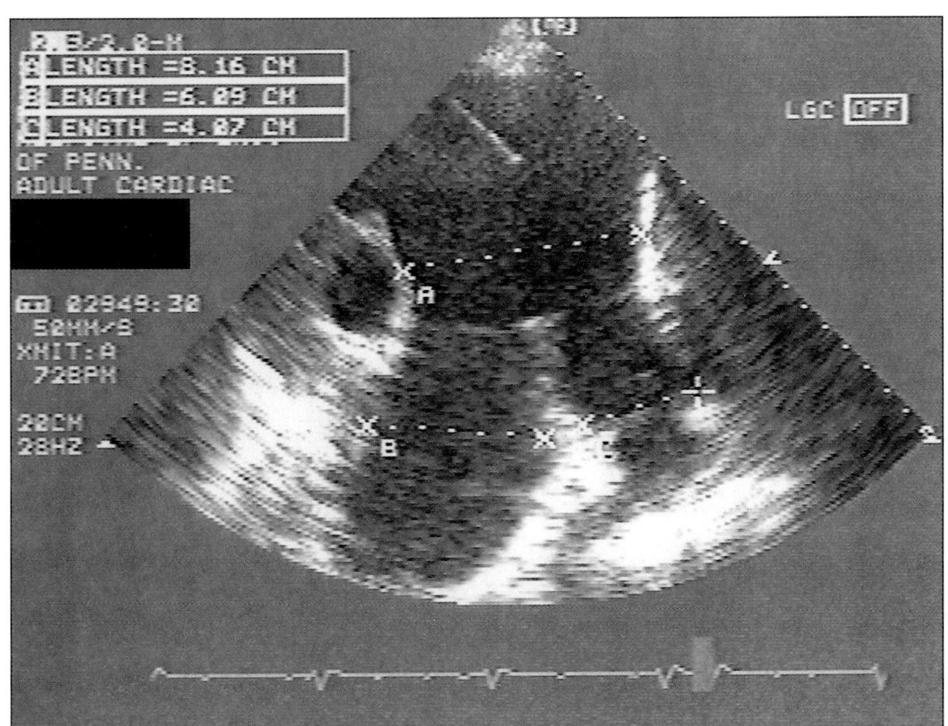

Figure 17.18
Echocardiographic pulmonary artery long-axis view demonstrating a complication of severe longstanding pulmonary hypertension – pulmonary artery (PA) dissection. Under chronic pressure overload, the vessels may become calcified and friable, and spontaneously develop a dissection, similar to the aorta. Note the dissection flap at the top of the image. The PA measures 8.2 cm at the bifurcation. This patient went on to bilateral lung transplantation shortly after this event.

diagnoses other than pulmonary embolism. However, in contrast to the high sensitivity and low specificity of radionucleotide lung scanning for clot detection, CT is limited by its low sensitivity for the detection of segmental and smaller clots. Published reports on spiral CT angiographic studies have indicated that spiral CT has a sensitivity of 95.5% (range 64–100%) and a specificity of 97.6% (range 89–100%) for the detection of pulmonary embolism.[93]

Magnetic resonance imaging (MRI)

MRI is also rapidly evolving as a noninvasive method of visualizing pulmonary artery thrombi.[94] As compared to CT, MRI does not require the use of iodinated intravenous contrast agents. Moreover, pulmonary vascular MRI for pulmonary emboli may easily be combined with MR venography for evaluation of the pelvic veins and the deep veins of the legs.

The sensitivity of MRI for the detection of pulmonary embolism varies with clot size and location; diagnostic accuracy is currently satisfactory only for segmental or larger clots. As for CT scanning, the inability of this technique to detect small, peripheral emboli may be of minor clinical importance if evaluation for deep vein thrombosis can be easily accomplished. At present, the accuracy of spiral CT scanning appears to be somewhat better than that of MRI. However, the role of MRI in diagnosing thromboembolic disease holds great promise because of technical advances that are both shortening image acquisition times (thereby decreasing the image degradation that occurs as a consequence of cardiac and respiratory motion) and enhancing vascular signal intensity[95] (Fig. 17.17).

Role of imaging in long-term management of pulmonary hypertension

The treatment of chronic pulmonary hypertension is focused on the primary cause of the disorder, if treatable. Some diseases are manageable to some degree, for example, nasal continuous positive airways pressure (CPAP) for sleep apnea, or thromboendarterectomy for thromboembolic pulmonary hypertension. While lung transplantation may be an option for some patients, systemic disorders preclude patients from candidacy in

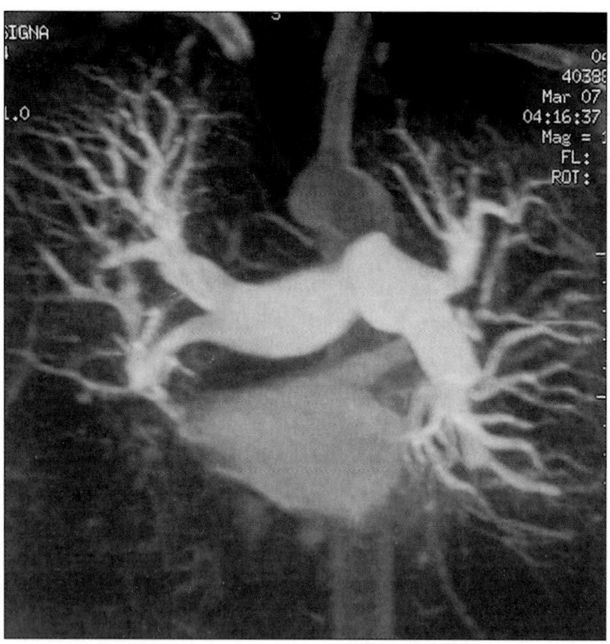

Figure 17.19
Reformatted ultrafast 3-D MR angiogram in a patient with chronic idiopathic pulmonary hypertension demonstrating enlarged central vessels and rapid tapering of the vessels in the periphery. This process, called 'pruning', represents progressive obliteration of the distal pulmonary vessels and arterioles, which leads to a correspoding increase in pulmonary vascular resistance.

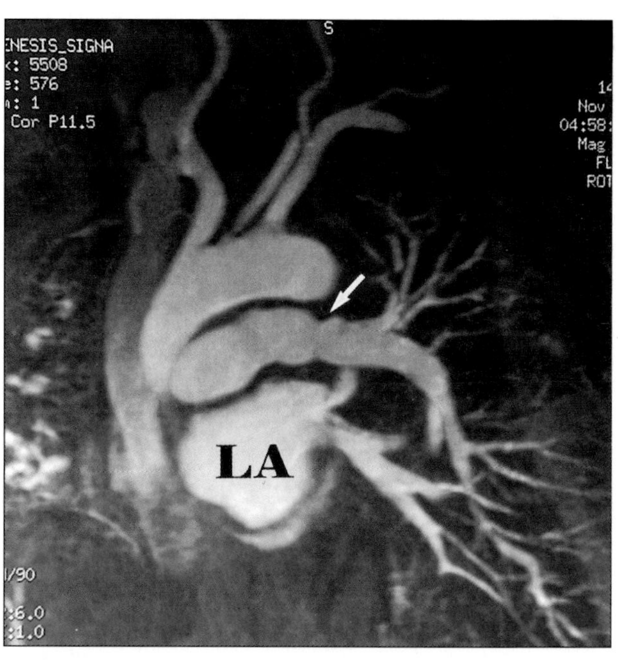

Figure 17.20
In a patient with an unexplained large ventilation–perfusion mismatch post-lung transplant, 3-D MR angiographic techniques were able to noninvasively demonstrate patency of the pulmonary veins, and a lack of high grade stenosis at the anastomotic site. The arrow points to the anastomosis, and the patent pulmonary veins are seen draining into the left atrium (LA).

most programs. Although many patients with collagen vascular disorders may initially improve on vasodilator therapy, often they return in 3–5 years with worsening of their pulmonary hypertension, having become refractory to oral drug therapy. Patients with severe pulmonary hypertension are frequently placed on systemic anticoagulation and possibly oxygen in an attempt to correct at least some of their abnormalities. Monitoring and following patients noninvasively during this chronic phase of their illness is of great importance. Most patients are followed with clincial examinations and echocardiography in an attempt to track the PA pressure over time. While echo is satisfactory for most patients, other imaging techniques have proven useful in certain circumstances. Complications of chronic pulmonary hypertension include pulmonary artery dissection (Fig. 17.18) and progressive obliteration of the pulmonary vascular bed (Fig. 17.19).

In those patients who undergo lung transplantation, imaging plays an important role in following their clinical course. MR angiographic techniques have proven useful in evaluating anastomotic sites in patients with unexplained large alveolar-arterial gradients (Fig. 17.20), and after complicated transplantations (Fig. 17.21).

Conclusions

Cor pulmonale and pulmonary hypertension may result from a diverse set of etiologies. Noninvasive imaging techniques are an important adjunct to the diagnosis and selection of therapy and the management of patients in the chronic phase of illness. Echocardiography remains the single most useful modality in the evaluation of patients with pulmonary hypertension, and provides important information early in the work-up of these disorders. Echo is particularly valuable in the evaluation of acutely ill patients, such as those with acute mitral regurgitation or acute pulmonary embolism. Nuclear medicine techniques continue to have an important role in the evaluation of suspected pulmonary embolism, both acute and chronic unresolved types. While CT may prove to be a surrogate

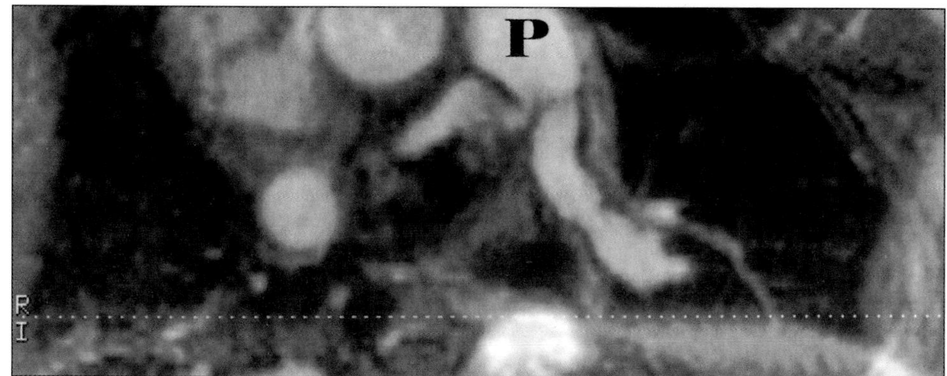

a

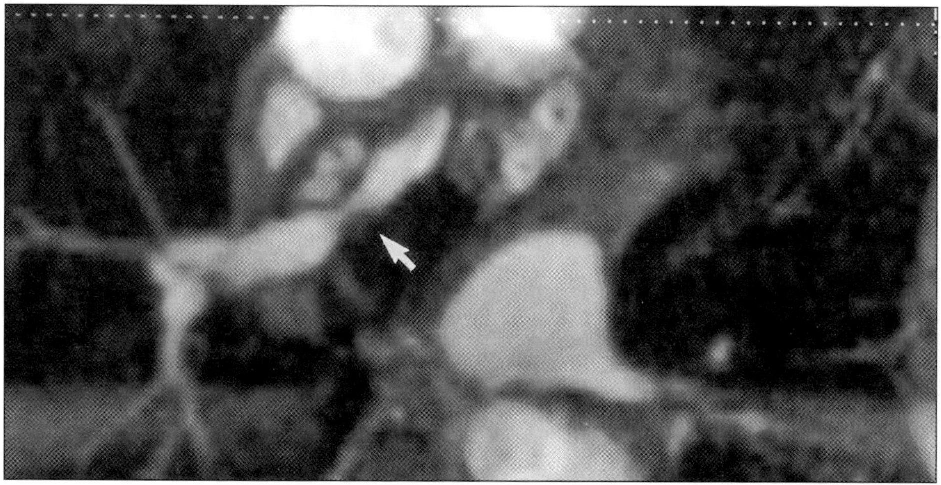

b

Figure 17.21
Post-transplant MR angiogram of the patient in Fig. 17.18 with the pulmonary artery dissection. The patient had graft material inserted to connect his native pulmonary artery (P) to the donor pulmonary arteries. While the left graft appears widely patent, the right graft has a mid-graft stenosis present (arrow).

for pulmonary angiography in some cases, the obligate radiation exposure and use of intravenous contrast injections may limit its utility in some patient populations. New methods such as MRI and MR angiography are providing both conventional and new information with less risk than some current techniques, and with further refinements they may prove even more useful. Recent concerns over the increased incidence of pulmonary hypertension and cardiac valvular disease in patients taking certain weight loss-promoting drugs (Phen-Fen) may further support interest in the role of noninvasive imaging in this disorder.[96]

Acknowledgments

The authors thank Bernadette Roberts and Robin Hall for assistance with manuscript preparation, and Ted Plappert and Martin St John Sutton for assistance with echocardiographic figures. The expertise of Drs Leon Axel, George Holland, and Alan Stolpen is appreciated with regard to MRI data acquisition and interpretation.

References

1 Palevsky HI: Exercise and the pulmonary circulation. In: Leff A, ed., *Cardiopulmonary Exercise Testing* (Orlando, FL: Grune and Stratton, 1986), 89–106.

2 Meyrick B, Reid L: Pulmonary hypertension: anatomic and physiologic correlations. *Clin Chem Med* 1983; 4: 199.

3 Palevsky H, Schloo B, Pietra G et al: Primary pulmonary hypertension: vascular structure, morphometry, and responsiveness to vasodilator agents. *Circulation* 1989; 80: 1207–21.

4 Loyd J, Atkinson J, Pietra G: Heterogeneity of pathologic lesions in familial primary pulmonary hypertension. *Am Rev Resp Dis* 1988; 138: 952–7.

5 Pietra G, Edwards W, Kay J et al: Histopathology of primary pulmonary hypertension: a qualitative and quantitative study of pulmonary blood vessels from 58 patients in the National Heart, Lung, and Blood Institute Primary Pulmonary Hypertension Registry. *Circulation* 1989; 60: 1198.

6 Fuster V, Steele P, Edwards W et al: Primary pulmonary hypertension: natural history and the importance of thrombosis. *Circulation* 1984; 70: 580–7.

7 Lerman A, Hildebrand FJ, Margulies K et al: Endothelin: a new cardiovascular regulatory peptide. *Mayo Clin Proc* 1990; 64: 1441.

8 Vanhoutte P: Endothelium and control of vascular function. State of the art. *Hypertension* 1989; 13: 658.

9 Haworth S. Pulmonary vascular disease in secundum atrial septal defect. *Am J Cardiol* 1983; 51: 265.

10 Heath D, Edwards J: The pathology of hypertensive pulmonary vascular disease. A description of six grades of structural changes in the pulmonary arteries with special reference to congenital cardiac septal defects. *Circulation* 1958; 18: 533.

11 Rabinovitch M, Keave J, Norwood W et al: Vascular structure in lung tissue obtained at biopsy correlated with pulmonary hemodynamic findings after repair of congenital heart defects. *Circulation* 1984; 69: 655.

12 Wood P: The Eisenmenger syndrome, or pulmonary hypertension with reversed central shunt. *BMJ* 1958; 2: 755.

13 Friedman W, Heiferman M: Clinical problems of postoperative pulmonary vascular disease. *Am J Cardiol* 1982; 50: 631.

14 McGregor C, Jamieson S, Baldwin J et al: Combined heart–lung transplantation for end-stage Eisenmenger's syndrome. *J Thorac Cardiovasc Surg* 1986; 91:443.

15 Heath D, Edwards J: Histologic changes in the lung in diseases associated with pulmonary venous hypertension. *Br J Dis Chest* 1959; 53: 8.

16 Harris P, Heath D: *The Human Pulmonary Ciculation* (New York: Churchill Livingstone, 1986), 702.

17 Haworth S: Pulmonary vascular disease in different types of congenital heart disease. Implications for interpretation of lung biopsy findings in early childhood. *Br Heart J* 1984; 52: 557.

18 Dexter L: Pulmonary vascular disease in acquired heart disease. In: Moser K, ed., *Pulmonary Vascular Diseases* (New York; Marcel Dekker, 1979), 427.

19 Dexter L: Physiologic changes in mitral stenosis. *N Eng J Med* 1986; 254: 829.

20 Magidson A: Cor triatriatum. Severe pulmonary arterial hypertension and pulmonary venous hypertension in a child. *Am J Cardiol* 1962; 9: 603.

21 Grossman W, McLaurin L, Stefadouros M: Left ventricular stiffness associated with chronic pressure and volume overloads in man. *Circ Res* 1974; 35: 793.

22 Benotti J, Grossman W, Cohn P: The clinical profile of restrictive cardiomyopathy. *Circulation* 1980; 61: 1206.

23 Lorell B, Grossman W: Profiles in constrictive pericarditis, restrictive cardiomyopathy, and cardiac tamponade. In: Grossman W, ed., *Cardiac Catheterization and Angiography*, 3rd edn (Philadelphia; Lea and Febiger, 1986).

24 Wagenvoort C: Pulmonary veno-occlusive disease: entity or syndrome. *Chest* 1976; 69: 82.

25 Asherson R, Oakley C: Pulmonary hypertension and systemic lupus erythematosus. *J Rheumatol* 1986; 13: 1.

26 Kobayashi H, Sano T, Fi K: Mixed connective tissue disease with fatal pulmonary hypertension. *Acta Pathol Jpn* 1982; 32: 1121.

27 Kline L, Ferrari V. Mechanical complications of respiratory failure. In: Carlson R, Geheb M, ed., *Principles and Practice of Medical Intensive Care* (Philadelphia: WB Saunders and Co., 1992).

28 Stupi A, Steen V, Owens G et al: Pulmonary hypertension in the CREST syndrome variant of systemic sclerosis (scleroderma). *Arthritis Rheum* 1986; 29: 515–24.

29 Fahey P, Utell M, Condemi J et al: Raynaud's phenomenon of the lung. *Am J Med* 1984; 76: 263.

30 Elliott C: Pulmonary physiology during pulmonary embolism. *Chest* 1992; 101(4) (suppl): 163S–171S.

31 Moser K: Pulmonary embolism. *Am Rev Resp Dis* 1977; 115: 829.

32 McIntyre K, Sasahara A: Hemodynamic and ventricular responses to pulmonary embolism. *Prog Cardiovasc Dis* 1974; 17: 175.

33 Sutton G, Hall R, Kerr I: Clinical course and late prognosis of treated subacute massive, acute minor, and chronic pulmonary thromboembolism. *Br Heart J* 1977; 39:1135.

34 Weir E, Archer S, Edwards J: Chronic primary and secondary thromboembolic pulmonary hypertension. *Chest* 1988; 93: 149S.

35 Cohen M, Fuster V, Williams W: Anticoagulation in the treatment of pulmonary hypertension. In: Fishman A, ed., *The Pulmonary Circulation: Normal and Abnormal Mechanisms, Management, and the National Registry.* (Philadelphia; University of Pennsylvania Press, 1990); 501.

36 Rich S, Levitsky S, Brundage B. Pulmonary hypertension from chronic pulmonary thromboembolism. *Ann Intern Med* 1988; 108: 425.

37 Daily P, Dembitsky W, Inersen S et al: Risk factors for pulmonary thromboendarterectomy. *J Thorac Cardiovasc Surg* 1990; 99: 670.

38 Moser K, Daily P, Peterson K et al: Thromboendarterectomy for chronic, major vessel thromboembolic pulmonary hypertension: immediate and long-term results in 42 patients. *Ann Intern Med* 1987; 107: 560–5.

39 Rich S, Dantzker D, Ayres S et al: Primary pulmonary hypertension: a national study, *Ann Intern Med* 1987; 107: 216.

40 Glanville A, Burke C, Theodore J et al: Primary pulmonary hypertension: length of survival in patients referred for heart–lung transplantation. *Chest* 1987; 91: 675.

41 D'Alonzo G, Barst R, Ayres S et al: Survival in patients with primary pulmonary hypertension. Results from a national prospective registry. *Ann Intern Med* 1991; 115: 343.

42 Voelkel N, Reeves J: Primary pulmonary hypertension. In: Moser K, ed., *Pulmonary Vascular Disease* (New York, Marcel Dekker, 1979), 573–628.

43 Gurtner H: Aminorex pulmonary hypertension. In: Fishman A, ed., *The Pulmonary Circulation: Normal and Abnormal Mechanisms, Management, and the National Registry* (Philadelphia: University of Pennsylvania Press, 1990), 397.

44 Gomez-Sanchez M, Saenz De La Calzada C, Gomez-Pajuelo C et al: Clinical and pathologic manifestations of pulmonary vascular disease in the toxic oil syndrome. *J Am Coll Cardiol* 1991, 18: 1539.

45 Mette S, Palevsky H, Pietra G et al: Primary pulmonary hypertension in association with human immunodeficiency virus infection: a possible viral etiology for some forms of hypertensive pulmonary arteriopathy. *Am Rev Resp Dis* 1992; 145: 1196.

46 Miller G, Sutton G: Clinical and haemodynamic findings in 23 patients studied by cardiac catheterization and pulmonary arteriography. *Br Heart J* 1970; 32: 518.

47 Spann JF, Buccino RA, Sonnenblick EH, Braunwald E: Contractile state of cardiac muscle obtained from cats with experimentally produced ventricular hypertrophy and heart failure. *Circ Res* 1967, 21: 341–54.

48 Staar I, Jeffers WA, Meade RH: The absence of conspicuous increments of venous pressure after severe damage to the right ventricle of the dog, with discussion of the relation between clinical congestive failure and heart disease. *Am Heart J* 1943; 26: 291–301.

49 Rodbard S, Wagner D: By-passing the right ventricle. *Proc Soc Exp Biol Med* 1949; 71: 69–70.

50 Bakos ACP: The question of the function of the right ventricle myocardium: an experimental study. *Circulation* 1950; 1: 724.

51 Guiha NH, Limas CJ, Cohn JN: Predominant right ventricular dysfunction after right ventricular destruction in the dog. *Am J Cardiol* 1974; 33(2): 254–8.

52 Tani M: Roles of the right ventricular free wall and ventricular septum in right ventricular performance and influence of the parietal pericardium during right ventricular failure in dogs. *Am J Cardiol* 1983; 52(1):196–202.

53 Cohn JN, Guiha NH, Broder MI, Limas CJ: Right ventricular infarction: clinical and hemodynamic features. *Am J Cardiol* 1974; 33: 209–14.

54 Alpert JS: Effect of right ventricular dysfunction on left ventricular function. *Adv Cardiol* 1986; 34: 25–34.

55 Wiedemann H, Matthay R: Cor Pulmonale. In: Braunwald E, ed., *Heart Disease. A Textbook of Cardiovascular Medicine.* 5th ed. (Philadelphia, WB Saunders, 1997); 1604–25.

56 Horan LG, Flowers NC, Havelda CJ: Relation between right ventricular mass and cavity size: an analysis of 1500 human hearts. *Circulation* 1981; 64(1):135–8.

57 Brinker JA, Weiss JL, Lappe DL et al: Leftward septal displacement during right ventricular loading in man. *Circulation* 1980; 61(3): 626–33.

58 Rushmer RF, Thal N: The mechanics of ventricular contraction. A cinefluorographic study. *Circulation* 1951; IV: 219–28.

59 Rushmer RF, Crystal DK: Changes in configuration of the ventricular chambers during the cardiac cycle. *Circulation* 1951; IV: 211–18.

60 Meier GD, Bove AA, Santamore WP, Lynch PR: Contractile function in canine right ventricle. *Am J Physiol* 1980; 239(6): H794–H804.

61 James TN: Anatomy of the crista supraventricularis: its importance for understanding right ventricular function, right ventricular infarction and related conditions. *J Am Coll Cardiol* 1985; 6(5): 1083–5.

62 Gentzler R, Briselli MF, Gault JH: Angiographic estimation of right ventricular volume in man. *Circulation* 1974; 50(2): 324–30.

63 Maddahi J, Berman DS, Matsuoka DT et al: A new technique for assessing right ventricular ejection fraction using rapid multiple-gated equilibrium cardiac blood pool scintigraphy. Description, validation and findings in chronic coronary artery disease. *Circulation* 1979; 60(3): 581–9.

64 Baker BJ, Scovil JA, Kane JJ, Murphy ML: Echocardiographic detection of right ventricular hypertrophy. *Am Heart J* 1983; 105(4): 611–4.

65 Hajduczok ZD, Weiss RM, Stanford W, Marcus ML: Determination of right ventricular mass in humans and dogs with ultrafast cardiac computed tomography. *Circulation* 1990; 82(1): 202–12.

66 Jain D, Zaret B: Assessment of right ventricular function: role of nuclear imaging techniques: *Cardiol Clin* 1992; 10: 23.

67 Linker D, Moritz W, Pearlman A: A new three-dimensional method of right ventricular volume measurement. In vitro validation. *J Am Coll Cardiol* 1986; 8: 101.

68 Mahoney L, Smith W, Noel M, Florentine M, Skorton D: Measurement of right ventricular volume using cine computed tomography. *Invest Radiol* 1987; 22(Jun): 451–5.

69 Boxt LM, Katz J, Kolb T, Czegledy FP, Barst RJ: Direct quantitation of right and left ventricular volumes with nuclear magnetic resonance imaging in patients with primary pulmonary hypertension. *J Am Coll Cardiol* 1992; 19(7): 1508–15.

70 Debatin JF, Nadel SN, Sostman HD, Spritzer CE, Evans AJ, Grist TM: Magnetic resonance imaging–cardiac ejection fraction measurements. Phantom study comparing four different methods. *Invest Radiol* 1992; 27(3): 198–204.

71 Pattynama PM, Willems LN, Smit AH, van der Wall EE, de Roos A: Early diagnosis of cor pulmonale with MR imaging of the right ventricle. *Radiology* 1992; 182(2): 375–9.

72 Dell'Italia LJ, Pearce DJ, Blackwell GG, Singleton HR, Bishop SP, Pohost GM: Right and left ventricular volumes and function after acute pulmonary hypertension in intact dogs. *J Appl Physiol* 1995; 78(6): 2320–7.

73 Dong SJ, Crawley AP, MacGregor JH et al: Regional left ventricular systolic function in relation to the cavity geometry in patients with chronic right ventricular pressure overload. A three-dimensional tagged magnetic resonance imaging study. *Circulation* 1995; 91(9): 2359–70.

74 Fayad ZA, Ferrari VA, Kraitchman DL, Young AA, Bloomgarden DC, Axel L: Right ventricular wall mechanics in normals and patients with pulmonary hypertension using magnetic resonance tissue tagging. IEEE, Computers in Cardiology. Vienna, Austria, 1995: 233–6.

75 Fayad ZA, Connick TJ, Axel L: An improved quadrature or phased-array coil for MR cardiac imaging. *Magnetic Resonance Med* 1995; 34: 186–93.

76 Chin BB, Bloomgarden DC, Xia W et al: Right and left ventricular volume and ejection fraction by tomographic gated blood-pool scintigraphy. *J Nuclear Med* (1997) 38(6): 942–8.

77 Skorton D, Schelbert H, Wolf G, Brundage B, ed. Marcus: Cardiac imaging. In: Braunwald E, ed., *Heart Disease*, 2nd edn (Philadelphia, WB Saunders Company, 1996).

78 St John Sutton M, Oldershaw P, Kotler M, eds: *Textbook of Echocardiography and Doppler in Adults and Children*, 2nd edn (Boston, Blackwell Scientific, 1996).

79 Steiner R, Levin D: Radiology of the heart. In: Braunwald E, ed., *Heart Disease: A Textbook of Cardiovascular Medicine* 5th edn (Philadelphia, WB Saunders Company, 1997).

80 Eysmann SB, Palevsky HI, Reichek N, Hackney K, Douglas PS: Two-dimensional and Doppler echocardiographic and cardiac catheterization correlates of survival in primary pulmonary hypertension. *Circulation* 1989; 80: 353–60.

81 Abascal VM, Wilkins GT, O'Shea JP et al: Prediction of successful outcome in 130 patients undergoing percutaneous balloon valvuloplasty. *Circulation* 1990; 82: 448–56.

82 McConnell M, Solomon S, Rayan M, Come P, Goldhaber S, Lee R: Regional right ventricular dysfunction detected by echocardiography in acute pulmonary embolism. *Am J Cardiol* 1996; 78(4): 469–73.

83 Come P: Echocardiographic evaluation of pulmonary embolism and its response to therapeutic interventions [review]. *Chest* 1992; 101(4) (suppl): 151S–162S.

84 Schena M, Clini E, Errera D, Quadri A: Echo-Doppler evaluation of left ventricular impairment in chronic cor pulmonale. *Chest* 1996; 109(6): 1446–51.

85 Moser K, ed: Pulmonary vascular obstruction due to embolism and thrombosis. In: Moser K, ed., *Pulmonary Vascular Disease* (New York, Marcel Dekker, 1979), 341–86.

86 Worsley D, Alavi A, Palevsky H, Kundel H: Comparison of diagnostic performance with ventilation-perfusion lung imaging in different patient populations. *Radiology* 1996; 199: 481–3.

87 Investigators TP: Value of the ventilation/perfusion scan in acute pulmonary embolism: results of the prospective investigation of pulmonary embolism diagnosis (PIOPED). *JAMA* 1990; 263: 2753–59.

88 Powe J, Palevsky H, McCarthy K, Alavi A: Usefulness of lung scanning in the evaluation of patients with pulmonary arterial hypertension. *Radiology* 1987; 164: 727.

89 Greenspan R: Pulmonary angiography and the diagnosis of pulmonary embolism. *Prog Cardiovasc Dis* 1994; 37: 93–105.

90 Auger W, Feullo P, Moser K et al: Chronic major-vessel thromboembolic pulmonary artery obstruction: appearance at angiography. *Radiology* 1992; 182: 393.

91 Nicod P, Peterson K, Levine M et al: Pulmonary angiography in severe chronic pulmonary hypertension. *Ann Int Med* 1987; 107: 565–8.

92 Goodman L, Curtin J, Mewissen M et al: Detection of pulmonary embolism in patients with unresolved clinical and scintigraphic diagnosis: helical CT versus angiography. *Am J Radiol* 1995; 164: 1369–74.

93 Van Erkel A, Van Rossum A, Bloem J, Kierit J, Pattynama P: Spiral CT angiography for suspect pulmonary embolism: a cost-effectiveness analysis. *Radiology* 1996; 201: 29–36.

94 Gefter W, Hatabu H, Holland G, Gupta K, Henschke C, Palevsky H: Pulmonary thromboembolism: recent developments in diagnosis with CT and MRI imaging. *Radiology* 1995; 197: 561–74.

95 Meaney JFM, Weg JG, Chenevert TL, Stafford-Johnson D, Hamilton BH, Prince MR: Diagnosis of pulmonary embolism with magnetic resonance angiography. *N Engl J Med* 1997; 336:1422–7.

96 Abenheim L, Moride Y, Brenot F et al: Appetite-suppressant drugs and the risk of primary pulmonary hypertension. Internal Primary Pulmonary Hypertension Group. *N Engl J Med* 1996; 355(9): 609–16.

18

Perioperative echocardiography

Marvin L Appel, James Ayd and Eugenie S Heitmiller

Introduction

Intraoperative echocardiography was initially performed during cardiac surgery by placing a transducer directly on the heart.[1] This required either a sterile transducer or a sterile sheath to enclose the transducer. There were many inherent problems and limitations with on-the-heart imaging or 'epicardial echocardiography', including the inability to continuously monitor the heart during surgery. With the development of transesophageal echocardiography (TEE), intraoperative monitoring using continuous TEE imaging has rapidly increased over the past 10 years and has tremendously enhanced our understanding of cardiovascular events during both cardiac and noncardiac surgical procedures. The indications for using perioperative TEE are listed in Table 18.1.

This chapter reviews the more common uses of TEE in the operating room and the intensive care unit. The images used for the figures in this chapter were obtained from TEE studies performed at The Johns Hopkins Medical Institutions.

Table 18.1 Common indications for perioperative echocardiography.

Operative	*ICU*
Intracardiac air or embolism	Inadequate chest wall study
Masses	Low cardiac output
Myxomas	Tamponade
Thrombus	Acute valve dysfunction
Ventricular function	Vegetations
Wall motion abnormalities (ischemia)	Atrial thrombus
Assess valve structure and function	
Assess shunts and septal repairs	
Aortic aneurysm and dissections	

Intracardiac air detection

Air can enter the venous circulation under a variety of intraoperative circumstances. One frequently discussed example is the sitting craniotomy, in which low venous pressure at the operative site and non-collapsible veins create the potential for massive amounts of air to be entrained. Papadopoulos et al[2] found air in the right atrium by TEE in 76% of sitting posterior fossa craniotomies and 22% of sitting cervical laminectomies. Other non-cardiac operative settings in which air can enter the venous system include: liver transplantation with veno-venous bypass,[3,4] total hip arthroplasty,[5] and radical retropubic prostatectomy.[6]

Traditional ways of detecting intravenous air include: precordial Doppler sounds, an increase in end-tidal nitrogen, a decrease in end-tidal carbon dioxide, oxygen desaturation, and the development of pulmonary hypertension and systemic hypotension. When these methods are compared with TEE, studies show TEE to be the most sensitive for detecting air.[7] This is due to the extremely intense reflection of ultrasound by air, a characteristic used to great advantage in contrast echocardiography. TEE could detect an average of 0.19 ml/kg of air injected slowly (infusion rates ranging from 0.001 to 0.01 ml/kg per min), compared to 0.24 ml/kg of air detected by precordial Doppler.[8] When agitated saline was injected into seated human volunteers, both TEE Doppler and two-dimensional TEE were found to be more sensitive than precordial Doppler in detecting air bubbles.[9] However, Koishi et al,[10] were able to increase the sensitivity of the precordial Doppler to the level of TEE with additional signal processing of the precordial Doppler signal. Of interest is the finding that the sensitivity of TEE for venous air does not depend upon the use of nitrous oxide, although this has been found to increase the sensitivity of the end-tidal carbon dioxide monitor and new-onset pulmonary hypertension for detection of air embolism.[11]

Several studies have demonstrated the usefulness of TEE for detecting the presence of a patent foramen ovale (PFO) and shunting (Fig. 18.1). The incidence of a PFO has been reported to be as high as 25% by autopsy studies,[12] as well as by adult TEE studies.[13–15] In one study, contrast TEE detected a PFO in 50 of 238 patients compared with 45 of 238 by transthoracic echocardiography.[15] Paradoxical blood-flow (right to left), with potential embolization, can occur under conditions that increase right-sided pressures, such as the presence of positive end-expiratory pressure (PEEP), pulmonary hypertension, tamponade, Valsalva and coughing.[16,17] Thus, using TEE as a preliminary screen could define patients at risk for paradoxical embolism and result in modification of surgical or anesthetic technique. Patients with congenital heart disease who possess larger shunts than those presenting with a PFO may be monitored using TEE for venous air that may arise from the surgical field or from intravenous infusion therapy.

TEE is a sensitive monitor for air remaining in the heart or great vessels during open heart procedures. In addition, some air may be detectable in the right upper pulmonary vein, left ventricular apex, left atrium and pulmonary artery during coronary artery bypass grafting.[18] At The Johns Hopkins Medical Institutions, when a TEE probe is in place intra-operatively, it is routinely used to monitor the heart during de-airing maneuvers. Intracardiac air appears as bright, floating echogenic foci within the heart chambers and as stretches of increased echogenicity (brightness) along the endocardial surfaces (Fig. 18.2). Although it is clear that air is detected readily by TEE, the importance of this capability may depend on the clinical setting. In the case of a seated neurosurgical procedure where a small amount of air may be the forerunner of a sudden large and devastating air embolism, detection of microbubbles by TEE may be crucial. On the other hand, during cardiac surgery the technique is perhaps overly sensitive, detecting microbubbles which thus far have not been shown to be of any clinical significance. It remains a possibility, however, that more sensitive neuropsychological testing will uncover subtle deficits that could be attributed to the presence of even small amounts of left ventricular microbubbles after open-heart surgery.

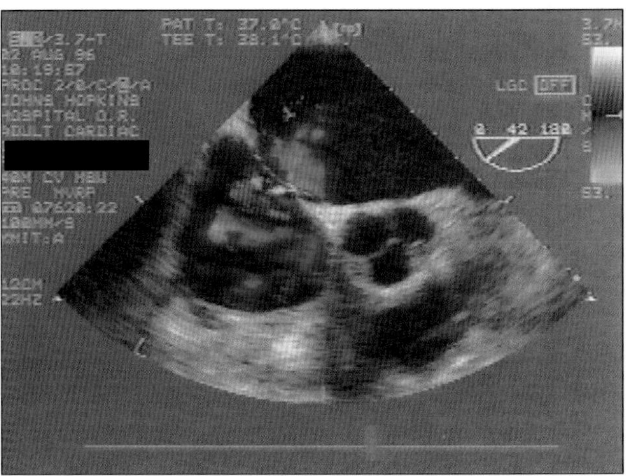

Figure 18.1
An omniplane color Doppler TEE scan of the basal short-axis view showing a small patent foramen ovale between the left atrium (at top of sector) and right atrium.

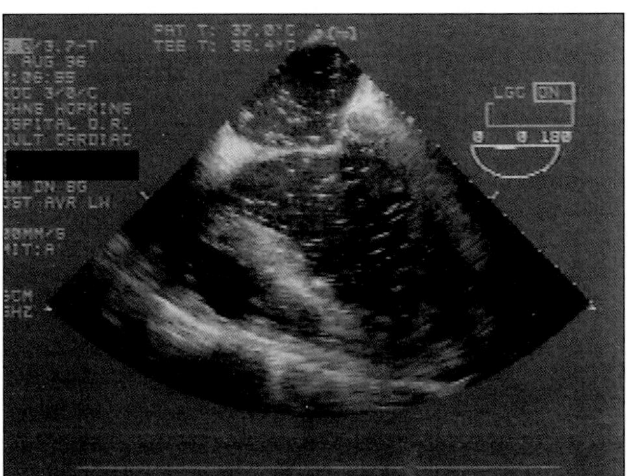

Figure 18.2
An omniplane 4-chamber TEE scan (horizontal plane) showing intracardiac air in the left heart chamber (left atrium at top of sector).

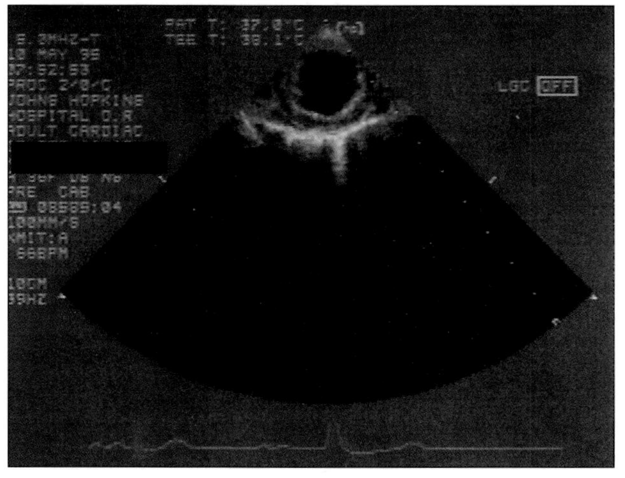

a

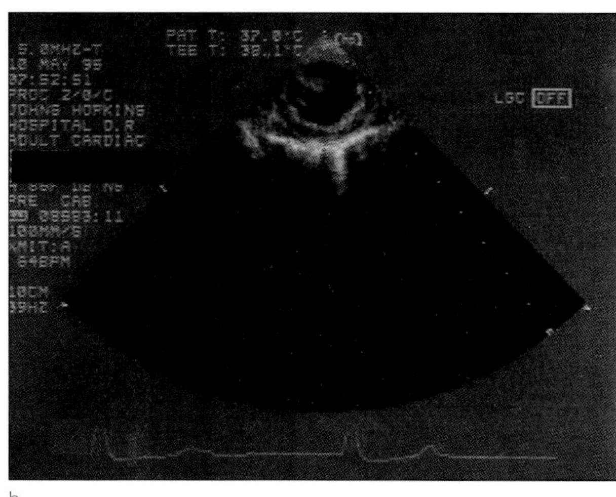

b

Figure 18.3
A single-plane TEE scan of the descending aorta displaying (a) moderate and (b) severe atheromatous changes.

TEE and disease of the thoracic aorta

Several studies have suggested that atheromatous disease detected by TEE of the aorta (Fig. 18.3) is associated with strokes and other embolic events in nonsurgical patients.[19–21] Two studies from the same group have correlated intraoperative assessment of aortic arch atheromas by TEE with the incidence of postoperative stroke.[22,23] Ribakove et al[22] performed TEE in 97 cardiac surgery patients, four of whom suffered intraoperative stroke. On the basis of palpation of the arch, all four stroke victims were felt to have mild atheromatous disease, but three of the four had mobile atheroma in the lumen seen on TEE. Of the 20 patients with protruding or mobile atheromata, 16 were felt to have mild atheromatous disease on the basis of palpation. Katz et al[23] reported that the surgeon's assessment of the aorta by palpation correlated with the degree of calcification seen on chest radiograph and on TEE, but not with the severity of atheromatous disease seen on TEE. This study found that the severity of aortic arch atheromata correlated with the incidence of intraoperative stroke, while a history of peripheral or cerebrovascular disease, presence of aortic calcification, age, duration of cardiopulmonary bypass, and presence of cardiac risk factors did not.

Despite the above findings, one study by Konstadt et al[24] demonstrated that biplane TEE did not detect severe atherosclerotic plaques in 5 of 14 patients who underwent epiaortic echocardiography. In addition, biplane TEE was unable to visualize a significant portion of the ascending aorta (because the large airways obstruct ultrasound transmission), and was able to visualize the aortic cannulation site in only 1 of 27 cardiac surgery patients studied. The authors concluded that TEE was not useful in guiding the placement of the aortic cannula in patients undergoing cardiopulmonary bypass. Thus far, no study has demonstrated an improved neurologic outcome when intraoperative TEE is used to modify the surgical procedure.

TEE has been used successfully in the evaluation of traumatic aortic injury. Smith et al[25] attempted TEE in 101 patients admitted to the emergency room with possible aortic rupture. The study could be completed in 93 of those patients; TEE was found to be 100% specific, 98% sensitive, and required less time and transport than the gold standard, aortography. There were no complications from TEE in this group of patients, with seven patients unable to tolerate the study and one patient with concurrent maxillofacial trauma that precluded attempting TEE. Buckmaster et al[26] reported a sensitivity of 100% and a specificity of 99% for TEE diagnosis of aortic rupture when performed in the operating room, emergency room, and intensive care unit (ICU), which compared favorably to a sensitivity of 73% and specificity of 99% for aortography judged against the ultimate intraoperative or post-mortem findings. TEE required an average of 30 min, compared with 74 min for aortography. Six of the 160 patients in this series did not tolerate TEE, and one developed aspiration pneumonitis. It is of interest to note that the presence of pre-existing atherosclerotic disease complicated the interpretation of the TEE studies.

TEE also has an important role in the evaluation of suspected aortic dissections. Previously, aortography was used to diagnose dissections. However, with the advent of TEE and magnetic resonance imaging (MRI), aortography has fallen out of favor. One study of 65 patients with aortic dissections (types I, II and III) all of whom preoperatively underwent both TEE and aortography, found a sensitivity of 77% for aortography and 97% for TEE. The two patients whose dissections did not appear on TEE had localized pathology in the ascending aorta that was obscured by the large airways.[27] Other reported sensitivities and specificities for single-plane TEE are 97% and 100%, respectively,[28] and for TTE are 99% and 98%, respectively.[29]

Studies comparing single-plane TEE and MRI have found MRI to be more sensitive and specific in diagnosing dissections. Laissey et al studied 41 patients with suspected aortic dissection with both biplane TEE and MRI.[30] The sensitivity and specificity of TEE were 86% and 90%, whereas for MRI both the sensitivity and specificity were 95%. It is noteworthy that in a subset of 10 patients who had undergone previous surgery for type A dissections, MRI was 100% sensitive and specific for recurrent dissection, while TEE was only 85% sensitive and 67% specific.[30] Another study of 53 patients with suspected aortic dissections reported a sensitivity and specificity of 100% for MRI, compared with a sensitivity of 100% and a specificity of 68% for TEE. The lower specificity of TEE resulted mainly from false-positive diagnoses of dissections in the ascending aorta.[31]

Despite the superior sensitivity and specificity of MRI over TEE in the diagnosis of aortic dissection, other considerations may sometimes favor the use of TEE. TEE requires less time than MRI and patient transport is unnecessary, making it more suitable for unstable patients.[30] One group has even suggested that the decrease in preoperative mortality of aortic dissection patients in their hands compared to earlier reports results from the faster progression to surgery that the initial evaluation with TEE permits.[32] Several of the studies already cited confirm that a principal weakness of TEE is the obscured view of the distal ascending aorta and proximal arch. The use of multiplane TEE and preoperative suprasternal and parasternal TEE mitigates this problem.[33] Additional information obtained from TEE, but not MRI, includes assessment of left ventricle (LV) function, regional wall motion abnormalities (RWMA), and a more accurate measure of aortic regurgitation. Even when the preoperative diagnosis of dissection is made by MRI, we routinely use intraoperative TEE in cases of aortic dissection to evaluate the degree of aortic regurgitation post-repair.

Intraoperative assessment of ventricular function

TEE can be used as an intraoperative monitor of volume status when rapid changes are anticipated. Iafrati et al[34] reported that TEE significantly altered the management of 9 of 17 patients undergoing thoracoabdominal aneurysm repair, and that concurrent pulmonary artery catheter monitoring failed to indicate hemodynamic derangements in six of these nine patients. The most common diagnosis made by TEE, but not by pulmonary artery catheter data, was a hyperdynamic and under-filled left ventricle. Similarly, Sutton and Cahalan[35] pointed out that left ventricular loading could be accurately assessed by TEE, but not by pulmonary artery catheter data, when left ventricular compliance was impaired, when right ventricular distension occurred, or when mitral valve disease was present.

Cheung et al[36] studied patients with either normal or reduced left ventricular function undergoing elective coronary artery bypass grafting (CABG), and found that left ventricular end-diastolic area (LVEDA), central venous pressure and pulmonary capillary wedge pressure all decreased linearly in response to graded acute hypovolemia induced by removing measured volumes of blood. The change in LVEDA was found to be 0.3 cm^2 per 1% of the estimated blood volume, and was the same regardless of left ventricular function. The baseline LVEDA was greater in patients with reduced left ventricular function, and the effect of acute hemorrhage might have been harder to detect visually by TEE. Although LVEDA is the preferred intraoperative estimate of left ventricle filling, many practitioners rely on left ventricular end-systolic cavity obliteration as a marker of hypovolemia. Leung and Levine[37] found that 80% of episodes of left ventricle cavity obliteration were associated with decreases in LVEDA (i.e. with decreased left ventricular filling), 10% were associated with increases in ejection fraction, and 10% were associated with small (<10%) increases in ejection fraction and small decreases in LVEDA.

Intracardiac masses

TEE is often used in the preoperative work-up of patients with intracardiac masses (Figs 18.4 and 18.5). Masses well visualized by TEE include thrombus[38–47] and myxomas.[48–53]

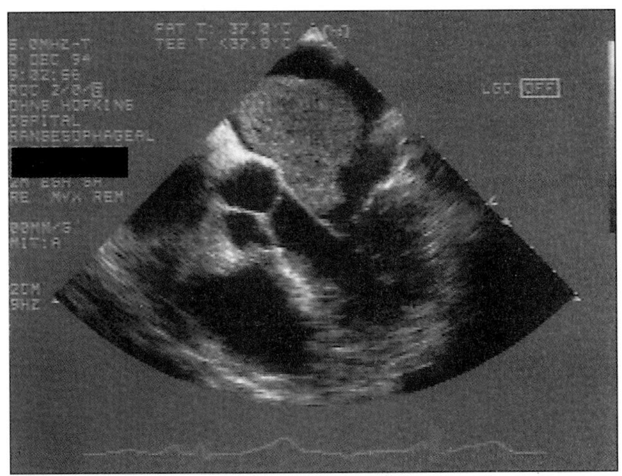

Figure 18.4
A 5-chamber single-plane TEE scan showing a large left atrial myxoma attached to the interatrial septum.

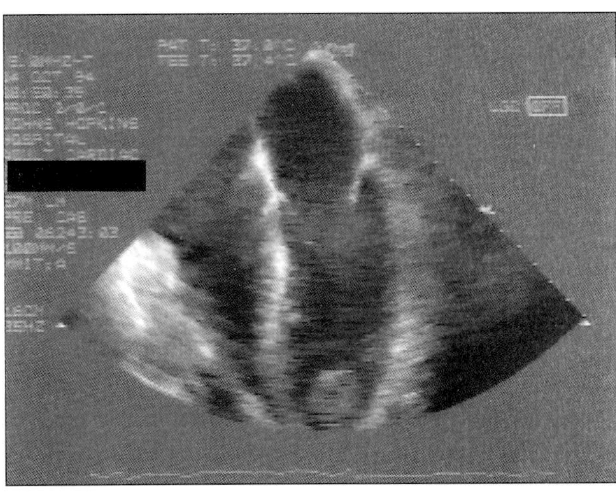

Figure 18.5
A 4-chamber single-plane TEE scan showing a large thrombus in the apex of the left ventricle.

Authors have also reported TEE visualization of intracardiac lymphoma,[54] primary left atrial leiomyosarcoma,[55] and intracardiac lipoma.[56] TEE has been shown to be superior to transthoracic echocardiography (TTE) in detecting left atrial thrombus,[45,57–59] cardiac sources of systemic emboli,[60,61] and in diagnosing thrombi and vegetations associated with indwelling central lines or pacing wires.[52] A series of six patients were reported to have TTE thought to be suggestive of right atrial mass lesions that on TEE were shown to be normal variants (Eustachian valves, Chiari network, thickened atrial septum).[63]

At The Johns Hopkins Medical Institutions, TEE is routinely used intraoperatively to verify the absence of residual intracardiac tumor following resection and to rule out valve or septum damage resulting from mass removal. Case reports have supported the use of TEE to assist in surgical decision-making, such as to guide the placement of right atrial purse string sutures in a patient with a large right atrial thrombosis of a peritoneovenous shunt[64] and to make the intraoperative diagnosis of pulmonary venous extension of a squamous cell lung cancer, resulting in modification of the operative procedure.[64,65] Preoperative work-up of this latter patient with TTE, chest radiography and chest computed tomography (CT) scan had not suggested the extent of the tumor.

Shunt lesions

Echocardiography provides valuable information when diagnosing shunt lesions (Fig. 18.6). There are several reports comparing the use of preoperative TTE and TEE in diagnosing the presence of intracardiac shunts.[66–71] Gorcsan et al[71] evaluated the impact of TEE as part of the preoperative evaluation of patients with severe pulmonary hypertension for lung transplantation. These patients had previously undergone right and left heart catheterizations, TTE, and radionucleotide ventriculography. The unsuspected TEE findings in their series (including PFO, atrial septal defect (ASD), ventricular septal defect (VSD), and double-outlet right ventricle) altered surgical therapy in 25% of patients studied. In a study of 41 patients with clinically suspected ASD, Kronzon et al[70] were able to visualize the ASD in all patients with TEE, but in only 33 (80%) with TTE. Six of the eight sinus venosus defects were missed with TTE.

In contrast to the differences in preoperative TTE and TEE, intraoperative epicardial echocardiography and TEE have been found to provide similar information. Roberson et al reported on the intraoperative use of single-plane TEE and epicardial echocardiography during ASD repair.[72] There were no differences in the findings using TEE or

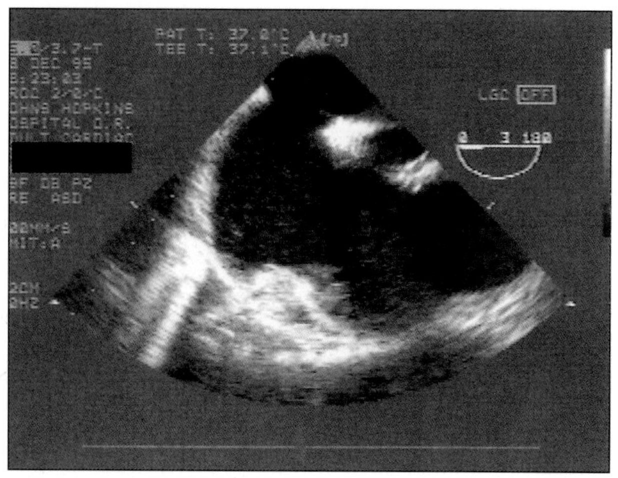

a

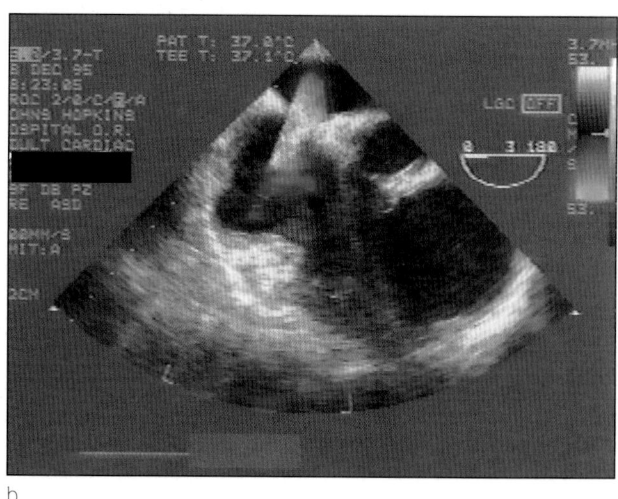

b

Figure 18.6
An atrial septal defect shown by: (a) an omniplane TEE scan (horizontal plane) and (b) color Doppler scan displaying shunting between the left and right atrium (left atrium at top of sector).

epicardial echocardiography in 13 patients. In 5 of 16 patients, findings on intraoperative echocardiography altered the surgical management. All of these findings involved structures that were obscured in the operative field by redundant valve tissue. Echocardiography documented successful repairs in all patients in this series before chest closure. It is noteworthy, however, that both TEE and epicardial echocardiography were unable to image anomalous pulmonary venous return (two complete and one partial) and an interrupted inferior vena cava in patients whose anatomy had been defined in the preoperative workup.[72]

The technology of the TEE probe has been rapidly advancing, and is being used with increasing frequency to evaluate the adequacy of shunt repairs in children. Pediatric biplane and multiplane TEE probes are now available for use in infants as small as 3 kg.[73] This technology has provided valuable information for the intraoperative management of these young patients.

Valvular heart disease

The use of intraoperative TEE during mitral valve replacements and repairs is standard practice at many institutions.[74–90] TEE is used during valve surgery to assess any of four possible intraoperative problems: paravalvular leaks, abnormal leaflet mobility, persistent intracardiac air, and circulatory impairment from other concurrent cardiac pathology.

In order to assess valve replacement, one must be familiar with the structure and function of the prosthetic valve. St Jude valves have a tiny gap at the center where the two disks meet and a gap at the periphery between the disk and the ring. This results in small, narrow regurgitant jets originating from within the valve ring (Fig. 18.7). As many as four jets can be seen. Bioprosthetic valves, such as the bovine pericardial valve, may have central jets, but these are smaller than those seen in mechanical valves. Small jets originating outside the valve ring (pinhole jets) (Fig. 18.8) may resolve spontaneously after protamine is given and do not necessitate revision of the valve replacement. Meloni et al[90] observed insignificant paraprosthetic jets in 14 of 27 mitral valve replacements with both mechanical and bioprosthetic valves.

Residual mitral regurgitation following mitral valve repair is evaluated by TEE prior to separation from cardiopulmonary bypass. If mitral regurgitation exceeds 'moderate', the repair may be revised or the mitral valve may be replaced (Fig. 18.9). The success rate of mitral valve repair depends in part on the initial pathology. Freeman et al[91] studied 143 patients undergoing mitral valve repair, and found that five needed further repair and five needed a mitral valve replacement on the basis of intraoperative TEE. Of the patients with isolated posterior mitral leaflet disease,

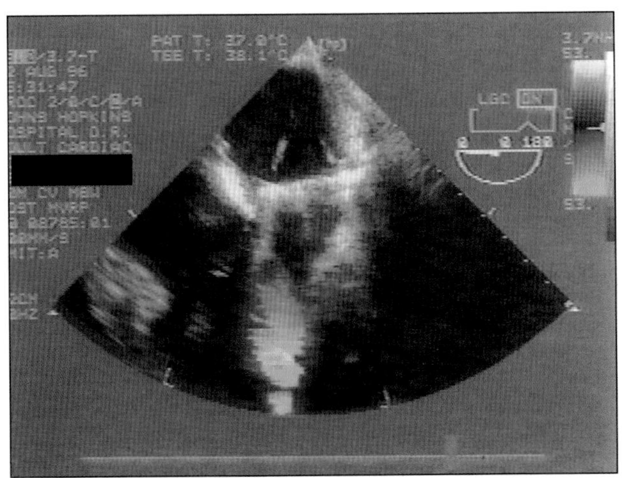

Figure 18.7
An omniplane color Doppler TEE scan (4-chamber view) showing two small regurgitant jets originating from within the valve ring of a St Jude prosthetic valve (left atrium at top of sector).

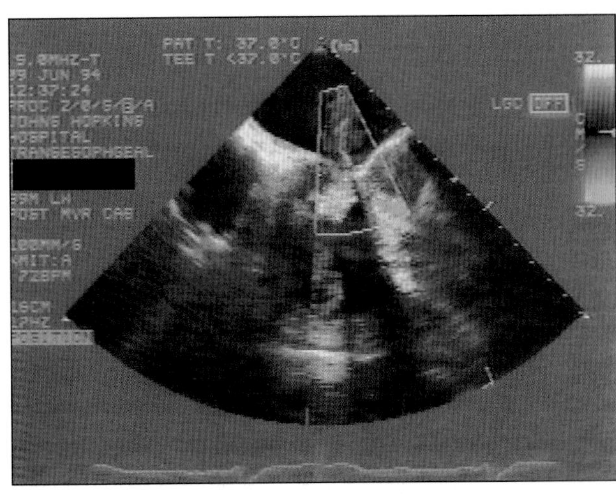

Figure 18.8
A single-plane 4-chamber TEE scan showing a small pinhole regurgitant jet into the left atrium after placement of a St Jude valve in the mitral position.

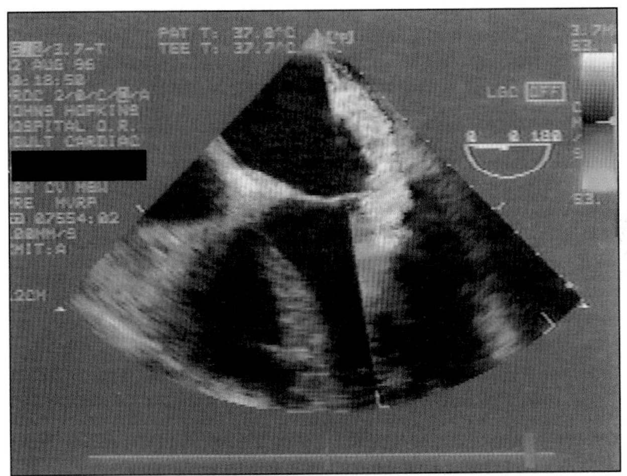

a

b

Figure 18.9
An omniplane TEE scan showing (a) severe mitral regurgitation pre-mitral valve repair and (b) moderate mitral regurgitation post-mitral valve repair. The patient went on to have a mitral valve replacement.

1.7% were left with moderate or worse mitral valve regurgitation following repair, compared with 22.5% of patients with anterior or bileaflet disease. In a different series of 50 patients undergoing isolated mitral valve repair, three required valve replacement or repeat repair on the basis of TEE.[92] Three of 36 patients who underwent a mitral valve repair in addition to another procedure had significant mitral valve regurgitation seen on TEE post-repair. Only one of the three patients needed a revision of the valve repair. The other two patients responded to measures to reduce systolic anterior motion of the mitral valve leaflet, which included increasing left ventricular volume, decreasing inotropy, and additional time on bypass to allow left ventricular recovery. The study concluded that

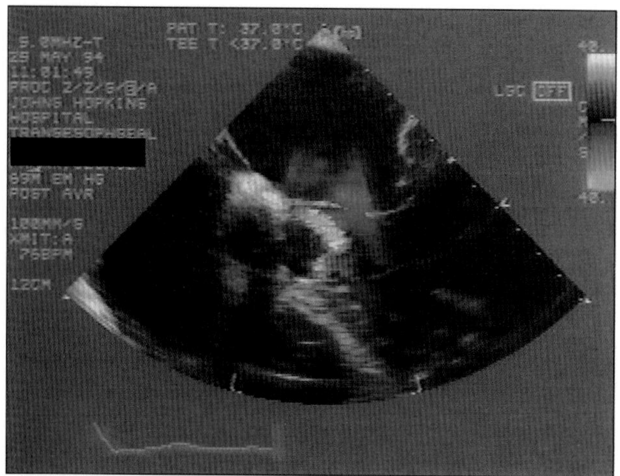

Figure 18.10
A single-plane color Doppler TEE scan showing a paravalvular leak around a St Jude valve in the aortic position.

intraoperative TEE was 'invaluable' during the post-bypass period.[92] DeSimone et al[93] reported that 2 of 10 patients undergoing mitral valve repair went on to valve replacement based on intraoperative TEE.

Some surgeons have employed intraoperative TEE to guide adjustable valve repairs. Gorton et al[94] found that adjusting a flexible mitral annuloplasty ring after it was sewn in place decreased residual mitral valve regurgitation in 9 of 20 patients. Kasegawa et al[95] adjusted the length of artificial chordae in anterior mitral leaflet repairs and checked the repair with TEE before typing down the sutures. DeSimone et al[96] reported the use of an adjustable tricuspid annuloplasty ring in 25 patients, where fine-tuning with TEE guidance decreased residual tricuspid valve regurgitation.

TEE has been found to be useful following aortic valve replacement for evaluating prosthetic valve dysfunction and paravalvular leak[97] (Fig. 18.10). It may also be used to assist in decision-making during aortic commissurotomy procedures. TEE was shown to help determine which commissurotomy patients ultimately required an aortic valve replacement due to aortic regurgitation.[93] Pretre and Faidutti[98] proposed that simple traumatic injuries involving only one cusp of the aortic valve are amenable to valve repair and that intraoperative TEE increased the safety of this approach. As experience with aortic valve repairs increases, the value of TEE in providing information which would affect the likelihood of a successful aortic valve repair will become more apparent.

Left ventricular outflow tract obstruction

Intraoperative echocardiography has been effective in guiding the surgical correction of left ventricular outflow tract obstruction (Fig. 18.11). When surgeons view the LV outflow tract using a transaortic approach, their direct visualization is limited. One study shows that findings on intraoperative TEE prompted a return to cardiopulmonary bypass in 8 of 27 patients. The echocardiographic findings included residual pressure gradient, ventricular septal defect and mitral valve dysfunction.[99] Another study using epicardial echocardiography in 50 patients reported that 20% of myectomy patients needed a second bypass run to correct residual gradients or mitral regurgitation.[100]

Ischemia detection

Initial studies on controlled reductions in coronary blood flow resulting in ischemia suggested that new, reversible RWMA appeared earlier and more reliably than ECG or hemodynamic changes. In dogs, for example, RWMA (measured by implanted transducers) appeared 1–10 min earlier than surface ECG changes following partial coronary artery occlusion. The smaller the disruption to coronary blood flow, the greater the delay in the appearance of ECG changes relative to RWMA.[101,102] The results in humans were similar. Hauser et al[102] used TTE to study patients undergoing percutaneous transluminal coronary angioplasty (PTCA) of stenotic vessels without collaterals. They found TTE detected RWMA with all balloon inflations, while ECG changes occurred only 30% of the time. Patients experienced angina in 41% of inflations. RWMA always occurred before either angina or ECG changes in instances when both were present. In a separate study using TTE on patients with uncollateralized, isolated left anterior descending coronary artery (LAD) lesions undergoing PTCA, RWMA appeared within 10 s after balloon inflation in all patients, while ST changes appeared at an average of 22 s in 90% of patients.[103]

The advent of TEE made it possible to compare intraoperative RWMA with ECG changes. Initial studies were done retrospectively,[104,105] with TEE and ECG recorded and analyzed off-line by blinded observers. Smith et al[104] studied 50 patients undergoing coronary artery bypass (CAB) surgery or major vascular surgery, and found that TEE detected 24 episodes of new RWMA. Only six of these 24 episodes generated diagnostic ECG changes, and in all six cases, the RWMA preceded the ECG changes. Leung et al[105] observed that 14% of new RWMA were accompanied by ECG changes, while 44% of ischemic ECG changes were accompanied by new RWMA. In that study, no significant hemodynamic changes were associated with

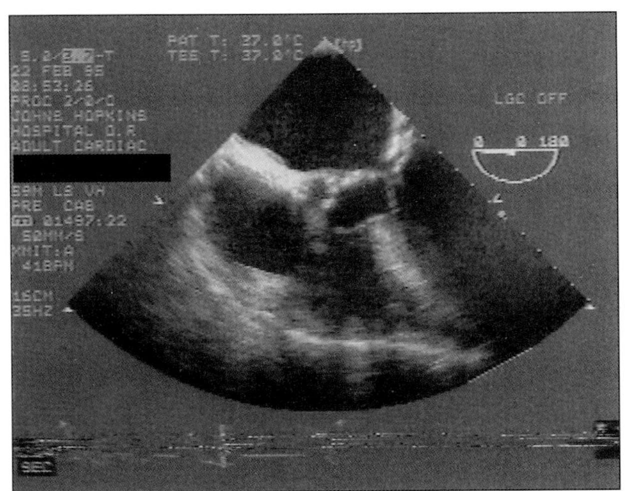

a

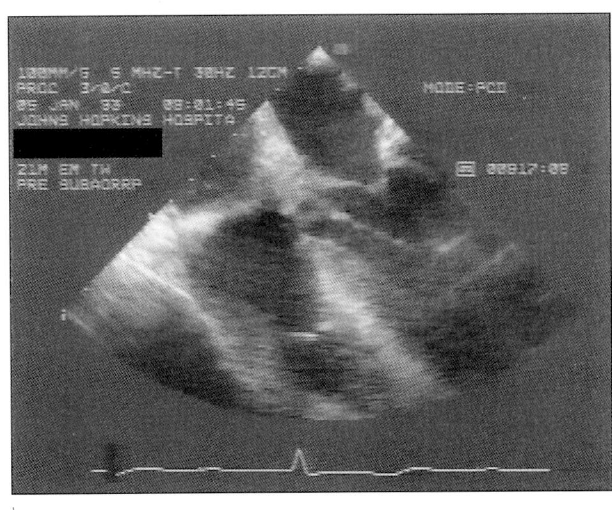

b

Figure 18.11
Left ventricular outflow obstruction seen by (a) an omniplane TEE scan showing systolic anterior motion of the mitral valve and (b) a single plane scan showing a subaortic membrane.

any of the RWMA or ECG changes. Both Smith et al and Leung et al found that new RWMA which persisted throughout the surgery were associated with adverse outcomes.

Consistent with the above studies is a case report of real-time monitoring of controlled ischemia in the operating room with TEE.[106] A vein graft was lacerated during pre-bypass dissection in a redo-CAB patient. It was noted that RWMA varied according to how much pressure the surgeon placed on the vein graft to stem bleeding during repair of the graft. Both the onset and resolution of ischemic ECG changes lagged minutes behind RWMA.

Although many current studies in the literature use RWMA as a gold standard for ischemia, or as one of a variety of markers for ischemia,[107–115] the intraoperative use of TEE as a real-time ischemia monitor may be problematic. Anesthesiologists were found to miss new intraoperative RWMA if the mid-papillary muscle short-axis view of the left ventricle was displayed continuously on a single screen.[114] If a divided screen was used to replay the baseline TEE and the current TEE simultaneously, RWMA recognition increased to 67%.[114]

Even if anesthesiologists could accurately detect all new RWMA while tending to other aspects of patient care, it is not clear that the improved detection of ischemia would affect the clinical outcome. Eisenberg et al[115] recorded 2-lead Holter ECG, 12-lead ECG and TEE during non-cardiac surgery in 285 patients. The Holter data were analyzed off-line, while the 12-lead ECG and the TEE data were analyzed in real time in the operating room. All results were unavailable to the patient care staff in the operating room. It was found that preoperative clinical data and off-line analysis of the Holter recordings predicted most of the postoperative cardiac complications, with TEE adding little predictive ability. However, in a univariate model, intraoperative ischemia increased the likelihood of postoperative cardiac complications. The off-line Holter analysis was most sensitive for ischemia, but the TEE was more sensitive than the 12-lead ECG when both were analyzed in real time. Although there are currently no outcome studies to support the use of TEE as an intraoperative ischemia monitor, its sensitivity is clearly superior to the routine monitors used presently.

Echocardiography in the intensive care unit

Echocardiography is used in the ICU to evaluate numerous clinical questions.[116–122] TEE has been shown to be safe and useful in the ICU, and can be used as an adjunct to TTE in patients who are difficult to image. Intubated patients receiving more than 10 cm of PEEP have uniformly poor TTE studies.[117] Patients who have undergone thoracic or cardiac surgical procedures may have dressings that interfere with TTE problems.[118] The reported frequencies of inadequate TTE studies in the ICU setting varies widely, from 5% to 75%.[119,120] TTE is often able to assess LV function and to detect pericardial effusion. When an echocardiogram is requested for other diagnoses (including hemodynamic instability, suspected cardiac source of emboli, suspected endocarditis, evaluation of valvular heart disease), several studies have shown that TEE more frequently answered the clinical question than TTE in patients who received both.[116,119,120–122] The general consensus is that ICU patients should first receive a TTE, because TTE will often successfully evaluate LV volume and function and the presence of pericardial effusion. If questions remain about the TTE findings, then TEE should be performed.

Complications of TEE

Many patients have undergone TEE without problems.[123–127] Studies examining the complication risk of TEE have been done mostly in nonoperative settings (i.e. outpatients, cardiac catheterization, and ICU patients). The risk of major complications has been reported to range from 0.18% to 0.5%, and the risk of death to be 0.04%.

A major concern is the existence of esophageal pathology. A history of dysphagia, esophageal strictures, esophageal tumors or previous esophageal surgery are usually contraindications to using TEE. One reported fatality associated with TEE was due to a bleeding complication resulting from a malignant lung tumor with esophageal infiltration.[123] A preliminary barium swallow has been recommended in some cases.[124] A hiatal hernia is not necessarily a contraindication unless it is severe, but it should be noted that due to the patient's anatomy, obtaining an adequate examination may be difficult or impossible.

The potential for gastrointestinal injury poses some concern, especially when the TEE probe is placed for intraoperative monitoring and is left for several hours. Animal and human studies have suggested that even prolonged pressure on the esophagus with a flexed probe does not result in histologic or gross injury.[128] However, the authors cautioned that potentially dangerous pressure may be generated in some cases in humans and that the TEE probe should not be fixed in a flexed position for prolonged periods. The potential of the TEE probe to damage the esophagus and upper gastrointestinal tract is illustrated by case reports of a Mallory–Weiss tear,[129] a hypopharynx perforation,[130] and a gastric laceration.[131] The Mallory–Weiss tear occurred during TEE monitoring in a patient who developed a coagulopathy while undergoing cardiac surgery.[129] The patient had a remote history of gastritis, but no known esophageal pathology, and the injury responded to conservative treatment. The patient with the hypopharynx perforation underwent surgical repair of the perforation after the completion of the cardiac surgical procedure.[130] Other case reports of upper gastrointestinal injury following intraoperative TEE include an esophageal perforation in a patient whose long history of dysphagia was unknown to the echocardiographer,[132] and kinking of the tip of the transesophageal probe which could be removed only with subsequent rigid esophagoscopy.[133]

Investigators have examined the association of intraoperative TEE and postoperative dysphagia. One study of 869 patients implicated TEE as an independent risk factor for postoperative swallowing dysfunction in cardiac surgery patients with a 7% incidence of dysphagia in patients who underwent intraoperative TEE compared to 4% in those who did not.[134] In contrast, a mixed prospective and retrospective study of 281 patients found no association between intraoperative TEE and dysphagia or upper gastrointestinal bleeding.[135]

Cervical disc disease also represents a relative contraindication because the TEE probe may exert undue continuous pressure on the posterior pharynx. Unilateral vocal cord paralysis has been reported when TEE has been used during operations with the patient in the sitting position with the neck flexed.[136] Recent experiences with smaller TEE probes has not reproduced this complication, although the safety of the larger omniplane probes now available has not been established for these types of operations.

Hemodynamic instability can accompany TEE examinations and, if easily corrected, may not always be reported as a complication. Stoddard and Longaker[137] retrospectively studied 566 patients; half were 70 years or older, and half were 50 years or younger. Most of the patients were not in an ICU. Transient hypotension developed in 5% of the elder group and in 1.5% of the younger group. In the elder group, one patient developed third degree heart block and another had a profound vasovagal reaction, while one of the younger patients had an episode of myocardial ischemia. At age 70 years or more, mechanical ventilation was an independent predictor of hypotension during TEE. A case of hypotension during intraoperative TEE in an infant with total anomalous pulmonary venous return has been reported; the hypotension was attributed to compression of the pulmonary venous confluence.[138]

Technical complications of intraoperative TEE studies include the inability to pass the TEE probe due to operator inexperience or patient anatomy,[123,124] placement of the TEE probe into the trachea,[139] and movement of an esophageal stethoscope placed adjacent to the TEE probe.[140] The esophageal stethoscope can be pushed into the stomach due to frictional contact with movement of the TEE probe, so it is usually advised that an esophageal stethoscope should *not* be used together with a TEE probe. Buckling of the tip of the TEE probe in the esophagus has been reported, even though the probe was able to be inserted without difficulty and the control knobs were in the release position.[133] In these patients, images could not be easily obtained, manipulation of the probe was difficult, resistance was felt when withdrawal of the probe was attempted and the knob controlling the flexion of the tip of the probe was fixed in the extreme anteflexion position.

In conclusion, the surface has barely been scratched of the potential applications of two-dimensional and Doppler echocardiographic techniques during the perioperative period. In particular, use of both echocardiography and Doppler in patients with congenital heart disease could allow intraoperative monitoring to a degree previously unavailable. Refinement of cardiac output measurements by Doppler, as well as increased acceptance of and familiarity with echocardiographic parameters, could decrease the need for invasive hemodynamic monitoring. Immediate assessment of surgical repairs could become commonplace. Three-dimensional imaging, myocardial textural analysis, and on-line tracking of cavity area are now commercially available. Intraoperative analysis of these exciting techniques remains for future investigators.

References

1 Strom J, Becker RM, Frishman W et al: Effects of hypothermic hyperkalemia arrest on ventricular performance during cardiac surgery: assessment of intraoperative echocardiography. *NY State J Med* 1978; **78**: 2210.

2 Papadopoulos G, Kuhly P, Brock M et al: Venous and paradoxical air embolism in the sitting position. A prospective study with transesophageal echocardiography. *Acta Neurochir* 1994; **126**: 140–3.

3 Murakana M, Shichino T, Hara Y et al: Prevention of venous air embolism related to veno-venous bypass during orthotopic liver transplantation. *Anesthesiology* 1992; **76**: 662–3 (letter).

4 Prager MC, Gregory GA, Ascher NL, Roberts JP: Massive venous air embolism during orthotopic liver transplantation. *Anesthesiology* 1990; **72**: 198–200.

5 Ereth MH, Weber JG, Abel MD et al: Cemented versus noncemented total hip arthroplasty—embolism, hemodynamics and intrapulmonary shunting. *Mayo Clin Proc* 1992; **67**: 1066–74.

6 Albin MS, Ritter RR, Reinhart R et al: Venous air embolism during radical retropubic prostatectomy. *Anes Analg* 1992; **74**: 151–3.

7 Akamatsu S, Terazawa E, Kagawa K et al: Evaluation of intraoperative transesophageal echocardiography. *J Cardiol* 1991; **26** (suppl) 103–8.

8 Glenski JA, Cucchiara RF, Michenfelder JD: Transesophageal echocardiography and transcutaneous O_2 and CO_2 monitoring for detection of venous air embolism. *Anesthesiology* 1986; **64**: 541–5.

9 Muzzu DA, Lasasso TJ, Black S et al: Comparison of a transesophageal and precordial ultrasonic Doppler sensor in the detection of venous air embolism. *Anes Analg* 1990; **70**: 103–4.

10 Koishi K, Sha M, Ohtaguro T et al: Power spectrum of experimental gas embolism in dogs and a new device for its detection. *Masui* 1993; **42**: 1541–7.

11 Losasso TJ, Black S, Muzzi DA et al: Detection and hemodynamic consequences of venous air embolism. Does nitrous oxide make a difference? *Anesthesiology* 1992; **77**: 148–52.

12 Hagen PT, Scholz DG, Edwards WD: Incidence and size of patent foramen ovale during the first ten decades of life: an autopsy study of 965 normal hearts. *Mayo Clin Proc* 1984; **59**: 17–20.

13 Bedell EA, Berge KH, Losasso TJ: Paradoxic air embolism during venous air embolism: transesophageal echocardiographic evidence of transpulmonary air passage. *Anesthesiology* 1994; **80**: 947–50.

14 Schwarz G, Fuchs G, Weihs W et al: Sitting position for neurosurgery: experience with preoperative contrast echocardiography in 301 patients. *J Neurosurg Anes* 1994; **6**: 83–8.

15 Hausmann D, Mugge A, Becht I, Daniel WG: Diagnosis of patent foramen ovale by transesophageal echocardiography and association with cerebral and peripheral embolic events. *Am J Cardiol* 1992; **70**: 668–72.

16 Konstadt SN, Louie EK, Black S et al: Intraoperative detection of patent foramen ovale by transesophageal echocardiography. *Anesthesiology* 1991; **74**: 212–16.

17 Langholz D, Louie EK, Konstadt SN et al: Transesophageal echocardiographic demonstration of distinct mechanisms for right to left shunting across a patent foramen ovale in the absence of pulmonary hypertension. *J Am Coll Cardiol* 1991; **18**: 1112–7.

18 Orihashi K, Matsuura Y, Hamanaka Y et al: Retained intracardiac air in open heart operations examined by transesophageal echocardiography. *Ann Thorac Surg* 1993; **55**: 1467–71.

19 Amerenco P, Cohen A, Tzourio C et al: Atherosclerotic disease of the aortic arch and the risk of ischemic stroke. *N Engl J Med* 1994; **331**: 1474–9.

20 Jones EF, Kalman JM, Calafiore P et al: Proximal aortic atheroma. An independent risk factor for cerebral ischemia. *Stroke* 1995; **26**: 218–24.

21 Tunick PA, Rosenzweig BP, Katz ES et al: High risk for vascular events in patients with protruding aortic atheromas: a prospective study. *J Am Coll Cardiol* 1994; **23**: 1084–90.

22 Ribakove GH, Katz ES, Galloway AC et al: Surgical implications of transesophageal echocardiography to grade the atheromatous aortic arch. *Ann Thorac Surg* 1992; **53**: 758–61.

23 Katz ES, Tunick PA, Risinek H et al: Protruding atheromas predict stroke in elderly patients undergoing cardiopulmonary bypass: experience with intraoperative transesophageal echocardiography. *J Am Coll Cardiol* 1992; **290**: 70–7.

24 Konstadt SN, Reich DL, Quintana C, Levy M: The ascending aorta: how much does transesophageal echocardiography see? *Anes Analg* 1994; **78**: 240–4.

25 Smith MD, Cassidy J, Souther S et al: Transesophageal echocardiography in the diagnosis of traumatic rupture of the aorta. *N Engl J Med* 1995; **332**: 356–62.

26 Buckmaster MJ, Kearney PA, Johnson SB et al: Further experience with transesophageal echocardiography in the evaluation of thoracic aortic injury. *J Trauma* 1994; **37**: 989–95.

27 Bansal RC, Chandrasekaran K, Ayala K, Smith DC: Frequency and explanation of false negative diagnosis of aortic dissection by aortography and transesophageal echocardiography. *J Am Coll Cardiol* 1995; **25**: 1393–401.

28 Ballal RS, Nanda NC, Gatewood R: Usefulness of transesophageal echocardiography in assessment of aortic dissection. *Circulation* 1991; **894**: 1903–14.

29 Erbel R, Engberding R, Daniel W et al: Echocardiography in diagnosis of aortic dissection. *Lancet* 1989; **I**: 457–61.

30 Laissey JP, Blanc F, Soyer P et al: Thoracic aortic dissection: diagnosis with transesophageal echocardiography versus MR imaging. *Radiology* 1995; **194**: 331–6.

31 Nienaber CA, Spielmann RP, von Kodolitsch Y et al: Diagnosis of thoracic aortic dissection: magnetic resonance imaging versus transesophageal echocardiography. *Circulation* 1992; **85**: 434–47.

32 Erbel R, Oelert H, Meyer J et al: Effect of medical and surgical therapy on aortic dissection evaluated by transesophageal echocardiography: implications for prognosis and therapy. *Circulation* 1993; **87**: 1604–15.

33 Blanchard DG, Kimura BJ, Dittrich HC, DeMaria AN: Transesophageal echocardiography of the aorta. *JAMA* 1994; **272**: 546–51.

34 Iafrati MD, Gordon G, Staples MH et al: Transesophageal echocardiography for hemodynamic management of thoracoabdominal aneurysm repair. *Am J Surg* 1993; **166**: 179–85.

35 Sutton DC, Cahalan MK: Intraoperative assessment of left ventricular function with transesophageal echocardiography. *Cardiol Clin* 1993; **11**: 389–98.

36 Cheung AT, Savino JS, Weiss SJ et al: Echocardiographic and hemodynamic indexes of left ventricular preload in patients with normal and abnormal ventricular function. *Anesthesiology* 1994; **81**: 376–87.

37 Leung JM, Levine EH: Left ventricular end-systolic cavity obliteration as an estimate of intraoperative hypovolemia. *Anesthesiology* 1994; **81**: 1102–9.

38 Cohen GI, Klein AL, Chan KL et al: Transesophageal echocardiographic diagnosis of right-sided cardiac masses in patients with central lines. *Am J Cardiol* 1992; **70**: 925–9.

39 Hwang JJ, Kuan P, Lin SC et al: Reappraisal by transesophageal echocardiography of the significance of left atrial thrombi in the prediction of systemic arterial embolization in rheumatic mitral valve disease. *Am J Cardiol* 1992; **70**: 769–73.

40 Guindo J, Montagud M, Carreras F et al: Fibrinolytic therapy for superior vena cava and right atrial thrombosis: diagnosis and follow-up with biplane transesophageal echocardiography. *Am Heart J* 1992; **124**: 510–13.

41 Kuo CT, Chiang CW, Lee YS et al: Left atrial ball thrombus in nonrheumatic atrial fibrillation diagnosed by transesophageal echocardiography. *Am Heart J* 1992; **123**: 1394–7.

42 Pasierski TJ, Alton ME, van Fossen DB et al: Right atrial mobile thrombus; improved visualization by transesophageal echocardiography. *Am Heart J* 1992; **123**: 802–3.

43 Fyfe DA, Kline CH, Sade RM et al: Transesophageal echocardiography detects thrombus formation not identified by transthoracic echocardiography after the Fontan operation. *J Am Coll Cardiol* 1991; **18**: 1733–7.

44 Aschenberg W, Schluter M, Kremer P et al: Transesophageal two-dimensional echocardiography for the detection of left atrial appendage thrombus. *J Am Coll Cardiol* 1986; **7**: 163–6.

45 Daniel WG, Nikutta P, Schroder E, Nellessen U: Transesophageal echocardiographic detection of left atrial appendage thrombi in patients with unexplained arterial embolism. *Circulation* 1986; **74**: (suppl II): 391.

46 Nellessen U, Daniel WG, Matheis G et al: Impeding paradoxical embolism from atrial thrombus: correct

diagnosis by transesophageal echocardiography and prevention by surgery. *J Am Coll Cardiol* 1985; **5**: 1002–4.

47 Goldman ME, Mindich BP: Intraoperative two-dimensional echocardiography: new application of an old technique. *J Am Coll Cardiol* 1986; **7**: 374–82.

48 Gorcsan J, Blanc MS, Reddy PS et al: Hemodynamic diagnosis of mitral valve obstruction by left atrial myxoma with transesophageal continuous wave Doppler. *Am Heart J* 1992; **124**: 1109–12.

49 Aru GM, Cattolica FS, Cardu G et al: A fractured and detached right atrial myxoma: an unusual and threatening condition detected by intraoperative transesophageal echocardiography. *J Thorac Cardiovasc Surg* 1992; **104**: 215–17.

50 Samdarshi TE, Mahan EF, Nanda NC et al: Transesophageal echocardiographic diagnosis of multicentric left ventricular myxomas mimicking a left atrial tumor. *J Thorac Cardiovasc Surg* 1992; **103**: 471–4.

51 Fyke FE: Transesophageal echocardiography and cardiac masses. *Mayo Clin Proc* 1991; **66**: 1101–9.

52 Rey M, Tunon J, Compres H et al: Prolapsing right atrial myxoma evaluated by transesophageal echocardiography. *Am Heart J* 1991; **122**: 875–7.

53 Mora F, Mindich BP, Guarino T, Goldman ME: Improved surgical approach to cardiac tumors with intraoperative two-dimensional echocardiography. *Chest* 1987; **91**: 142–4.

54 Moore JA, DeRan BP, Minor R et al: Transesophageal echocardiographic evaluation of intracardiac lymphoma. *Am Heart J* 1992; **124**: 514–16.

55 Nguyen KT, Mak K, Sanfilippo AJ et al: Primary left atrial leiomyosarcoma simulating pulmonary thromboembolism. *Can Assn Radio J* 1993; **45**: 48–51.

56 Tuna IC, Julsrud PR, Click RL et al: Tissue characterization of an unusual right atrial mass by magnetic resonance imaging. *Mayo Clin Proc* 1991; **66**: 498–501.

57 Mugge A, Daniel WG, Haverich A et al: Diagnosis of noninfective cardiac mass lesions by two-dimensional echocardiography: comparison of the transthoracic and transesophageal approaches. *Circulation* 1991; **83**: 70–8.

58 Kronzon I, Tunick PA, Glassman E et al: Transesophageal echocardiography to detect atrial clots in candidates for percutaneous transseptal mitral balloon valvuloplasty. *J Am Coll Cardiol* 1990; **16**: 1320–2.

59 Mugge A, Daniel WG, Hausmann D et al: Diagnosis of left atrial appendage thrombi by transesophageal echocardiography: clinical implications and follow-up. *Am J Card Imag* 1990; **4**: 173–9.

60 Dressler FA, Labovitz AJ: Systemic arterial emboli and cardiac masses. Assessment with transesophageal echocardiography. *Cardiol Clin* 1993; **11**: 447–60.

61 Pearson AC, Labovitz AJ, Tatineni S, Gomez CR: Superiority of transesophageal echocardiography in detecting cardiac source of embolism in patients with cerebral ischemia of uncertain etiology. *J Am Coll Cardiol* 1991; **17**: 66–72.

62 Cohen GI, Klein AL, Chan KL et al: Transesophageal echocardiographic diagnosis of right-sided cardiac masses in patients with central lines. *Am J Cardiol* 1992; **70**: 925–9.

63 Alam M, Sun I, Smith S: Transesophageal echocardiographic evaluation of right atrial mass lesions. *J Am Soc Echocardiogr* 1991; **4**: 331–7.

64 Holman WL, Coghlan CH, Dodson MR et al: Removal of massive right atrial thrombus guided by transesophageal echocardiography. *Ann Thorac Surg* 1991; **52**: 313–15.

65 Suriani R, Konstadt S, Camunas J, Goldman M: Transesophageal echocardiographic detection of left atrial involvement of a lung tumor. *J Cardiothor Vas Anes* 1993; **7**: 73–5.

66 Chen WJ, Chen JJ, Lin SC et al: Detection of cardiovascular shunts by transesophageal echocardiography in patients with pulmonary hypertension of unexplained cause. *Chest* 1995; **107**: 8–13.

67 Belkin RN, Pollack BD, Ruggiero ML et al: Comparison of transesophageal and transthoracic echocardiography with contrast and color flow Doppler in the detection of patent foramen ovale. *Am Heart J* 1994; **128**: 520–5.

68 Konstantinides S, Kasper W, Geibel A et al: Detection of left-to-right shunt in atrial septal defect by negative contrast echocardiography: a comparison of transthoracic and transesophageal approach. *Am Heart J* 1993; **126**: 909–17.

69 deBelder MA, Tourikis L, Griffith M et al: Transesophageal contrast echocardiography and color flow mapping: methods of choice for the detection of shunts at the atrial level? *Am Heart J* 1992; **124**: 1545–50.

70 Kronzon I, Tunick PA, Freedberg RS et al: Transesophageal echocardiography is superior to transthoracic echocardiography in the diagnosis of sinus venosus atrial septal defect. *J Am Coll Cardiol* 1991; **17**: 537–42.

71 Gorcsan J, Edwards TD, Ziady GM et al: Transesophageal echocardiography to evaluate patients with severe pulmonary hypertension for lung transplantation. *Ann Thorac Surg* 1995; **59**: 717–22.

72 Roberson DA, Muhiudeen IA, Silverman NH et al: Intraoperative transesophageal echocardiography of atrioventricular septal defect. *J Am Coll Cardiol* 1991; **18**: 537–45.

73 Fyfe DA, Ritter SB, Snider RA et al: Guidelines for transesophageal echocardiography in children. *J Am Soc Echocardiogr* 1992; **5**: 640–4.

74 Goldman ME, Mindich BP: Intraoperative two-dimensional echocardiography: new application of an old technique. *J Am Coll Cardiol* 1986; **7**: 374–82.

75 Mindich BP, Goldman ME, Fuster V et al: Improved intraoperative evaluation of mitral valve operations utilizing two-dimensional contrast echocardiography. *J Thorac Cardiovasc Surg* 1985; **90**: 112–18.

76 Johnson ML, Holmes JH, Spangler RD, Paton BC: Usefulness of echocardiography in patients undergoing mitral valve surgery. *J Thorac Cardiovasc Surg* 1972; **64**: 922–34.

77 Drexler M, Oelert H, Dahm M et al: Assessment of successful valve reconstruction by intraoperative transesophageal echocardiography. *Circulation* 1986; **74**: II-390.

78 Freeman WK, Schaff HV, Khandheria BK et al: Intraoperative evaluation of mitral valve regurgitation and repair by transesophageal echocardiography: incidence and significance of systolic anterior motion. *J Am Coll Cardiol* 1992; **20**: 599–609.

79 Reichert SL, Visser CA, Moulijn AC et al: Intraoperative transesophageal color-coded Doppler echocardiography for evaluation of residual regurgitation after mitral valve repair. *J Thorac Cardiovasc Surg* 1990; **100**: 756–61.

80 Wolfe WG, Kisslo J: The utility of transesophageal echocardiography and Doppler color flow imaging in patients undergoing cardiac/valve surgery. *J Am Coll Cardiol* 1990; **15**: 363–72.

81 Castello R, Lenzen P, Aguirre F et al: Quantitation of mitral regurgitation by transesophageal echocardiography with Doppler color flow mapping: correlation with cardiac catheterization. *J Am Coll Cardiol* 1992; **19**: 1516–21.

82 Herrera CJ, Chaudhry FA, DeFrino PF et al: Value and limitations of transesophageal echocardiography in evaluating prosthetic or bioprosthetic valve dysfunction. *Am J Cardiol* 1992; **69**: 697–9.

83 Dzavik V, Cohen G, Chan KL: Role of transesophageal echocardiography in the diagnosis and management of prosthetic valve thrombosis. *J Am Coll Cardiol* 1991; **18**: 1829–33.

84 Chen YT, Kan MN, Chen JS: Detection of prosthetic mitral valve leak: a comparative study using transesophageal echocardiography, transthoracic echocardiography, and auscultation. *J Clin Ultrasound* 1990; **18**: 557–61.

85 Sheikh KH, Bengtson JR, Rankin JS et al: Intraoperative transesophageal Doppler color flow imaging used to guide patient selection and operative treatment of ischemic mitral regurgitation. *Circulation* 1991; **84**: 594–604.

86 Kyo S, Takamoto S, Matsumura M et al: Immediate and early postoperative evaluation of results of cardiac surgery by transesophageal two-dimensional Doppler echocardiography. *Circulation* 1987; **76**: V-113.

87 Maurer G, Czer LSC, Chauz A et al: Intraoperative Doppler color flow mapping for assessment of valve repair for mitral regurgitation. *Am J Cardiol* 1987; **60**: 333–7.

88 Seward JB, Khandheria BK, Edwards WD et al: Biplanar transesophageal echocardiography: anatomic correlations, image orientation, and clinical applications. *Mayo Clin Proc* 1990; **65**: 1193–213.

89 Takamoto S, Kyo S, Adachi H et al: Intraoperative color flow mapping by real-time two-dimensional Doppler echocardiography for evaluation of valvular and congenital heart disease and vascular disease. *J Thorac Cardiovasc Surg* 1985; **90**: 802–12.

90 Meloni L, Aru G, Abbruzzese PA et al: Regurgitant flow of mitral valve prostheses: an intraoperative transesophageal echocardiographic study. *J Am Soc Echocardiogr* 1994; **7**: 36–46.

91 Freeman WK, Schaf HV, Khandheria BK et al: Intraoperative evaluation of mitral valve regurgitation and repair by transesophageal echocardiography: incidence and significance of systolic anterior motion. *J Am Coll Cardiol* 1992; **20**: 599–609.

92 Guyton SW, Paull DL, Anderson RP: Mitral valve reconstruction. *Am J Surg* 1992; **163**: 497–501.

93 DeSimone R, Lange R, Saggau W et al: Intraoperative transesophageal echocardiography for the evaluation of mitral, aortic and tricuspid valve repair. A tool to optimize surgical outcome. *Eur J Cardiovasc Surg* 1992; **6**: 665–73.

94 Gorton ME, Piehler JM, Killen DA et al: Mitral valve repair using a flexible and adjustable annuloplasty ring. *Ann Thorac Surg*1993; **55**: 860–3.

95 Kasegawa H, Kamata S, Hirata S et al: Simple method for determining proper length of artificial chordae in mitral valve repair. *Ann Thorac Surg* 1994; **57**: 237–8.

96 DeSimone R, Lange R, Tanzeem A et al: Adjustable tricuspid valve annuloplasty assisted by intraoperative transesophageal color Doppler echocardiography. *Am J Cardiol* 1993; **71**: 926–31.

97 Deutsch HJ, Curtius JM, Leischik R et al: Diagnostic value of transesophageal echocardiography in cardiac surgery. *Thorac Cardiovasc Surg* 1991; **39**: 199–204.

98 Pretre R, Faidutti B: Surgical management of aortic valve injury after nonpenetrating trauma. *Ann Thorac Surg* 1993; **56**: 1426–31.

99 Stevenson JG, Sorensen GK, Gartman DM et al: Left ventricular outflow tract obstruction: an indication for intraoperative transesophageal echocardiography. *J Am Soc Echocardiogr* 1993; **6**: 525–35.

100 Marwick TH, Stewart WJ, Lever HM et al: Benefits of intraoperative echocardiography in the surgical management of hypertropic cardiomyopathy. *J Am Coll Card* 1992; **20**: 1066–72.

101 Battler A, Froelicher VG, Gallagher KP et al: Dissociation between regional myocardial dysfunction and ECG changes during ischemia in the conscious dog. *Circulation* 1980; **62**: 735–44.

102 Hauser AM, Gangadharan V, Ramos RG et al: Sequence of mechanical, electrocardiographic and clinical effects of repeated coronary artery occlusion in human beings: echocardiographic observations during coronary angioplasty. *J Am Coll Cardiol* 1985; **5**: 193–7.

103 Wohlgelemter D, Jaffe CC, Cabin HS et al: Silent ischemia during coronary occlusion produced by balloon inflation: relation to regional myocardial dysfunction. *J Am Coll Cardiol* 1987; **10**: 491–8.

104 Smith JS, Cahalan MK, Benefiel DJ et al: Intraoperative detection of myocardial ischemia in high-risk patients: electrocardiography versus two-dimensional transesophageal echocardiography. *Circulation* 1985; **72**: 1015–21.

105 Leung JM, O'Kelly B, Browner WS et al: Prognostic importance of postbypass regional wall-motion abnormalities in patients undergoing coronary artery bypass graft surgery. SPI Research Group. *Anesthesiology* 1989; **71**: 16–25.

106 Hong YW, Orihashi K, Cochran T et al: Detection of myocardial ischemia by transesophageal echocardiography during vein graft repair. *J Cardiothorac Vas Anes* 1991; **5**: 489–501.

107 Kamp O, deCock CC, van Eenige MJ, Visser CA: Influence of pacing-induced myocardial ischemia on left atrial regurgitant jet: a transesophageal echocardiographic study. *J Am Coll Cardiol* 1994; **23**: 1584–91.

108 Saada M, Catoire P, Bonnet F et al: Effect of thoracic epidural anesthesia combined with general anesthesia on segmental wall motion assessed by transesophageal echocardiography. *Anes Analg* 1992; **75**: 329–35.

109 Leung JM, Hollengerg M, O'Kelly BF et al: Effects of steal-prone anatomy on intraoperative myocardial ischemia. The SPI Research Group. *J Am Coll Cardiol* 1992; **20**: 1205–12.

110 Harris SN, Gordon MA, Urban MK et al: The pressure rate quotient is not an indicator of myocardial ischemia in humans. An echocardiographic evaluation. *Anesthesiology* 1993; **78**: 242–50.

111 Keupski WC, Layug EL, Reilly LM et al: Comparison of cardiac morbidity between aortic and infrainguinal operations. The SPI Research Group. *J Vasc Surg* 1992; **15**: 354–63.

112 Leung JM, Goehner P, O'Kelly BF et al: Isoflurane anesthesia and myocardial ischemia: comparative risk versus sufentanil anesthesia in patients undergoing coronary artery bypass graft surgery. The SPI Research Group. *Anesthesiology* 1991; **74**: 838–47.

113 Mangano DT, London MJ, Tubau JF et al: Dipyridamole thallium-201 scintigraphy as a preoperative screening test. A reexamination of its predictive potential. The SPI Research Group. *Circulation* 1991; **84**: 493–502.

114 Saada M, Cahalan MK, Lee E et al: Real-time evaluation of echocardiograms. *Anesthesiology* 1989; **71**: A344 (abstract).

115 Eisenberg MJ, London MJ, Leung JM et al: Monitoring for myocardial ischemia during noncardiac surgery. A technology assessment of transesophageal echocardiography and 12-lead electrocardiography. SPI Research Group. *JAMA* 1992; **268**: 210–16.

116 Chenzbraun A, Pinto FJ, Schnittger I: Transesophageal echocardiography in the intensive care unit: impact on diagnosis and decision-making. *Clin Cardiol* 1993; **17**: 438–44.

117 Parker MM, Cunnion RE, Parrillo JE: Echocardiography and nuclear cardiac imaging in the critical care unit. *JAMA* 1985; **254**: 2935–9.

118 Kyo S, Takamoto S, Matsumura M et al: Immediate and early postoperative evaluation of results of cardiac surgery by transesophageal two-dimensional Doppler echocardiography. *Circulation* 1987; **76**: V-113.

119 Vignon P, Mentec H, Terre S et al: Diagnostic accuracy and therapeutic impact of transthoracic and transesophageal echocardiography in mechanically ventilated patients in the ICU. *Chest* 1993; **106**: 1829–34.

120 Khoury AF, Afridi I, Quinones MA, Zoghbi WA: Transesophageal echocardiography in critically ill patients: feasibility, safety, and impact on management. *Am Heart J* 1994; **127**: 1363–71.

121 Hwang JJ, Shuy KG, Chen JJ et al: Usefulness of transesophageal echocardiography in the treatment of critically ill patients. *Chest* 1993; **104**: 861–6.

122 Foster E, Schiller NB: The role of transesophageal echocardiography in critical care: UCSF experience. *J Am Soc Echocardiogr* 1992; **5**: 368–74.

123 Daniel WG, Erbel R, Kasper W et al: Safety of transesophageal echocardiography. A multicenter survey of 10,419 examinations. *Circulation* 1991; **83**: 817–21.

124 Chan KL, Cohen GI, Sochowski RA, Baird MG: Complications of transesophageal echocardiography in ambulatory adult patients: analysis of 1500 consecutive examinations. *J Am Soc Echocardiogr* 1991; **4**: 577–82.

125 Ritter SB: Transesophageal real-time echocardiography in infants and children with congenital heart disease. *J Am Coll Cardiol* 1991; **18**: 569–80.

126 Kearney PA, Smith DW, Johnson SB et al: Use of transesophageal echocardiography in the evaluation of traumatic aortic injury. *J Trauma* 1993; **34**: 696–701.

127 Shapiro MJ, Yanofsky SD, Trapp J et al: Cardiovascular evaluation in blunt thoracic trauma using transesophageal echocardiography. *J Trauma* 1991; **31**: 835–40.

128 O'Shea JP, Southern JF, D'Ambra MN et al: Effects of prolonged transesophageal echocardiographic imaging and probe manipulation on the esophagus: an echocardiographic–pathologic study. *J Am Coll Cardiol* 1991; **17**: 1426–9.

129 Dewhirst WE, Stragand JJ, Fleming BM: Mallory–Weiss tear complicating intraoperative transesophageal echocardiography in a patient undergoing aortic valve replacement. *Anesthesiology* 1990; **72**: 777–8.

130 Spahn DR, Schmid S, Carrel T et al: Hypopharynx perforation by a transesophageal echocardiography probe. *Anesthesiology* 1995; **82**: 581–3.

131 Latham P, Hodgins LR: A gastric laceration after transesophageal echocardiography in a patient undergoing aortic valve replacement. *Anes Analg* 1995; **81**: 641–2.

132 Yasick A, Samra SK: An unusual complication of transesophageal echocardiography. *Anes Analg* 1995; **81**: 657–8.

133 Kronzon I, Cziner DG, Katz ES et al: Buckling of the tip of the transesophageal echocardiography probe: a potentially dangerous technical malfunction. *J Am Soc Echocardiogr* 1992; **5**: 176–7.

134 Hogue CW Jr, Lappas GD, Creswell LL et al: Swallowing dysfunction after cardiac operations. Associated adverse outcomes and risk factors including intraoperative transesophageal echocardiography. *J Thorac Cardiovasc Surg* 1995; **110**: 517–22.

135 Hulyalkar AR, Ayd J: Low risk of gastroesophageal injury associated with transesophageal echocardiography during cardiac surgery. *Cardiothorac Vasc Anes* 1993; **7**: 175–7.

136 Cucchiara RF, Nugent M, Seward JB, Messick JM: Air embolism in upright neurosurgical patients: detection and localization by two-dimensional transesophageal echocardiography. *Anesthesiology* 1984; **60**: 353–5.

137 Stoddard MF, Longaker RA: The safety of transesophageal echocardiography in the elderly. *Am Heart J* 1993; **125**: 1358–62.

138 Frommelt PC, Stuth EA: Transesophageal echocardiography in total anomalous pulmonary venous drainage: hypotension caused by comparession of the pulmonary venous confluence during probe passage. *J Am Soc Echocardiogr* 1994; **7**: 652–4.

139 Fagan LF Jr, Weiss R, Castello R, Labovita AJ: Transtracheal placement and imaging with a transesophageal echocardiographic probe. *Am J Cardiol* 1991; **67**: 909–10.

140 Humphrey LS: Esophageal stethoscope loss complicating transesophageal echocardiography. *J Cardiothorac Anes* 1988; **2**: 356.

19

Aortic dissection

Christopher M Kramer

Introduction

Pathophysiology

Aortic dissection is precipitated by a tear in the aortic intima which allows blood to separate the intima from the adventitia in a course along the aortic media.[1] In the classic study by Hirst et al,[2] 4% of patients had no intimal tear, but more recent studies suggest that essentially all cases are associated with such a tear.[3] Of the tears, 70% occur in the ascending aorta just above the aortic valve, 10% in the arch, 20% in the descending aorta, and <2% in the abdominal aorta.[4]

Classification

The degeneration of the aortic media, with or without cystic changes, is associated with most of the cases of aortic dissection. Most authors refer now to the general process of 'medial degeneration'[5,6] rather than the older more specific term 'cystic medial necrosis'.[7] Approximately 70% of patients with acute aortic dissection have a history of systemic hypertension.[3,5,8–10] Other associated disorders include connective tissue diseases such as Marfan's syndrome,[11] Ehlers–Danlos syndrome,[12] bicuspid aortic valves,[3] aortic coarctation,[13,14] pregnancy,[15] trauma,[16] and iatrogenic damage from aortic catheterization[17] or cardiac surgery.[18,19]

Pathophysiology

Two types of classification schemes have been developed (Fig. 19.1); the first by Debakey et al,[20] and a second more recently by Daily et al[21] which has been termed the 'Stanford' classification. The Debakey classification recognizes three types based on the site of intimal tear and the extent of the dissection. Debakey types I and II begin in the ascending aorta with type I extending into the descending aorta and type II remaining limited to the ascending aorta. Debakey type III dissections originate in the descending aorta and either remain superior to the diaphragm (subtype A) or extend below the diaphragm (subtype B). The

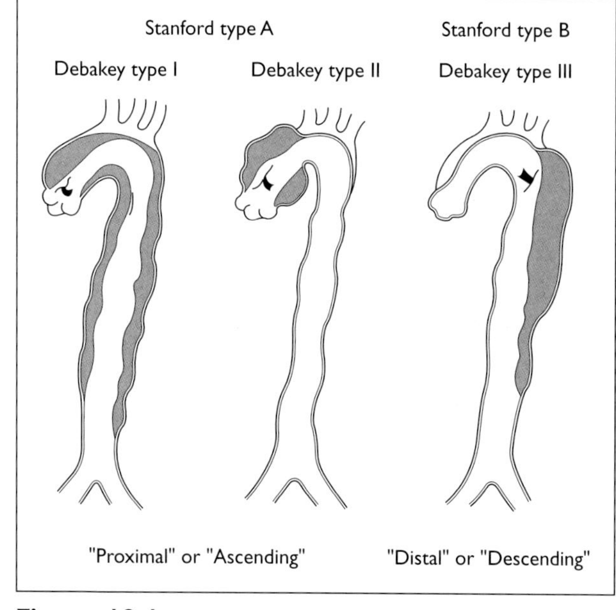

Figure 19.1
Diagram of the types of aortic dissection and the two types of classification schemes in clinical usage: Debakey and Stanford.

Stanford classification is based solely on the involvement or lack thereof of the ascending aorta. Stanford type A dissections involve the ascending aorta and Stanford type B dissections do not. Temporal distinctions are also important as the prognosis may depend on the time prior to presentation.[1,22] Dissections that present within 2 weeks of onset are termed acute and those that present after 2 weeks are classified as chronic. Of patients with untreated dissection, 75% do not live beyond 2 weeks of symptom onset.[5]

Angiography

Aortic angiography has been the invasive method of choice for many years in the diagnosis of aortic dissection.[22,23] The diagnostic accuracy has been reported to be 95–99%.[1] It has been used as the 'gold standard' in several studies of the sensitivity and specificity of noninvasive imaging techniques.[24,25] Retrograde aortic catheterization (Fig. 19.2) yields the most optimal results, and can be performed in critically ill patients.[26,27] Digital subtraction angiography has been used to diagnose dissection,[28] but is associated with reduced spatial resolution, poorer visualization of aortic branch detail, and motion artifacts that may make this technique less appealing in the setting of acute dissection.[29]

Diagnostic criteria

Both direct and indirect signs of aortic dissection are available using aortography.[30] Direct diagnostic signs include visualization of the intimal flap and a true and false lumen (Figs 19.2 and 19.3). Indirect signs that may be suggestive and helpful in management of the patient are compression of the true lumen by the false lumen, severity of aortic regurgitation, branch vessel abnormalities, and involvement of proximal coronary arteries.[31,32] In one study of 52 patients, a false lumen was seen in 87% of cases, whereas the site of intimal tear was seen in only 56% of cases.[33]

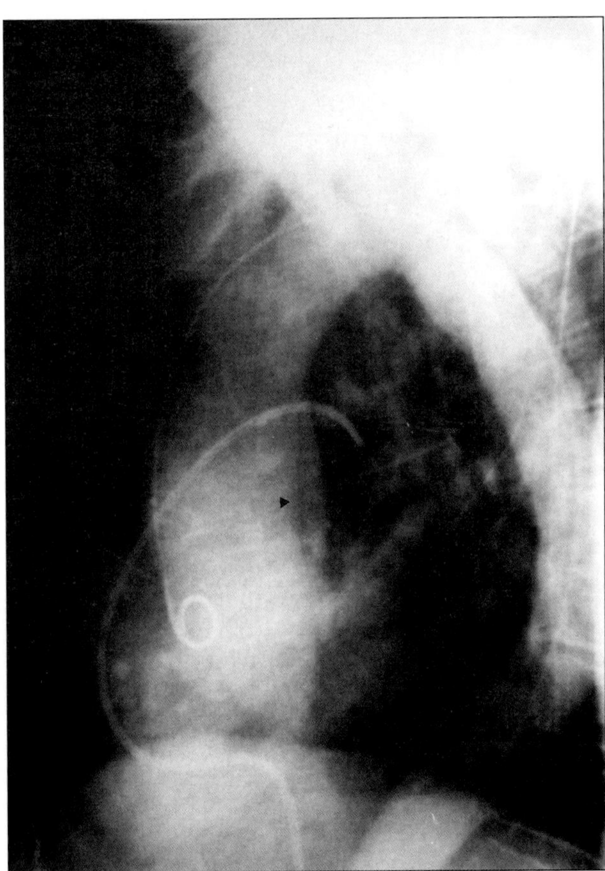

Figure 19.2
Aortic angiogram in the left anterior oblique plane from a retrograde approach showing an intimal flap in the ascending aorta (arrow).

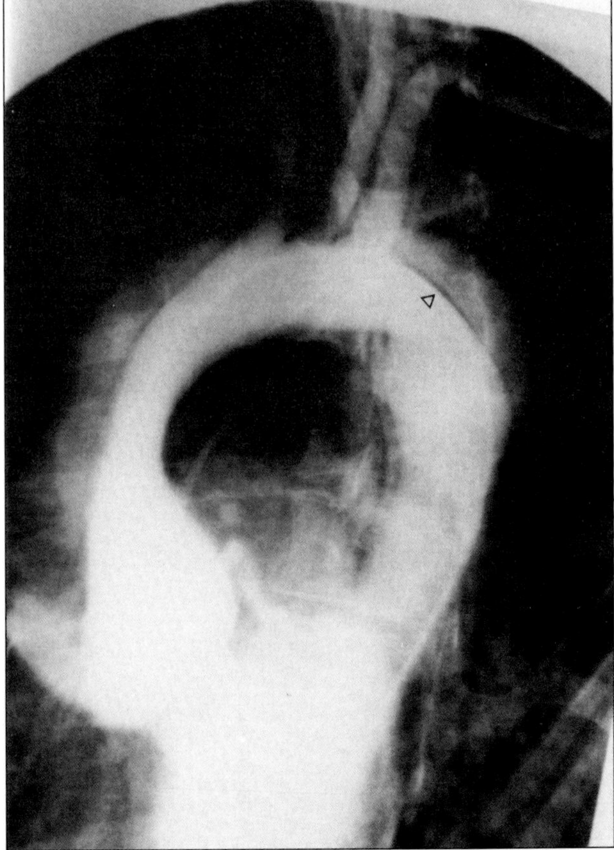

Figure 19.3
Angiogram of the aorta demonstrating an intimal flap extending from the aortic root into the arch (arrow) and descending aorta.

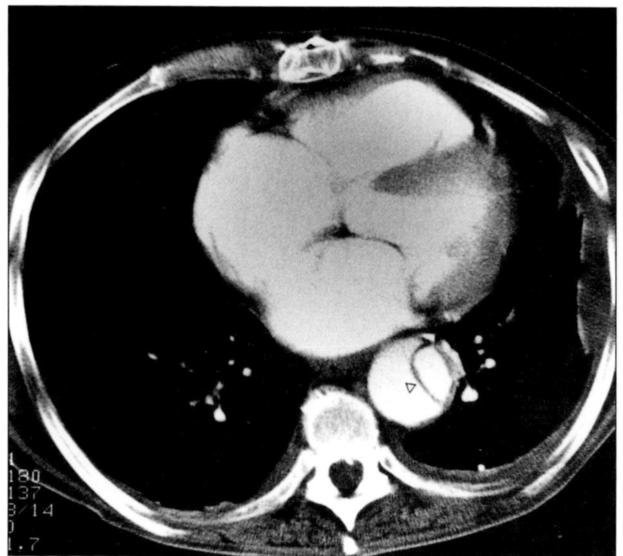

Figure 19.4
Computed tomographic image demonstrating an intimal flap in the descending thoracic aorta (arrow).

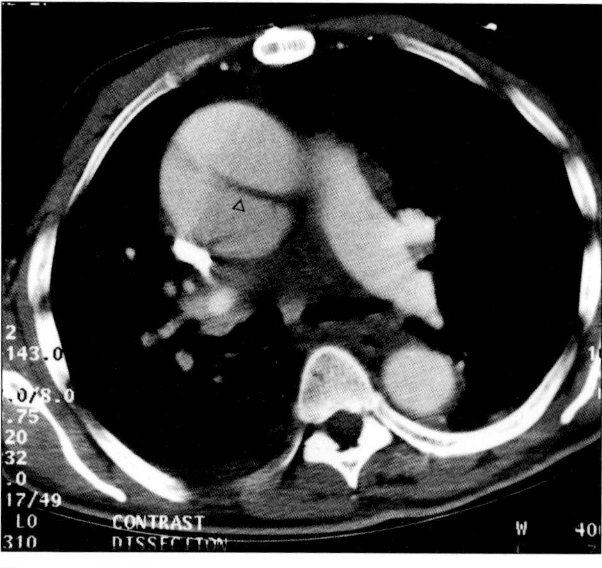

Figure 19.5
CT image showing a markedly dilated ascending aorta. An intimal flap within the ascending aorta is demonstrated (arrow).

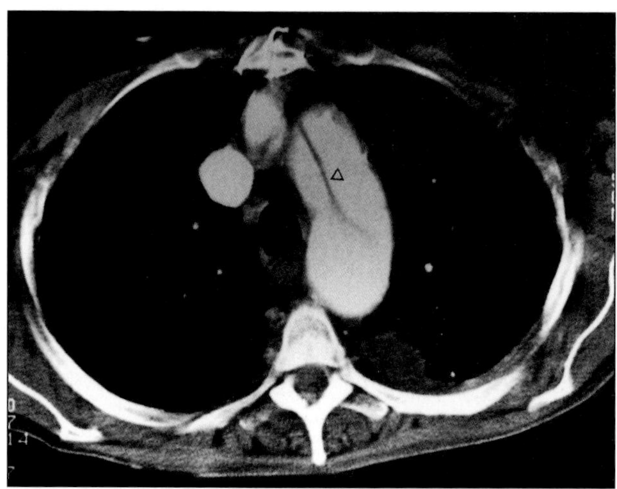

Figure 19.6
CT image of the aortic arch depicting an intimal flap within the arch (arrow). The flap is also seen in the ascending aorta lying just to the left of the arch.

Limitations

Disadvantages of aortography include the false negative rate which has varied, depending on the study, from as low as 2% to as high as 23%.[34–36] Causes of false negative aortograms include nonvisualization of the intimal flap due to simultaneous and equal opacification of true and false lumen, presence of intramural hematoma or thrombosis of the false lumen, or a perpendicular angle of the X-ray beam relative to the flap.[1,23,32] Other potential disadvantages are the risks of the contrast dye, especially in patients who may have underlying renal insufficiency or renal involvement. In addition, there are the potential delays of assembling the catheterization team and of the transportation to the angiographic suite.[30] In one comparative study of transesophageal echocardiography (TEE) and angiography in 70 patients with dissection,[37] the examination time was significantly shorter for TEE (9 min versus 48 min on average), and there was a trend to improved sensitivity with TEE. Rizzo et al have suggested that the mortality associated with aortic dissection has been reduced with the use of noninvasive imaging techniques due to the avoidance of the risks and delays associated with invasive angiography and coronary arteriography.[38]

Computed tomography

Computed tomography (CT) and its variants, including helical or spiral CT and ultrafast CT, have been used to diagnose aortic dissection noninvasively. Typically, serial short-axis sections are obtained throughout the chest, and then sites are chosen for single-level dynamic scanning. Unenhanced imaging can reveal displaced calcification, an intimal flap (Fig. 19.4), thrombosed false lumen, pericardial or pleural fluid or blood, and dilatation of the aorta (Fig. 19.5). With standard CT scanning, different boluses of contrast material during dynamic imaging are usually given to visualize the aorta at three important sites: the aortic root, mid ascending aorta (Fig. 19.5), and aortic arch (Fig. 19.6).

Enhanced imaging is more useful for delineating the intimal flap, true and false lumen and their anatomic relationship, branch involvement and extraluminal fluid or blood.[39] Internally displaced calcification can suggest dissection.[40] Acute thrombosis of the false lumen may be hyperdense on unenhanced CT,[40] and this finding is often diagnostic of dissection.

Accuracy

Overall accuracy of CT scanning for diagnosing acute aortic dissection from several series is approximately 95% with sensitivity ranging from 67% to 100%, and specificity from 96% to 100%.[24,25,35,41–45] False-negatives and false-positives have been reported, and in one study[41] the type of dissection was misclassified in 33% of positives. Newer techniques such as ultrafast CT and spiral scanning may improve upon the sensitivity and specificity of these techniques.[46]

Ultrafast CT

Ultrafast CT has some advantages over conventional CT.[47] Because of millisecond image acquisition, all imaging can be performed during bolus contrast administration, significantly reducing the time in the scanner. Faster scan times also limit patient and respiratory motion artifact. Flow mode imaging can be used to determine direction and sequence of flow in the true and false lumen.[48] In one study by Hamada et al, 17 patients with Stanford type A dissection were imaged by ultrafast CT.[49] In two patients the false lumen was thrombosed, and the sensitivity for determining the intimal tear was 93% in the remaining 15 patients. An intimal tear in the aortic arch was missed.

Spiral CT

A newly developed imaging modality known as spiral or helical CT has been used in the diagnosis of aortic dissection.[50] The entire thoracic aorta can be imaged faster and with less contrast volume. The images can be reconstructed in other planes or in three dimensions. Zeman et al studied 23 patients with suspected aortic dissection; all seven true dissections were identified and one false-positive was found (specificity 93%). In three of the seven patients with dissection, the multiplanar re-formation or three-dimensional views improved the ability to determine the intimal flap.

Limitations

Potential problems with CT assessment of dissection include the lack of visibility of the intimal tear, especially in type A dissections,[45] and the lack of distinction between the density of true and false lumen depending upon the windowing used.[51] Other causes of inability to distinguish true and false lumen include similar blood flow in both lumen or thrombosed false lumen.[52] Intimal flaps can be simulated by cardiac movement, calcification or a high-contrast interface,[39] but these can be recognized if they are seen on one level only. Major limitations are the inability to adequately demonstrate aortic regurgitation and the difficulty in assessing branches of the aortic arch or coronary artery involvement, because CT is limited to axial scanning. False internal displacement of calcification can occur through volume averaging of a thick slice including angulated calcification, commonly at sites of tortuosity of the aorta. In addition, in chronic dissection the false lumen may develop atheromatous disease quickly and may calcify.[53] False-positive identification of a false lumen is possible by enhancement of contiguous vessels or misidentification of the normal sinus of Valsalva. Hyperdensity of the aortic wall has been used to diagnose dissection in the absence of anemia, although advanced age and calcification has been shown to cause this finding.[54] Fluid in the superior preaortic or retroaortic pericardial recess can also mimic acute dissection.[39]

Magnetic resonance imaging (MRI)

MRI began to be used in the early 1980s to diagnose aortic dissection.[55–57] The technique is noninvasive and does not require contrast material or ionizing radiation. Images can be obtained, unlike in CT, in multiple planes which enables localization of the intimal flap (Fig. 19.7) and delineates involvement of branch vessels and coronary arteries.[55]

Spin echo imaging

In standard T1-weighted spin-echo imaging, rapidly moving blood produces a signal void while slow moving or stationary blood produces a signal (Fig. 19.8).[32] In the setting of different flow velocities in true or false lumens, the intimal flap will be delineated by regions of low and high signal on either side (Fig. 19.9). Criteria used to make the diagnosis are a visible intimal flap with identification of true and false lumen. Sensitivity for detection of aortic dissection is generally >90%[56–58] and in recent studies was 98–100%.[24,25] The sensitivity was 85% and specificity 100% for identifying the

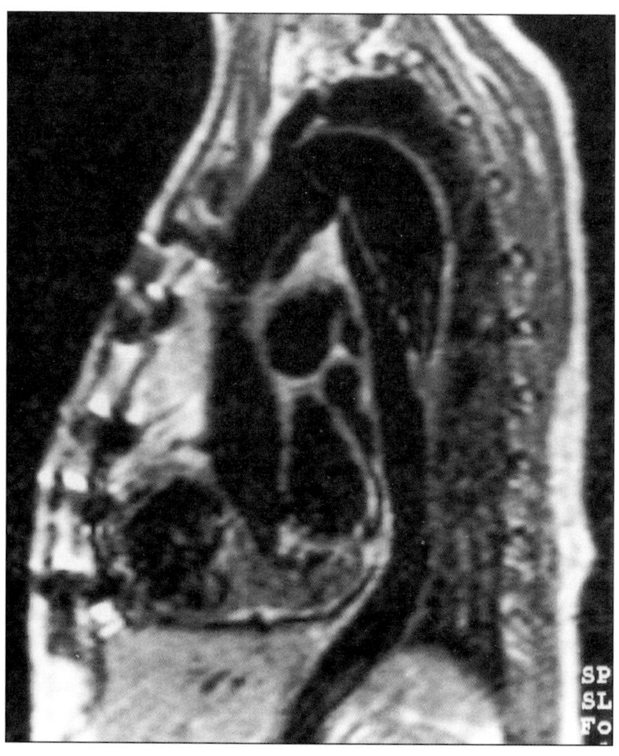

Figure 19.7
T1-weighted spin echo MR image in a parasagittal plane of a complex intimal flap involving the ascending aorta, aortic arch, and descending aorta.

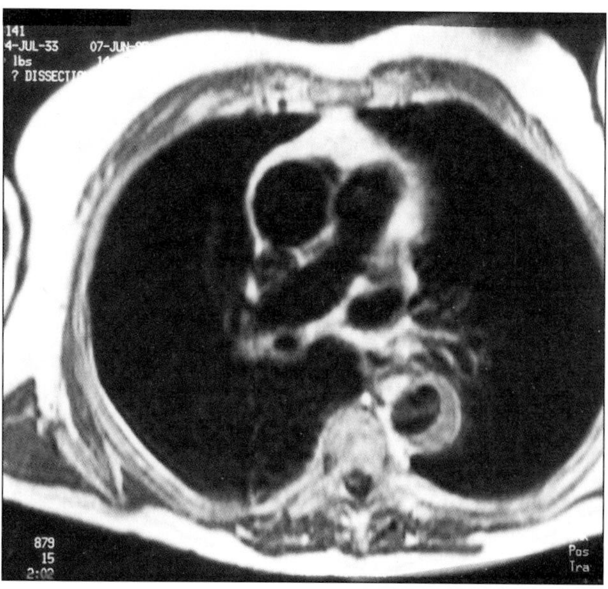

Figure 19.9
T1-weighted spin echo MR image in an axial plane demonstrating an intimal flap in the descending aorta with a thrombosed false lumen.

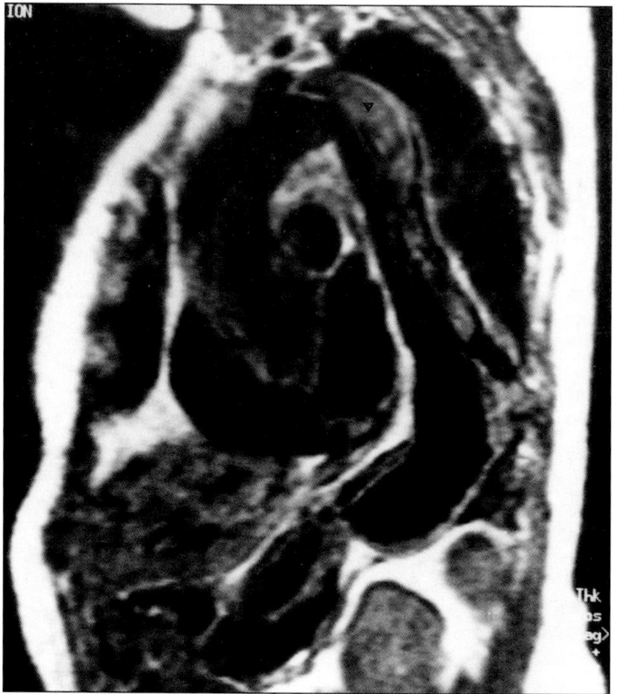

Figure 19.8
T1-weighted spin echo MR image in a parasagittal plane of an intimal flap with two lumens in the aortic arch and descending thoracic aorta. Sluggish flow is seen in the false lumen as evidenced by the brighter signal (arrow).

entry site in Nienaber's early study, and sensitivity and specificity were both 100% for demonstrating thrombus and pericardial effusions.

When compared directly to TEE in a recent study, MRI has a higher sensitivity for an intimal flap (95% versus 86%), and was able to detect the inferior extent of the dissected lumen.[59] Chung et al[60] demonstrated the ability to visualize the entry tears as discontinuity in the intimal flap and a flow void in the false lumen caused by flow across the entry site in eight of nine patients, all confirmed by operation or aortography. MRI has also identified so-called aortic cobwebs which are, by pathologic assessment, residual pieces of media that are incompletely torn during the dissection and appear to create a third lumen.[61] MRI has been used to diagnose aortic dissection in asymptomatic patients with abnormal chest X-rays[62] or in asymptomatic patients with Marfan's syndrome on routine examination.[63]

Cine MRI

Cine MRI techniques can be used in the diagnosis of aortic dissection. Cine images are electrocardiographically gated and can detect motion of the intimal flap (Figs 19.10 and 19.11), flow of blood within the true and false lumen, and aortic regurgitation.[64] In the study of Nienaber et al the

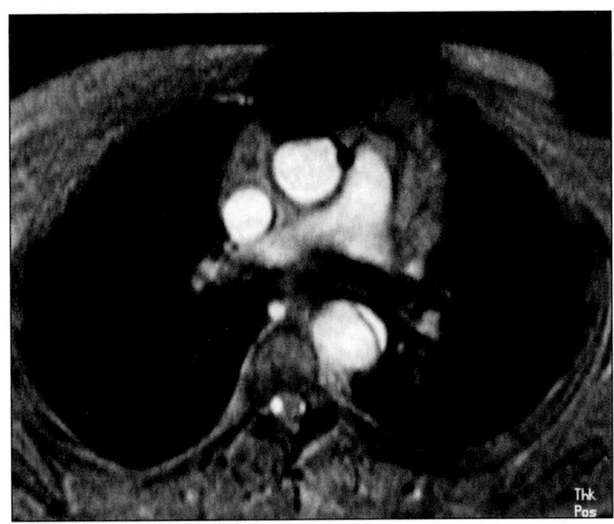

Figure 19.10
Gradient echo cine MR image at end-diastole with an intimal flap visualized in the descending aorta.

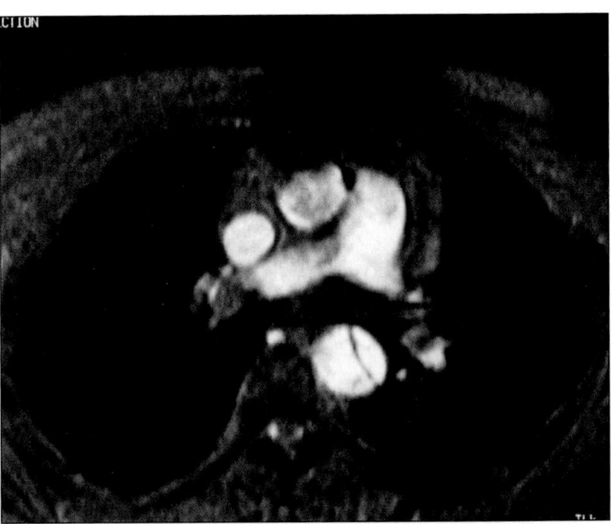

Figure 19.11
Gradient echo cine MR image at end-systole in the same plane as Figure 19.10. Note that the intimal flap has moved from right to left, identifying the true lumen as the lumen on the right of the image.

sensitivity of cine MRI for demonstrating aortic regurgitation was 83% in a group of patients with dissection, although some cases could not be completed due to the length of scanning time and patient safety issues.[25] Contrast-enhanced Turbo-FLASH MRI has been used to localize the entry and re-entry sites pre- and postoperatively.[65]

Velocity-encoded MRI

Recently, the technique of velocity-encoded cine MRI has been applied to patients with aortic dissection.[66,67] This technique allowed identification of the intimal flap (Fig. 19.12)[66] and quantification of flow within the true and false lumen.[67] Rumancik et al have used spin echo phase images to differentiate thrombus from blood flow in various cardiovascular conditions including aortic dissection in which they demonstrated thrombosed false lumen.[68]

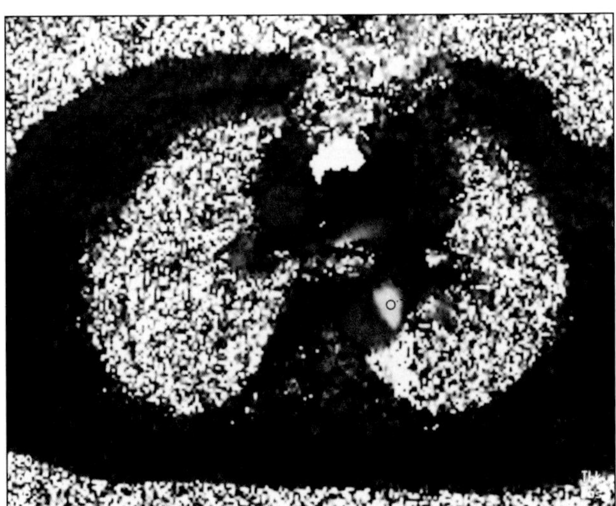

Figure 19.12
Velocity-encoded cine MR image in the same patient as Figures 19.10 and 19.11 showing high velocity flow (bright signal) in the true lumen on the right of the descending aorta (see circle) and lower velocity flow (darker signal) in the false lumen on the left.

Limitations

A study by Solomon et al[69] identified many of the pitfalls of MRI in aortic dissection. Most (77%) of the artifacts identified would be correctly classified as such by imaging oblique planes or the same plane in a cine mode. The more complicated artifacts included the effects of motion (respiratory, cardiac, and/or the patient), the origins of arch vessels mimicking intimal flap, the superior pericardial recess imitating ascending dissection, and fibrosing mediastinitis. Pernes et al were unable to make the diagnosis in four cases with thrombosed false lumen out of a group of 30 with dissection. In these four patients the diagnosis was made by CT which demonstrated displaced calcification.[70] Additionally, there are other important limitations of MRI in potentially ill patients with aortic dissection. MRI becomes quite complex in patients who are hemodynamically unstable, on ventilators, or require intravenous medications. Monitoring of vital signs in the bore of the scanner where the patient is inaccessible for up to 45 min is difficult. Newer monitoring systems and open superconducting magnets may alleviate some of these shortcomings.[71] Other limitations include patients with claustrophobia, pacemakers, aneurysm clips, older cardiac valvular prostheses, and metallic ocular implants.[72]

Two-dimensional echocardiography

Both M-mode and two-dimensional echocardiography have been used to diagnose aortic dissection.[73–75] Early in the development of the techniques, the sensitivity was reported to be about 80%[76,77] rising as high as 100% when all of the dissections involved the proximal ascending aorta.[78] False-negative echocardiograms mostly occur in the setting of Debakey type III dissections as the descending thoracic aorta cannot often be well visualized on transthoracic imaging. A retrospective study of 67 patients by Khanderia et al demonstrated a sensitivity of 79% and positive predictive accuracy of 91%.[79] More recent prospective data yielded a sensitivity of 59%.[25] Specificity ranges from 63% to 96% in published studies.[80] In the study of Granato et al, there were five false-positives yielding a specificity of 88%.[78] Mathew and Nanda[75] developed criteria for the diagnosis of ascending aortic dissection which include a prominent, flap-like motion of the inner dissected wall (Fig. 19.13) or a marked parallel widening of ≥15 mm in either or both aortic walls. Another clinically useful finding on two-dimensional scanning is the presence of pericardial effusion.[78]

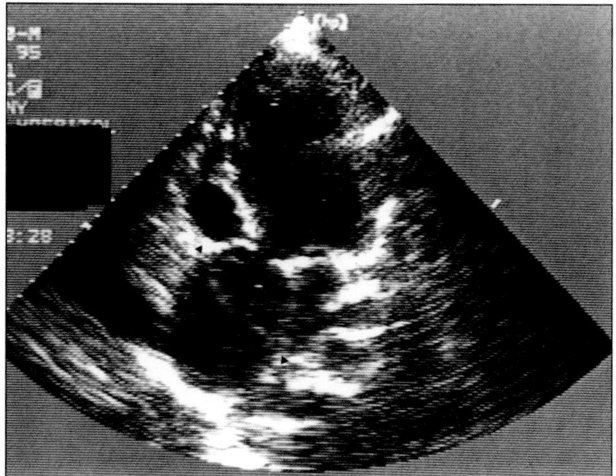

Figure 19.13
Two-dimensional echocardiographic image in the apical long axis demonstrating an intimal flap (between the arrows) and a dilated ascending aorta.

Doppler techniques

Pulse Doppler techniques have been employed to assess flow within true and false lumen.[75] Color Doppler assessment of 16 patients with proven aortic dissection enabled correct identification of thrombosis in one lumen as absence of flow, and in 75% of the cases demonstrated direct visualization of communication between true and false lumen.[81] In addition, color Doppler was used to correctly diagnose the severity of aortic regurgitation in seven of the patients.

Limitations

Limitations of transthoracic echocardiography include the lack of visualization of the descending thoracic aorta and the poor quality of images in approximately 10% of patients due to obesity, chronic lung disease, mechanical ventilation, or chest wall deformities.[1,80] In addition, involvement of the proximal coronary arteries cannot be assessed.

TEE

TEE has eliminated many of the shortcomings of transthoracic echocardiography (TTE) in the diagnosis of aortic dissection. Image quality is improved due to proximity of the probe to the aorta. Multiple imaging planes are available, especially with the more recently developed omniplane TEE probes. Acutely ill patients can be imaged at the bedside or in the operating room without compromising either care or monitoring of the patient.

The first report of the use of TEE to diagnose a type B aortic dissection not visualized by TTE was by Borner et al in 1984.[82] In a subsequent study of 18 patients with dissection confirmed by angiography or at surgery, only six patients were diagnosed by TTE and the remaining 12

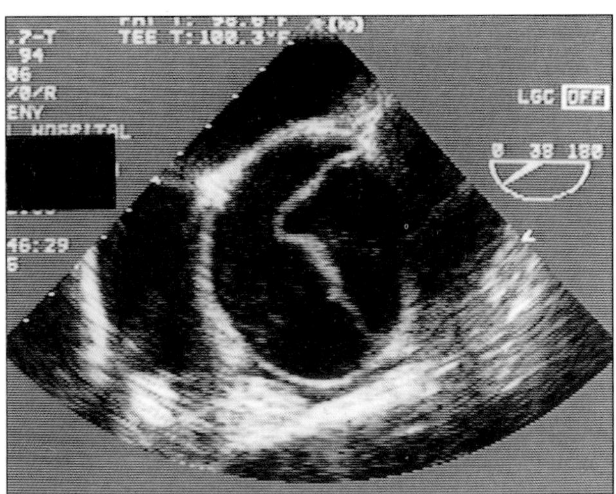

Figure 19.14
Multiplane TEE image of an intimal flap in the ascending aorta at end-diastole.

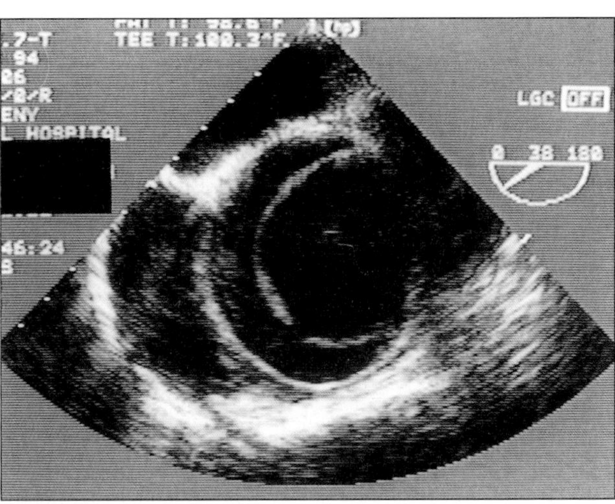

Figure 19.15
Multiplane TEE image of the same intimal flap as Figure 19.14 during systole. The true lumen is to the right of the flap as the flap has been pushed to the left during systole.

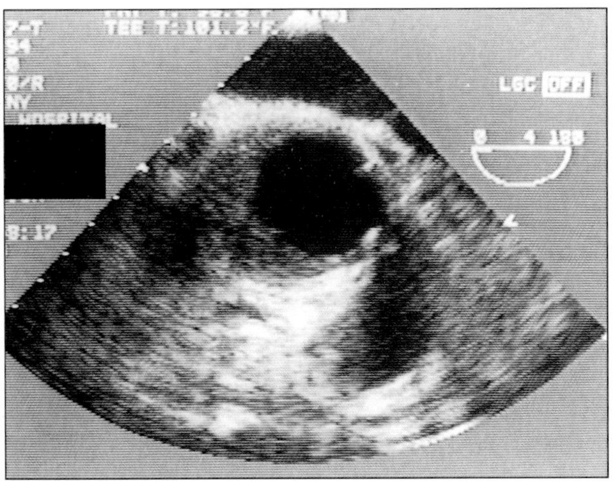

Figure 19.16
Multiplane TEE image of the ascending aorta with a dissection with true lumen to the right and thrombus in the false lumen to the left.

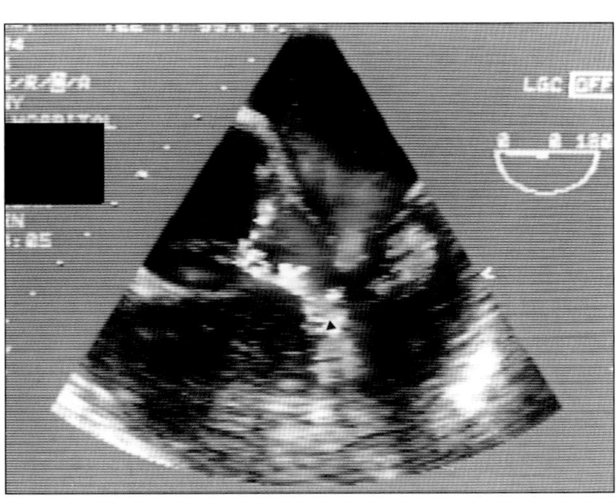

Figure 19.17
Multiplane TEE image with color Doppler of the left ventricle, aortic valve, and mitral valve during diastole. The blue color seen in the left ventricular outflow tract is aortic regurgitation (arrow).

required TEE for correct identification (Figs 19.14 and 19.15).[83] Erbel et al[84] confirmed the superiority of TEE to TTE in a study of 21 patients and described the finding of spontaneous echocardiographic contrast with mural thrombus in the false lumen (Fig. 19.16). In this study, TTE correctly identified only five of nine type A dissections and 1 of 12 type B dissections. CT did not identify an intimal flap in four patients and aortography was also negative in four patients. Another study by Hashimoto et al[85] confirmed the superiority of TEE with Doppler to TTE, demonstrating improved sensitivity and ability to detect the entry site (100% for TEE and only 42% for TTE). This study also identified the presence of thrombus in the false lumen, aortic regurgitation (Fig. 19.17), and pericardial effusion.

In a multicenter study of 164 patients with suspected dissection, 82 of whom were positive, Erbel et al[35]

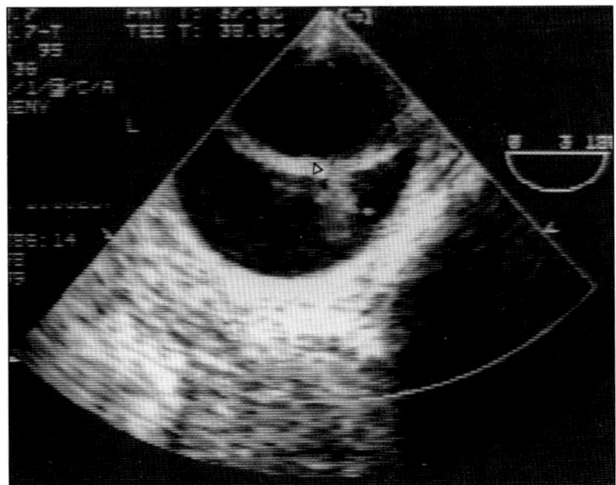

Figure 19.18
Multiplane TEE image with color Doppler of the descending thoracic aorta with an entry site visualized within the intimal flap (arrow) with flow between the two lumens.

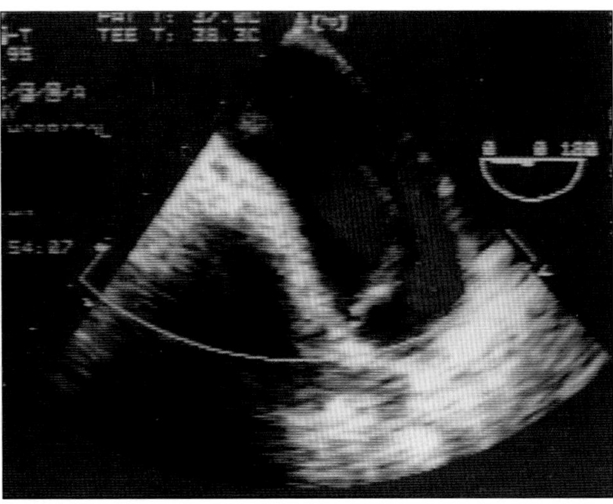

Figure 19.19
Multiplane TEE image with color Doppler of the arch and descending thoracic aorta with an intimal flap seen and flow documented by color Doppler (the blue seen in the image) in both lumens.

demonstrated an overall sensitivity of 99% for TEE and a specificity of 98%. The two false-positives were patients with aortic ectasia. This and previous studies had not used a standard for comparison of TEE findings. The study by Ballal et al[41] compared TEE findings to aortography, surgery, or autopsy in positive studies (34 patients) and to aortography in negative studies. The sensitivity and specificity were 97% and 100%, respectively. However, five patients could not have the DeBakey class of their dissection classified. TEE did, however, identify coronary artery involvement correctly in six of seven patients and correctly described a communication between lumens, thrombus in the false lumen, two cases of false aneurysm formation, and all cases of moderate to severe aortic regurgitation. One explanation for the rare false-negatives has been image interference in localized DeBakey type II dissections from the trachea and mainstem bronchi as shown in 2 of 65 patients in the study by Bansal et al[36] in which the diagnosis of dissection was confirmed by aortography.

Prospective studies

Recently, controlled prospective studies of noninvasive imaging techniques in patients with suspected dissection have been reported. In the study by Nienaber et al,[24] 53 patients were studied with MRI versus TEE; all were compared to aortography and 34 were compared to surgery or autopsy. The sensitivity for both MRI and TEE was 100%, although specificity was much lower for TEE (68% versus 100%). The reason for the low specificity may have been the use of monoplane probes in this study and the number of artifacts seen in the ascending aorta from echoes from atheromatous vessels or calcified aortic disease mimicking an intimal flap.[85] The sensitivity and specificity for demonstrating the entry site were 75% and 100%, respectively, and for demonstrating thrombus, 64% and 100%, respectively. Aortic regurgitation was identified 100% of the time, but with a 10% false-positive rate. In a subsequent study of 110 patients, Nienaber et al[25] demonstrated a sensitivity and specificity in the diagnosis of dissection of 98% and 77%, respectively, with very similar accuracy to their previous study for entry site (Fig. 19.18), thrombus, aortic insufficiency, and pericardial effusion. One reviewer[30] suggested that specificity would be improved by separating diagnostic categories into definite and probable. A definite diagnosis would be reserved for cases in which in addition to an intimal flap, another echocardiographic feature such as site of entry, Doppler flow characteristics (Fig. 19.19), thrombus, etc., was demonstrated.

Multiplane TEE

Most of the aforementioned studies were performed with monoplane TEE probes. In the late 1980s biplane probes became available, and in a study by Adachi et al[86] biplane TEE was shown to be more accurate than monoplane in the visualization of the entry site because of the addition

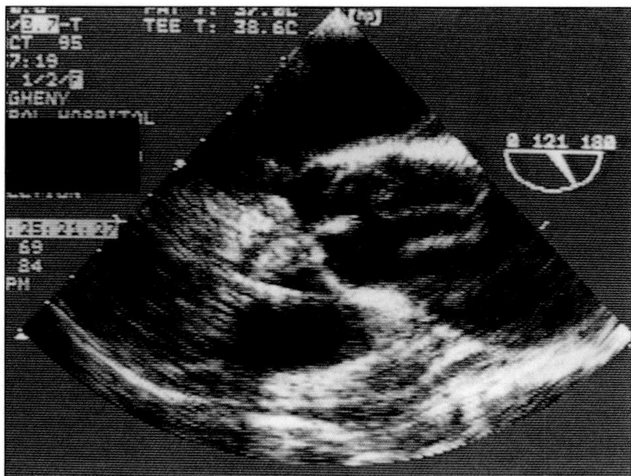

Figure 19.20
Multiplane TEE image in the longitudinal plane of a complex intimal flap in the ascending aorta extending to the aortic valve.

of the longitudinal view of the aorta (Fig. 19.20). The same group compared single-plane with biplane TEE in 200 consecutive patients, 30 of whom had aortic dissection.[87] They found that longitudinal scanning was slightly superior as three cases with an entry site were missed with horizontal scanning.

Some authors have recommended TEE as the single mode of diagnosis for suspected dissection.[80,88] In the study by Banning et al,[80] 45 patients underwent TEE, about half with a biplane probe. Dissection was confirmed in 22 and TEE was 96% specific for the proximal extent. No patient without dissection on TEE required examination of their aorta at 2-year follow-up, although no other imaging modality was performed to substantiate the TEE findings in this study.

Establishing prognosis

TEE has been used to establish prognosis in the setting of aortic dissection by The European Cooperative Study Group on Echocardiography.[89] They studied 168 patients with proven aortic dissection at the start of medical or surgical therapy, and at a mean of 10 months' follow-up. Survival rates in type I, II and III dissections were 52%, 69%, and 70%, respectively. A high mortality rate of 52% was found in patients with fluid extravasation, pleural effusion, pericardial tamponade, periaortic effusion, and mediastinal hematoma. The highest rate of reoperation was found in patients with type III dissections that dissected antegradely because of lack of intimal flap resection in the descending aorta. Thrombus formation in the false lumen was regarded as a good prognostic sign easily recognized by TEE. The limitation of biplane TEE in this setting was the lack of visualization of the distal ascending aortic arch due to the position of the trachea and its bifurcation.

Intraoperative TEE

Intraoperative TEE is an important method of assessing operative management of aortic dissection.[90] Problems with distal aortic perfusion and leakages from anastomotic sites can be identified. The involvement of aortic arch branch vessels and their adequate perfusion can be assessed by a combination of transesophageal, epicardial, and transcutaneous Doppler imaging.[91] Intraoperative TEE is also potentially useful in the diagnosis of cases where aortic dissection is complicating other cardiac surgery, often due to cannulation site injury.[92]

Limitations

One shortcoming of TEE is its inability to assess disease in the abdomen and pelvis.[93] Rarely, false-positive findings by TEE have been noted due to unusual anatomic relationships in the chest.[94] Even TEE examinations that are negative for dissection may identify important aortic disease such as aneurysm, atheroma, masses, and thrombus.[95]

Intravascular ultrasound

In recent years, advances in ultrasound technology have created the ability to mount transducers on intravascular catheters. In one recent multicenter study,[96] 28 patients with suspected aortic dissection underwent intravascular ultrasound imaging of the aorta which was compared to angiography and at least one noninvasive imaging method (CT or TEE). The entire aorta was imaged quickly (10 min on average) without complications, and the sensitivity and specificity were 100%—23 patients had dissection and five patients did not. In addition, the entire extent of the dissection, involvement of aortic branches, and the presence of intramural hematoma could all be assessed. In six patients intravascular ultrasound was able to delineate the distal extent of dissection as far as the bifurcation of the abdominal aorta, a finding not obtainable by TEE. Intravascular ultrasound was not able to evaluate communications between true and false lumen or coronary artery involvement, and was relatively insensitive to thrombus in the false lumen. Similarly, in another study of 15 patients,[97] intravascular ultrasound was 100% sensitive for detection of an intimal flap and was efficacious at identifying involvement of abdominal aortic branch vessels. The accuracy of detection of the intimal tear site was lower. With the advent of endoluminal stenting of aortic dissection, intravascular ultrasound may have a role for evaluation of stent deployment.[98]

Comparative techniques

The various imaging modalities have different strengths and weaknesses in the diagnosis of aortic dissection (see Table 19.1 for a summary).

Many factors must be taken into account when choosing an imaging modality in any given patient. Firstly, the expertise of the institution in the different imaging techniques is an important consideration. The diagnostic accuracy of the technique is likewise important. MRI or TEE are the most sensitive. The availability and safety profile of each modality and the severity of the patient's illness are other variables that influence the choice of procedure. In the critically ill patient, MRI is less feasible due to lack of adequate monitoring in most scanners. TEE if available, can be performed quite rapidly and safely in an intensive care or operating room setting and is quite accurate. MRI has an equally good profile in its diagnostic accuracy, and in the stable or postoperative patient may be the imaging modality of choice. CT scanning, which may be the only available option in the community setting, is still a reasonable choice as a screening test. Aortography is losing ground to the newer modalities due to potential delays in performing the test, the associated risks—including its invasiveness and use of contrast dye—and its limitation in diagnostic accuracy.

Table 19.1

	Aortography	CT	MRI	TEE
Sensitivity	++	++	+++	+++
Specificity	+++	+++	+++	+++
Site of intimal tear	++	+	+++	+++
Differentiate lumen	++	++	+++	+++
Presence of thrombus	+++	++	+++	++
Presence of aortic regurgitation	+++	–	++	+++
Pericardial effusion	–	++	+++	+++
Branch vessel involvement	+++	+	++	+
Coronary artery involvement	+++	–	+	++
Bedside procedure	No	No	No	Yes

Related aortic pathology

Intramural hemorrhage

Aortic intramural hemorrhage without definitive evidence of intimal rupture has been demonstrated in up to 10% of autopsy studies.[2] Various imaging techniques have been used to diagnose this entity, distinct from classic aortic dissection.

Yamada et al[100] first described MRI and CT findings in 14 patients with aortic dissection without intimal rupture. MRI revealed a region of higher signal intensity along the aortic wall, whereas CT showed a nonenhanced crescentic area along the wall. These patients had repeat imaging at 1 year that showed normalization of these areas. Of the patients, two died and had autopsies confirming intramural hemorrhage in the absence of an intimal tear. In a CT study of eight patients, Williams and Farrow[101] showed that in follow-up, two of the patients with intramural hemorrhage developed ulceration of the hemorrhage. In the study by Wolff et al[102] using MRI on 64 patients with aortic dissection, nine or 14% had aortic wall thickening on T1-weighted images as the only sign of dissection, and six of these had had false-negative angiograms.

In two studies of TEE in aortic dissection, 13% of aortic dissection cases were documented to have intramural hemorrhage without an intimal flap.[103,104] In the prospective study by Mohr-Kahaly et al,[103] 114 patients were found to have aortic dissection over a 5-year period. Of these patients, 15 had localized thickening of the aortic wall with medial displacement of intimal calcification, and the diagnosis was confirmed pathologically in seven of these and by CT or MRI in the remaining eight. Five of these 15 patients progressed to typical aortic dissection by follow-up TEE and four progressed to aortic rupture within a week. A larger study of 195 patients studied by TEE over 10 years[104] demonstrated a subgroup of 25 patients (12.8%) with intramural hemorrhage. In 32% of patients this syndrome progressed to dissection, aortic rupture, or pericardial tamponade within 24–72 h. Mortality within 30 days in type A intramural hemorrhage treated medically was 80% versus 20% with medical therapy, prompting these authors to recommend immediate surgical therapy for intramural hemorrhage of the ascending aorta.

Penetrating atherosclerotic ulcers

Penetrating atherosclerotic ulcers of the thoracic aorta may produce a clinical syndrome and presentation very similar to that of classic aortic dissection, involving an ulceration of an atheromatous plaque through the intima and into the media

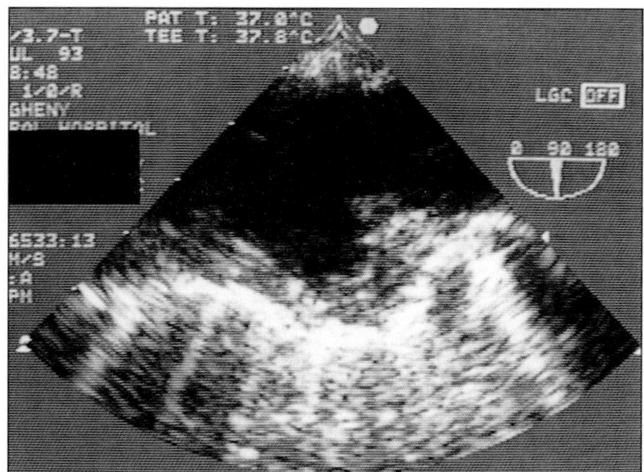

Figure 19.21
Longitudinal multiplane TEE image of the descending thoracic aorta demonstrating an ulcer penetrating into the media.

(Fig. 19.21) that may dissect locally or rupture.[105] Stanson et al[106] described the findings in 16 patients (2.3% of 684 patients who underwent thoracic aortography over 8 years) as an ulcer with a clearly defined entry site often with associated intimal calcification and adjacent hematoma, occasionally associated with a large saccular aneurysm. The ulcer size was 5–20 mm in diameter and 5–30 mm in depth with a uniform distribution throughout the descending thoracic aorta. Fifteen of the 16 patients demonstrated adjacent intramural hematoma ranging from 7 cm long to the entire descending thoracic aorta. CT was used in 10 cases to confirm the diagnosis. Fourteen of the 16 patients underwent surgical repair with graft placement. Another study suggested the incidence of penetrating atherosclerotic ulcers may be as high as 10.6% (5 of 47) in patients examined by CT for significant aortic abnormalities.[107] CT was used by Kazerooni et al to diagnose penetrating atherosclerotic ulcer; typical findings were hematoma (16 patients), displaced calcification (13), pleural or extrapleural fluid (7), mediastinal fluid (4), and thick or enhancing aortic wall (6).[108]

A recent study with longer follow-up suggested a benign prognosis for penetrating atherosclerotic ulcer. Harris et al[109] reviewed 29 ulcers in 18 patients diagnosed by CT in 17, MRI in 9, and aortography in 5. Ten patients were followed up; five were found to progress to saccular pseudoaneurysm and two to fusiform aneurysm. No progression to dissection, rupture, or death over 1–7 years' follow-up were noted, and only one ulcer was resected.

Post-surgery

After successful operative repair of aortic dissection, patients remain at risk of recurrent dissection and aneurysm formation.[110] Controversy exists over the prognostic implications of patency or thrombosis of the false lumen. Various imaging modalities have been used to follow such a patient. Aortography[111] and CT[112] have been used to follow patients after repair, but both techniques may not identify a thrombosed false lumen. The two were compared in one study in which the extent of dissection and thrombosis of the false lumen were better identified by CT.[114]

TEE

TEE with color Doppler has been shown to be quite useful in the follow-up of patients after surgical or medical therapy of aortic dissection.[114] These authors used TEE to demonstrate the persistence of a false lumen in 71% of patients after surgery and 82% after medical therapy with documentation of flow patterns within the false lumen. Persistent intimal tears with flow across them were seen, as were extension of the dissection, localized dilatation, mediastinal hematoma, and aortic regurgitation.

MRI

MRI has come into favor for this indication. White et al[115] published the initial experience with MRI after surgical repair. In 11 patients (nine with type A dissections, two with type B), these investigators found all patients to have aneurysmal dilatation beyond the graft, a residual intimal flap in 10 patients (Fig. 19.22), and in two-thirds of cases of a persistent dissection of the abdominal aorta, a visceral vessel originating from the false lumen. The techniques used included spin echo techniques as well as phase contrast to differentiate slow flow from thrombus. Fedriga and colleagues studied 28 patients with type A dissections and found abnormalities in 23 including further aortic dilatation in 9, recurrent dissection in 2, and residual intimal flap in 15 (Fig. 19.23).[116] MRI was compared with TEE in one study, and found to be better at visualizing anastomotic sites and arch vessels and better at serial studies.[117] TEE was better suited for demonstrating small entry sites.

MRI and CT have been used to study patients who have undergone wrapping of the native aorta around the ascending graft, a newer operation that may be associated with reduced surgical risk. Pucillo et al used MRI to assess 10 patients after type A dissection repair and found lumen compromise in two patients due to probable thrombus between the graft and native wrapped aorta.[118] In one study, MRI and CT were compared in evaluating such

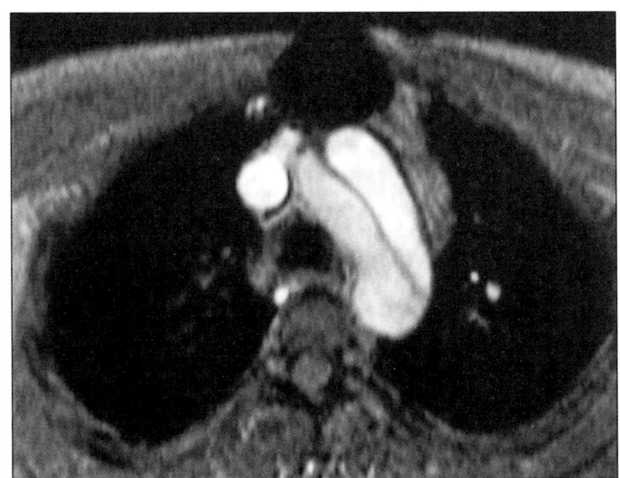

Figure 19.22
Gradient echo cine MR image in the axial plane in a postoperative patient. Note the signal void from the sternal wires in the anterior chest wall. Residual dissection with an intimal flap and flow (high signal) in both lumens is seen in the aortic arch.

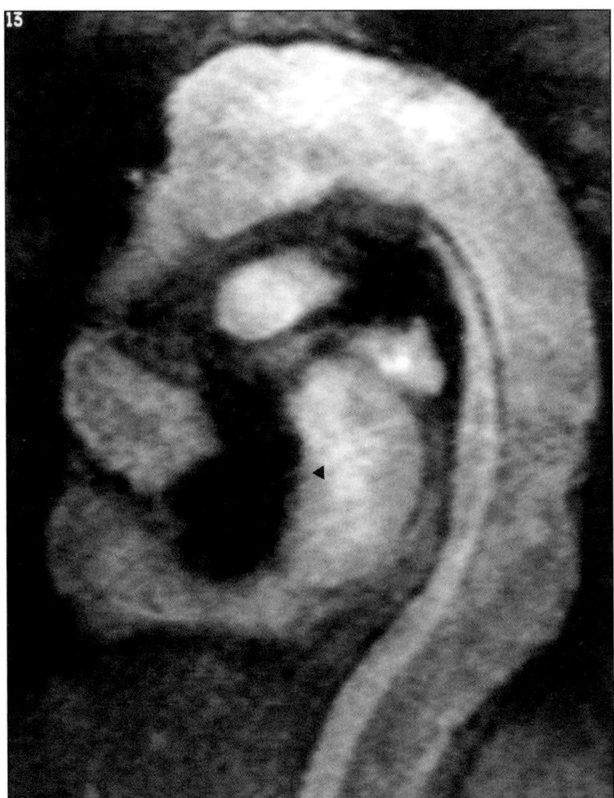

Figure 19.23
Gradient echo cine MR image in a parasagittal plane in a patient with Marfan's syndrome after composite graft placement with a mechanical prosthesis in the aortic position. Note the signal void around the metal portions of the valve (arrow). A residual intimal flap in the descending aorta is seen with flow in both lumens.

grafts.[119] MRI was more sensitive for perigraft thickening and for a residual intimal flap than CT. Gradient echo techniques were found to be useful in differentiating slow flow from thrombus.

References

1 DeSanctis RW, Doroghazi RM, Austen WG et al: Aortic dissection. *N Engl J Med* 1987; **317**: 1060–7.

2 Hirst AE Jr, Johns VJ Jr, Kime SW Jr: Dissecting aneurysm of the aorta: a review of 505 cases. *Medicine* 1958; **37**: 217–79.

3 Larson EW, Edwards WD: Risk factors for aortic dissection: a necropsy study of 161 cases. *Am J Cardiol* 1984; **53**: 849–55.

4 Roberts WC: Aortic dissection: anatomy, consequences, and causes. *Am Heart J* 1981; **101**: 195–214.

5 Hirst AE, Gore I: The etiology and pathology of aortic dissection. In: Doroghazi RM, Slater EE, eds, *Aortic Dissection* (McGraw-Hill: New York, 1983); 13–54.

6 Hirst AE, Gore I: Is cystic medionecrosis the cause of dissecting aortic aneurysm? *Circulation* 1976; **53**: 915–16.

7 Erdheim J: Medionecrosis aortae idiopathica cystica. *Virchow Arch (A)* 1930; **276**: 187–229.

8 Lindsay J Jr, Hurst JW: Clinical features and prognosis in dissecting aneurysm of the aorta: a re-appraisal. *Circulation* 1967; **35**: 880–8.

9 Slater EE, DeSanctis RW: The clinical recognition of dissecting aortic aneurysm. *Am J Med* 1976; **60**: 625–33.

10 Wilson SK, Hutchins GM: Aortic dissecting aneurysms: causative factors in 204 cases. *Arch Pathol Lab Med* 1982; **106**: 175–80.

11 Pyeritz RE, McKusick VA: The Marfan syndrome: diagnosis and management. *N Engl J Med* 1979; **300**: 772–7.

12 McFarland W, Fuller DE: Mortality in Ehlers–Danlos syndrome due to spontaneous rupture of large arteries. *N Engl J Med* 1964; **271**: 1309–10.

13 Abbott ME: Coarctation of the aorta of the adult type. *Am Heart J* 1929; **3**: 574.

14 Reifenstein GH, Levine SA, Gross RE: Coarctation of the aorta: a review of 104 autopsied cases of the 'adult type', 2 years of age or older. *Am Heart J* 1947; **33**: 146–68.

15 Pedowitz P, Perell A: Aneurysms complicated by pregnancy. I. Aneurysms of the aorta and its major branches. *Am J Obstet Gynecol* 1957; **73**: 720–35.

16 Parmley LF, Mattingly TM, Manion WC et al: Nonpenetrating traumatic injury of aorta. *Circulation* 1958; **17**: 1086.

17 Kantrowitz A, Wasfie T, Freed PS et al: Intraaortic balloon pumping 1967 through 1982: analysis of complications in 733 patients. *Am J Cardiol* 1986; **57**: 976–83.

18 Murphy DA, Craver JM, Jones EL et al: Recognition and management of ascending aortic dissection complicating cardiac surgical operations. *J Thorac Cardiovasc Surg* 1983; **85**: 247–56.

19 Muna WF, Spray TI, Morrow AG et al: Aortic dissection after aortic valve replacement in patients with valvular aortic stenosis. *J Thorac Cardiovasc Surg* 1977; **74**: 65–9.

20 DeBakey ME, Henly WS, Cooley DA et al: Surgical management of dissecting aneurysms of the aorta. *J Thorac Cardiovasc Surg* 1965; **49**: 130–49.

21 Daily PO, Trueblood W, Stinson EB et al: Management of acute aortic dissections. *Ann Thorac Surg* 1970; **10**: 237–47.

22 Eagle KA, DeSanctis RW: Aortic dissection. *Curr Probl Cardiol* 1989; **14**: 225–78.

23 Slater EE, DeSanctis RW: The clinical recognition of dissecting aortic aneurysm. *Am J Med* 1976; **60**: 625–33.

24 Nienaber CA, Spielmann RP, von Kodolitsch Y et al: Diagnosis of thoracic aortic dissection: magnetic resonance imaging versus transesophageal echocardiography. *Circulation* 1992; **85**: 434–47.

25 Nienaber CA, von Kodolitsch, NV et al: The diagnosis of thoracic aortic dissection by noninvasive imaging procedures. *N Engl J Med* 1993; **328**: 1–9.

26 Kirschner LP, Twigg HL, Conrad PW: Retrograde catheter aortography in dissecting aortic aneurysms. *Am J Roentgenol* 1968; **102**: 349–53.

27 Stein HL, Steinberg I: Selective aortography, the definitive technique for diagnosis of dissecting aneurysm of the aorta. *Am J Roentgenol* 1968; **102**: 333–48.

28 Guthaner DR, Miller DC: Digital subtraction angiography of aortic dissection. *Am J Roentgenol* 1983; **141**: 157–61.

29 Sanders C: Current role of conventional and digital aortography in the diagnosis of aortic disease. *J Thorac Imag* 1990; **5**: 48–59.

30 Cigarroa JE, Isselbacher EM, DeSanctis RW et al: Diagnostic imaging in the evaluation of suspected aortic dissection. *N Engl J Med* 1993; **328**: 35–43.

31 Hayashi K, Meaney TF, Zelch JV: Aortographic analysis of aortic dissection. *Am J Roentgenol* 1974; **122**: 769–82.

32 Petasnick JP: Radiologic evaluation of aortic dissection. *Radiology* 1991; **180**: 297–305.

33 Earnest F IV, Muhm JR, Sheedy PF II: Roentgenographic findings in thoracic aortic dissection. *Mayo Clin Proc* 1979; **54**: 43–50.

34 Eagle KA, Quertermous T, Kritzer GA et al: Spectrum of conditions initially suggesting aortic dissection but with negative aortograms. *Am J Cardiol* 1986; **57**: 322–6.

35 Erbel R, Engberding R, Daniel W et al: Echocardiography in diagnosis of aortic dissection. *Lancet* 1989; **I**: 457–61.

36 Bansal RC, Chandrasekaran K, Ayala K et al: Frequency and explanation of false negative diagnosis of aortic dissection by aortography and transesophageal echocardiography. *J Am Coll Cardiol* 1995; **25**: 1393–401.

37 Chirillo F, Cavallini C, Longhini C et al: Comparative diagnostic value of transesophageal echocardiography and retrograde aortography in the evaluation of thoracic aortic dissection. *Am J Cardiol* 1994; **74**: 590–5.

38 Rizzo RJ, Aranki SF, Aklog L et al: Rapid noninvasive diagnosis and surgical repair of acute ascending aortic dissection. *J Thorac Cardiovasc Surg* 1994; **108**: 567–75.

39 Demos TC, Posniak HV, Marsan RE: CT of aortic dissection. *Semin Roentgenol* 1989; **24**: 22–37.

40 Heiberg E, Wolverson MK, Sundaram M et al: CT characteristics of aortic atherosclerotic aneurysm versus aortic dissection. *J Comput Assist Tomogr* 1985; **9**: 78–88.

41 Ballal RS, Nanda NC, Gatewood R et al: Usefulness of transesophageal echocardiography in assessment of aortic dissection. *Circulation* 1991; **84**: 1903–14.

42 Gross SC, Barr I, Eyler WR et al: Computed tomography in dissection of the thoracic aorta. *Radiology* 1980; **136**: 135–9.

43 Oudkerk M, Overbosch E, Dee P: CT recognition of acute aortic dissection. *Am J Roentgenol* 1983; **131**: 671–6.

44 Thorsen MK, San Dretto MA, Lawson TL et al: Dissecting aortic aneurysms: accuracy of computed tomographic diagnosis. *Radiology* 1983; **148**: 773–7.

45 Vasile N, Mathieu D, Ketia K et al: Computed tomography of thoracic aortic dissection: accuracy and pitfalls. *J Comput Assist Tomogr* 1986; **10**: 211–15.

46 Hartnell G, Costello P: The diagnosis of thoracic aortic dissection by noninvasive imaging procedures. *N Engl J Med* 1993; **328**: 1637 (letter).

47 Thompson BH, Stanford W: Utility of ultrafast computed tomography in the detection of thoracic aortic aneurysms

and dissections. *Semin Ultrasound CT MRI* 1993; **14**: 117–28.

48 Bleiweis MS, Georgiou D, Brundage BH: Ultrafast CT and the cardiovascular system. *Int J Card Imag* 1992; **8**: 289–302.

49 Hamada S, Takamiya M, Kimura K et al: Type A aortic dissection: evaluation with ultrafast CT. *Radiology* 1992; **183**: 155–8.

50 Zeman RK, Berman PM, Silverman PM et al: Diagnosis of aortic dissection: value of helical CT with multiplanar reformation and three-dimensional rendering. *Am J Roentgenol* 1995; **164**: 1375–80.

51 Godwin JD, Breiman RS, Speckman JM: Problems and pitfalls in the evaluation of thoracic aortic dissection by computed tomography. *J Comput Assist Tomogr* 1982; **6**: 750–6.

52 Mugge A, Daniel WG, Laas J et al: False-negative diagnosis of proximal aortic dissection by computed tomography or angiography and possible explanations based on transesophageal echocardiographic findings. *Am J Cardiol* 1990; **65**: 528–9.

53 Hachiya J, Nitatori T, Yoshino A: CT of calcified chronic aortic dissection simulating atherosclerotic aneurysm. *J Comput Assist Tomogr* 1991; **17**: 374–8.

54 Landay MJ, Virolainan H; 'Hyperdense' aortic wall: potential pitfall in CT screening for aortic dissection. *J Comput Assist Tomogr* 1991; **15**: 561–4.

55 Geisinger MA, Risius B, O'Donnell JA et al: Thoracic aortic dissections: magnetic resonance imaging. *Radiology* 1985; **155**: 407–12.

56 Amparo EG, Higgins CV, Hricak H et al: Aortic dissection: magnetic resonance imaging. *Radiology* 1985; **155**: 399–406.

57 Kersting-Sommerhoff BA, Higgins CV, White RD et al: Aortic dissection: sensitivity and specificity of MR imaging. *Radiology* 1988; **166**: 651–5.

58 Goldman AP, Kotler MN, Scanlon MH: The complementary role of magnetic resonance imaging, Doppler echocardiography, and computed tomography in the diagnosis of dissecting thoracic aneurysm. *Am Heart J* 1986; **111**: 970–81.

59 Laissy J-P, Blanc F, Soyer P et al: Thoracic aortic dissection: diagnosis with transesophageal echocardiography versus MR imaging. *Radiology* 1995; **194**: 331–6.

60 Chung JW, Park JH, Kim HC et al: Entry tears of thoracic aortic dissections: MR appearance on gated SE imaging. *J Comput Assist Tomogr* 1994; **18**: 250–5.

61 Williams DM, Joshi A, Dake MD et al: Aortic cobwebs: an anatomic marker identifying the false lumen in aortic dissection-imaging and pathologic correlation. *Radiology* 1994; **190**: 167–74.

62 Friese KK, Steffens JC, Caputo GR et al: Evaluation of painless aortic dissection with MR imaging. *Am Heart J* 1991; **122**: 1169–73.

63 Banki JHZ, Meiners LC, Barentsz JO et al: Detection of aortic dissection by magnetic resonance imaging in adults with Marfan's syndrome. *Int J Card Imag* 1992; **8**: 249–54.

64 Sechtem U, Plugfelder PW, Cassidy MM et al: Mitral or aortic regurgitation: quantification of regurgitant volumes with cine MR imaging. *Radiology* 1988; **167**: 425–30.

65 Fischer U, Vosshenrich R, Kopka L: Dissection of the thoracic aorta: pre- and postoperative findings on turbo-Flash MR images obtained in the plane of the aortic arch. *Am J Roentgenol* 1994; **163**: 1069–72.

66 Bogren HG, Underwood MA, Firmin DN et al: Magnetic resonance velocity mapping in aortic dissection. *Br J Radiol* 1988; **61**: 456–62.

67 Chang J-M, Friese K, Caputo GR et al: MR measurement of blood flow in the true and false channel in chronic aortic dissection. *J Comput Assist Tomogr* 1991; **15**: 418–23.

68 Rumancik WM, Naidich DP, Chandra R et al: Cardiovascular disease: evaluation with MR phase imaging. *Radiology* 1988; **166**: 63–8.

69 Solomon SL, Brown JJ, Glazer HS et al: Thoracic aortic dissection: pitfalls and artifacts in MR imaging. *Radiology* 1990; **177**: 223–8.

70 Pernes JM, Grenier P, Desbleds MT et al: MR evaluation of chronic aortic dissection. *J Comput Assist Tomogr* 1987; **11**: 975–81.

71 Schenck JF, Jolesz FA, Roemer PB et al: Superconducting open-configuration MR imaging system for image-guided therapy. *Radiology* 1995; **195**: 805–14.

72 Shellock FG, Curtis JS: MR imaging and biomedical implants, materials, and devices: an updated review. *Radiology* 1991; **180**: 541–50.

73 Nanda NC, Gramiak RE, Shah PM: Diagnosis of aortic root dissection by echocardiography. *Circulation* 1973; **48**: 506–13.

74 Brown OR, Popp RL, Kolster FE: Echocardiographic criteria for aortic root dissection. *Am J Cardiol* 1975; **36**: 17–20.

75 Mathew T, Nanda NC: Two-dimensional and Doppler echocardiographic evaluation of aortic aneurysm and dissection. *Am J Cardiol* 1984; **54**: 379–85.

76 Victor MF, Mintz GS, Kotler MN et al: Two dimensional echocardiographic diagnosis of aortic dissection. *Am J Cardiol* 1981; **48**: 1155–9.

77 McLeod AA, Monaghan MJ, Richardson PJ et al: Diagnosis of acute aortic dissection by M-mode and cross-sectional echocardiography; a five-year experience. *Eur Heart J* 1983; **4**: 196–202.

78 Granato JE, Dee P, Gibson RS: Utility of two-dimensional echocardiography in suspected ascending aortic dissection. *Am J Cardiol* 1985; **56**: 123–9.

79 Khanderia BK, Tajik AJ, Taylor CL et al: Aortic dissection: review of value and limitations of two-dimensional echocardiography in a six-year experience. *J Am Soc Echocardiogr* 1989; **2**: 17–24.

80 Khanderia BK: Aortic dissection: the last frontier. *Circulation* 1993; **87**: 1765–8.

81 Iliceto S, Nanda NC, Rizzon P et al: Color Doppler evaluation of aortic dissection. *Circulation* 1987; **75**: 748–55.

82 Borner N, Erbel R, Bran B et al: Diagnosis of aortic dissection by transesophageal echocardiography. *Am J Cardiol* 1984; **54**: 1157–8.

83 Engberding R, Bender F, Grosse-Heitmeyer W et al: Identification of dissection or aneurysm of the descending thoracic aorta by conventional and transesophageal two-dimensional echocardiography. *Am J Cardiol* 1986; **59**: 717–19.

84 Erbel R, Borner N, Steller D et al: Detection of aortic dissection by transoesophageal echocardiography. *Br Heart J* 1987; **58**: 45–51.

85 Hashimoto S, Kumada T, Osakada G et al: Assessment of transesophageal Doppler echography in dissecting aortic aneurysm. *J Am Coll Cardiol* 1989; **14**: 1253–62.

86 Adachi H, Kyo S, Takamoto S et al: Early diagnosis and surgical intervention of acute aortic dissection by transesophageal color flow mapping. *Circulation* 1990; **82** (suppl IV): 19–23.

87 Omoto R, Kyo S, Matsumara M et al: Evaluation of biplane color Doppler transesophageal echocardiography in 200 consecutive patients. *Circulation* 1992; **85**: 1237–47.

88 Banning AP, Masani ND, Ikram S et al: Transesophageal echocardiography as the sole diagnostic investigation in patients with suspected thoracic aortic dissection. *Br Heart J* 1994; **72**: 461–5.

89 Erbel R, Oelert H, Meyer J et al: Effect of medical and surgical therapy on aortic dissection evaluated by transesophageal echocardiography. *Circulation* 1993; **87**: 1604–15.

90 Kyo S, Takamoto S, Omoto R et al: Introperative echocardiography for diagnosis and treatment of aortic dissection. *Herz* 1992; **6**: 377–89.

91 Pinto FJ, Bolger AF: Doppler echocardiographic diagnostic advances in aortic dissection using transesophageal and intraoperative epicardial approaches. *Semin Thorac Cardiovasc Surg* 1993; **5**: 17–26.

92 Katz ES, Tunick PA, Colvin SB et al: Aortic dissection complicating cardiac surgery: diagnosis by intraoperative biplane transesophageal echocardiography. *J Am Soc Echocardiogr* 1993; **6**: 217–22.

93 Wiet SP, Pearce WH, McCarthy WJ et al: Utility of transesophageal echocardiography in the diagnosis of disease of the thoracic aorta. *J Vasc Surg* 1994; **20**: 613–20.

94 Kronzon I, Demopoulos L, Schrem SS et al: Pitfalls in the diagnosis of thoracic aortic aneurysm by transesophageal echocardiography. *J Am Soc Echocardiogr* 1990; **3**: 145–8.

95 Chan K-L: Usefulness of transesophageal echocardiography in the diagnosis of conditions mimicking aortic dissection. *Am Heart J* 1991; **122**: 495.

96 Weintraub AR, Erbel R, Gorge G et al: Intravascular ultrasound imaging in acute aortic dissection. *J Am Coll Cardiol* 1994; **24**: 495–503.

97 Yamada E, Matsumura M, Kyo S et al: Usefulness of a prototype intravascular ultrasound imaging in evaluation of aortic dissection and comparison with angiographic study, transesophageal echocardiography, computed tomography, and magnetic resonance imaging. *Am J Cardiol* 1995; **75**: 161–5.

98 Cavaye DM, White RA, Lerman RD et al: Usefulness of intravascular ultrasound imaging for detecting experimentally induced aortic dissection in dogs and for determining the effectiveness of endoluminal stenting. *Am J Cardiol* 1992; **69**: 705–7.

99 Goldstein SA, Mintz GS, Lindsay J: Aorta: comprehensive evaluation by echocardiography and transesophageal echocardiography. *J Am Soc Echocardiogr* 1993; **6**: 634–59.

100 Yamada T, Tada S, Harada J: Aortic dissection without intimal rupture: diagnosis with MR imaging and CT. *Radiology* 1988; **168**: 347–52.

101 Williams MP, Farrow R: Atypical patterns in the CT diagnosis of aortic dissection. *Clinical Radiology* 1994; **49**: 686–9.

102 Wolff KA, Herold CJ, Tempany CM et al: Aortic dissection: atypical patterns seen at MR imaging. *Radiology* 1991; **181**: 489–95.

103 Mohr-Kahaly S, Erbel R, Kearney P et al: Aortic intramural hemorrhage visualized by transesophageal echocardiography:

findings and prognostic implications. *J Am Coll Cardiol* 1994; **23**: 658–64.

104 Nienaber CA, von Kodolitsch Y, Petersen B et al: Intramural hemorrhage of the thoracic aorta: diagnostic and therapeutic implications. *Circulation* 1995; **92**: 1465–72.

105 Cooke JP, Kazmier FJ, Orszulak TA: The penetrating aortic ulcer: pathologic manifestations, diagnosis, and management. *Mayo Clin Proc* 1988; **63**: 718–25.

106 Stanson AW, Kazmier FJ, Hollier LH et al: Penetrating atherosclerotic ulcers of the thoracic aorta: natural history and clinicopathologic correlations. *Ann Vasc Surg* 1986; **1**: 15–23.

107 Hussain S, Glover JL, Bree R et al: Penetrating atherosclerotic ulcers of the thoracic aorta. *J Vasc Surg* 1989; **9**: 710–17.

108 Kazerooni EA, Bree RL, Williams DM: Penetrating atherosclerotic ulcers of the descending thoracic aorta: evaluation with CT and distinction from aortic dissection. *Radiology* 1992; **183**: 759–65.

109 Harris JA, Bis KG, Glover JL: Penetrating atherosclerotic ulcers of the aorta. *J Vasc Surg* 1994; **19**: 90–9.

110 Miller DC, Stinson EB, Oyer PE et al: The operative treatment of aortic dissection: experience with 125 patients over a sixteen-year period. *J Thorac Cardiovasc Surg* 1979; **78**: 365–82.

111 Guthanar DF, Miller DC, Silverman JF et al: Fate of the false lumen following surgical repair of aortic dissections: an angiographic study. *Radiology* 1979; **133**: 1–8.

112 Mathieu D, Keita K, Loisance D et al: Postoperative CT follow-up of aortic dissection. *J Comput Assist Tomogr* 1986; **10**: 216–18.

113 Hendrickx PH, Reifer P, Prokop M, et al: Intravenous DSA and dynamic computed tomography for post-operative follow-up of type A aortic dissection. *Eur J Radiol* 1989; **9**: 158–62.

114 Mohr-Kahaly S, Erbel R, Rennollet H: Ambulatory follow-up of aortic dissection by transesophageal two-dimensional and color-coded Doppler echocardiography. *Circulation* 1989; **80**: 24–33.

115 White RD, Ullyot DJ, Higgins CB: MR imaging of the aorta after surgery for aortic dissection. *Am J Roentgenol* 1988; **150**: 87–92.

116 Fedriga E, Gordini V, Pellegrini A et al: Postoperative MR follow-up of type A aortic dissection. *J Comput Assist Tomogr* 1993; **17**: 873–7.

117 Deutsch HJ, Sechtem U, Meyer H et al: Chronic aortic dissection: comparison of MR imaging and transesophageal echocardiography. *Radiology* 1994; **192**: 645–50.

118 Pucillo AL, Schechter AG, Moggio RA et al: Postoperative evaluation of ascending aortic prosthetic conduits by magnetic resonance imaging. *Chest* 1990; **97**: 106–10.

119 Rofsky NM, Weinreb JC, Grossi EA et al: Aortic aneurysm and dissection: normal MR imaging and CT findings after surgical repair with the continuous-suture graft-inclusion technique. *Radiology* 1993; **186**: 195–201.

Index

Page numbers in italics indicate figures.